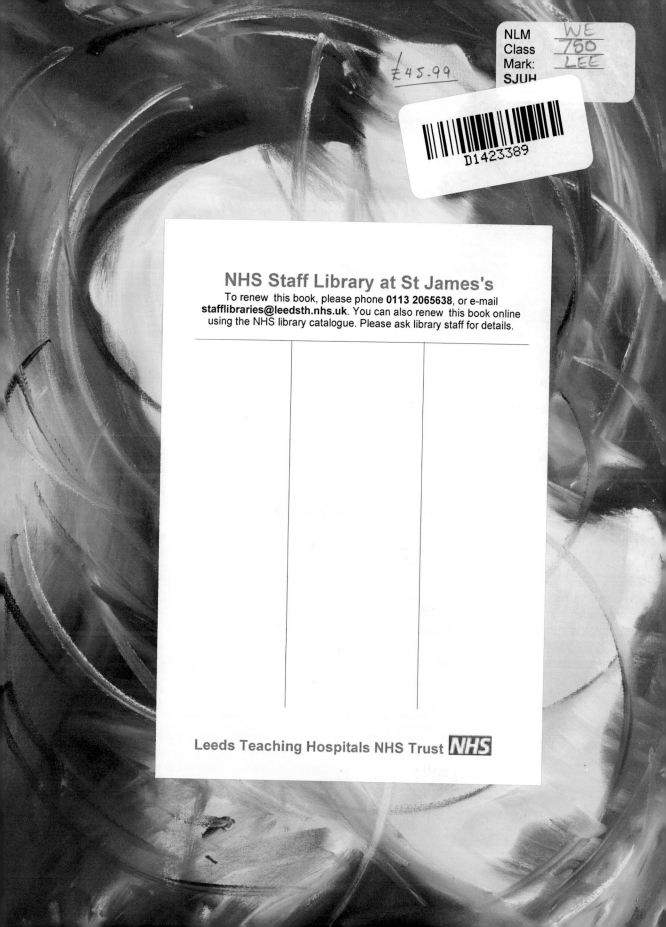

The Pelvic Girdle

This edition is dedicated to my good friend, Carol. Thank you for reminding me to listen to my heart.
Nameste, Diane

Nameste is a symbol of gratitude and respect whereby
I honor the place in you in which the entire universe dwells;
it is the place of love, truth, light and peace.
When we honor this place within each other, we are one.

For Elsevier

Publisher: *Sarena Wolfaard*
Development Editor: *Helen Leng*
Project Manager: *Gopika Sasidharan*
Designer/Design Direction: *Stewart Larking*
Illustration Manager: *Bruce Hogarth*

The Pelvic Girdle

An Integration of Clinical Expertise and Research

FOURTH EDITION

Diane Lee BSR FCAMPT CGIMS

Diane Lee & Associates, Consultants in Physiotherapy,
Discover Physio,
White Rock, BC, Canada

Major contributor

Linda-Joy Lee PhD BSc(PT) BSc FCAMPT CGIMS MCPA

Synergy Physiotherapy,
Discover Physio,
North Vancouver, BC, Canada

Contributor

Andry Vleeming PhD PT

Clinical Anatomist and Founder, Spine and Joint Center, Rotterdam,
The Netherlands

Foreword by

Mark A Jones BSc (Psych), PT, MAppSc (Manipulative Therapy)

Program Director, Senior Lecturer, Master of Musculoskeletal and Sports Physiotherapy,
School of Health Sciences, University of South Australia

Cover artwork – Scott Kish, BSc (KIN) (1995) specializing in human anatomy and visual information processing.
www.KishStudio.com
Photographer – Goran Basaric
Medical illustrator – Frank Crymble

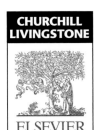

CHURCHILL LIVINGSTONE

ELSEVIER

Edinburgh   London   New York   Oxford   Philadelphia   St Louis   Sydney   Toronto   2011

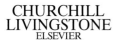

© 2011 Elsevier Ltd. All rights reserved.

First edition 1989
Second edition 1999
Third edition 2004
Fourth edition 2011

ISBN 9780443069635

British Library Cataloguing in Publication Data
A catalogue record for this book is available from the British Library

Library of Congress Cataloging in Publication Data
A catalog record for this book is available from the Library of Congress

Notices
Knowledge and best practice in this field are constantly changing. As new research and experience broaden our understanding, changes in research methods, professional practices, or medical treatment may become necessary.

Practitioners and researchers must always rely on their own experience and knowledge in evaluating and using any information, methods, compounds, or experiments described herein. In using such information or methods they should be mindful of their own safety and the safety of others, including parties for whom they have a professional responsibility.

With respect to any drug or pharmaceutical products identified, readers are advised to check the most current information provided (i) on procedures featured or (ii) by the manufacturer of each product to be administered, to verify the recommended dose or formula, the method and duration of administration, and contraindications. It is the responsibility of practitioners, relying on their own experience and knowledge of their patients, to make diagnoses, to determine dosages and the best treatment for each individual patient, and to take all appropriate safety precautions.

To the fullest extent of the law, neither the Publisher nor the authors, contributors, or editors, assume any liability for any injury and/or damage to persons or property as a matter of products liability, negligence or otherwise, or from any use or operation of any methods, products, instructions, or ideas contained in the material herein.

ELSEVIER your source for books, journals and multimedia in the health sciences

www.elsevierhealth.com

Working together to grow libraries in developing countries

www.elsevier.com | www.bookaid.org | www.sabre.org

ELSEVIER | BOOK AID International | Sabre Foundation

The Publisher's policy is to use paper manufactured from sustainable forests

Printed in China

Contents

Foreword vii

Preface ix

Acknowledgments xi

Abbreviations xiii

1. Historical and contemporary perspectives on the pelvic girdle 1
   Diane Lee, Andry Vleeming

2. The evolution of myths and facts and the pelvic girdle 3
   Diane Lee

3. The structure of the lumbopelvic–hip complex 5
   Diane Lee

4. The functional lumbopelvic–hip complex 47
   Diane Lee, Linda-Joy Lee

5. The impaired lumbopelvic–hip complex 91
   Diane Lee, Linda-Joy Lee

6. Pregnancy and its potential complications 129
   Diane Lee

7. Clinical practice – the reality for clinicians 147
   Linda-Joy Lee, Diane Lee

8. Techniques and tools for assessing the lumbopelvic–hip complex 173
   Diane Lee, Linda-Joy Lee

9. Clinical reasoning, treatment planning, and case reports 255
   Diane Lee, Linda-Joy Lee

10. Techniques and tools for addressing barriers in the lumbopelvic–hip
    complex 283
    Diane Lee, Linda-Joy Lee

11. Tools and techniques for 'waking up' and coordinating the deep and
    superficial muscle systems 323
    Linda-Joy Lee, Diane Lee

12. Training new strategies for posture and movement 367
    Linda-Joy Lee

References 409

Index 425

Foreword

This 4th edition of *The Pelvic Girdle* is an excellent evidence-based clinicians' book. Diane and LJ provide both the research basis underpinning their approach to lumbopelvic-hip complex assessment and management, and their experience-based evidence in the form of case studies. Clinicians will enjoy their critical yet practical presentation of anatomy, kinematics, and motor-control research clearly linked to assessment and management with acknowledgment of where research substantiation is still lacking. They also rightly highlight an issue which is salient and has been of interest to me personally concerning the limitations of existing research that historically has not captured sufficient population assessment and intervention details to guide therapists adequately in their recognition and management of the multitude of patient problems and presentations seen in practice (Jones et al. 2006). Clinicians are regularly faced with the daunting challenge of maintaining best practice based on best evidence when the evidence is still largely not available or incomplete. Even when primary research studies (or systematic reviews) testing therapeutic interventions are available, very few studies provide sufficient detail and justification of the assessments and treatments (e.g. what precisely was done including details of positions, dosage, sequence, and progression; who did it including level of procedural competence; what was the therapeutic environment including associated explanations, instructions, verbal cues, and advice) to enable clinicians to replicate the assessments and management with confidence. By presenting research and experience-based evidence Diane and LJ provide readers with both the science and the art of pelvic girdle assessment and management.

Readers are taken through a systematic process of assessment, differential diagnosis, clinical reasoning and passive and dynamic treatment selection and progression. However, from a clinical perspective this is much more than simply a 'how to' book. While presentation of how to assess and manage the relevant factors associated with disability from lumbo-pelvic-hip complex impairment and pain are clearly articulated, this is superbly achieved within

a broader holistic biopsychosocial philosophy of practice, evident within their 'The Integrated Systems Model' and associated 'Integrated Model of Function'. The physiotherapist is portrayed as a teacher, facilitator, and coach who empower his/her patient to understand, take responsibility, and learn to self manage. Assessment and management procedures are biomedically presented with their research basis alongside psychosocial considerations highlighting the importance of a therapeutic environment that enhances awareness, understanding, positive emotions, learning, and neuroplasticity. The neuroscience of learning tells us that implicitly learned (unconscious) beliefs, postures, movement, and motor control can be difficult to change. To these ends, explicit strategies for facilitating cortical reorganization (i.e. learning) are presented with respect to patient perspectives, activating deep muscles, promoting co-contraction of the deep muscle system and integrating the deep and superficial muscle systems. Strategies and procedures to 'Release, Align, Connect, and Move' are provided, again in the context of patient cases, which illustrate the learning and reinforcement of neural networks from supported to upright postures and meaningful function. The attention given to describing and demonstrating, via video clips, the manner in which assessments and interventions are delivered (technically, educatively, behaviorally, and humanistically) is impressive providing the reader with a 'fly on the wall' view of how Diane and LJ practice.

A unique and effective aspect of this book is the presentation of both diagnostic and narrative clinical reasoning. Their 'Clinical Puzzle' tool provides an excellent means of representing assessment findings regarding both the person (including the sensorial experience, cognitions, and emotions) and his/her problem(s) across different systems (e.g. articular, neural, myofascial, visceral) influencing function, and performance. This is not only effective in the context of this book but also provides readers with a takeaway means of reflecting critically on their own patient assessments and reasoning. The importance of attending to activities that are meaningful to the patient through both the examination and subsequent management is emphasized. Common clinical patterns are highlighted along with effective treatment strategies while the uniqueness of individual patient presentations, and hence tailored management, are stressed.

Lastly, the various formats used to present both research and experience-based knowledge, including strategic use of questions to promote self reflection, fact boxes summarizing key points, interest boxes highlighting useful resources, high-quality diagrams and photographs, patient cases with associated clinical reasoning, and generous use of video clips (more that 240 in total!) all contribute to maximizing reader understanding and learning. The continual use of clinical examples in particular successfully engages the reader promoting deeper learning and application to practice creating an experiential learning package akin to good university-based and continuing education courses.

Mark A. Jones

Jones M., Grimmer K., Edwards I., et al. 2006. Challenges of applying best evidence to physiotherapy. The Internet Journal of Allied Health Sciences and Practice July, Vol 4(3).

From Diane. . .

Frequently, I am asked, 'Is there anything new in the subsequent editions of this text and is it worth purchasing the latest edition?' If you are asking this question as you peruse this book, the answer is a resounding YES! The byline for the 4th edition of *The Pelvic Girdle* reflects the focus of this edition – *An Integration of Clinical Expertise and Research*. I'd like to take a moment to acknowledge a major contributor to this edition, Linda-Joy (LJ) Lee. LJ and I have been working/traveling/learning together since 1999 and it would have been impossible to update this edition without her involvement, as this work is now as much hers as mine. I am grateful for her acceptance of my invitation to join me in this edition as she was 'in the thick' of her PhD at the time and I am sure she could have done without this extra work. She is a clinical expert, respected researcher, and a good friend.

So what's new in this edition? As always, the research pertaining to lumbopelvic–hip (LPH) function and impairment has been reviewed and integrated clinically and, like past editions, many techniques are described and illustrated for assessing and treating specific impairments in the LPH complex. Although much of this is new or updated, the additional feature of this edition that we are very excited to present is The Integrated Systems Model and the essential knowledge/skills necessary for the development of clinical expertise.

In the preface of the 1st edition (1989) I wrote:

In 1980, it was my good fortune to have the opportunity to study with one of the leaders in manipulative therapy, Mr. Cliff Fowler. Over the ensuing years I was shown how to treat people, not conditions, how to integrate academic knowledge with clinical experience and how to learn from every patient's story. . . The intent of this text is to assist the clinician in the development of a logical approach to the examination and treatment of the lumbopelvic–hip region based on the known anatomy, physiology and biomechanics.

This remains the intent of this text. There are two parts to this edition:

Part 1: Theoretical concepts and research pertaining to disability and pain in the lumbopelvic–hip complex – Chapters 1–6, and Part 2: The clinical application of The Integrated Systems Model for disability and pain in the lumbopelvic–hip complex – Chapters 7–12.

The Pelvic Girdle, 4th edition, continues to strive to provide the busy clinician with the latest evidence and the clinical tools/knowledge to immediately impact and enhance daily practice. It is hoped that The Integrated Systems Model and its Clinical Puzzle will facilitate improved clinical reasoning, hypothesis development and testing, and subsequent prescriptive treatment that is effective. It is highly unlikely that there will ever be enough research evidence to meet the needs of a busy clinician who is faced with patients presenting with a wide and variable range of single and multiple impairments every day. Clinical expertise (knowing how to do the right thing at the right time) comes from disciplined, reflective practice and it is hoped that this text will help more clinicians become expert in this field.

We all strive to be a clinical expert and I cannot find better words to end the preface of this 4th edition of *The Pelvic Girdle* than to quote Ian Edwards from Chapter 10 – Clinical reasoning and expert practice – a chapter he co-wrote with Mark Jones in *Expertise in Physical Therapy Practice* (editors Jensen, Gwyer, Hack & Shepard, 2007).

I have come to learn that it is not only what experts do but also who they are, as members and representatives of a practicing community, which leads to their peers attributing this term to them. The kind of practice that experts embody (including technical, interactive, teaching, collaborative, predictive, and ethical skills) represents what is collectively agreed to as being good for a particular practicing community. Experts, in this understanding, evoke both qualities and questions in those they mentor and teach. Expert practice also dictates a call to become a certain kind of clinician or therapist and not just to acquire a particular expertise or knowledge base (though that is certainly part of it). In all of this, such apparently "non-teachable" constructs (at least in a formal sense) as "passion," "motivation," "drive," and "love of one's work" are nurtured.

And now, it is done. I hope you enjoy the 4th edition of *The Pelvic Girdle*.

Diane Lee, White Rock, BC, Canada (2010)

From LJ...

The process of writing is an amazing catalyst for clarity, discovery, and growth. I recently read a quote attached to a Yogi tea bag:

'To learn, read.

To know, write.

To master, teach.'

As I considered these words and the journey of writing the 4th edition of *The Pelvic Girdle* with Diane, I recall the many emails and discussions back and forth that crystalized and clarified our ideas, our language, and that consolidated The Integrated Systems Model. Taking pen to paper (or fingers to keyboard), we know on a deeper level what it is we do with our patients, and the power of what we teach. I have also come to know a greater appreciation for what we share in our work together. The definition of 'synergy' describes it well: 'the interaction of two or more forces so that their combined effect is greater than the sum of their individual effects.' It is a rare thing.

I am also keenly aware of the unique and immense contributions that Diane has made over the history of the past three editions of *The Pelvic Girdle*. It is an incredible honor to share this journey with Diane and I am deeply grateful for the privilege.

This book is about facilitating change. Although our patients present with many different problems and symptoms, all of them seek help to make something different in their bodies. And because everything is connected, changing their experience of their bodies involves treating the whole person – mind, body, spirit. As many of you who have been on courses with us know, we do expect to facilitate change, and lasting change, every day in clinical practice. Discoveries in neuroscience on the amazing adaptability of the human brain have helped us, in this edition, better describe the underlying mechanisms behind what we do, why change is possible for all patients of all ages, and how we as clinicians can optimize neuroplasticity to facilitate a journey to better health. I hope you are inspired to let go of barriers you once thought were fixed, consider the endless possibilities, and enjoy the journey through the book as you Discover how to help your patients Move better, Feel better, and Be better.

Linda-Joy Lee, North Vancouver, BC, Canada (2010)

Acknowledgments

From Diane...

There are many people without whose support this edition would never have been completed and to whom I owe my heartfelt thanks. To Cliff Fowler, the first clinical expert to influence my path, and who continues to be passionate and in love with his work, I am forever grateful. Thanks to Carol Ingle, to whom I have dedicated this edition, who took on much more administrative work to grant me the time to write and, together with LJ, provided continual encouragement when I was so ready to accept 'less than the best' this edition could be. Thanks to Chelsea Lee, who used her fine editing skills, honed through the recent acquisition of her university degree in English (2009), to improve the grammar, and correct the punctuation, in every chapter. This edition truly reads much better thanks to her contribution. To my family, Tom, Michael & Chelsea, who waited so patiently for me to come back into the family fold, to my father Jim Hazell, for whom each day is a gift, who waited for a phone call or a visit, and to the associate physiotherapists and all the team at Diane Lee & Associates, who held the fort so well in my extended absence, I owe all of you my heartfelt gratitude; I look forward to coming back.

Diane Lee, White Rock, BC, Canada (2010)

From LJ...

There are so many people to thank that I cannot list them all here. Diane, an amazing clinician, teacher, person, and friend, thank you for your flexibility, understanding, and grace with our multiple revisions of timelines as I have juggled the responsibilities in my life. To my administrative team, Julie Block and Brenda Smit, for their efficiencies and expertise that allow me freedom to write and work on other projects knowing things on the home front are running smoothly. To Dad, Mija, Mark, Marnie & the rest of my family, to Bill, Julie, Karen, Katie, Tina, Anna, and my friends, who have all graciously taken the snippets of time left over between PhD, book, clinic, and training, all the while providing encouragement, love, laughter, and moral support to keep going. To the associate physiotherapists at Synergy Physio – Gillian, Jason, Philippa, Shawna – you are an amazing team and I am so grateful for your enthusiastic support of my endeavors even though it means there are limited windows of time for you. Thank you for your flexibility, and for supporting each other and the clinic in growth in my absences. To Professor Paul Hodges, for your understanding and flexibility in the PhD process, and much more for the immense learning journey and opportunities with you and your team at UQ. You have challenged and refined my thinking and writing, and I am grateful for all the experiences and growth you have fostered. I'm also thankful for my Canadian manual therapy roots, the founders of our postgraduate system, my instructors and examiners, the many skilled clinicians that I have discussed and practiced with – I have learned much from you all. Finally, to my patients, thank you for sharing your stories and your journeys with me. You are the inspiration for it all.

Linda-Joy Lee, North Vancouver, BC, Canada (2010)

Abbreviations

ABLR	active bent leg raise		**OE**	obturator externus
AM	adductor magnus		**OI**	obturator internus
AP	anteroposterior		**OLS**	one leg standing
ARA	anorectal angle		**P4**	posterior pelvic pain provocation
ASIS	anterior superior iliac spine		**PF(M)**	pelvic floor (muscle)
ASLR	active straight leg raise		**PGP**	pelvic girdle pain
ATFP	arcus tendineus fascia pelvis		**PHE**	prone hip extension
BB	backward bending		**PICR**	path of the instantaneous center of rotation
BOS	base of support		**PIIS**	posterior inferior iliac spine
CNS	central nervous system		**PIVM**	passive intervertebral motion
COM	center of mass		**PNF**	proprioceptive neuromuscular facilitation
CPR	clinical prediction rule		**PRPGP**	pregnancy-related pelvic girdle pain
CT	computed tomography		**PS**	pubic symphysis
DISH	diffuse idiopathic skeletal hyperostosis		**PSIS**	posterior superior iliac spine
DIV	doppler imaging of vibration		**PU**	a point halfway between the cranial aspect of the pubic symphysis and the superior aspect of the umbilicus
dMF	deep fibers of multifidus			
DRA	diastasis rectus abdominis		**R1**	point in the joint's range where the first resistance to movement is felt
EIA	external iliac artery			
EIV	external iliac vein		**R2**	end point of the joint's range
EMG	electromyogram		**RA**	rectus abdominis
EO	external oblique		**RACM**	release, align, connect, move
ER	external rotation		**RCT**	randomized controlled trial
ES	erector spinae		**RF**	rectus femoris
FAI	femoral acetabular impingement		**RHL**	right harder than left
FB	forward bending		**ROLS**	right one leg standing
FLT	failed load transfer		**ROM**	range of motion
HALAT	high acceleration, low amplitude thrust		**RSA**	roentgen stereophotogrammetric analysis
HIV	human immunodeficiency virus		**RTUS**	real-time ultrasound
IAP	intra-abdominal pressure		**SAW**	stretch with awareness
ILA	inferior lateral angle		**SI**	sacroiliac
IMS	intramuscular stimulation		**SIJ**	sacroiliac joint
IO	internal oblique		**sMF**	superficial fibers of multifidus
IPT	intrapelvic torsion		**SR**	systematic review
IPTL	intrapelvic torsion left		**SUI**	stress urinary incontinence
IPTR	intrapelvic torsion right		**TFL**	tensor fascia latae
IR	internal rotation		**TLF**	thoracolumbar fascia
LA	linea alba		**TrA**	transversus abdominis
LBP	low back pain		**TVT**	transvaginal tape
LHR	left harder than right		**U**	a point just superior to the umbilicus
LOLS	left one leg standing		**UI**	urinary incontinence or ultrasound imaging
LPH	lumbopelvic–hip		**UUI**	urge urinary incontinence
MRI	magnetic resonance imaging, the use of nuclear magnetic resonance of protons to produce proton density images		**UX**	a point halfway between the superior aspect of the umbilicus and the xyphoid process
			VAS	visual analog scale
MS	manubriosternal		**VL**	vastus lateralis
MUI	mixed urinary incontinence		**vs**	versus
MVA	motor vehicle accident			
MVC	maximal voluntary contraction			
NZ	neutral zone			

Historical and contemporary perspectives on the pelvic girdle

1

Diane Lee   Andry Vleeming

The first medical practitioners to record interest in the pelvic girdle were the obstetricians of Hippocrates' era. Hippocrates (460–377 BC) and Vesalius (AD 1543) felt that under normal conditions the sacroiliac joints (SIJ) were immobile; however, others (Paré 1643) felt that motion was apparent during pregnancy (Weisl 1955). This view was upheld until De Diemerbroeck (1689) demonstrated that mobility of the SIJ could occur apart from pregnancy. Since the 17th century, a controversy has existed as to the anatomy of the SIJ, the quantity (if any) of its mobility, its role in the transference of loads from the low back to the lower extremity, as well as its contribution to lumbopelvic pain. Theories and myths abound when the topic involves the pelvic girdle. The SIJ has been implicated as the cause of many symptoms, including sciatica; in fact, at the turn of the 20th century, Albee (1909), and Goldthwait & Osgood (1905) proposed that sciatica developed from direct pressure on the lumbosacral plexus as it crossed the anterior aspect of the SIJ. This pressure was thought to be caused by 'subluxed, relaxed or diseased sacroiliac joints' (Meisenbach 1911). Treatment consisted of manipulative reduction of the sacrum followed by immobilization (in plaster) in spinal hyperextension for 6 months. Following Mixter & Barr's (1934) discovery of prolapsed intervertebral discs and the clinical ramifications of pressure on the lumbosacral nerve roots intra-spinally, the SIJ fell out of the limelight. In the mid-1950s, impairments of this articulation were regarded as rare (Cyriax 1954).

Research over the last 60 years has provided important information pertaining to the anatomy and function of the pelvic girdle. In 1992, the first Interdisciplinary World Congress on Low Back and Pelvic Pain (Vleeming et al 1992b) presented the current state of knowledge in this area; most of the knowledge was empirical. It was clear that more research was needed to understand the biomechanics of the pelvic girdle, to develop valid differential diagnostic tests, and to determine the most effective way to treat lumbopelvic pain and disability.

Since this first congress five more have taken place (La Jolla 1995, Vienna 1998, Montreal 2001, Melbourne 2004, Barcelona 2007) and each has helped to develop more scientific evidence for the diagnosis and treatment of the lumbopelvis. Although we have a clearer understanding of the role of the pelvic girdle in lumbopelvic pain, much work still needs to be done.

The aim of this chapter is to take you on a journey that will look at some historical perspectives pertaining to the pelvic girdle, as well as the journey of a researcher (Andry Vleeming) and a clinician (Diane Lee) who came together to try to understand and foster some contemporary perspectives based on a combination of science and clinical expertise (Fig. 1.1). We have decided to write this chapter in an informal way (rather like an interview) and we hope you enjoy the 'dialogue' approach. The complete interview can be found online . Sit back with a glass of wine or a cup of tea/coffee and take a journey with us back in time.

© 2011, Elsevier Ltd.
DOI: 10.1016/B978-0-443-06963-5.00001-8

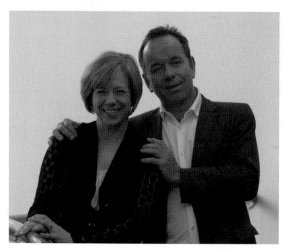

Fig. 1.1 • Diane Lee and Andry Vleeming, 2009.

The evolution of myths and facts and the pelvic girdle

2

Diane Lee

CHAPTER CONTENTS

Myths, facts & the pelvis 3

This chapter was published in its original form as Chapter 13 in: Vleeming A, Mooney V, Stoeckart R eds. Movement, Stability & Lumbopelvic Pain: Integration of Research and Therapy, 2nd edition (Lee 2007a). It has been modified for this text and is reproduced, in part, with permission from Vleeming A and the publisher Churchill Livingstone, Elsevier.

Myths, facts & the pelvis

For various reasons, the pelvis, and in particular the sacroiliac joint, has been a source of mystery to many clinicians and researchers. The mobility of the pelvic joints is difficult to measure objectively, especially in the weight bearing position and while many clinicians of multiple disciplines insist they can feel motion at the sacroiliac joint both during active and passive motion (myself included) it has been a difficult task to prove. The intent of this chapter is to discuss some of the past and present commonly held myths and hopefully clarify some of the reasons why they have evolved and what needs to be done to establish whether a myth is fact or fiction. Check online to learn more about the myths and facts pertaining to the following questions.

Does the sacroiliac joint cause low back pain?
Can we reliably identify patients who have painful sacroiliac joints?
Does the sacroiliac joint move?
Can we reliably detect motion at the sacroiliac joint?
Can we reliably detect when motion is not being controlled in the pelvic girdle?
How effective are our treatment protocols?
The future

© 2011, Elsevier Ltd.
DOI: 10.1016/B978-0-443-06963-5.00022-5

The structure of the lumbopelvic–hip complex

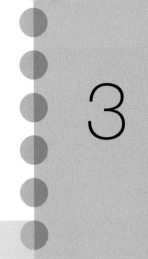

3

Diane Lee

CHAPTER CONTENTS

Evolution of the pelvic girdle 5
Comparative anatomy of the pelvic girdle 6
Embryology, development, and structure
of the human pelvic girdle 8

Evolution of the pelvic girdle[1]

The human lumbopelvic–hip complex, although in many respects unique in the animal world for its evolutionary adaptation to orthograde bipedalism, is based on a design originating almost half a billion years ago. The earliest evidence of habitual upright gait is now known to date to as early as 6 million years ago (Lovejoy 2007). This chapter will briefly outline the evolutionary steps that have facilitated human gait. Subsequently, the changes in human structure and posture as a result of bipedalism will be described.

The pelvic girdle first appeared as a pair of small cartilaginous elements lying in the abdomen of the primitive fish (Encyclopedia Britannica 1981, Gracovetsky & Farfan 1986, Nelson & Jurmain 1985, Romer 1959, Stein & Rowe 1982, Young 1981). The 'fin fold' theory maintains that lateral folds formed in the ancient fish to prevent rolling and buckling of the undulating body. As the folds contributed to propulsion and steering, they gradually began to fragment. From this fragmentation, two paired lateral fins were formed: the pectoral and pelvic fins. The pectoral fin was the primary propeller and was the largest and the most stable of the two. As stability was not a functional requirement of the pelvic girdle, axial attachment and attachment between the two sides was unnecessary.

With migration onto land, the pelvic fin rapidly developed into the powerhouse of locomotion and consequently an increase in stability of the pelvic girdle was required. The pectoral fin (and its later development of the forelimb) was relegated to the role of steering, resulting in a reversal of the original roles.

The pelvic girdle has evolved towards increased stability both at the pubic symphysis and at the sacroiliac joints (SIJ). The original innominate bone contained two elements, which together formed the puboischium. During the stabilization process, the puboischium enlarged and united with the opposite side via the puboischial symphysis. Intrapelvic stability was subsequently increased; however, stability between the primitive innominate bone and the axial skeleton was also required. A dorsal projection developed on the puboischium directed towards the axial skeleton, which ultimately formed the ilium.

Simultaneously, the costal element of the axial skeleton enlarged and fused with one (or more) pre-anal vertebra to form the sacrum. The iliac projection of the primitive innominate bone and the enlarged costal process of the primitive sacrum formed the first SIJ. The initial union was ligamentous. Thus, direct articulation between the axial and appendicular skeletons occurred. At this stage, the pelvic girdle had a full inventory of the elements that are present today in all tetrapods.

The number of vertebrae that contribute to the sacrum varies from species to species and depends

---

[1]The evolution section of this chapter was written in collaboration with James Meadows MCPA MCSP FCAMT as part of the first edition of this text and has been updated by the principal author (Diane Lee) for subsequent editions.

© 2011, Elsevier Ltd.
DOI: 10.1016/B978-0-443-06963-5.00003-1

on the degree of stability or mobility required at the SIJ. Many amphibians and reptiles have only one or two sacral vertebrae, whereas higher mammals have five. The extreme of sacral development is found in the bird where the synsacrum includes the fusion of the sacral, lumbar, and caudal thoracic vertebrae. This, together with the huge sternum, provides the stability necessary for anchoring the muscles that move the wings.

As the locomotive pattern of the vertebrates progressed from crawling to the linear-limb quadripedal and bipedal gait of the advanced mammals, the role of the ilium became more significant. The bone provided the major pelvic attachment for the limb musculature as well as the articular surface for the SIJ.

Comparative anatomy of the pelvic girdle

The structure of the human pelvic girdle reflects the adaptation required for bipedal gait (Basmajian & Deluca 1985, Farfan 1978, Goodall 1979, Keagy & Brumlik 1966, Nelson & Jurmain 1985, Rodman & McHenry 1980, Stein & Rowe 1982, Swindler & Wood 1982, Tuttle 1975, Williams 1995) (Fig. 3.1). The surface area of the ilia has increased, whereas the length of the ischium and the pubis has decreased. The posterior muscles have lost some bulk, secondary to the increased stability of the SIJ. Sufficient mobility of the SIJ has been maintained for bipedalism. In contrast to humans,

the great apes have a virtually immobile lumbar spine with only two to three mobile segments (Lovejoy 2007) and a very small erector spinae. Lovejoy (2007) feels that a mobile lumbar spine is crucial for upright walking and that early hominids had to reverse the prior changes that rendered the lumbar spine stable in order to walk bipedally.

The sacrum

The sacrum has increased in size, thus accommodating the increased osseous attachment of the gluteus maximus muscle. The articular surface of the SIJ has also increased in size, which facilitates the increased compression produced in bipedal stance. The surface itself has become more incongruous, which aids intrapelvic stability.

The innominate

The ilia have undergone dramatic changes in response to bipedalism. The bone has twisted such that the lateral aspect is now directed anteriorly. The gluteus medius and minimus muscles have migrated anteriorly and their function has subsequently changed. In the ape, the gluteus medius and minimus muscles are femoral extensors, whereas in humans they act as femoral abductors (Fig. 3.2) and thus prevent a Trendelenburg gait.

In addition to the reorientation of the ilium, a fossa has developed (the iliac fossa) that increases

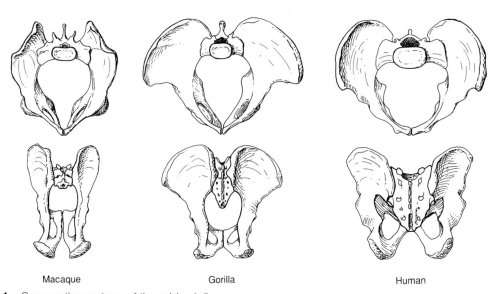

| Macaque | Gorilla | Human |

Fig. 3.1 • Comparative anatomy of the pelvic girdle. Redrawn from Stein & Rowe, 1982.

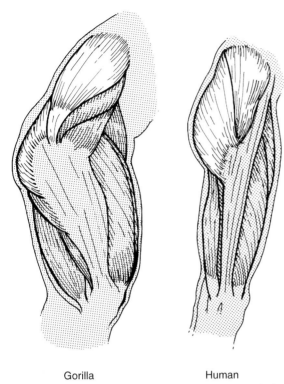

Gorilla   Human

Fig. 3.2 • The gluteus medius and minimus muscles in the gorilla function as femoral extensors, whereas in humans they act as femoral abductors.

the surface area available for the attachment of the gluteal and iliacus muscles. This, therefore, compensates for the reduction in extensor power caused by the anterior migration of the gluteus medius and minimus muscles. The iliac fossa also facilitates the enlargement of the iliacus muscle, which plays a significant role in the maintenance of our erect posture.

The anatomical changes in the ischium reflect the alteration in function of the hamstrings (see below). Although these muscles are still involved in femoral extension, constant activity is not a requirement of bipedal stance in the human. Subsequently, the ischial body and tuberosity have become reduced in both length and width (see Fig. 3.1). The vertical dimension of the pubic symphysis has also decreased with the evolution of efficient bipedal gait.

The acetabulum

The acetabulum has become deeper as well as reoriented in an anterolateral direction. This reorientation projects the femoral neck anteriorly and

together with the angle of inclination ensures that the leg adducts at heel strike to place the foot beneath the acetabulum. The ligaments of the hip joint are extensive in comparison to those of the ape, where they are almost non-existent.

Comparative posture

The vertebral column of humans, in comparison to other primates, differs primarily in its posture. Our vertebral column and innominates have rotated posteriorly through 90° to bring the head above the feet (Fig. 3.3). The sacral base is no longer horizontal as it is in non-human mammals, but neither has it rotated through 90° (Abitbol 1995, 1997). The angle of the sacral promontory with the fifth lumbar vertebra is acute. Consequently, the spine is organized into a vertical column, even though the orientation of the sacrum facilitated a more horizontal row. Caudally, the lumbosacral angle and lumbar lordosis developed. This curve was compensated for by the development of a thoracic kyphosis.

In all non-human primates, the lumbar spine is kyphotic. However, it is possible for a non-human primate to achieve a lumbar lordosis as was witnessed by Goodall (1979) in her Gombe Stream Reserve study. One ape in this study contracted poliomyelitis as an infant, which affected the function of one arm. As the characteristic 'knuckle walk' was not possible, the animal had developed a bipedal gait for locomotion. To facilitate this, a marked lumbar lordosis had developed. However, the attachment of the gluteal muscles in the ape prevents simultaneous extension of the lumbar spine and the femur and, as neither the osseous nor the myofascial structure had changed, an increase in both hip and knee flexion had to occur in order to maintain the line of gravity within the base of support.

The bipedal posture of the ape depends on the massive gluteal and hamstring muscles, the major role of which is to stabilize the pelvic girdle and the trunk on the flexed hips. Constant activity in both muscle groups is required as the line of gravity of the bipedal ape falls considerably anterior to the coronal axis of the hip joint. Consequently, the attachments of the posterior muscles in the ape are widespread and the ischial body and tuberosity are massive. Conversely in humans, the line of gravity falls slightly posterior to the coronal axis of the hip joint and therefore the requirements for postural balance are both reduced and reversed. According to Abitbol (1997), erect posture can be effortless when the center of the SIJ (biauricular line) and the center

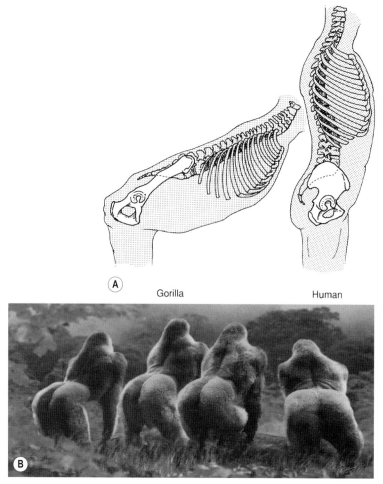

Gorilla   Human

Fig. 3.3 • (A) Posterior rotation of the vertebral column and the innominates has led to the development of lumbosacral lordosis and thoracic kyphosis. (B) Posture of a gorilla.

of the acetabulum (biacetabular line) form a vertical line when the sagittal plane of the pelvis is viewed laterally. The body weight is more efficiently balanced and tends to extend the pelvic girdle on the femora. To prevent this, slight recruitment of the psoas major muscle is required to maintain the optimal bipedal posture (Andersson et al 1995). Only intermittent activity is required from the hamstrings, and consequently the ischial body and tuberosity have become considerably reduced in size.

Summary

The human lumbopelvic–hip complex has developed from the primate pelvic girdle, which evolved for an arboreal lifestyle. The current vertebral curvatures are relatively recent; the early hominids and even Neanderthals had different vertebral curvatures. The curves are interdependent and any factor that causes a change in one results in a compensatory change in all others. The major structural changes in humans appear to have evolved to facilitate the most bioenergetically efficient gait among terrestrial tetrapods.

Embryology, development, and structure of the human pelvic girdle

The earliest record of anatomical data pertaining to the pelvic girdle is credited to Bernhard Siegfried Albinus (1697–1770) and William Hunter (1718–1783)

(Lynch 1920). These anatomists were the first to demonstrate that the SIJ was a true synovial joint, a finding confirmed by Meckel in 1816. Von Luschka, in 1854, was the first to classify the joint as diarthrodial. Further anatomical studies conducted by Albee in 1909 on 50 postmortem specimens confirmed that the joint was lined with a synovial membrane and contained by a well-formed articular capsule. His findings were confirmed by Brooke in 1924. It was not until 1938 (Schunke 1938) that the variations in the articular cartilage lining the iliac surface were noted. In 1957, Solonen conducted a comprehensive study of the osteology and arthrology of the pelvic girdle, from which some findings will be reported later in this chapter.

The pelvic girdle supports the abdomen and the organs of the lower pelvis and also provides a dynamic link between the thorax, the lumbar spine, and the lower limbs. It is a closed osteoarticular ring composed of four or five bones, which include the two innominates, the sacrum, the one or two bones that together form the coccyx, as well as four or five joints including the two sacroiliac, the sacrococcygeal, often an intercoccygeal, and the pubic symphysis. The lumbar spine and hip add another seven bones (five lumbar vertebrae and two femora) and 17 joints (15 lumbar and two hip) to create the lumbopelvic–hip complex. The reader is referred to other anatomy texts for a detailed review of the development and structure of the lumbar spine and development of the hip joint.

Osteology of the pelvic girdle

The development of the sacrum

The word 'sacrum' comes from the Latin word *sacer* meaning sacred (see online Chapter 1 🖱 for an in-depth discussion by Dr. Andry Vleeming on the origin of the word sacrum). It is thought that the sacrum was the last bone to decay after death and, as such, must be sacred. Fryette (1954) credits the 'ancient Phallic Worshipers [for naming] the base of the spine the Sacred Bone.'

> Little wonder that the ancient Phallic Worshipers named the base of the spine the Sacred bone. It is the seat of the transverse center of gravity, the keystone of the pelvis, the foundation of the spine. It is closely associated with our greatest abilities and disabilities, with our greatest romances and tragedies, our greatest pleasure and pains.
>
> Fryette 1954.

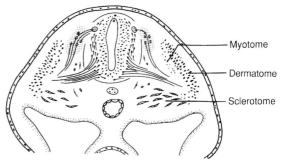

Fig. 3.4 • Differentiation of the mesodermal somite into sclerotome, myotome, and dermatome. Redrawn from Williams, 1995.

The bone is derived from the fusion of five mesodermal somites. During the fourth embryonic week, 42–44 pairs of somites arise from the paraxial mesoderm. Although not consistently, the sacrum evolves from the 31st to the 35th somites, each of which divides into three components: the sclerotome, myotome, and dermatome (Fig. 3.4). The sclerotome multiplies and migrates both ventrally and dorsally to surround the notochord and the evolving spinal cord. Subsequently, each sclerotome divides into equal cranial and caudal components separated by a sclerotomic fissure, which in the sacrum progresses to develop a rudimentary intervertebral disc composed of fibrocartilage. The adjacent sclerotomic segments then fuse to form the centrum of the sacral vertebral body. The dorsal aspect of the sclerotome, which has migrated posteriorly, forms the vertebral arch (the neural arch is part of this), whereas the ventrolateral aspect becomes the costal process (ala of the sacrum) (Fig. 3.5). This process appears in the upper two or three sacral segments only and is responsible for forming the auricular sacral surface.

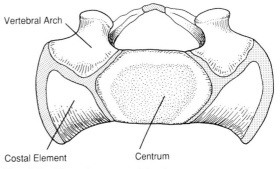

Fig. 3.5 • The sclerotome of the future sacrum differentiates into three parts – the centrum, the vertebral arch, and the costal element or process.

Chondrification of the sacrum precedes ossification and begins during the sixth embryonic week (Rothman & Simeone 1975). The primary ossification centers for the centrum and each half of the vertebral arch appear between the 10th and the 20th week, whereas the primary centers for the costal elements appear later, between the sixth and the eighth month. The three components of the sacral segment (see Fig. 3.5), the costal element, the vertebral arch, and the centrum, remain separated by hyaline cartilage up until 2–5 years of age when the costal element (ala of the sacrum) unites with the vertebral arch. This unit then fuses to the centrum and to the other vertebral arch in the eighth year.

The conjoined costal element, vertebral arch, and centrum of each sacral segment remain separated from those above and below by hyaline cartilage laterally and by fibrocartilage medially (Fig. 3.6A,B) (Rohen & Yokochi 1983). A cartilaginous epiphysis extends the entire length of the lateral aspect of the sacrum. Fusion of the sacral segments occurs after puberty in a caudocranial direction with the simultaneous appearance of secondary ossification centers for the centrum, spinous process, transverse processes, and costal elements. The adjacent margins of the sacral vertebrae ossify after the 20th year. However, the central portion of the intervertebral disc can remain unossified even after middle life.

The adult sacrum

The adult sacrum is a large triangular bone situated at the base of the spine wedged between the two innominates. It is formed by the fusion of five sacral vertebrae, and the vertebral equivalents are easily recognized. The sacrum is highly variable both between individuals and between the left and right sides of the same bone. In spite of this, certain anatomical features remain consistent and only those that are essential to the description and evaluation of function will be described here.

The cranial aspect of the first sacral vertebra (Fig. 3.7) (the sacral base), consists of the vertebral body anteriorly (the anterior projecting edge being the sacral promontory) and the vertebral arch posteriorly. Laterally, the costal elements fuse with the transverse processes of the first sacral vertebra (Fig. 3.5) to form the alae of the sacrum. Variations have been noted (Grieve 1981) in the height of the sacral alae as well as the body of the S1 vertebra.

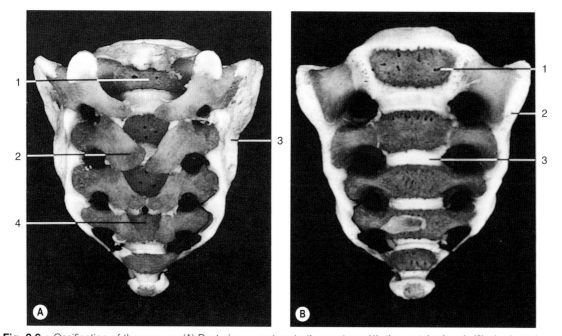

Fig. 3.6 • Ossification of the sacrum. (A) Posterior aspect: note the centrum (1), the vertebral arch (2), the lateral epiphysis (3), and the sacral canal (4). (B) Anterior aspect: note the centrum (1), the lateral epiphysis (2), and the intervertebral disc (3). Reproduced with permission from Rohen & Yokochi and the publisher F K Schattauer, 1983.

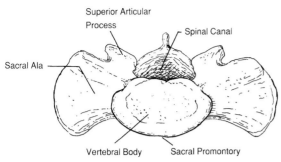

Fig. 3.7 • The cranial aspect of the first sacral vertebra, the sacral base.

The orientation of the superior articular processes of the S1 vertebra is also variable (see below).

The posterior surface of the sacrum (Fig. 3.8) is convex in both the sagittal and the transverse planes. The spinous processes of the S1 to S4 vertebrae are fused in the midline to form the median sacral crest. Lateral to the median sacral crest, the fused laminae of the S1 to S5 vertebrae form the intermediate sacral crest. The laminae and inferior articular processes of the S5 (and occasionally the S4) vertebra remain unfused in the midline. They project caudally to form the sacral cornua, and together with the posterior aspect of the vertebral body of the S5 vertebra form the sacral hiatus. The lateral sacral crest represents the fused transverse processes of the S1 to S5 vertebrae. Between this crest and the intermediate sacral crest lie the dorsal sacral foramina, which transmit the dorsal sacral ramus of each sacral spinal

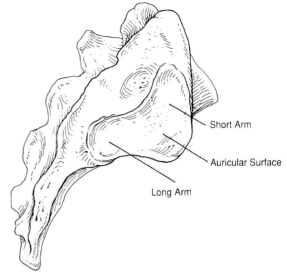

Fig. 3.9 • The lateral aspect of the sacrum.

nerve. There are three deep depressions in the lateral sacral crest at the levels of the S1, S2, and S3 vertebrae. These depressions contain the strong attachments of the interosseous sacroiliac ligament (Figs 3.8, 3.25).

The lateral sacral crest fuses with the costal element to form the lateral aspect of the sacrum (Fig. 3.9). Superiorly, the lateral aspect of the sacrum is wide, whereas inferiorly the anteroposterior dimension narrows to a thin border that curves medially to join the S5 vertebral body. This angle is called

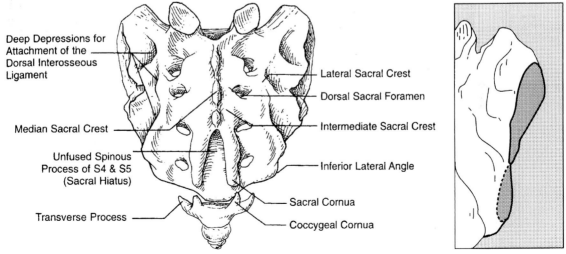

Fig. 3.8 • The posterior aspect of the sacrum and coccyx. Inset: the orientation of the three components of the auricular surface, shaped like a propeller. Redrawn from Vleeming et al, 2007.

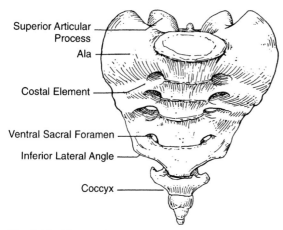

Superior Articular Process

Ala

Costal Element

Ventral Sacral Foramen

Inferior Lateral Angle

Coccyx

Fig. 3.10 • The anterior aspect of the sacrum and coccyx.

the inferior lateral angle (ILA) of the sacrum (Figs 3.8, 3.10). The articular surface of the sacrum is auricular in shape (L-shaped) and is contained entirely by the costal elements of the first three sacral segments.

The short arm of the L-shaped surface (see Fig. 3.9) lies in the vertical plane and is contained within the first sacral segment. The long arm lies in the antero-posterior plane within the second and third sacral segments. The contours of the articular surface are reported (Kapandji 1970, Solonen 1957, Vleeming et al 1990a, Weisl 1954, 1955) to be highly variable, depending on the age of the individual studied. Solonen (1957) noted that there were numerous depressions, elevations, and other irregularities to the SIJ surface. Vleeming et al (1990a) confirmed that these 'ridges and grooves' involve both the cartilage and the underlying bone, and are complementary on both sides of the joint. The geometry of the ridges and grooves is variable between individuals both of the same age and of different ages (Fig. 3.11) (Vleeming et al 1990b).

The anterior surface of the sacrum (see Fig. 3.10) is concave in both the sagittal and the transverse planes. In the midline, four interbody ridges represent the sclerotomic fissures, which are not always completely fused. Lateral to the fused vertebral bodies are four ventral sacral foramina that transmit the ventral ramus of each sacral spinal nerve as well as the segmental ventral sacral artery. The costal elements project laterally from the middle of each vertebral body between the ventral sacral foramina and fuse with those above and below, as well as with the transverse processes posteriorly to form the lateral aspect of the sacrum.

The orientation of the articular surface of the sacrum in both the coronal and the transverse planes has been studied by Solonen (1957) and a summary of his findings is presented in Table 3.1. These observations represent the common findings but variations were also noted. The stereometric drawings of two pelves studied by Solonen are illustrated in Figure 3.12A,B. Vleeming et al (1995b, 2007) describe the orientation of the three components of the auricular surface as resembling those of a propeller (see Fig. 3.8 inset).

Fryette (1954) examined 23 sacra and subsequently classified the bone into three types: A, B, and C (Fig. 3.13). This classification depends on the orientation of the sacral articular surface in the coronal plane, which he found to correlate with the orientation of the superior articular processes of the S1 vertebra. The Type A sacrum narrows inferiorly at S1 and S2 and superiorly at S3. The orientation of the superior articular processes in this group is in the coronal plane. The Type B sacrum narrows superiorly at S1 and the orientation of the superior articular processes in this group is in the sagittal plane. The Type C sacrum narrows inferiorly at S1 on one side (Type A) and superiorly at S1 on the other (Type B). The orientation of the superior articular processes is in the coronal plane on the Type A side and in the sagittal plane on the Type B.

Clinical consideration. The plane of the SIJ is highly variable in both the coronal and the transverse planes as well as in the shape of the articulating surfaces. As clinicians, this anatomical uncertainty requires consideration when evaluating the passive mobility of the SIJ (see Chapter 8).

The adult coccyx

The coccyx (see Figs 3.8, 3.10) is represented by four fused coccygeal segments, although the first is commonly separate. The bone is roughly triangular and the base bears an oval facet, which articulates with the inferior aspect of the S5 vertebral body. The first coccygeal segment contains two rudimentary transverse processes as well as two coccygeal cornua that project superiorly to articulate with the sacral cornua.

The development of the innominate

The word 'innominate' comes from the Latin derivative *innominatus*, meaning 'having no name.' During the seventh embryonic week it appears as three

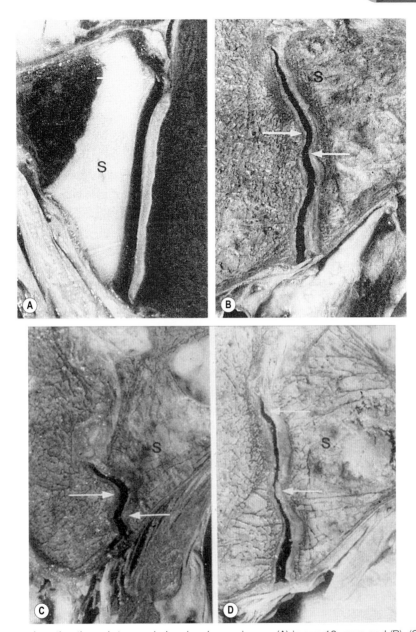

Fig. 3.11 • A coronal section through two embalmed male specimens; (A) is age 12 years and (B), (C), and (D) are over 60 years. Note the planar nature of the sacroiliac joint in the young and the presence and variety of ridges and grooves in the old. S, Reproduced with permission from Vleeming et al and the publisher Spine, 1990a.

bones (the ilium, the ischium, and the pubis), which are derived from a small proliferating mass of mesenchyme from the somatopleure in the developing limb bud. Three primary ossification centers appear before birth: one for the ilium above the sciatic notch during the eighth intrauterine week, one for the ischium in the body of the bone during the fourth month, and one for the pubis in the superior ramus between the fourth and fifth months. At birth, the iliac crest, the acetabular fossa, and the inferior ischiopubic ramus are cartilaginous (Fig. 3.14). The latter ossifies during the seventh to eighth year.

Table 3.1 Orientation of the articular surface of the sacrum in the coronal and transverse planes as described by Solonen (1957) and as shown graphically in Figure 3.12

Coronal plane

90% of the specimens narrowed inferiorly at S1	Fig. 3.12A,B
85% of the specimens examined narrowed inferiorly at S2	Fig. 3.12B
80% of the specimens examined narrowed superiorly at S3	Fig. 3.12A

Transverse plane

S1 and S2 narrow posteriorly	
S3 narrows anteriorly	

The iliac crest and the acetabular fossa develop secondary ossification centers during puberty but can remain unossified until 25 years of age.

The adult innominate

The three parts of the innominate – the ilium, the ischium and the pubis – fuse in the adult to form the innominate (Fig. 3.15). Only the anatomical features pertinent to the description and evaluation of function will be described here.

The adult ilium. The ilium is a fan-like structure forming the superior aspect of the innominate and contributing to the superior portion of the acetabulum (Figs 3.15, 3.16). The iliac crest is convex in the sagittal plane and sinusoidal in the transverse plane such that the anterior portion is concave medially, whereas the posterior portion is convex medially. The curve reversal occurs in the same coronal plane as the short arm of the L-shaped articular surface. The anterior superior iliac spine (ASIS) and the posterior superior iliac spine (PSIS) are at either end of the iliac crest. Inferior to the PSIS, the ilium curves

irregularly to end at the posterior inferior iliac spine (PIIS). This is often the site of an accessory SIJ (Solonen 1957, Trotter 1937).

Several anatomical points are worthy of note on the medial aspect of the ilium. The articular surface lies on the posterosuperior aspect of the medial surface. Like the sacrum, the articular surface is L-shaped, with the axis of the short arm in the craniocaudal plane, whereas the long arm has an anteroposterior axis. A variety of elevations, depressions, ridges, and furrows have been reported and these develop with age (Vleeming et al 1990b) (see Fig. 3.11). Superior to the articular surface, the medial aspect of the ilium is very rough and affords attachment to the strong interosseous sacroiliac ligament, which has been noted (Colachis et al 1963) to remain intact when the sacrum and the innominate are forced apart in cadavers. The SIJ cannot be palpated given the depth of the articulation and this point should be noted when studying the anatomy.

Anteriorly, the arcuate line of the ilium appears at the angle between the short and the long arms of the articular surface and projects anteroinferiorly to reach the iliopectineal eminence, a point at which the ilium and the pubis unite. This line between the SIJ and the iliopectineal eminence represents a line of force transmission from the vertebral column to the lower limb and is reinforced by subperiosteal trabeculae (Kapandji 1974).

The adult pubis. The inferomedial aspect of the innominate is formed by the pubis, which articulates with the pubis of the opposite side via the pubic symphysis (Fig. 3.16). It joins the ilium superiorly via the superior pubic ramus, which constitutes the anterior one-fifth of the acetabulum. Inferiorly, the inferior pubic ramus projects posterolaterally to join the ischium on the medial aspect of the obturator foramen. The lateral surface of the pubis is directed towards the lower limb and affords attachment for many of the medial muscles of the thigh. The pubic tubercle is located at the lateral aspect of the pubic crest approximately 1cm lateral to the midsymphyseal line.

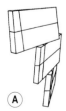 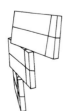 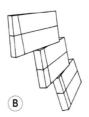 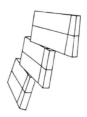

(A) (B)

Fig. 3.12 • Steriometric drawings of two pelves studied by Solonen (1957) illustrating the variation found in the orientation of the sacral articular surface. Redrawn with permission from Solonen and the publisher Acta Orthopaedica Scandinavica, 1957.

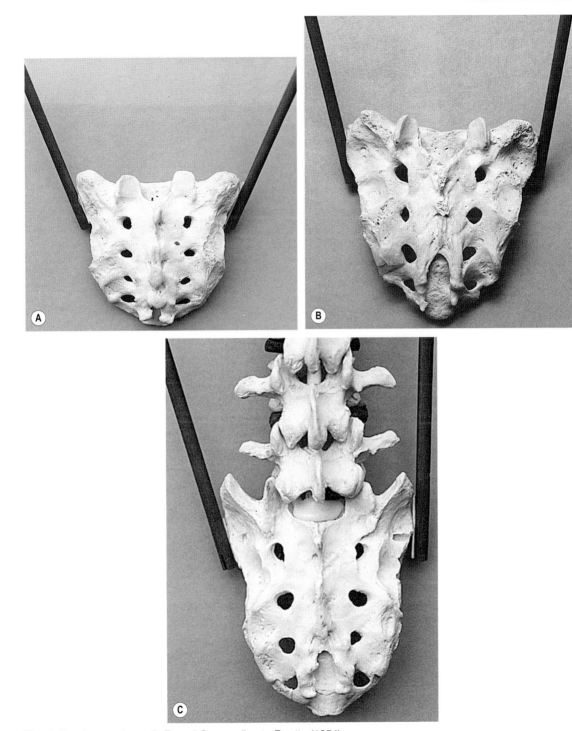

Fig. 3.13 • Sacrum types A, B, and C according to Fryette (1954).

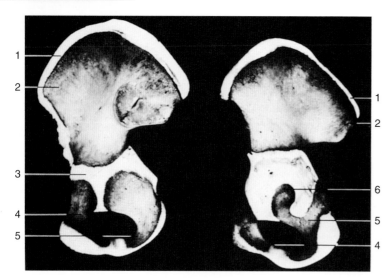

Fig. 3.14 • Ossification of the innominate bone. Note the cartilage of the iliac crest (1), the ilium (2), the cartilage separating the ilium, pubis, and ischium (3), the pubis (4), the ischium (5), and the acetabulum (6). Reproduced with permission from Rohen & Yokochi and the publisher F K Schattauer, 1983.

The adult ischium. The inferolateral one-third of the innominate is formed by the ischium. The upper part of the body of the ischium forms the floor of the acetabulum as well as the posterior two-fifths of the articular surface of the hip joint. From the lower part of the body, the ischial ramus projects anteromedially to join the inferior ramus of the pubis. The ischial tuberosity is a roughened area on the posterior and inferior aspect of the ischial body and is the site of strong muscular and ligamentous attachments. Superior to the tuberosity, the ischial spine projects medially. This process is also

the site of ligamentous and muscular attachments (see Figs 3.16, 3.28, 3.29).

The adult acetabulum. The acetabulum (see Figs 3.14, 3.15, 3.17) is formed from the fusion of the three bones that make up the innominate. It is roughly the shape of a hemisphere and projects in an anterolateral and inferior direction (approximately 45° and 15° anterior) (Anda et al 1986, Reikeras et al 1983). The lunate surface represents the articular portion of the acetabulum, whereas the non-articular portion constitutes the floor, or the acetabular fossa. This fossa is continuous with

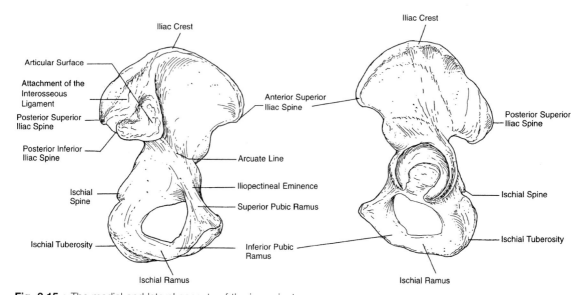

Fig. 3.15 • The medial and lateral aspects of the innominate.

Fig. 3.16 • The ligaments of the pelvic girdle viewed from the anterior aspect.

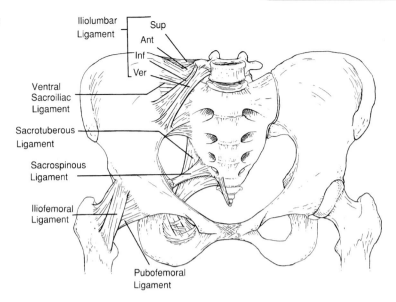

Iliolumbar Ligament
Sup
Ant
Inf
Ver
Ventral Sacroiliac Ligament
Sacrotuberous Ligament
Sacrospinous Ligament
Iliofemoral Ligament
Pubofemoral Ligament

the acetabular notch located between the two ends of the lunate surface. Optimal anteversion of the acetabulum is thought to be essential for maintaining a normal relationship with the femoral head to avoid femoral impingement during functional tasks (Siebenrock et al 2003). Normal range of acetabular anteversion is 15–20°, decreased anteversion is 10–14°, and increased anteversion is 21–25° (Tonnis & Heinecke 1999).

The blood supply of the innominate. The nutrient supply for the innominate is derived from the iliac branches of the obturator and iliolumbar vessels as well as the superior gluteal vessels (Williams 1995).

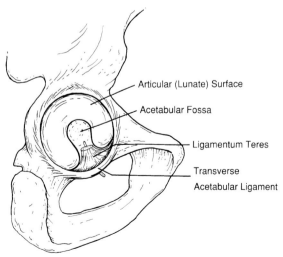

Articular (Lunate) Surface
Acetabular Fossa
Ligamentum Teres
Transverse Acetabular Ligament

Fig. 3.17 • The acetabulum.

The adult femora

Clinically, it is important to note that the angle of inclination of the femoral neck to the shaft of the femur, as well as the angle of anteversion between the femoral neck and the coronal plane, is highly variable. This variability will be reflected in both the pattern and the range of motion available at the hip joint (Kapandji 1970, Torry et al 2006). Anteversion of the femur is important for both static and dynamic function of the hip and anteversion of the femur is known to diminish with age (Fabry 1997). The femoral head forms two-thirds of a sphere and is flattened in the area where the acetabulum applies the greatest load. In the neutral anatomical position, the anterior part of the femoral head should not engage the acetabulum (Shindle et al 2006).

Arthrology of the pelvic girdle

The development of the SIJ

Intrauterine development. The development of the SIJ commences during the eighth week of intrauterine life (Bellamy et al 1983, Schunke 1938). As in other synovial joints, a trilayer structure initially appears in the mesenchyme between the ilium and the costal element of the sacrum. Cavitation begins both peripherally and centrally by the 10th week, and by the 13th week the enlarged cavities are separated by fibrous septae. These findings are not consistent with Walker's (1984, 1986) study of 36 fetuses in which she noted that cavitation did not begin until the 32nd week (Fig. 3.18A,B). The stage at which cavitation is complete and the fibrous bands disappear is controversial. Bellamy et al (1983) state that the cavity is fully developed by the eighth month and that the fibrous septae soon disappear, whereas Walker (1986) notes that unlike most synovial joints, which show complete cavitation by the 12th week, the SIJ remains separated by fibrous bands at birth and she questions their persistence in some joints into adulthood. Bowen & Cassidy (1981) report that the 10 specimens studied in this age group did not contain the fibrous septae previously noted in late fetal life. Schunke (1938) was the first to describe these intra-articular bands and felt that they disappeared in the first year of life.

The synovium of the joint develops from the mesenchyme at the edges of the primordial cavity, as does the articular capsule, which is thin and pliable at this stage (Bowen & Cassidy 1981). All investigators note the macroscopic and microscopic differences between the cartilage that lines the articular surfaces of the ilium and the sacrum (Bowen & Cassidy 1981, Kampen & Tillmann 1998, McLauchlan & Gardner 2002, Schunke 1938, Walker 1986) (Plate 1).

The ilium is lined with a type of fibrocartilage that is bluer, duller, and more striated than the hyaline cartilage that lines the sacrum; this difference is noted

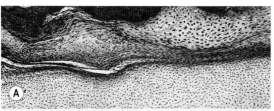

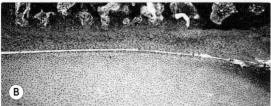

Fig. 3.18 • Cavitation of the sacroiliac joint. (A) Sacroiliac joint of a fetus at 16 weeks of gestation. Note the proximity of the iliac bone to the joint surface, the partial cavitation of the joint, and the presence of a fibrous band connecting the two surfaces. (B) Sacroiliac joint of a fetus at 34 weeks of gestation. Note that cavitation is almost complete except for a few loose fibrous bands. Reproduced with permission from Walker and the publisher JOSPT, 1986.

from birth, although Kampen & Tillmann (1998) report that the cartilage lining the ilium becomes more hyaline with maturation. The depth of the cartilage is also different with the sacral cartilage being two to five times thicker than the iliac cartilage (Bowen & Cassidy 1981, Kampen & Tillman 1998, MacDonald & Hunt 1951, McLauchlan & Gardner 2002, Schunke 1938, Walker 1986). All note that the corresponding articular surfaces were smooth and flat in the young, and Bowen & Cassidy (1981) note that, during handling of the fetal pelves, the joint was capable of gliding in a multitude of directions.

The first decade (0–10 years). Bowen & Cassidy (1981) studied seven pelves in this age group and reported that the surfaces of the SIJ remain primarily flat (Plate 2), with the major restraint to passive motion being provided by the very strong interosseous ligaments. The articular cartilage remains as noted prenatally.

The second and third decades (11–30 years). The availability of cadavers for investigation in this age group is limited; therefore the data obtained are based on few specimens. Sashin's (1930) investigation of age-related intra-articular changes is perhaps the most extensive; 42 specimens in his study belonged to this age group. The study of Resnick et al (1975) included only two specimens, MacDonald & Hunt's (1951) seven, Bowen & Cassidy's (1981) seven, and Walker's (1986) none.

Early in the second decade the SIJ appears planar (see Fig. 3.11A). However, by the beginning of the third decade, all specimens manifest a convex ridge that runs along the entire length of the articular surface of the ilium apposed to a corresponding sacral groove (Bowen & Cassidy 1981, Vleeming et al 1990a). The iliac fibrocartilaginous surface is duller, rougher, and intermittently coated with fibrous plaques (Plate 3). The deep articular cartilage is microscopically normal, but the superficial layers are fibrillated and some crevice formation and erosion occurs by the end of the third decade. The sacral hyaline cartilage takes on a yellowish hue, although macroscopic changes are not evident at this stage. The collagen content of the fibrous capsule increases, thus reducing its extensibility. Shibata et al (2002) investigated age-related changes (joint space narrowing, sclerosis, osteophytes, cysts, and erosion) of the SIJ via computed tomography (CT) and found changes beginning in the third decade.

The fourth and fifth decades (31–50 years). Several investigators (Bowen & Cassidy 1981, Faflia et al 1998, Schunke 1938, Shibata et al 2002, Walker

1984, 1986) feel that the changes noted in the articular surfaces during this stage represent a degenerative process. The changes occur earlier in males (fourth decade) than females (fifth decade). Vleeming et al (1990a,b) feel that, since these changes are asymptomatic in most, they reflect a functional adaptation secondary to an increase in body weight during puberty and not a degenerative process. They studied the effects of the cartilage texture on the friction coefficient of the joint (Vleeming et al 1990b) and found that, together with the development of ridges and grooves, the fibrillated surface increased friction and thus stability of the SIJ. This was felt to reflect an adaptation to bipedalism.

The articular surfaces increase in irregularity with marked fibrillation occurring on the iliac side by the end of the fourth decade (Plate 4). Plaque formation and peripheral erosion of cartilage progress to subchondral sclerosis of bone on the iliac side. The joint space contains flaky, amorphous debris. The articular capsule thickens but still permits the translatory motion noted in the second and third decades (Bowen & Cassidy 1981). Bony hypertrophy with some lipping of the sacral articular margins was noted in some specimens in the fifth decade. Shibata et al (2002) found degeneration to be more frequent in this age group and found sclerosis to be common on the upper and middle anterior of the articular surface of the ilium, whereas osteophytes were common on the anterior surface of the sacrum. Women showed more advanced

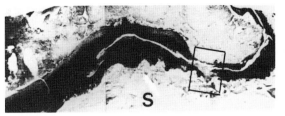

Fig. 3.19 • Sacroiliac joint of a male, 60 years of age. Note the variability in the depth of both the sacral (S) and the iliac cartilage at different sites. Reproduced with permission from Walker and the publisher JOSPT, 1986.

signs of degeneration and parous women tended to progress faster than nulliparous.

The sixth and seventh decades (51–70 years). At this stage (Figs 3.19, 3.20A,B), the articular surfaces become totally irregular with deep erosions occasionally exposing the subchondral bone. Peripheral osteophytes enlarge and often bridge the margins of the joint. Fibrous interconnections between the articular surfaces are commonplace; however, 'when stressed, all specimens maintained some degree of mobility, although this was restricted when compared with the younger specimens' (Bowen & Cassidy 1981). Vleeming et al (1992c) found that, even in old age, small movements of the SIJ are possible and felt that ankylosis of this joint was not normal. Faflia et al (1998) also noted that ankylosis of the SIJ was rare and, like Shibata et al (2002), found joint changes in all subjects imaged in this age group. Interestingly,

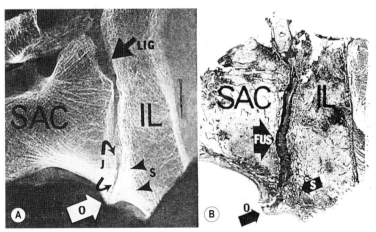

Fig. 3.20 • (A) This radiograph of a coronal section through the sacroiliac joint of a cadaver over 70 years of age illustrates narrowing of the joint space (J), sclerosis of the bone (S), and osteophyte formation (O) secondary to the degenerative process. Note the space for the interosseous ligament (LIG). SAC indicates the sacrum and IL the ilium. (B) This photomicrograph reveals the thickened trabeculae in the sclerotic region (S), an area of fibrous intra-articular fusion (FUS), and the previously noted osteophyte (O). SAC indicates the sacrum and IL the ilium. Reproduced with permission from Resnick et al and the publishers J. B. Lippincott, 1975.

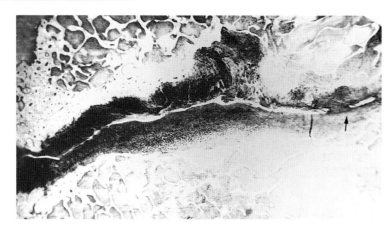

Fig. 3.21 • Sacroiliac joint of a female, 81 years of age. Note the erosion of the articular cartilage and the intra-articular fibrous connection (arrow). Reproduced with permission from Walker and the publisher JOSPT, 1986.

Faflia et al (1998) found a higher prevalence of asymmetrical non-uniform SIJ narrowing and extensive subchondral sclerosis in obese and multiparous women when age-matched to men, normal-weighted women, and non-multiparous women.

The eighth decade (over 70 years). Intra-articular fibrous connections are more often the rule with some periarticular osteophytosis present (Plate 5, Fig. 3.21). Cartilaginous erosion and plaque formation are extensive and universal, filling the joint space with debris. Consequently, the joint space is markedly reduced. Intra-articular bony ankylosis is rarely reported and usually thought to be associated with ankylosing spondylitis (Fig. 3.22). Schunke (1938) reports that the average age of the specimens with bony ankylosis is considerably less than that in those without fusion, confirming a probable pathological cause. Dar et al (2008) recently imaged 287 men and women (3D CT imaging) between the ages of 22 and 93. They found extra-articular fusion present in 27.7% of the males and 2.3% of the females and noted that the fusions were age-dependent in the men, increasing from 5.8% in the 20–39 age group to 46.7% in the over 80 age group. The extra-articular fusions were all found in the superior aspect of the joint.

The adult SIJ

The SIJ (Figs 3.23a,b, 3.24, Video 3.1 🖱) has been classified as a synovial joint or diarthrosis (Bowen & Cassidy 1981), an amphiarthroses (Gerlach & Lierse 1992), and a symphysis (Puhakka et al 2004). The shape, as well as the articular cartilage, have been previously described. The joint capsule is composed of two layers, an external fibrous layer that contains abundant fibroblasts, blood vessels, and collagen fibers, and an inner synovial layer. Anteriorly, the capsule is clearly distinguished from the overlying ventral sacroiliac ligament, whereas posteriorly the fibers of the capsule and the deep interosseous ligament are intimately blended. Inferiorly, the capsule blends with the periosteum of the contiguous sacrum and innominates.

Like other synovial joints, the SIJ capsule is supported by overlying ligaments and fascia, some of which are the strongest in the body. They include the ventral sacroiliac, interosseous sacroiliac, long dorsal sacroiliac, sacrotuberous, sacrospinous, and iliolumbar ligaments.

The ventral sacroiliac ligament (see Fig. 3.16) is the weakest of the group and is little more than a

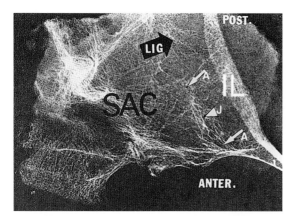

Fig. 3.22 • This radiograph of a transverse section (ANTER is the anterior aspect of the pelvis and POST is the posterior aspect) through the sacroiliac joint (J) illustrates the intra-articular ankylosis (A) of ankylosing spondylitis. Note the ossification of the interosseous ligament (LIG). SAC indicates the sacrum and IL the ilium. Reproduced with permission from Resnick et al and the publisher J. B. Lippincott, 1975.

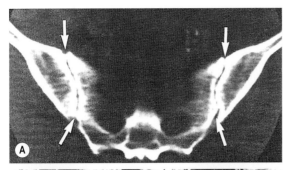

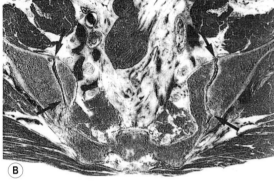

Fig. 3.23 • A computed tomography scan (A) with a photograph of the corresponding anatomical section (B) through the synovial portion of a cadaveric sacroiliac joint (arrows). Reproduced with permission from Lawson et al and the publisher Raven Press, 1982.

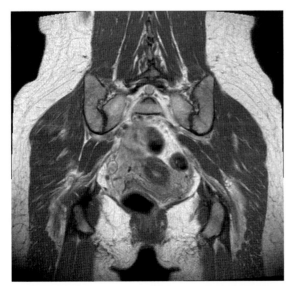

Fig. 3.24 • MRI of a coronal slice through the sacroiliac joint. Note the anterior synovial and posterior ligamentous portions of the joint. See Video 3.1 🖱 to watch several MRI coronal slices from anterior to posterior.

thickening of the anterior and inferior parts of the joint capsule (Bowen & Cassidy 1981, Williams 1995).

The ligaments of the SIJ. The interosseous sacro-iliac ligament is the strongest of the group and completely fills the space between the lateral sacral crest and the iliac tuberosity (see Figs 3.20, 3.24, 3.25A,B). The fibers are multidirectional and can be divided into a deep and a superficial group. The deep layer attaches medially to three fossae on the lateral aspect of the dorsal sacral surface (see Fig. 3.8) and laterally to the adjacent iliac tuber-osity. The superficial layer of this ligament is a fibrous sheet that attaches to the lateral sacral crest at S1 and S2 and to the medial aspect of the iliac crest. This structure is the primary barrier to direct palpation of the SIJ in its superior part and its density makes intra-articular injections extremely difficult.

The long dorsal sacroiliac ligament (Fig. 3.26) attaches medially to the lateral sacral crest at S3 and S4 and laterally to the posterior superior iliac spine and the inner lip of the iliac crest. It lies poste-rior to the interosseous ligament and is separated from it by the emerging dorsal branches of the sacral

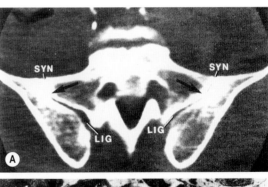

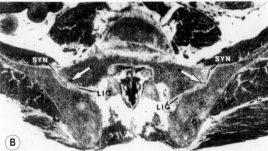

Fig. 3.25 • A computed tomography scan (A) with a photograph of the corresponding anatomical section (B) through the sacroiliac joint. Note the depth of the synovial portion (SYN) of the joint and the interosseous ligament (LIG). Reproduced with permission from Lawson et al and the publishers Raven Press, 1982.

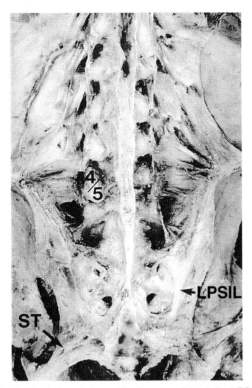

Fig. 3.26 • A dorsal view of the female pelvic girdle. LPSIL, the long dorsal sacroiliac ligament; 4/5, the zygapophyseal joint between L4 and L5; ST, the sacrotuberous ligament. Reproduced with permission from Willard et al and the publisher Churchill Livingstone, 1997.

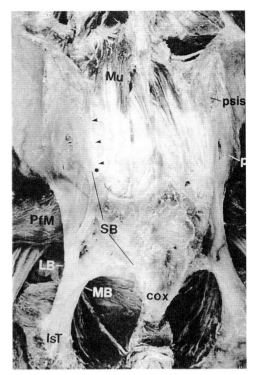

Fig. 3.27 • A dorsal view of the male pelvic girdle, ligaments intact and all but the deepest laminae of multifidus (Mu) removed. The arrowheads mark the long dorsal ligament beneath the lateral band (LB) of the sacrotuberous ligament. The medial band (MB) of the sacrotuberous ligament traverses the ischial tuberosity (IsT) and the coccyx (cox). The superior band of the sacrotuberous ligament (SB) runs superficial to the long dorsal ligament to connect the coccyx with the PSIS. Tendons of the multifidus (Mu) pass between the superior band and the long dorsal ligament to insert into the body of the sacrotuberous ligament. Reproduced with permission from Willard et al and the publisher Churchill Livingstone, 1997.

spinal nerves and blood vessels. It can be palpated directly caudal to the PSIS as a thick band and at this point it is covered by the fascia of the gluteus maximus muscle. Medially, fibers of this ligament attach to the deep lamina of the posterior layer of the thoracolumbar fascia and the aponeurosis of the erector spinae muscle (Vleeming et al 1996). At a deeper level, connections have been noted between the long dorsal ligament and the multifidus muscle (Willard 1997, 2007). Laterally, fibers blend with the superior band of the sacrotuberous ligament.

The sacrotuberous ligament is composed of three large fibrous bands, the lateral, medial, and superior (Figs 3.27, 3.28, 3.29) (Willard 1997, 2007). The lateral band connects the ischial tuberosity and the posterior inferior iliac spine and spans the piriformis muscle from which it receives some fibers. The medial band (inferior arcuate band) attaches to the transverse tubercles of S3, S4, and S5 and the lateral margin of the lower sacrum and coccyx. These fibers run anteroinferolaterally to reach the ischial tuberosity. The

fibers of this band spiral such that those arising from the lateral aspect of the ischial tuberosity insert into the caudal part of the sacrum, whereas those from the medial aspect of the ischial tuberosity attach cranially (Vleeming et al 1996). The superior band runs superficial to the interosseus ligament and connects the coccyx with the PSIS. The gluteus maximus also attaches to the sacrotuberous ligament and its contraction can increase the tension in the sacrotuberous ligament (Vleeming et al 1989a,b).

Phylogenetically, the sacrotuberous ligament represents the tendinous insertion of the biceps femoris muscle in lower vertebrates (Williams 1995). In some humans, this ligament still receives some fibers from

Fig. 3.28 • The biceps femoris muscle (BFM) has been found to alter tension in the sacrotuberous ligament (STL) through its indirect (attaching to the ischial tuberosity first) and, in some, direct (bypassing the ischial tuberosity) connection to the ligament. Reproduced with permission from Vleeming et al, 1989b.

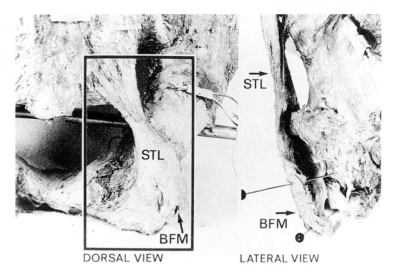

DORSAL VIEW   LATERAL VIEW

the biceps femoris muscle (Fig. 3.28) (Vleeming et al 1989a, 1995b). The fibers of the biceps femoris muscle can completely bridge the ischial tuberosity, attaching directly into the sacrotuberous ligament.

The tendons of the deep laminae of the multifidus muscle can also blend into the superior surface of the sacrotuberous ligament (Fig. 3.27) (Willard 2007). The ligament is pierced by the perforating cutaneous nerve (S2, S3), which subsequently winds around the inferior border of the gluteus maximus muscle to supply the skin covering the medial and inferior part of the buttock, perhaps a source of paresthesia when entrapped.

The sacrospinous ligament (see Figs 3.16, 3.29) attaches medially to the lower lateral aspect of the sacrum and the coccyx. Laterally, the apex of this triangular ligament attaches to the ischial spine of the innominate; proximally, fibers blend with the capsule of the SIJ (Willard 2007). It is closely connected to the coccygeus muscle, of which it may represent a degenerated part (Williams 1995).

Up to five bands of the iliolumbar ligament: anterior, superior, inferior, vertical (Fig. 3.16), and posterior (Fig. 3.30) have been described (Bogduk 1997, Pool-Goudzwaard et al 2001).

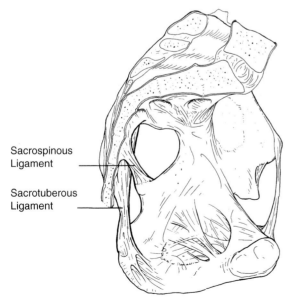

Sacrospinous Ligament

Sacrotuberous Ligament

Fig. 3.29 • A sagittal section of the pelvic girdle illustrating the anchoring effect of the sacrotuberous ligament on the sacral base.

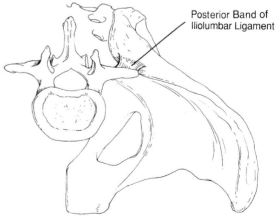

Posterior Band of Iliolumbar Ligament

Fig. 3.30 • A transverse section of the lumbosacral junction illustrating the attachment of the posterior band of the iliolumbar ligament.

- The anterior or ventral band attaches to the anteroinferior aspect of the entire length of the transverse process of the L5 vertebra. It blends with the superior band anterior to the quadratus lumborum muscle to attach to the anterior margin of the iliac crest.
- The superior band arises from the tip of the transverse process of the L5 vertebra. Laterally, the band divides to envelop the quadratus lumborum muscle before inserting onto the iliac crest.
- The posterior band also arises from the tip of the transverse process of the L5 vertebra. Laterally, it inserts onto the iliac tuberosity posteroinferiorly to the superior band. A direct attachment of this dorsal band attaches to the deep ventral layer of the thoracolumbar fascia.
- The inferior band arises both from the body and the inferior border of the transverse process of the L5 vertebra. Inferiorly, the fibers cross the ventral sacroiliac ligament obliquely to attach to the iliac fossa.
- The vertical band arises from the anteroinferior border of the transverse process of the L5 vertebra. These fibers descend vertically to attach to the posterior aspect of the arcuate line.

Willard (2007) reports that the individual bands of the iliolumbar ligament are highly variable in number and form, but consistently arise from the transverse processes of the L4 and L5 vertebrae blending inferiorly with the sacroiliac ligaments and laterally with the iliac crest. Previous descriptions of the evolution of this ligament from the quadratus lumborum muscle in the second decade of life (Luk et al 1986) have been refuted with the discovery of this ligament in the fetus (Hanson & Sonesson 1994, Uhtoff 1993). Although it is known that the iliolumbar ligament is an important structure for stabilization of the lumbosacral junction (Chow et al 1989, Leong et al 1987, Yamamoto et al 1990), Pool-Goudzwaard et al (2003) have also shown that the anterior, or ventral, band of the iliolumbar ligament plays an important role in restricting sagittal mobility of the SIJ.

The nerve supply of the sacroiliac joint. The most extensive study of the macroscopic innervation of the SIJ was done in 1957 by Solonen. He examined 18 joints in nine cadavers and found that posteriorly all of the joints were innervated from branches of the posterior rami of the S1 and S2 spinal nerves. Bradlay (1985) reported that the dorsal sacroiliac ligaments receive supply from the lateral divisions of the dorsal rami of the L5, S1, S2, and S3 spinal nerves. This was later confirmed by Grob et al (1995). According to Willard (2007), the dorsal sacral plexus (S1, S2, S3) forms in the sacral gutter inferior to the sacral attachment of multifidus and superficial to the sacrotuberous ligament and divides into medial and lateral divisions. The medial divisions supply multifidus, while the lateral divisions pass either through or under the long dorsal ligament where they are flattened to a very thin layer. These branches innervate the posterior aspect of the SIJ. Anteriorly, Solonen (1957) found that the articular innervation was not always consistent or necessarily symmetrical. Of the 18 specimens examined, all of the joints were innervated by branches from the ventral rami of the L5 spinal nerve, 17 from L4, 11 from S1, 4 from S2, 1 from L3, and 15 received innervation from the superior gluteal nerve. Grob et al (1995) were unable to confirm any innervation from the ventral rami. Fortin et al (1999) concur with Grob et al and feel that the SIJ is innervated only from the dorsal rami S1–4. They suggest that the investigators who have reported innervation of the joint from ventral rami have mistaken blood vessels for nerves as both are imaged with the same staining technique. The wide distribution of innervation is reflected clinically in the variety of pain patterns reported by patients with SIJ dysfunction (Fortin et al 1994a).

The blood supply of the sacrum and SIJ. The nutrient arteries and veins for the sacrum arise from the lateral and median sacral system. The lateral sacral vessels arise from the posterior trunk of the internal iliac and descend over the anterolateral aspect of the sacrum. The two longitudinal arteries give off anterior central branches, which course medially to anastomose with the median sacral artery. The anterior central branches send feeder vessels into the centrum of the sacrum. At the level of the ventral sacral foramina, spinal branches supply the cauda equina as well as the contents of the sacral canal. The foraminal branch, after passing through the dorsal sacral foramina, supplies the posterior aspect of the medial and intermediate sacral crests and also the posterior musculature and SIJ. Venous drainage is via vessels that accompany the arteries and subsequently drain into the common iliac system (Williams 1995).

The adult sacrococcygeal joint

The sacrococcygeal joint is classified as a symphysis, although synovial joints have been found at this articulation. Maigne (1997) examined nine specimens and found one fibrocartilaginous disc, four synovial joints, and four mixed (part synovial and part fibrocartilaginous). All of the specimens were older and it is not known if the sacrococcygeal joint can change from one form to another during a lifetime. The supporting ligaments include the ventral sacrococcygeal ligament, dorsal sacrococcygeal ligament, and the lateral sacrococcygeal ligament.

The ventral sacrococcygeal ligament represents the continuation of the anterior longitudinal ligament of the vertebral column. The dorsal sacrococcygeal ligament has two layers. The deep layer attaches to the posterior aspect of the body of the S5 vertebra and the coccyx (analogous to the posterior longitudinal ligament), whereas the superficial layer bridges the margins of the sacral hiatus and the posterior aspect of the coccyx, thus completing the sacral canal. Laterally, the intercornual ligaments, or the lateral sacrococcygeal ligaments, connect the sacral and coccygeal cornua.

The adult intercoccygeal joint

The intercoccygeal joint is classified as a symphysis in the young as the first two segments are separated via a fibrocartilaginous disc. With time, the joint usually ossifies; however, it occasionally remains synovial.

The development of the pubic symphysis

The pubic symphysis is a non-synovial joint, which contains a thick fibrocartilaginous disc between thin layers of hyaline cartilage. The symphysis is present by the end of the second month of gestation (Gamble et al 1986) with thick cartilaginous end-plates at birth (9–10mm) that become thin (200–400μm) with skeletal maturity. The secondary ossification centers appear in early puberty and by mid-adolescence the joint has reached its mature size.

The adult pubic symphysis

This joint contains a fibrocartilaginous disc (Figs 3.31, 3.32, Video 3.2), has neither synovial tissue nor fluid, and therefore is classified as a symphysis – a Greek term for 'growing together' (Gamble et al 1986). The osseous surfaces are covered by a thin layer of hyaline cartilage but they are separated by the fibrocartilaginous disc. The posterosuperior aspect of the disc often contains a cavity, which is not seen before the age of 10 years (Williams 1995).

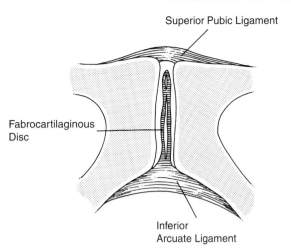

Fig. 3.31 • A coronal section through the pubic symphysis. Redrawn from Kapandji, 1974.

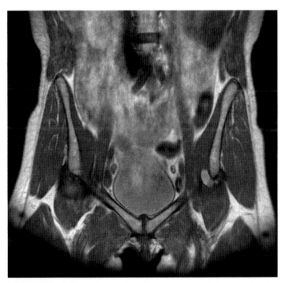

Fig. 3.32 • MRI coronal slice through the pubic symphysis. See Video 3.2 to watch several MRI coronal slices merge from anterior to posterior .

This is a non-synovial cavity and may represent a chronological degenerative change. The supporting ligaments of this articulation (Figs 3.31, 3.33) include the superior pubic ligament, inferior arcuate ligament, posterior pubic ligament, and the anterior pubic ligament.

The superior pubic ligament is a thick fibrous band that runs transversely between the pubic tubercles of the pubic bones. Inferiorly, the arcuate ligament blends with the fibrocartilaginous disc to attach to

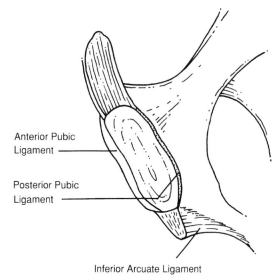

Anterior Pubic
Ligament

Posterior Pubic
Ligament

Inferior Arcuate Ligament

Fig. 3.33 • A sagittal section through the fibrocartilaginous disc of the pubic symphysis. Redrawn from Kapandji, 1974.

the inferior pubic rami bilaterally. According to Gamble et al (1986) this ligament provides most of the joint's stability. The posterior pubic ligament (Fig. 3.33) is membranous and blends with the adjacent periosteum, whereas the anterior ligament of the pubic symphysis is very thick and contains both transverse and oblique fibers (Kapandji 1974). It receives fibers from the aponeurotic expansion of the abdominal musculature as well as the adductor longus muscle, which decussates across the joint (Fig. 3.34).

The nerve supply of the pubic symphysis. The pubic symphysis is innervated from branches from the pudendal and genitofemoral nerves (Gamble et al 1986).

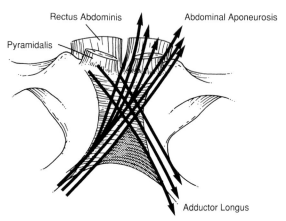

Rectus Abdominis

Abdominal Aponeurosis

Pyramidalis

Adductor Longus

Fig. 3.34 • The anterior aspect of the pubic symphysis. Redrawn from Kapandji, 1974.

The pubic symphysis and aging

In the fourth decade, smooth undulations appear along the margins of the joint and the bone begins to compact. This process continues and, in the sixth decade, the superior and inferior edges of the symphysis are clearly demarcated on X-ray, with a dense sclerotic streak present. This sclerosis continues and marginal osteophytes may appear (Gamble et al 1986).

The adult hip joint

The hip joint (Fig. 3.35A,B) is classified as an unmodified ovoid synovial joint (MacConaill & Basmajian 1977). The head of the femur forms roughly two-thirds of a sphere and, except for a small fovea, is covered by hyaline cartilage, which decreases in depth toward the periphery of the surface. The acetabulum has been described. The lunate surface of the acetabulum (see Fig. 3.17) is lined with hyaline cartilage, whereas the non-articular portion (the acetabular fossa) is filled with loose areolar tissue and covered with synovium. The acetabulum is deepened by a fibrocartilaginous labrum that is triangular in shape on cross-section. The base of the labrum attaches to the rim of the acetabulum. However, inferiorly it is deficient at the acetabular notch, which is bridged by the transverse acetabular ligament. The apex of the labrum is lined with articular cartilage and lies inside the hip joint as a free border; the capsule of the joint attaches to the labrum at its peripheral base, thus creating a circular recess. The anterior and superior aspect of the labrum is thought to be the most innervated portion containing receptors sensitive to pain and pressure (Hunt et al 2007). It is thought that the acetabular labrum contributes to both stability of the hip joint as well as preservation of its integrity by assisting in the distribution of the load during weight bearing (Hunt et al 2007). In addition, it helps to limit the expression of fluid from the joint space, and has an important sealing function (Shindle et al 2006).

The capsule and ligaments of the hip joint. The articular capsule encloses the joint and most of the femoral neck. Medially, it attaches to the base of the acetabular labrum and extends 5–6cm beyond this point onto the innominate. Inferiorly, the medial attachment is to the transverse acetabular ligament. Laterally, the capsule inserts onto the femur anteriorly along the entire extent of the trochanteric line, posteriorly to the femoral neck above the trochanteric crest, superiorly to the base of the femoral neck,

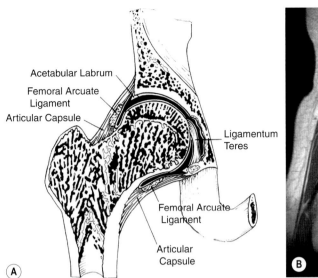

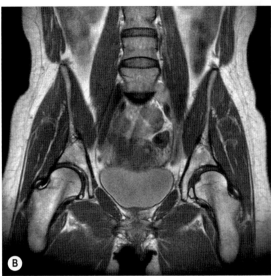

Fig. 3.35 • (A) A coronal section through the hip joint. (B) A coronal MRI slice through the hip joints.

and inferiorly to the femoral neck above the lesser trochanter. The superficial bands of the capsular fibers are predominantly longitudinal, whereas the deep bands are circular (Hewitt et al 2002). The ligaments, which are intimately blended with and support the capsule, include the iliofemoral ligament, pubofemoral ligament, the ischiofemoral ligament, and the femoral arcuate ligament. There are two intra-articular ligaments: the ligamentum teres and the transverse acetabular ligament. Hewitt et al (2002) tested some of these ligaments to failure in tension and also noted the stiffness value (force/displacement) at the point of failure.

The iliofemoral ligament (see Figs 3.16, 3.36, 3.37) is extremely strong and reinforces the anterior aspect of the hip joint. It is triangular in shape and attaches to the anterior inferior iliac spine at its apex. Inferolaterally, it diverges into two bands: the lateral iliotrochanteric band, which inserts onto the superior aspect of the trochanteric line, and the medial inferior band, which inserts onto the inferior aspect of the trochanteric line. Together, these two bands form an inverted Y, the center of which is filled with weaker ligamentous tissue. Hewitt et al (2002) noted that both bands of the iliofemoral ligament resisted a greater tensile force than the ischiofemoral and femoral arcuate ligaments and failed with the least amount of displacement. This ligament exhibits the greatest stiffness and prevents anterior translation during extension and external rotation (Shindle et al 2006).

The pubofemoral ligament (see Figs 3.16, 3.37) attaches medially to the iliopectineal eminence, the superior pubic ramus, and the obturator crest and membrane. Laterally, it attaches to the anterior surface of the trochanteric line. The capsule of the hip joint is unsupported by any ligament between the pubofemoral ligament and the inferior band of the iliofemoral ligament; however, the tendon of the psoas major muscle crosses the joint at this point, contributing to its dynamic support. A bursa is located here

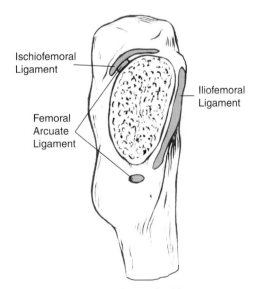

Fig. 3.36 • Medial view of the proximal femur. Redrawn from Hewitt et al, 2002.

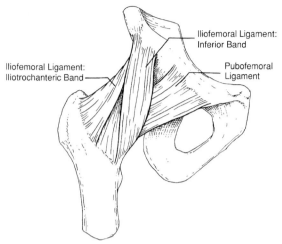

Fig. 3.37 • The ligaments of the anterior aspect of the hip joint.

between the tendon of the psoas muscle and the capsule and occasionally will communicate directly with the synovial cavity of the hip joint. Hewitt et al (2002) did not test this ligament in their study and, although most authors feel that the pubofemoral ligament limits abduction, it is recognized that the ligaments of the hip joint do not function independently (Torry et al 2006).

The ischiofemoral ligament (Fig. 3.38) arises medially from the ischial rim of the acetabulum

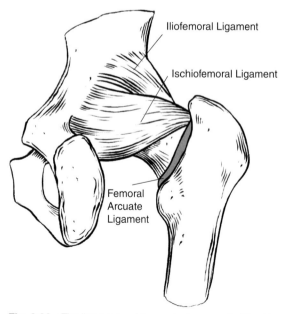

Fig. 3.38 • The ligaments of the posterior aspect of the hip joint.

and its labrum. Laterally, the fibers spiral supero-anteriorly over the back of the femoral neck to insert anterior to the trochanteric fossa deep to the ilio-femoral ligament. Some fibers from this ligament also run transversely to blend with those forming the femoral arcuate ligament (Hewitt et al 2002). The ischiofemoral ligament primarily restricts internal rotation of the hip as well as adduction of the flexed hip. This ligament failed under lower tensile loads than the iliofemoral ligament and exhibited greater displacement at the point of failure (less stiff) (Hewitt et al 2002).

The femoral arcuate ligament was previously called the zona orbicularis and some changes in its anatomy have been noted (Hewitt et al 2002). The fibers are circular and located in the deep posterior capsule (see Figs 3.35A, 3.38). It originates at the greater trochanter and passes deep to the ischiofemoral ligament posteriorly to insert inferiorly at the lesser trochanter. It does not cross the hip joint but rather functions to tense the capsule at the limits of extension and flexion. In tension studies (Hewitt et al 2002), this ligament exhibited the least amount of stiffness and failed at the lowest force.

The ligamentum teres (see Figs 3.17, 3.35A) attaches laterally to the anterosuperior part of the fovea of the femoral head, medially via three bands to either end of the lunate surface of the acetabulum inferiorly, and to the upper border of the transverse acetabular ligament.

The transverse acetabular ligament is a continuation of the acetabular labrum inferiorly and converts the acetabular notch into a foramen through which the intra-articular vessels pass to supply the head of the femur. In addition to the ligamentous support, the hip joint is dynamically stabilized by numerous muscles.

The nerve supply of the hip joint. The hip joint is innervated by branches from the obturator nerve (L2, L3, L4), the nerve to the quadratus femoris (L2, L3, L4), and the superior gluteal nerve (L5, S1) (Grieve 1986). As well, the joint receives branches from the nerves that supply the muscles crossing the joint. The hip joint is principally derived from the L3 segment of mesoderm with contributions from L2 to S1, hence the potential for a variety of patterns of pain referral.

The blood supply of the hip joint. The hip joint is supplied by the obturator, the medial and lateral femoral circumflex, and the superior and inferior gluteal arteries and veins (Crock 1980, Grieve 1981, Singleton & LeVeau 1975). The acetabular fossa, its contents as well as the head of the femur, receive supply from the acetabular branch of the obturator and medial femoral circumflex vessels via the ligamentum teres. The vascular anatomy is inconsistent and rarely sufficient to sustain the viability of the head of the femur following interruption of other sources of supply.

Myology of the pelvic girdle

There are 35 muscles that attach directly to the sacrum and/or innominate and together with the ligaments and fascia contribute to motion control and function of the pelvic girdle, which will be discussed in detail in Chapter 4. It is not the intent of this text to describe the anatomy of each of these muscles, but rather to highlight certain muscles and their fascial connections to facilitate later discussions.

The muscles of the abdominal wall

Transversus abdominis (TrA). Transversus abdominis (Fig. 3.39) is the deepest abdominal muscle and its anatomy has received recent attention (Urquhart et al 2005, Urquhart & Hodges 2007). This deep abdominal arises from the lateral one-third of the inguinal ligament, the anterior two-thirds of the inner lip of the iliac crest, the lateral raphe of the thoracolumbar fascia (and through this to the lumbar spine, more detail on this attachment below), and the inner surface of the lower six costal cartilages interdigitating with the costal fibers of the diaphragm. From this broad attachment, the muscle

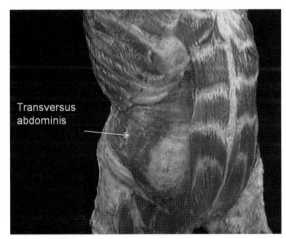

Transversus abdominis

Fig. 3.39 • The deepest abdominal is transversus abdominis. Note the extensive fascial attachment medially. Reproduced with permission from Acland and the publisher Lippincott Williams & Wilkins, 2004.

runs transversely around the trunk where its upper and middle fibers blend with the fascial envelope of the rectus abdominis, reaching the linea alba in the midline through a complex aponeurosis to be described below. The lower fibers, together with the lower fibers of the internal oblique (IO), join to form the conjoint tendon that attaches to the inguinal ligament and pubic crest.

Urquhart et al (2005) have noted differences in the fiber orientation of the upper, middle, and lower regions of transversus abdominis. The fibers in the upper region (from the sixth costal cartilage to the inferior border of the rib cage) were oriented superomedially; those in the middle region (from the inferior border of the rib cage to a line connecting the superior borders of the iliac crest) were oriented inferomedially; and those in the lower region (from the iliac crest line to the pubic symphysis) were oriented inferomedially (more so than the middle region). In this same dissection study (Urquhart et al 2005), regional variations in the thickness of transversus abdominis were noted in that the upper region of TrA was thicker than the lower and middle regions. In addition, intramuscular septa between the regions were found.

Anatomical variations of transversus abdominis have also been noted (for a literature review of this topic see Urquhart & Hodges 2007):

- Occasional fusion of TrA with the IO.
- Complete or partial detachment of TrA from the iliac crest.
- No attachment of TrA to the lateral raphe of the thoracolumbar fascia.
- TrA may stop above the anterior superior iliac spine.
- TrA may be completely absent.

According to Urquhart & Hodges (2007) these variations are rare; 96% of specimens in Urquhart et al's (2005) study found TrA to extend below the iliac crest. Clinically, it is very rare not to see transversus abdominis below the iliac crest when imaging the abdominal wall via ultrasound (author's personal observation). The transversus abdominis is innervated by the anterior primary rami of T6–T12 and L1 (Standring 2008).

In summary, the upper fibers of TrA are the thickest and are oriented horizontally; the middle fibers are less thick and are oriented inferomedially; and the lower fibers are the thinnest and are oriented the most inferomedially. Urquhart & Hodges (2007) suggest that the differences in the regional morphology of TrA support different functions for each part of the muscle. They suggest that, although all of TrA may contribute to increasing intra-abdominal pressure, the upper region may play a bigger role in stabilization of the rib cage, the middle region may facilitate stabilization of the lumbar spine through its connections to the thoracolumbar fascia, and the lower fibers may contribute to stabilization of the pelvis. The function of TrA will be covered in greater detail in Chapter 4.

Internal oblique (IO). The IO (Fig. 3.40) lies between the external oblique and the transversus abdominis and arises from the anterior two-thirds of the intermediate line of the iliac crest, the lateral two-thirds of the inguinal ligament, and the lateral raphe of the thoracolumbar fascia (TLF). Barker (2005) found that the IO consistently attaches to the TLF below L3 confirming the findings of Knox (2002). Like TrA, the IO also has regional differences in its morphology with upper, middle, and lower fibers. The upper and middle fibers of the IO are oriented superomedially, whereas the lowest fibers are oriented inferomedially. At the level of the ASIS, the IO fibers orient horizontally (Urquhart et al 2005). The fibers arising from the posterior aspect of the iliac crest ascend laterally from their point of origin to reach the tips of the 11th and 12th ribs, and the 10th rib near the costochondral junction. The fibers arising from the middle aspect of the iliac crest ascend to reach the costal cartilages of the seventh to ninth ribs, whereas those from the anterior aspect of the iliac crest blend with the fascial envelope of the rectus

abdominis reaching the linea alba in the midline through a complex aponeurosis (to be described below). The fibers arising from the inguinal ligament arch inferomedially to blend with the aponeurosis of transversus abdominis and attach to the pubic crest. Similar to TrA, Urquhart et al (2005) found regional differences in the thickness of IO with the upper fibers being thicker than the lower. IO is also thicker than TrA in the lower region. The internal oblique muscle is innervated by the ventral rami of the lower six thoracic and first lumbar spinal nerves (Standring 2008).

External oblique (EO). The external oblique (Fig. 3.41) is the largest abdominal with eight digitations arising from the external surfaces and inferior borders of the lower eight ribs (ribs 5–12) interdigitating with fibers of serratus anterior and latissimus dorsi. The upper attachments of the external oblique arise close to the costochondral joints, the middle attachments to the body of the ribs, and the lowest to the tip of the cartilage of the 12th rib. Inferiorly, the posterior fibers descend vertically to attach to the outer lip of the anterior half of the iliac crest. The upper and middle fibers descend inferomedially to blend with the fascial envelope of the rectus abdominis reaching the linea alba in the midline through a complex aponeurosis (to be described below). Whereas anatomy texts (Williams 1995) do not mention any attachment of the EO to the TLF, Knox (2002) found that the EO muscle sheath blended with the dorsal aponeurosis of the TrA and thus to the TLF, whereas Barker (2005) found a consistent attachment of the posterior fibers of EO to the lateral raphe of the TLF above the level of L3. Urquhart et al (2005) also noted regional variations in the thickness of the EO, with its middle region being the thickest.

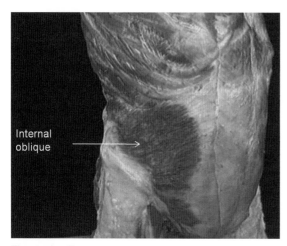

Fig. 3.40 • The middle layer of the abdominal wall, the internal oblique. Reproduced with permission from Acland and the publisher Lippincott Williams & Wilkins, 2004.

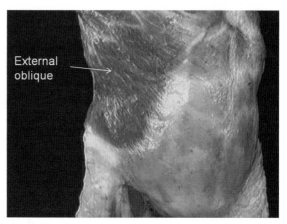

Fig. 3.41 • The external oblique. Reproduced with permission from Acland and the publisher Lippincott Williams & Wilkins, 2004.

When comparing thickness of the middle region only, the EO is thicker than TrA, but thinner than IO. The EO muscle is innervated by the ventral rami of the lower six thoracic spinal nerves (Standring 2008).

Rectus abdominis (RA). The RA muscle (Figs 3.42, 3.43) is a long muscular strap just lateral to

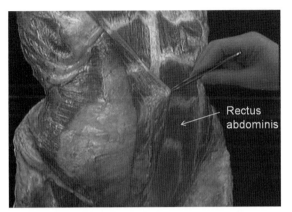

Fig. 3.42 • The rectus abdominis with the internal and external oblique removed. Reproduced with permission from Acland and the publisher Lippincott Williams & Wilkins, 2004.

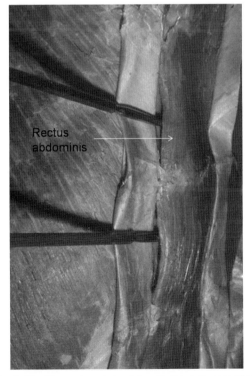

Fig. 3.43 • The rectus abdominis with the external oblique attached. Reproduced with permission from Porterfield & DeRosa, 1998.

the anterior midline of the abdomen. It arises from the pubic crest and tubercle as well as the ligaments of the symphysis pubis (see Fig. 3.34). The aponeurotic expansions of this muscle interdigitate anterior to the symphysis to form a dense network of fibers, thus contributing to the stability of this joint (Kapandji 1974, Williams 1995). The RA inserts into the fifth to seventh costal cartilages (sometimes as high as the third costal cartilage) and the xyphoid process. Three horizontal tendinous bands separate the muscle and receive attachment from the external oblique (Fig. 3.43) (DeRosa 2001). The rectus abdominis is enclosed in a fascial sheath formed by the decussating aponeurosis of the external and internal oblique muscles as well as the aponeurosis of the transversus abdominis. The medial borders of the RA connect through this bilaminar aponeurosis, collectively known as the linea alba (to be described below). The nerve supply is through the ventral rami of the lower six or seven thoracic spinal nerves (Standring 2008).

Pyramidalis. This triangular muscle is located anterior to the inferior aspect of the RA muscle and is enclosed within its sheath (see Fig. 3.34). The base attaches to the pubic crest as well as to the pubic symphysis, whereas the apex blends with the linea alba midway between the umbilicus and the pubis. This muscle is innervated by the subcostal nerve, which is the ventral ramus of the T12 spinal nerve.

The linea alba and the aponeurosis of the rectus sheaths

The linea alba. Past descriptions of the linea alba and the aponeuroses of the rectus sheaths were derived from macroscopic examination (Askar 1977, Rizk 1980, Williams 1995). These descriptions led to the belief that the aponeuroses of the abdominal muscles decussated across the midline linea alba to join with the aponeuroses of the opposite side (Fig. 3.44). More recent studies using confocal laser scanning microscopy have revealed that these descriptions are not accurate. Axer et al (2000, 2001) used this method to investigate the morphological configuration of the collagen fibrils in the medial rectus sheaths, as well as the linea alba along its entire length (from xyphoid to pubic symphysis) in both men and women. Although there was some individual variation, a general pattern of fibril arrangement was present.

Essentially, the linea alba can be divided into three zones in its anteroposterior dimension and four regions in its craniocaudal dimension.

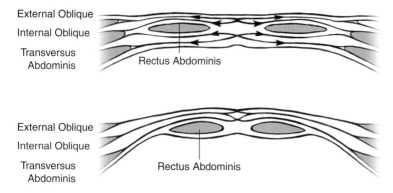

External Oblique
Internal Oblique
Transversus
Abdominis
Rectus Abdominis

External Oblique
Internal Oblique
Transversus
Abdominis
Rectus Abdominis

Fig. 3.44 • Traditional macroscopic illustrations of the contribution and morphology of the aponeuroses of the abdominal muscles to the rectus sheaths and the linea alba above (top) and below (bottom) the umbilicus. Redrawn from Williams, 1995.

Anteroposteriorly, there is a superficial ventral zone of obliquely arranged fibrils, an intermediate zone of transverse fibrils, and a thin dorsal zone of oblique fibrils (Fig. 3.45). Craniocaudally, there are four different regions categorized according to the morphological characteristics of the collagen fibrils. The first, or supraumbilical, region has a fibril scheme as described (Fig. 3.45). The second, or umbilical, region has circular collagen fibril bundles of the navel, which interweave with the fibril bundles of the linea alba. The third region is called the transition zone, where oblique fibrils predominate and the layer of transverse fibrils is smaller. This region corresponds to the region where the fibril bundles of the dorsal rectus sheath become distributed onto the ventral rectus sheaths. The fourth, or infra-arcuate, region is the most caudal and has the same architectural scheme of fibril orientation as the supraumbilical region.

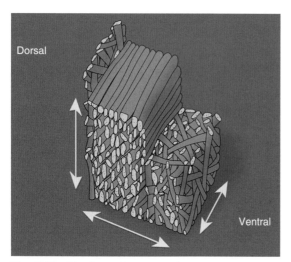

Dorsal

Ventral

Fig. 3.45 • The linea alba as seen by confocal laser scanning microscopy. Redrawn from Axer et al, 2001.

Axer et al (2001) also found that the mean diameter (thickness) of the fibril bundles was smaller in the supraumbilical region (linea alba was thus thinner) and suggests that this may have a role on why primary hernias are found only in the supraumbilical and umbilical regions of the linea alba and not the infraumbilical region. Clinically, diastasis RA (Chapter 6) can involve all four regions of the linea alba.

There are significant differences between men and women in the number of fibers in the linea alba regionally (Gräßel et al 2005) and also in the relative compliance in either the transverse or oblique plane(s). Women have more transverse fibers relative to oblique fibers in the infraumbilical region (60.4% vs 39.6%), whereas men have more oblique fibers relative to transverse (62.5% vs 37.5%).

For both sexes, the highest compliance of the linea alba was in the longitudinal direction (craniocaudal) and the least in the transverse direction in the infraumbilical region. Women have more transversely oriented fibers in the infraumbilical region than men (60.4% vs 37.5%). On compliance testing, the infraumbilical region of the female subjects had the least compliance of all regions in the transverse plane. One female subject in this study was nulliparous and her fiber orientation distribution and compliance in the transverse plane were similar to that of the male group. Gräßel et al (2005) hypothesize that the linea alba adapts to increases in intra-abdominal pressure during pregnancy by increasing fiber size and number. There is no evidence yet to support this hypothesis.

The rectus sheaths. The aponeuroses of the EO, IO, and TrA form the sheaths that envelop the left and right RA muscles. According to Gray's Anatomy (Williams 1995) (Fig. 3.44):

At the lateral margin of the Rectus, the aponeurosis of the Obliquus internus divides into two lamellæ, one of which passes in front of the Rectus, blending with the aponeurosis of the Obliquus externus, the other, behind it, blending with the aponeurosis of the Transversus, and these, joining again at the medial border of the Rectus, are inserted into the linea alba. This arrangement of the aponeurosis exists from the costal margin to midway between the umbilicus and symphysis pubis, where the posterior wall of the sheath ends in a thin curved margin, the **linea semicircularis,** the concavity of which is directed downward: below this level the aponeuroses of all three muscles pass in front of the Rectus. The Rectus, in the situation where its sheath is deficient below, is separated from the peritoneum by the transversalis fascia. Since the tendons of the Obliquus internus and Transversus only reach as high as the costal margin, it follows that above this level the sheath of the Rectus is deficient behind, the muscle resting directly on the cartilages of the ribs, and being covered merely by the tendon of the Obliquus externus.

Axer et al (2000, 2001) did not investigate the lateral sheath of the rectus, but only the medial sheath, and found an interesting orientation of collagen fibrils. Three different regions were described for the medial sheath of RA (Figs 3.46, 3.47), the supraumbilical, transition, and infra-arcuate. In the supraumbilical region (Fig. 3.46), the medial ventral rectus sheath contains mainly obliquely oriented fibril bundles, which intermingle with each other, whereas the medial dorsal rectus sheath contains

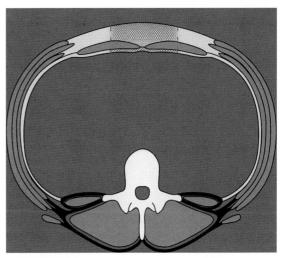

Fig. 3.47 • A graphic representation of the morphology of the medial rectus sheath, linea alba, and thoracolumbar fascia at the level of L4. The lateral aspect of the rectus sheaths as well as the fascial morphology contributing to these sheaths has been left absent on purpose as Axer et al (2000, 2001) did not investigate the orientation of the collagen fibers in this region.

mainly fibrils that are oriented transversely. They do not note whether the IO aponeuroses split around the RA in this region. In the second region, the transition zone (below the umbilicus), the dorsal transverse bundles begin to move to the ventral side of the rectus sheath. This transition is not sudden but rather occurs over a few centimeters (Axer et al 2000, 2001). In the infra-arcuate region (Fig. 3.47), the dorsal sheath of the rectus contains only a few thin collagen fibers, whereas the ventral sheath continuously becomes thicker. They suggest that there is no such thing as an arcuate line or linea semicircularis, and that the arcuate line is really a zone of transition of fibers with a high degree of variability.

The muscles of the back

Multifidus. In the lumbosacral region, the deepest fibers of multifidus (laminar fibers) arise from the posteroinferior aspect of the lamina and articular capsule of the zygapophyseal joint and insert onto the mammillary process two levels below (Bogduk 1997) (Figs 3.27, 3.48, 3.49). The remainder of the muscle arises medially from the spinous process, blending laterally with the laminar fibers. Inferiorly, the superficial fascicles of multifidus insert *three* levels below, such that those arising from the L1

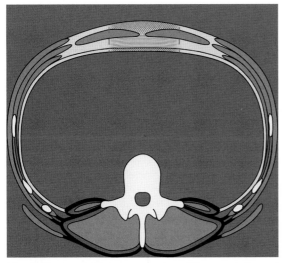

Fig. 3.46 • A graphic representation of the morphology of the medial rectus sheath, linea alba, and thoracolumbar fascia at the level of L2. The lateral aspect of the rectus sheaths as well as the fascial morphology contributing to these sheaths has been left absent on purpose as Axer et al (2000, 2001) did not investigate the orientation of the collagen fibers in this region.

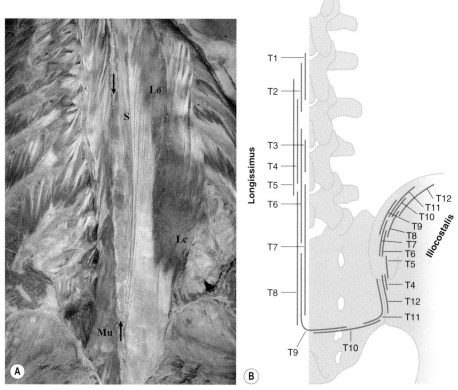

Fig. 3.48 • (A) Longissimus thoracis pars thoracis (Lo), iliocostalis lumborum pars thoracis (Ic), and superficial fibers of multifidus (Mu) can be clearly seen in this beautiful dissection of Willard. S, Reproduced with permission from Willard and the publisher Churchill Livingstone, 1997. (B) Posteroanterior view of the lumbar vertebral column showing the range and extent of the attachment sites of individual fascicles of the thoracic portions of the iliocostalis lumborum and the longissimus thoracis. The junction between longissimus and iliocostalis occurs constantly at the base of the posterior superior iliac spine. The numbers indicate the vertebral level of the rostral attachment of each fascicle. Redrawn from MacIntosh & Bogduk, 1991.

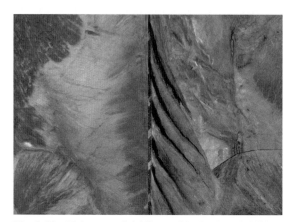

Fig. 3.49 • Right: superficial fibers of the lumbar multifidus. Left: thoracolumbar fascia. Reproduced with permission from Gracovetsky (personal library).

vertebra insert onto the mammillary processes of the L4, L5, and S1 vertebrae as well as the medial aspect of the iliac crest. Inferiorly, the fibers from the spinous process of the L2 vertebra (superficial multifidus) insert onto the mammillary processes of the L5 and S1 vertebrae and the posterior superior iliac spine (PSIS) of the innominate. The fibers from the spinous process of the L3 vertebra insert onto the S1 articular process, the superolateral aspect (costal element) of the S1 and S2 segments, and the iliac crest. The fibers from the spinous process of the L4 vertebra insert onto the lateral sacral crest and the area of bone between this crest and the dorsal sacral foramina, whereas those from the L5 vertebra insert onto the intermediate sacral crest inferiorly to S3. Within the pelvis, the multifidus muscle also attaches to the deep laminae of the posterior thoracolumbar fascia at a raphe that separates it from the gluteus maximus muscle (Willard 1997, 2007). Willard (2007) notes that this raphe is anchored into the capsule of the SIJ. Tendinous slips of the multifidus pass beneath the posterior sacroiliac ligaments to blend with the sacrotuberous ligament (see Fig. 3.27). Hides et al (1995a) note that the cross-sectional area of multifidus increases progressively from L2 to L5 and, although the size varies between subjects, the intrasubject between side measurements suggest that the mutifidus is symmetrical (Hides et al 2008).

The fascicles are innervated by the medial branch of the dorsal ramus such that all of the fascicles that arise from the same spinous process are innervated by the same nerve regardless of the inferior extent of their insertion (Bogduk 1983, 1997). MacDonald et al (2006) conducted an extensive literature review for multifidus and pooled the results from multiple studies that investigated its fiber composition, noting that both the deep and superficial fibers of multifidus have a greater percentage of type I than type II muscle fibers. This suggests that fiber type is not the only factor responsible for the differential activation in function and dysfunction noted in the deep and superficial fibers (Chapters 4, 5).

Erector spinae (ES). ES is a collective name for several separate muscles that 'erect the spine.' Although they may be collectively grouped anatomically, current research suggests that they function quite differently (Chapter 4). Bogduk (1997) has divided the erector spinae according to the regional attachments as follows:

- Longissimus thoracis pars lumborum.
- Longissimus thoracis pars thoracis.
- Iliocostalis lumborum pars lumborum.
- Iliocostalis lumborum pars thoracis.

Longissimus thoracis pars lumborum. The lumbar component of longissimus thoracis arises from five muscle fascicles, the deepest of which is from the L5 vertebra overlapped by those from L4, then L3, L2, and finally L1 (Bogduk 1997). Medially, these laminae arise from the accessory and the medial end of the dorsal surface of the transverse processes. The fibers from the L1 to L4 vertebrae insert via a common tendon into the medial aspect of the lumbar intramuscular aponeurosis, which attaches inferiorly to the medial aspect of the PSIS just lateral to the fascicle from L5.

Longissimus thoracis pars thoracis. The thoracic component of longissimus thoracis is the largest part of the ES group in the thoracic spine and forms the bulk of the paravertebral muscle mass adjacent to the spine. It arises from the ribs and transverse processes of T1–T12 and descends to attach via the aponeurosis of the ES to the spinous processes of the lumbar spine and sacrum (Fig. 3.48A,B). Each fascicle descends a variable length with those from the upper thorax reaching to L3, whereas the lower fascicles bridge the lumbar spine completely. Note the specificity of the distal attachment to the lumbar and sacral spinous processes according to MacIntosh & Bogduk (1991) in Figure 3.48B.

Iliocostalis lumborum pars lumborum. The lumbar component of iliocostalis lumborum arises as four overlapping fascicles from the tips of the transverse processes of the L1 to L4 vertebrae (lateral to the longissimus thoracis pars lumborum) and from the middle layer of the thoracolumbar fascia. Inferiorly, the muscle inserts onto the iliac crest lateral to the PSIS.

Iliocostalis lumborum pars thoracis. The thoracic component of iliocostalis lumborum is large and the most lateral part of the ES muscle group. Fascicles from the inferior borders of the angles of the lower seven to eight ribs originate lateral to the attachment of iliocostalis thoracis and descend to attach to the ilium and sacrum with the thoracic component of the longissimus thoracis to form the aponeurosis of ES (Fig. 3.48A,B). These thoracic fascicles have no attachment to the lumbar vertebra bridging the gap between the thorax and the pelvis. Note the specificity of the distal attachment to the iliac crest and sacrum according to MacIntosh & Bogduk (1991) in Figure 3.48B.

The ES aponeurosis is derived from the tendons of the longissimus thoracis pars thoracis and iliocostalis lumborum pars thoracis. This muscle is innervated from the lateral and intermediate branches of the segmental dorsal spinal rami.

Quadratus lumborum. This muscle is not quite rectangular (or quadrate) and lies deep to the ES and lateral to psoas. It arises from the transverse process of L5, the split superior band of the iliolumbar ligament and the adjacent iliac crest. The most lateral fibers ascend to insert into the lower anterior aspect of the medial half of the 12th rib. The medial fibers ascend superomedially to attach to the anterior surfaces of each of the lumbar transverse processes above L5. Bogduk (1997) notes that there are also other obliquely directed fibers that arise from each of the lumbar transverse processes and ascend superolaterally to attach to the 12th rib. These fibers intermingle with those ascending superomedially from the iliac crest. Quadratus lumborum is innervated from the ventral rami of the 12th thoracic through to the 4th lumbar nerves.

Thoracolumbar fascia

The thoracolumbar fascia is a critical structure when considering how loads are transferred between the trunk and the lower extremity (Barker et al 2004, Barker 2005, Barker et al 2006, Barker & Briggs 1999, 2007, Vleeming et al 1995a). Several muscles attach to this fascia and can affect tension within it, including the transversus abdominis, internal oblique, external oblique, gluteus maximus, latissimus dorsi, ES, multifidus, and biceps femoris. In addition, recent research has found a variable amount of α-smooth muscle actin (smooth muscle-like cells also known as myofibroblasts) in all fascial tissue including the thoracolumbar fascia (Schleip et al 2005) and it is now widely accepted that fascia has contractile capability. Fascia is a highly sensorial tissue containing Golgi, Pacini, Ruffini, and interstitial receptors, which when stimulated can decrease muscle tone (Golgi), provide proprioceptive and interoceptive feedback (Pacini and interstitial), inhibit overall sympathetic activity (Ruffini), and increase vasodilation and plasma extrusion (interstitial) (Schleip 2008). Schleip describes the sensory role of fascia as providing the ability 'to feel yourself and your relationship to the environment.' Fascial research is revealing exciting new findings suggesting that fascia is not just connective tissue that supports and transmits forces, but rather has a huge messenger role and is capable of dynamic contractile behavior.

The macroscopic anatomy of the thoracolumbar fascia is complex (Barker 2005, Barker & Briggs 1999, 2007, Bogduk 1997, Vleeming et al 1995a) (see Figs 3.46, 3.47). There are three layers to the fascia: the anterior, middle, and posterior. The anterior layer is thin (with minimal tensile strength) (Barker 2005) and covers the anterior aspect of the quadratus lumborum muscles. It attaches medially to the anterior aspect of the transverse processes and blends with the intertransverse ligaments. It also joins the middle layer at the lateral raphe.

The middle layer is posterior to the quadratus lumborum. It arises medially from the tips of the transverse processes and intertransverse ligaments and inferiorly to the iliac crest and iliolumbar

ligament. It is much thicker than the anterior layer and extends a mere 2–3cm laterally before it fuses with the posterior layer to form the lateral raphe. In the lower lumbar spine, this layer attaches to the transversus abdominis, internal oblique, and latissimus dorsi. Above L3 it remains attached to the transversus abdominis, latissimus dorsi, and external oblique; however, it is no longer attached to the internal oblique (Barker et al 2004).

There are two laminae that comprise the posterior layer of the thoracolumbar fascia, which are increasingly fused below T12 (Barker & Briggs 2007). The combined laminae of the posterior layer of the thoracolumbar fascia is as thick as the middle layer and extends approximately 7cm lateral to the spinous processes of the lumbar spine.

The superficial lamina of this layer is predominantly derived from the aponeurosis of the latissimus dorsi muscle (Fig. 3.50), and contains oblique fibers that run caudomedially. In the midline, strong connections

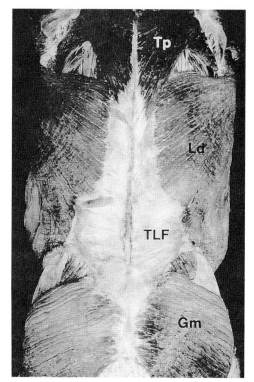

Fig. 3.50 • A posterior view of the thoracolumbar fascia (TLF) illustrates the attachments of latissimus dorsi (Ld) and gluteus maximus (Gm) into the superficial lamina of the posterior layer. Note the small attachment of the lower fibers of the trapezius muscle (Tp). Reproduced with permission from Willard and the publisher Churchill Livingstone, 1997.

attach the fascia to the supraspinal ligaments and the spinous processes of the lumbar vertebrae cranial to L4. According to Willard (1997, 2007), the posterior border of the ligamentum flavum becomes the supraspinous ligament, which in turn is anchored to the thoracolumbar fascia (Figs 3.51, 3.52). Through these attachments, tension of the thoracolumbar fascia is transmitted to the ligamentum flavum and, according to Willard (1997, 2007), assists in the alignment of the lumbar vertebrae. The superficial laminae also receive some fibers from the external oblique above L3 (Barker 2005) and the lower trapezius muscles (Vleeming et al 1995a). Caudal to L4, midline connections are very loose and actually cross the midline to reach the opposite iliac crest and sacrum. Over the sacrum, the superficial lamina blends with the fascia of the gluteus maximus. These fibers run in a caudolateral direction from a medial attachment to the median sacral crest, and occasionally as far cranial as the L4 spinous process (Fig. 3.53).

The deep lamina of the posterior layer is also complex with several muscular connections (Fig. 3.54A,B). The fibers run in a caudolateral direction attaching medially to the interspinous ligaments and caudally to the PSIS, iliac crest, and posterior sacroiliac ligaments. Above the pelvis, the deep lamina of the posterior layer attaches to the lateral raphe and blends with the middle layer of the thoracolumbar fascia.

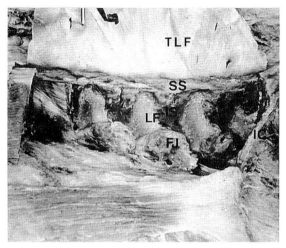

Fig. 3.51 • Dorsolateral view of the lumbar spine. The thoracolumbar fascia (TLF) blends with the supraspinous ligament (SS) and interspinous ligament and ligamentum flavum (LF). IC is the iliac crest. Reproduced with permission from Willard and the publisher Churchill Livingstone, 1997.

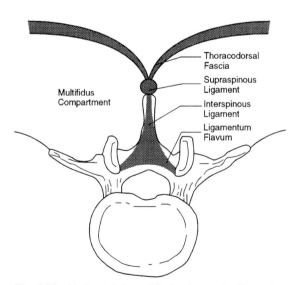

Fig. 3.52 • Horizontal view of the lumbar region illustrating the ligamentum flavum/interspinous ligament/supraspinous ligament/thoracolumbar fascia connections. Redrawn from Willard, 1997.

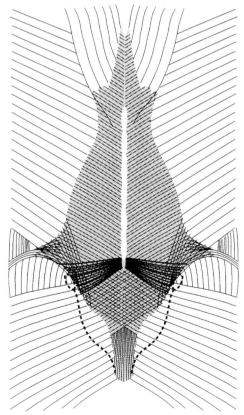

Fig. 3.53 • The superficial lamina of the thoracolumbar fascia. Redrawn from Vleeming et al, 1997.

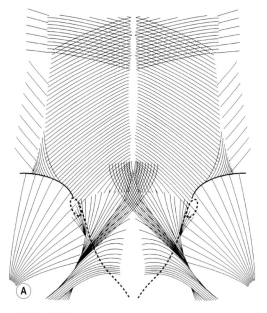

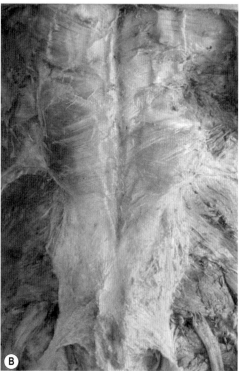

Fig. 3.54 • (A) The deep lamina of the thoracolumbar fascia. Redrawn from Vleeming et al, 2007. (B) The deep lamina of the thoracolumbar fascia forms the roof of multifidus and blends with the sacrotuberous ligament. Reproduced with permission from Vleeming et al, 2007.

Over the pelvis, some fibers blend with the deep fascia of the erector spinae muscle (forming the roof over the sacral multifidus) and the sacrotuberous ligament.

The muscles and fascia of the pelvic floor

The pelvic floor is not really a floor at all (other than the fact that it is at the bottom of the abdominal canister and therefore analogous to the bottom of a room). A floor has two dimensions – width and length – whereas the structures of the bottom of the abdominal canister have three: width, length, and height (or depth). Perhaps the pelvic diaphragm is a better inclusive term for all of the structures that comprise the bottom of the abdominal canister. The proposal is that this three-dimensional diaphragm extends from the left to the right greater trochanter (Fig. 3.55A,B,C) and is comprised of several muscles as well as an extensive complex fascial support system. The levator ani (pubovisceralis, pubococcygeus, iliococcygeus, and puborectalis) and the obturator internus are significant parts of this diaphragm and will be described in detail below, as will the piriformis, ischiococcygeus, and iliacus (muscles that form the back wall of the inner pelvis). In addition, a detailed description of the integrated endopelvic fascial system will be described. The reader is referred to other anatomy texts and/or *Primal Pictures Interactive Pelvis and Perineum* (2003) for descriptions of the urogenital diaphragm, urethral sphincteric muscles, and the anal sphincter muscles.

Levator ani. According to Ashton-Miller & DeLancey (2007), the levator ani is comprised of the following parts:

- The relatively flat iliococcygeus (Fig. 3.55B, 3.56A,B), which originates from the medial aspect of the ischial spine and the posterior part of the arcus tendineus levator ani fascia bilaterally (see below). The muscle forms a horizontal sheet that covers the posterior aspect of the pelvis. Fibers from this muscle attach to the anterior aspect of the coccyx.

- The obliquely oriented pubococcygeus and the more medial puborectalis originate from the inner surface of the pubic bone, 2.5–4cm above the arcus tendineus levator ani fascia (Figs 3.56A,B, 3.57). The posterior fibers of the pubococcygeus arise from the anterior half of this fascia. Pubococcygeus passes posteriorly and attaches to

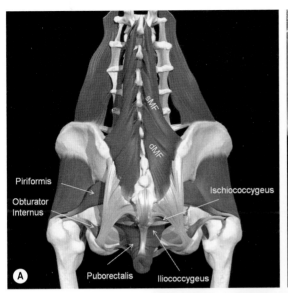

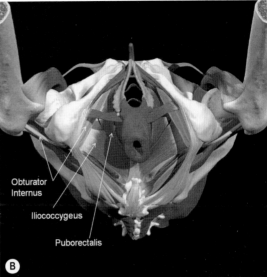

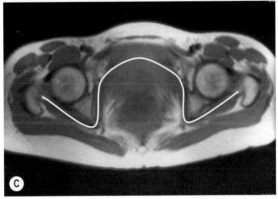

Fig. 3.55 • (A) A posterior view of the pelvic diaphragm. Picture from Primal Pictures, 2003. dMF = deep multifidus at the lumbosacral junction; sMF = superficial multifidus from L2 spinous process to the iliac crest. (B) An inferior perspective of the pelvic diaphragm. Picture from Primal Pictures, 2003. (C) An MRI of the pelvic diaphragm. In all three figures, note the connection between the left and right obturator internus and the fascia that connects it to the levator ani in the midline.

a midline raphe posterior to the rectum. Through this raphe, fibers unite and continue posteriorly from the anorectal flexure to attach to the anterior aspect of the last two coccygeal segments. The puborectalis passes posteriorly lateral to the urethra, vagina (females), and rectum to unite with its counterpart to form a muscular sling at the anorectal flexure; there is no posterior osseus attachment.

- Puboviscernlis has been used to describe a muscle that includes both pubococcygeus and puborectalis (DeLancey 1994); more recently, it has been used to describe three smaller muscles,

none of which is pubococcygeus or puborectalis (Ashton-Miller & DeLancey 2007). In this latest anatomical description of the levator ani, the term puboviscernlis is used to describe three smaller muscles (Fig. 3.56B), which all originate from the pubic bone medial to puborectalis. They include: pubovaginalis, which inserts into the lateral aspect of the vaginal wall, puboperineus, which inserts into the perineal body, and puboanalis, which inserts into the intersphincteric groove of the anal canal (Fig. 3.57).

The urogenital hiatus is an opening in the anterior part of the levator ani through which the urethra

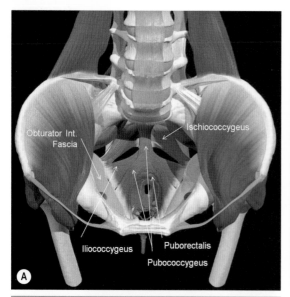

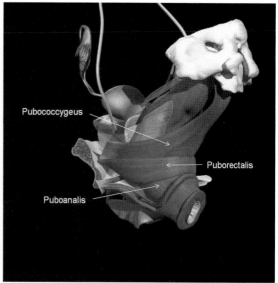

Fig. 3.57 • A posterolateral view of the detailed anatomy of the medial aspect of the pelvic diaphragm. Picture from Primal Pictures, 2003.

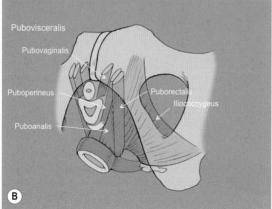

Fig. 3.56 • (A) The middle part of the pelvic diaphragm (the levator ani) arises predominantly from the fascia overlying the obturator internus. (B) Detailed illustration of puboviscerals (pubovaginalis, puboperineus, puboanalis), puborectalis, and iliococcygeus. Redrawn from Ashton-Miller & DeLancey, 2007.

and vagina (in females) pass. This hiatus is supported anteriorly by the pubic bones and the levator ani muscle and posteriorly by the perineal body and the external anal sphincter. The levator ani muscles comprise primarily type I (slow twitch) fibers, although each group also has a smaller proportion of type II (fast twitch) fibers. The levator ani takes origin off of the arcus tendineus levator ani fascia, which is a thickening of the fascia overlying obturator internus. Through the connections of the obturator internus muscles (see below) the levator ani is indirectly connected to each greater trochanter, hence the

concept of the functional pelvic diaphragm extending from femur to femur (see Fig. 3.55A,B,C). The anteromedial portion of the levator ani is supplied by branches of the pudendal nerve, whereas the posterolateral region is supplied directly from the sacral plexus S3 and S4 (Williams 1995).

The endopelvic fascia. This connective tissue matrix is actually a fibromuscular layer that includes fibroblasts, smooth muscle cells, and elastin, as well as type III collagen, all of which is loosely organized to form an elastic fibromuscular layer that supports the urethra and invests the vaginal walls and rectum laterally, superiorly, and inferiorly (Cundiff & Fenner 2004). Laterally, this fascia attaches the vagina and rectum to the arcus tendineus fascia pelvis (ATFP) (Figs 3.58, 3.59), which is a thickening of the fascia over the obturator internus. Anteriorly near its origin at the pubic bone, the ATFP is a well-defined fibrous band that broadens into an aponeurotic sheet posteriorly attaching to the ischial spine and blending medially with the endopelvic fascia and the levator ani muscles. At the apex of the vagina, the fascia between it and the rectum (rectovaginal fascia or septum) thickens to become the cardinal and uterosacral ligaments that insert into the presacral fascia at S2, S3, and S4. Therefore, the vagina and rectum are suspended laterally to the ATFP and posterosuperiorly to the presacral fascia. The perineal body is also attached to this complex fascia through the rectovaginal fascia, and

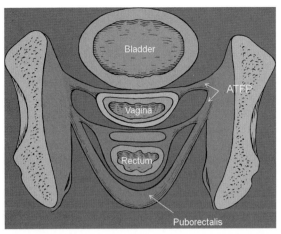

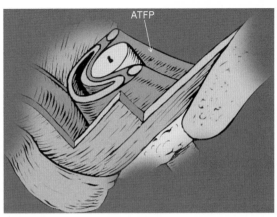

Fig. 3.58 • The vagina and rectum are supported laterally by fascial connections to the arcus tendineus fascia pelvis (ATFP). Redrawn from Retzky & Rogers, 1995.

Fig. 3.60 • The hammock of support for the urethra depends on the integrity of the endopelvic fascia and its lateral extensions to the arcus tendineus fascia pelvis (ATFP). Redrawn from DeLancey, 1994.

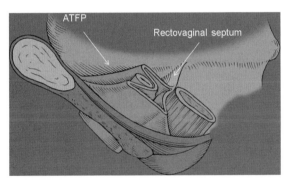

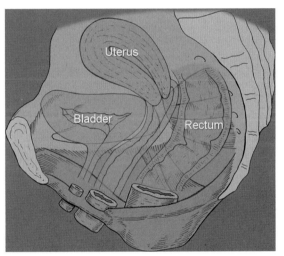

Fig. 3.59 • The rectovaginal fascia or septum connects the vagina to the rectum in the midline and extends laterally to attach to the arcus tendineus fascia pelvis (ATFP). Redrawn from Leffler et al, 2001.

Fig. 3.61 • The relationship between the myofascia of the functional pelvic diaphragm and the pelvic organs.

is thus suspended from the presacral fascia and lateral pelvic walls. The urethra rests in a hammock created by the endopelvic fascia, which is suspended between the left and right ATFPs (Fig. 3.60). This complex fibro-muscular matrix is actively supported by the levator ani and together this complex plays a vital role in the support of the pelvic organs (Chapter 4) (Fig. 3.61).

Obturator internus. The obturator internus arises from the medial two-thirds of the obturator mem-brane and the pelvic margins of the obturator foramen (see Figs 3.55A,B,C, 3.56A). Overlying this muscle is the thickened ATFP and, above this thickening, a thin fascial layer extends and is continuous with the fascia of iliacus. Below, the fascial covering of the obturator internus blends with the fascia of the levator ani. Laterally, the muscle fibers coalesce to form a tendon

that exits the inner pelvis through the lesser sciatic notch to insert into an impression on the medial sur-face of the greater trochanter along with the superior and inferior gemelli. The obturator internus is sup-plied by the ventral rami of L5, S1, and S2.

The muscles of the deep back wall of the pelvis

The deep back wall of the pelvis is comprised of the ischiococcygeus, piriformis, and iliacus muscles (Fig. 3.62A), which lies in the same plane

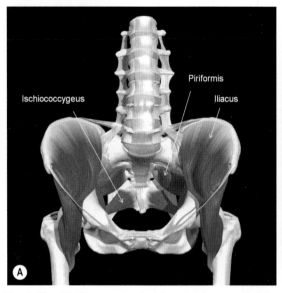 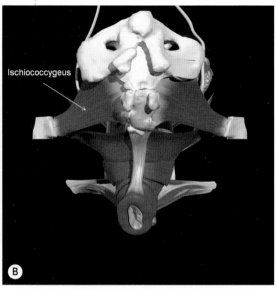

Fig. 3.62 • (A) The muscles that form the back wall of the internal pelvis include the iliacus, piriformis, and ischiococcygeus. Picture from Primal Pictures, 2003. (B) Ischiococcygeus (also known as coccygeus) lies in the same frontal plane as piriformis (90° to iliococcygeus), deep and contiguous to the sacrospinous ligament. Picture from Primal Pictures, 2003.

as the piriformis (another muscle of the deep back wall).

Ischiococcygeus. The ischiococcygeus (see Figs 3.55A,B, 3.62A,B) arises from the ventral aspect of the sacrospinous ligament and the ischial spine, and inserts into the apex of the sacrum between S4 and S5. This muscle is supplied by ventral rami of the sacral plexus, S3 and S4.

Piriformis. Piriformis (see Figs 3.55A,B, 3.62A) arises from the anterior aspect of the S2, S3, and S4 segments of the sacrum as well as the ventral capsule of the SIJ, the anterior aspect of the PIIS of the ilium, and often the upper part of the sacrotuberous ligament. It exits the pelvis through the greater sciatic foramen to attach to the greater trochanter of the femur. The nerve supply is from the ventral rami of L5 and S1.

Iliacus. Iliacus (see Figs 3.56A, 3.62A) arises from the upper two-thirds of the iliac fossa, the inner lip of the iliac crest, the ventral sacroiliac ligament, and the ala of the sacrum. Much of the muscle conjoins with the lateral aspect of the tendon of psoas to insert into the lesser trochanter, and a portion inserts directly into the capsule of the hip joint. Iliacus is supplied by a branch of the femoral nerve, L2 and L3.

The diaphragm and psoas

Diaphragm. The diaphragm is a modified half-dome that separates the thorax from the abdominal cavity (Fig. 3.63A,B,C). It has an extensive attachment to the xyphoid, internal surface of the lower six ribs (interdigitating with the transversus abodminis), and lumbar spine. Pickering & Jones (2002) suggest that the diaphragm is more correctly characterized as two separate muscles with a crural portion and a costal portion. This suggestion arises from the embryology of the muscle whereby the costal component is derived from myoblasts originating in the body wall (likely from the third, fourth, and fifth cervical segments), whereas crura develop from the mesentery of the esophagus.

The crura of the diaphragm arise from the anterolateral aspect of the bodies and intervertebral discs of L1–L3 on the right and L1–L2 on the left (Fig. 3.64). Laterally, fibers arise from the medial and lateral arcuate ligaments, which are thick bands of fascia that arch over the psoas major and quadratus lumborum. From this circumferential origin, fibers converge onto a central tendon – a thin, strong aponeurosis of collagen fibers. The nerve supply to the diaphragm is interesting in that the motor fibers

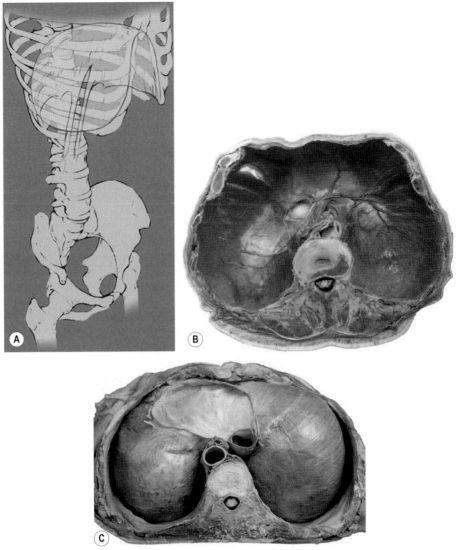

Fig. 3.63 • (A) A three-dimensional graphic representation of the respiratory diaphragm. (B) An actual anatomical dissection of the diaphragm viewed from below. Picture from Primal Pictures, 2003. (C) An actual anatomical dissection of the diaphragm viewed from above. Picture from Primal Pictures, 2003.

for both the costal and crural fibers are from the phrenic nerve (C3, C4), whereas the sensory supply comes from the lower six or seven intercostal nerves (T6–T12).

Psoas. Psoas is a very deep muscle lying in the back of the abdomen just lateral to the vertebral bodies of the lumbar spine (Fig. 3.64) and consists of a series of overlapping segmental fascicles (Bogduk et al 1992). The anterior fibers arise from the intervertebral discs between T12–L1 and L4–5 the adjacent vertebral bodies and from tendinous arches over the narrow waist of the vertebral bodies of L1 to L4. The posterior fibers arise from the anteromedial aspect of all the lumbar transverse processes. The fascicle length throughout the muscle was remarkably consistent (short segmental and long multisegmental fibers do *NOT* exist), although the fibers from the transverse process were noted to be smaller in size than those from the vertebrae. From its origin, each fascicle descends to insert into the psoas tendon, which winds

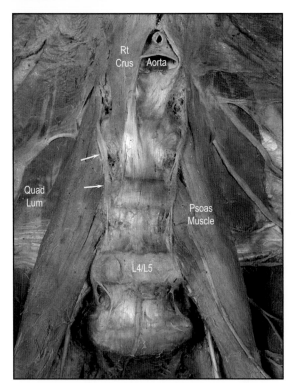

Fig. 3.64 • Anatomical dissection of the deep abdomen showing the attachments of the crus of the diaphragm and the psoas muscles (arrows). Quad Lum = quadratus lumborum. Reproduced with permission from Willard and the publisher Elsevier, 2007.

medially to insert onto the lesser trochanter of the femur. Inferiorly, the psoas tendon receives most of the fibers of iliacus on its lateral side.

Gibbons et al (2002) note that the anterior and posterior parts of psoas are innervated differently. They found the anterior fascicles were supplied by branches of the femoral nerve from L2, L3, and L4, whereas the posterior fascicles were innervated by branches of the ventral rami as classically described in anatomical texts.

The muscles of the hip

The reader is referred to standard anatomy texts to review the morphology of the superficial hip flexors (rectus femoris, tensor fascia lata, sartorius), the long and short adductors (pectineus, adductor brevis, adductor longus, adductor magnus, gracilus), the hamstrings (semimembranosus, semitendinosis, biceps femoris), deep external rotators not previously described (obturator externus, the gemelli, quadratus femoris), the gluteal group (gluteus maximus, gluteus medius, gluteus minimus), and the fascia of the lower extremity.

Neurology – sensory receptors

Accurate information from mechanoreceptors is required by the central nervous system so that the activity of the motor units essential for position, motion, and control of joint motion is coordinated. This mechanism protects the joint from excessive motion and coordinates the timing of motor recruitment such that movements and loads are produced and controlled in an efficient and safe manner.

Mechanoreceptors are located in multiple body tissues and have been classified according to their appearance, location, and function (Table 3.2) (Freeman & Wyke 1967, Rowinski 1985, Wyke 1981). Essentially, there are receptors in all layers of the articular capsule (Indahl et al 1995, 1999, McLain & Pickar 1998), in all ligaments and fascia (Indahl et al 1995, Schleip 2008, Yahia et al 1992), and within all parts of the muscles. Some have a low threshold for discharge and are slow in adapting. They report on static position of the joint, muscle length, muscle tone, and intra-articular pressure. Others have a low threshold for discharge and adapt very quickly. These receptors report dynamic changes in the environment including changes in joint position (direction, quantity, and velocity). The receptors that have a high threshold for discharge adapt very slowly and are protective. The effect of these receptors is to reflexively inhibit further muscle contraction and prevent further stretch of the joint capsule. Both large-diameter myelinated and non-myelinated axons are found in the ventral portion of the SIJ capsule as well as the dorsal periarticular ligaments (Fortin et al 1999, Grob et al 1995, Sakamoto et al 1999, Vilensky et al 2002).

Nociceptors are located throughout almost all of the body. They respond to extremes of mechanical deformation and/or chemical irritation (potassium ions, lactic acid, polypeptide kinins, 5-hydroxytryptamine, acetylcholine, norepinephrine, prostaglandins, histamine) and are high threshold, non-adapting receptors. These receptors contribute to the perception of pain (nociception); however, the afferent input can be significantly altered both peripherally and centrally.

The central effects of articular mechanoreceptor activity are threefold: pain suppression, reflex, and perceptual.

Pain suppression

Pain suppression via mechanoreceptor activity was proposed by Melzack & Wall (1965) to be part of a spinal gating theory whereby the activation of these

Table 3.2 Location and behavior of sensory receptors (adapted from Schleip 2008 and Yahia et al 1992)

	Golgi	Paccini	Ruffini	Interstitial or free nerve endings	Muscle spindle
Location	Musculotendinous junction Fascia Peripheral ligaments Joint capsule Close to bone	Deep capsule Spinal ligaments Musculotendinous junction Fascia	Peripheral ligaments Dura mater Outer layers of capsule Fascia	Most abundant receptor in whole body Found everywhere High density in periosteum	Intrafusal muscle fiber NOT found in fascia or other connective tissue
Stimulated by	Slow deep stretch close to attachments combined with active movement (ART)	Rapid pressure changes such as: high velocity manipulation Recoil techniques Vibration Rocking, shaking or rhythmic joint mobilizations	Slow mechanical pressure with lateral shear	50% are high threshold 50% are low threshold Techniques that stimulate periosteum and septi associated with bone, interosseus membranes Sensitized by neurotransmitters	Stretching muscle directly or by increased gamma activity
Response	Decreases muscle tone	Proprioceptive feedback	Decreases sympathetic activity	Increases vasodilation Plasma extrusion Interoception Mechanoreception and Nociception	Increases extrafusal muscle fiber contraction and inhibits antagonist muscle

receptors prevented the transmission of nociceptive activity to the higher centers. Melzack's (2001, 2005) current thoughts on pain mechanisms and spinal gating are a bit more complicated than this and will be covered in greater detail in Chapter 7.

Reflex effects

Depolarization of the afferent fibers from the low threshold articular mechanoreceptors reaches the fusimotor neurons polysynaptically, thus contributing to the gamma feedback loop from the muscle spindle both at rest and during joint motion. 'By this means the articular mechanoreceptors exert reciprocally coordinated reflexogenic influences on muscle tone and on the excitability of stretch reflexes in all the striated muscles' (Wyke 1981). When this capsular reflex is activated, the discharging receptors facilitate the muscles antagonistic to the occurring movement. When the high threshold articular mechanoreceptors are discharged, the reflex effect is projected polysynaptically to the alpha-motoneurons and results in local muscular inhibition. Nociceptors affect the discharge from the alpha-motoneuron pool and can distort the normal, coordinated, mechanoreceptor reflex system (Gandevia 1992).

Perceptual effects

Afferent input from the articular mechanoreceptors travels polysynaptically via the posterior and dorsal spinal columns to reach the paracentral and parietal regions of the cerebral cortex, thus contributing significantly, though not solely, to both postural and kinesthetic awareness.

The observation that capsulectomy of the hip joint performed in the course of hip replacement surgery does not result in total loss of postural sensation at the hip, leaves no doubt that while joint capsule mechanoreceptors contribute to awareness of static joint position, they are not the sole source of perceptual experience, and other recent studies suggest that their contribution in this regard is supplementary to and coordinated with that provided by the inputs from cutaneous and myotatic [muscle spindle] mechanoreceptors.

Wyke 1981.

Fascia is a highly sensorial tissue containing the greatest number of mechanoreceptors in all the body including Golgi, Pacini, Ruffini, and interstitial receptors (Table 3.2), which when stimulated can decrease muscle tone (Golgi), provide proprioceptive and interoceptive feedback (Pacini and interstitial), inhibit overall sympathetic activity (Ruffini) and increase vasodilation and plasma extrusion (interstitial) (Schleip 2008). In addition, recent research has found a variable amount of α-smooth muscle actin (smooth muscle-like cells also known as myofibroblasts) in all fascial tissue (Schleip et al 2005) and it is now widely accepted that fascia has contractile capability. The complex interplay between the sensory and motor systems helps to explain the wide effect that manual therapy techniques (Chapter 10) and movement training (Chapters 11, 12) can have on interoception (how do I feel my body?), proprioception (where am I in relation to myself and my environment?), and function (what do I need and want to do?).

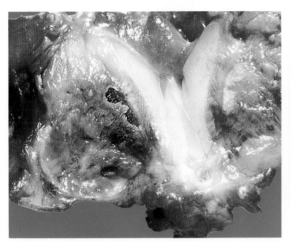

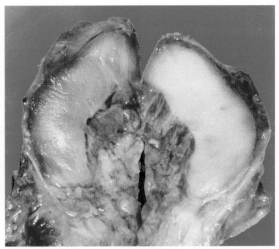

Plate 1 • Sacroiliac joint of a fetus at 37 weeks of gestation. Note that the fibrocartilage lining the articular surface of the ilium is bluer than the hyaline cartilage lining the articular surface of the sacrum.

Plate 2 • Sacroiliac joint of a male, 3 years of age (the sacral surface is on the right). Note the blue, dull fibrocartilage lining the articular surface of the ilium.

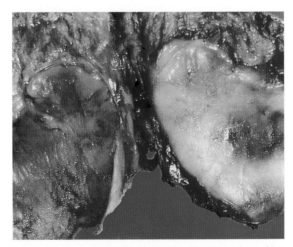

Plate 3 • Sacroiliac joint of a male, 17 years of age (the sacral surface is on the right). Note the dull, rough fibrocartilage lining the articular surface of the ilium.

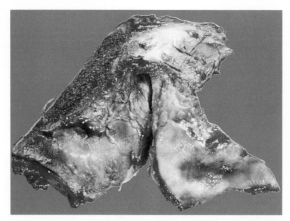

Plate 4 • Sacroiliac joint of a male, 40 years of age (the sacral surface is on the right).

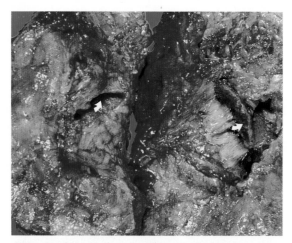

Plate 5 • Sacroiliac joint of a female, 72 years of age (the sacral surface is on the left). Note the marked loss of articular cartilage on both sides of the joint as well as the presence of an accessory sacroiliac joint (arrows). Plates 1–5 are reproduced with permission from Bowen & Cassidy and the publishers Harper and Rowe, 1981.

The functional lumbopelvic–hip complex

4

Diane Lee   Linda-Joy Lee

CHAPTER CONTENTS

Introduction – stability, what is it? 49
The integrated model of function
revisited 52
    Form closure theory 53
    Force closure theory 71
    Motor control theory 74
    Emotional states 85
The integrated biomechanics of the
lumbopelvic–hip complex 85
    Forward bending 86
    Backward bending 87
    Lateral bending 87
    Squat 87
    Walking 88
    Lifting 89
Summary 89

Authors' note

Chapters 4 and 5 have probably been the most difficult to update as there has been an incredible amount of conflicting, if not confusing, research published in the last 6 years pertaining to lumbopelvic pain and stability. Is transversus abdominis an important muscle to train or not? Is bracing the abdominal wall with a strong multiple muscle co-contraction strategy a better way to stabilize the trunk than a gentle abdominal hollow? Does the sacroiliac joint really move in the weight bearing position or are we just feeling soft tissue motion?

When you closely consider each research paper, and reflect on the things it did or did not measure, and how it measured these things (methods), who it measured them on (subjects and inclusion criteria), and not just read the conclusions, the relevance of the research to the bigger picture pertaining to function and dysfunction of the lumbopelvic–hip complex starts to make more sense.

Back pain has been compared (Lee 2006) to the fable by John Godfrey Saxe, The Blind Men and the Elephant, and recently Reeves et al (2007) used the fable to describe the current confusion in the use of the word 'stability.'

In research, focus is often necessarily limited to only one small part of the elephant. Confounding variables to the study are strictly controlled such that a clinician reading the paper may ask:

1. 'What relevance does this have to clinical practice?' Or, they may react;
2. 'This not the way we work.' Or they may note that;
3. 'No muscle operates in isolation so who cares, and how important is 50ms anyway?'

On some level, it is all very important, and relevant, but only if we consider the work as it pertains to the bigger picture, the whole elephant, or the patient with lumbopelvic–hip disability with or without pain. At the same time, it is important to keep in mind the limitations of the research and not draw conclusions that the study has no ability to make. Review articles and chapter contributions really help to understand the view of the elephant through the filter of certain researcher(s), as these writings give them an opportunity to fully explain and tell the story of not only their own research but also how it relates to others. We've had many 'aha' moments

DOI: 10.1016/B978-0-443-06963-5.00004-3

The Blind Men and the Elephant (Fig. 4.1)
A Fable by John Godfrey Saxe

It was six men of Indostan
To learning much inclined
Who went to see the Elephant
(Though all of them were blind)
That each by observation
Might satisfy his mind

The first approached the elephant
And happening to fall
Against his broad and sturdy side
At once began to bawl
'God bless me! – but the Elephant
Is very like a wall!'

The Second, feeling of the tusk,
Cried: 'Ho! – what have we here
So very round and smooth and sharp?
To me 'tis mighty clear
This wonder of an Elephant
Is very like a spear!'

The Third approached the animal
And happening to take
The squirming trunk within his hands
Thus boldly up and spake;
'I see,' quoth he, 'the Elephant
Is very like a snake!'

The Fourth reached out his eager hand
And felt about the knee
'What most this wondrous beast is like
Is mighty plain' quoth he;
''Tis clear enough the elephant
Is very like a tree!'

The Fifth, who chanced to touch the ear,
Said: 'E'en the blindest man
Can tell what this resembles most;
Deny the fact who can,
This marvel of an Elephant
Is very like a fan!'

The Sixth no sooner had begun
About the beast to grope,
Than, seizing on the swinging tail
That fell within his scope
'I see,' quoth he, 'the Elephant
Is very like a rope!'

And so these men of Indostan
Disputed loud and long
Each in his own opinion
Exceeding stiff and strong,
Though each was partly in the right, And all were in
the wrong!

MORAL
So, oft in theologic wars
The disputants, I ween,
Rail on in utter ignorance
Of what each other mean,
And prate about an Elephant
Not one of them has seen!

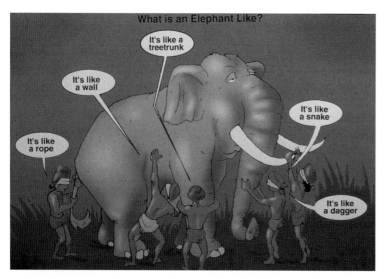

Fig. 4.1 • The Blind Men and the Elephant. Each man perceives the elephant through his own 'filter,' much like the various healthcare disciplines view 'back pain' (Lee 2006) or as Reeves et al (2007) note 'stability.'

while reading such articles and chapters and encourage you to look them up. At the Sixth Interdisciplinary World Congress on Low Back and Pelvic Pain in Barcelona (November 2007), Diane presented a paper titled 'Clinical Expertise in Evidence-based Practice for Pelvic Girdle Pain – Show Me the Patient!' (Lee 2007b) and following this Dr. Jacek Cholewicki, moderator of the session, asked her one question, 'Diane, would you be prepared to change your mind?' If the evolution of this book from 1989 to 2010 is any testimony, the answer is yes, our minds are changing all the time as we learn more from the scientific evidence (research) and our clinical and personal life experiences. For now, these two chapters present a summary, not a detailed analysis, of the current state of knowledge on the functional and impaired LPH complex; it is evident there is still much to discover.

Introduction – stability, what is it?

The primary function of the lumbopelvic–hip (LPH) complex is to transfer loads safely while fulfilling the movement and control requirements of any task in a way that ensures that the objectives of the task are met, musculoskeletal structures are not injured, either in the short or long term, and that the organs are supported/protected in concert with optimal respiration. Optimal function will, therefore, require both mobility and stability. Panjabi (1992a,b) proposed that for a system to be stable there must be optimal function of three interdependent systems, the passive, active, and control systems (Fig. 4.2). But what does 'a stable system' mean? The word 'stability' is often used ambiguously in both the literature pertaining to biomechanics, as well as in exercise training and rehabilitation. Recently, Reeves et al (2007), writing from a biomechanical perspective, expressed a fear that the word 'stability' had the potential to become an elephant much like the one in the famous fable by John Godfrey Saxe.

Stability is one of the most fundamental concepts to characterize and evaluate any system. Stability, one could argue, is a term that appears to change depending upon the context, and as such appears to have unstable definitions. The ambiguity of this term in spinal biomechanics should not be surprising, given that even in more established disciplines in engineering, there is

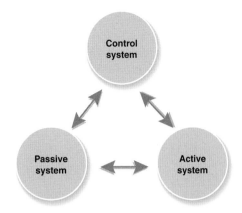

Fig. 4.2 • The conceptual model of Panjabi (1992a,b) illustrating the components that provide stability.

no absolute definition of stability. However, numerous definitions have emerged, each rigorously defined. So like the elephant, stability is an entity with many parts.

Reeves et al 2007.

This is supported by the range of seemingly contradictory models and data in the scientific literature in the field of spinal stability. Much debate has occurred between scientists and clinicians in regards to 'what muscles are most important to stabilize the spine?' and 'what are the best exercises to stabilize the spine?' A recent Google™ search on the words 'core stability' resulted in about 4,170,000 search results. Clearly, spinal stability has become a popular concern and multiple opinions abound. But is it possible that we are searching for simple recipes and answers to assess and treat a complex system? As Reeves et al (2007) highlight, 'stability is an entity with many parts.' Depending on the methodology, and the underlying assumptions and models used to design the studies, the resulting data illuminate different components of what stability is. So what are the many parts of 'stability'?

It is well established that the osseoligamentous spine is inherently unstable; that is, without muscular support the spine (T1–sacrum) will buckle, under a compression load of only 20N (Lucas & Bresler 1961), whereas the lumbar spine alone can support 90N of compression load (Crisco & Panjabi 1991). Thus, a focus on how to prevent buckling of the spine led to models of stability that focused around which muscles could best work as 'guy wires' to support and buttress the spine. These studies have provided information that is based on modeling the spine in a static sense.

> In a static sense, stability is assured if the spine maintains or returns to an equilibrium position (i.e. point of minimum potential energy) if perturbed. In an unstable system, perturbation would induce movement away from an equilibrium position.
>
> Hodges & Cholewicki 2007.

Many studies have shown that to prevent buckling of the spine and provide static stability under load, co-contraction of multiple segmental and multisegmental muscles around the trunk (the active system in Panjabi's model) is necessary (Fig. 4.3A) (Bergmark 1989, Cholewicki et al 1997, Cholewicki & McGill 1996, Cholewicki & van Vliet 2002, Crisco & Panjabi 1991, Crisco et al 1992, Grenier & McGill 2007, McGill et al 2003, McGill & Cholewicki 2001). Muscle co-contraction stiffens the joints of the spine. In static conditions, if the only thing the spine is required to do is to resist buckling, a stiff spine is a stable spine. As the more superficial, multisegmental muscles have a greater capacity to stiffen the spine, rehabilitation approaches based on static definitions of stability have recommended training co-contraction bracing of multisegmental trunk muscles at various intensities to increase spinal stiffness in order to prevent and treat low back pain and injury (McGill 2002, McGill & Stuart 2004). However, these same models also suggest that, if just one segment lacks muscular support, the spine is as

unstable as if it had no muscles at all (Cholewicki & McGill 1996, Crisco & Panjabi 1991) (Fig. 4.3B), which supports that the deep segmental muscles also play an important role. Indeed, anatomically, the deep muscles of the spine are more suited to provide selective segmental control of translation (a potential component of buckling) without the cost of multisegmental compression (which reduces mobility) and torque production that would be generated by using superficial muscles (Hodges & Cholewicki 2007).

However, it is necessary to ask, whether a stiff spine is a more functional spine. Does a stiff spine provide optimal function and performance of the body as a whole? Clearly, the prevention of buckling in a static sense (maintaining an equilibrium position) does not encompass the broad range of functions required of the human spine, not to mention the integrated role of the spine within the human body (Hodges & Cholewicki 2007, Reeves et al 2007). The spine needs not only to resist buckling, but also to allow movement at all segments to provide range of motion of the trunk, often as the body moves through space. Translation at each segment must be controlled not only in static tasks, but also during movement and under changing demands. Many studies of responses of the trunk muscles provide data that are not consistent with predictions from static models; these studies show that movement of the spine, and alternating activity in the trunk muscles, rather than simple stiffening of the spine, are

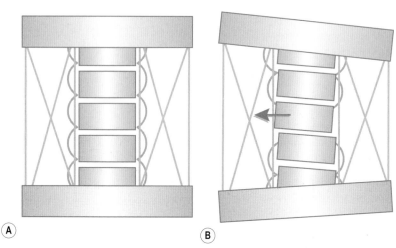

Ⓐ Ⓑ

Fig. 4.3 • (A) Euler model – multiple segmental and multisegmental muscles co-contract to prevent buckling of a system under load and a minimal level of co-contraction is required for static stability. (B) However, if just one segment lacks support the system will buckle as if it had no muscles at all.

required to control postural equilibrium, dampen perturbations, and allow for key functions such as respiration (Aruin & Latash 1995, Belenkii et al 1967, Bouisset & Zattara 1981, Hodges et al 1999, Hodges & Cholewicki 2007, Hodges & Richardson 1997). Indeed, many studies show that better *function* is often supported by a *less* stiff spine (Mok et al 2007, Reeves et al 2006, 2007). Thus, static models provide information about only one part of spinal stability, only one part of the elephant. As Reeves et al (2007) note,

> stability has to be defined both for static conditions in which the system is in equilibrium, as well as for dynamic situations in which the system is moving along some trajectory.

A broader definition of spinal stability is needed. Given that the human form is a dynamic entity and that all tasks (even standing still or sitting) involve some movement, consideration must be given to how systems are dynamically stabilized. Hodges & Cholewicki (2007) define stability of a dynamic system as

> the ability to maintain the desired trajectory despite kinetic, kinematic or control disturbances.

This definition considers the multiple factors (load demands, mobility requirements, predictability, and real or perceived risk) of any task (Fig. 4.4), and the multiple functions the spine must support and allow (e.g. respiration and continence) during any task. It encompasses static situations where the desired trajectory is to maintain one equilibrium position. It also allows for the consideration of complex relationships and interactions between the body and environments that are also dynamic and in flux. Note that what is required for spinal

stability varies according to the requirements of the task, 'the desired trajectory.' 'Stability depends on the system and the task being performed' (Reeves et al 2007). Clearly, there is not 'one way,' or one exercise, to stabilize the spine that can be applied across all functional tasks or contexts.

This broader view, and definition, of stability allows us to see the elephant, and understand the many different findings from scientific studies, as parts of a larger whole. It also provides an explanation for the wide variety of approaches that clinicians report to be effective with patients; different approaches are addressing different subgroups of patients with LPH disability and pain (see Chapter 7), and training different parts of stability. What is clear from the data is that all muscles are important for functional control of the spine and to look for 'the best exercise' to stabilize the spine is far too narrow an approach to take for such a dynamic, complex system. The central nervous system (CNS) uses different muscles for different purposes, and different overall strategies of muscle synergies, in order to achieve different goals. Recent research demonstrates that there is significant redundancy in the neuromuscular system and therefore a large degree of adaptability (i.e. potential for multiple strategies for any task). To ensure stability of the spine during both static and dynamic tasks, we need multiple strategies from which to choose. In situations of high load and low predictability, it is optimal to use a simple stiffening strategy with co-contraction of multiple trunk muscles, but in many other tasks, such as during gait and where movement is required, the control system stabilizes the spine using movements and phasic muscle activity rather than simply stiffening the system (Aruin & Latash 1995, Bouisset & Zattara 1981, Cholewicki et al 1991, Hodges et al

Fig. 4.4 • Stability of a dynamic system requires the maintenance of the desired trajectory despite kinetic, kinematic, or control disturbances (Hodges & Cholewicki 2007). There are multiple factors to consider for every task including the level of the load, the mobility requirements, the predictability of the task, and the level of either real or perceived risk.

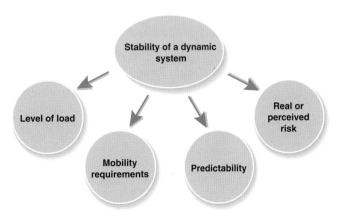

1999, 2000, 2003b, Saunders et al 2004a, van Dieen & de Looze 1999). For optimal function and performance, the CNS needs to be able to choose from multiple strategies, and apply them appropriately to the task, individual, and context.

> Motor control of spinal stability requires an integrated system that has sensors to detect the status of the body, a control system to interpret the requirements of stability and plan appropriate responses, and the muscles to execute the response.
>
> Hodges et al 2003b.

> Stability results from highly coordinated muscle activation patterns involving many muscles, and the recruitment patterns must continually change, depending on the task.
>
> McGill et al 2003.

Given the significant confusion around the word 'stability,' we have chosen to primarily use the word 'control' in the remainder of this book to facilitate clarity; however, where the term 'stability' is used, it is intended with the broader definition of Hodges & Cholewicki (2007). The remainder of this chapter uses the framework of the Integrated Model of Function (see below) to review the current understanding of the underlying anatomical, biomechanical, and neurophysiological mechanisms for stability of the functional LPH complex from interpretation of the scientific evidence. Further discussion of the relationship between LPH/spinal stability and total body performance occurs in the section on motor control.

The integrated model of function revisited

The Integrated Model of Function began as a framework for discussing the pelvis in both function and dysfunction (Fig. 4.5) (Lee 2004, Lee & Lee 2004a, Lee & Vleeming 1998, 2004, 2007). The

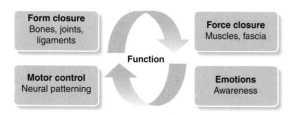

Fig. 4.5 • The Integrated Model of Function (Lee & Vleeming 1998, 2004, 2007).

original model sought to explain how form and force closure, together with motor control and emotional states, influence how loads are transferred through the LPH complex (Fig. 4.6). Several anatomical, biomechanical, and neurophysiological studies have investigated how forces are controlled when loads are applied to the LPH complex. What follows is our (Diane Lee & Linda-Joy Lee) updated perspective on the relevant research pertaining to this model.

One component of the Integrated Model of Function is form closure; the original definition is:

> Form closure refers to a stable situation where no extra forces are needed to maintain the state of the system, given the actual load distribution.
>
> Snijders et al 1993a.

Form closure, therefore, refers to how the joint's structure (the passive system) resists translation and shear forces when the joint is loaded.

A second component of the model is force closure; the original definition is:

> In the case of force closure, extra forces are needed to keep the object in place. Here friction must be present.
>
> Snijders et al 1993a.

The role of the deep and superficial muscles of the trunk and their related fascia (abdominal, thoracolumbar, endopelvic) in providing force closure to the LPH complex has been the topic of several studies, some of which will be considered later in this chapter. It is thought that a joint with less form closure requires more force closure for loads to be effectively controlled.

The third component of the Integrated Model of Function, motor control, encompasses the neural mechanisms for stability and movement of the LPH complex, and incorporates findings from studies that focus on the timing of muscle activity and the various patterns of muscle co-contraction during functional tasks in both predictable and unpredictable conditions. It is now well supported that all muscles are important for function, that there is significant redundancy in the neuromuscular system, and that the CNS can use a variety of muscle coactivation strategies for the same task.

The term 'force closure mechanism' encompasses two components of this model, force closure and motor control, as optimal function of the neuromuscular system (motor control) and the myofascial system (force closure) is required for provision of the 'extra forces to keep the object in place.'

Emotional states, the fourth component of the Integrated Model of Function, are influenced by past

Fig. 4.6 • The functional lumbopelvic–hip complex is one that effectively transfers loads through integrated kinetic chains and simultaneously protects the organs of the pelvis and preserves continence. This picture was on the cover of the third edition of this text and was chosen for its representation of optimal function of integrated kinetic chains through a stable platform, the pelvis.

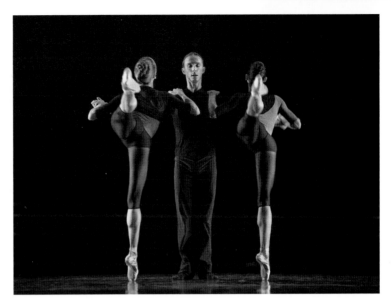

experiences, beliefs, fears, and attitudes, and significantly impact motor control and consequently affect strategies for function.

Form closure theory

Form closure theory pertains to how a joint's structure, orientation, and shape contribute to its potential mobility and ability to resist shear, or translation, when loaded (Fig. 4.7). All joints have a variable amount of form closure and the joint's anatomy and capsular/ligamentous compliance will dictate

how much additional compression, or support (force closure (Fig. 4.8)), is needed to ensure that integrity of the system is maintained when loads are increased. The anatomy, or form, of the lumbar spine, pelvic girdle, and hip has been described in detail in Chapter 3. What follows is a discussion on how the form of the joint contributes to its mobility and ability to resist to shear/translation.

All joints have a variable number of degrees of freedom of motion and variable amplitude of motion for each degree of freedom. Each degree, or direction, of motion can be divided into two zones: the neutral zone and the elastic zone (Panjabi 1992b)

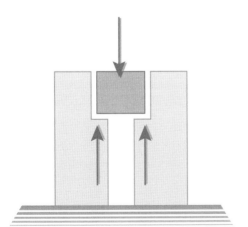

Fig. 4.7 • A schematic representation of form closure redrawn from Snijders et al 1993a and Vleeming et al 1990a,b.

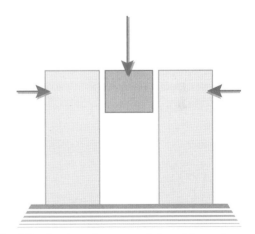

Fig. 4.8 • A schematic representation of force closure redrawn from Snijders et al 1993a and Vleeming et al 1990a,b.

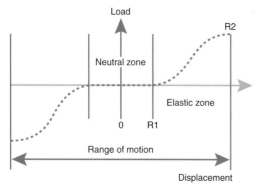

Fig. 4.9 • The zones of articular motion: the neutral zone is from 0–R1 and is the zone where the capsule and ligaments cannot control motion between the joint's surfaces. The elastic zone is from R1–R2, and is the zone where the capsule and ligaments provide a non-linear resistance to movement of the joint surfaces.

(Fig. 4.9). The neutral zone of motion is the range where the joint's capsule or ligaments provide no resistance to movement; it is the zone where the joint surfaces can freely translate relative to one another. The elastic zone of motion is the range where the capsule and ligaments provide resistance to the movement; the slope of this resistance is non-linear and depends on the compliance of the joint's connective tissue and its architecture, or form. The bones, joints, capsule, ligaments, and fascia comprise the passive system in Panjabi's model (1992a,b) (see Fig. 4.2), although many would question that fascia is a passive

structure (Chapter 3). Several things can influence a joint's mobility including:

1. intra-articular swelling;

2. subluxation;

3. capsular fibrosis or laxity;

4. adhesions of the ligaments to the capsule or laxity of the ligaments;

5. hypertonicity or hypotonicity of the muscles that cross the joint;

6. an increase or decrease in cross-sectional area of muscles surrounding the joint;

7. increased/decreased fascial tension secondary to hypertonicity/hypotonicity of muscles, or loss of cross-sectional area of muscles that do not necessarily cross the joint but create tension/slack in the fascia that does cross the joint.

Form closure – the lumbar spine

Newton's second law states that the motion of an object is directly proportional to the applied force and occurs in the direction of the straight line in which the force acts. Translation occurs when a single net force causes all points of the object to move in the same direction over the same distance. Rotation occurs when two unaligned and opposite forces cause the object to move around a stationary center or axis (Bogduk 1997). In mechanical terms, the lumbar vertebrae have the potential for 12 degrees of freedom (Levin 1997) (Fig. 4.10), as motion can occur in a

Fig. 4.10 • Each lumbar motion segment has the potential for 12 degrees of freedom of motion.

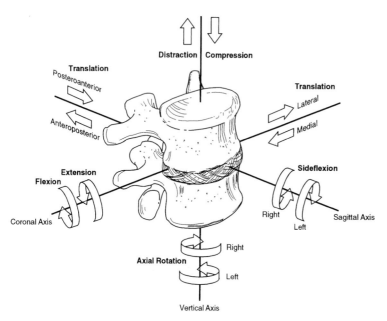

positive and negative direction along and about three perpendicular axes. However, this mechanical model does not account for the structural and neurophysiological factors that modify and restrict the actual motion that can occur in the lumbar spine (Chapter 5). Clinically, the lumbar spine appears to exhibit four degrees of freedom of motion: flexion, extension, rotation/sideflexion right, and rotation/sideflexion left (Bogduk 1997, Cholewicki et al 1996, Pearcy & Tibrewal 1984, Vicenzino & Twomey 1993). Throughout the spine, flexion/extension is an integral part of forward/backward bending of the head or trunk, whereas rotation/sideflexion occurs during any other motion. The shape of the zygapophyseal joints of the lumbar spine facilitates sagittal (flexion/extension) and coronal (sideflexion) plane motions, while resisting excessive motion in the transverse plane (rotation). Compression, torsion, and shear (translation) are part of sagittal, coronal, and transverse plane motions and form closure assists in controlling these forces. A recent systematic review and meta-analysis to determine the effect of age on the range of motion of the lumbar spine found that, although there are age-related reductions in flexion, extension, and lateral flexion (primarily from 40 to 50 years of age and after 60), there is very little age effect on lumbar rotation (Intolo et al 2009).

Kinematics – flexion/extension of the lumbar segment

In the lumbar spine, the coronal axis for sagittal plane motion is dynamic rather than static and moves forward with flexion such that flexion couples with a small degree (1–3 mm) of anterior translation (Fig. 4.11A,B) (Bogduk 1997, Gracovetsky et al 1981, Gracovetsky & Farfan 1986, Rousseau et al 2006, White & Panjabi 1978). Conversely, extension couples with posterior translation during backward bending of the trunk. A smooth lumbar curve is produced when the kinematics for sagittal plane motion is physiological and optimal (Fig. 4.12A,B). During flexion, the inferior articular processes of the superior vertebra glide superiorly and anteriorly along the superior articular processes of the inferior vertebra/sacrum (Bogduk 1997). During extension, the inferior articular processes of the superior vertebra glide inferiorly and posteriorly along the superior articular processes of the inferior vertebra/sacrum. The total amplitude of this glide is about 5–7 mm and there should be no coupling of axial rotation or sideflexion during sagittal plane motion (Cholewicki et al 1996).

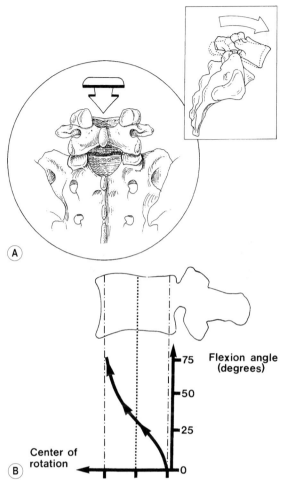

Fig. 4.11 • (A) Flexion couples with a small amount of anterior translation at L5–S1. The anterior translation is limited, in part, by the orientation of the superior articular process of S1. (B) The coronal axis for flexion moves anterior with increasing degrees of flexion; therefore anterior translation couples with forward sagittal rotation or flexion.

When flexion couples with posterior translation (Fig. 4.13A), or extension couples with anterior translation (Fig. 4.13B), a hinge, or kink, in the curve is palpable and often visible; these kinematics are non-physiological in that the direction of translation is the reverse of what should be occurring during the osteokinematic motion.

Kinematics – rotation/sideflexion of the lumbar segment

Motion coupling of the vertebral column during rotation or lateral bending of the trunk was first recorded by Lovett in 1903. He noted that when a flexible rod

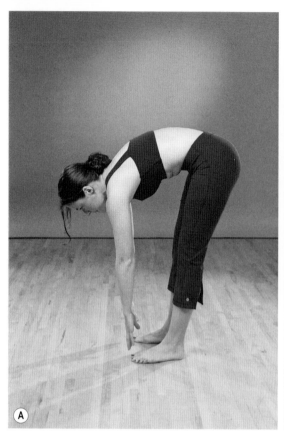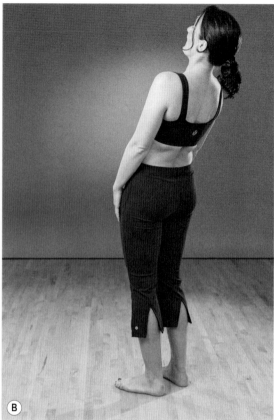

Fig. 4.12 • (A) A smooth even curve should occur in the lumbar spine when the strategy for forward bending is optimal. (B) Similarly, a smooth even curve should occur in backward bending.

was bent in one plane it could not bend in another without twisting. The direction of the bend and twist has been a controversial issue. In 1984, Pearcy & Tibrewal reported on a three-dimensional radiographic study of lumbar motion during rotation and lateral bending of 10 men under 30 years of age. Their findings of coupled motion (Fig. 4.14) were consistent with those of Gracovetsky & Farfan (1986) and Cholewicki et al (1996) except at the lumbosacral junction where lateral bending coupled with ipsilateral rotation. L4–L5 was often transitional and followed the movement pattern of either L3–L4 or L5–S1. Pearcy & Tibrewal did not investigate the coupling of motion when lateral bending was introduced from a position of flexion or extension, although Cholewicki et al (1996) note that a small amount of flexion was coupled with lateral bending when lateral bending was introduced first in the experimental model.

According to Bogduk (1997), 3° of *pure* axial rotation of a lumbar motion segment is possible.

At this point, all of the fibers of the annulus fibrosus that are aligned in the direction of the rotation are under stress, the sagittal component of the contralateral zygapophyseal joint is compressed, and the ipsilateral zygapophyseal joint capsule is tensed. The axis for this motion is vertical through the posterior part of the vertebral body. After 3° of rotation, the axis shifts to the impacted zygapophyseal joint and the upper vertebra pivots about this new axis. The vertebral body swings posterolaterally, imposing a lateral translation force on the intervertebral disc. The impacted inferior articular process swings backwards and medially, further stretching the capsule and ligaments. Further rotation can result in failure of any of the stressed or compressed components. Thirty-five percent of the resistance to rotation is provided by the intervertebral disc and 65% by the posterior elements of the neural arch (Bogduk 1997).

Bogduk (1997) supports Pearcy & Tibrewal's (1984) model of motion coupling and concurs that

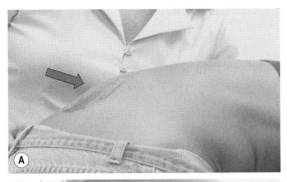

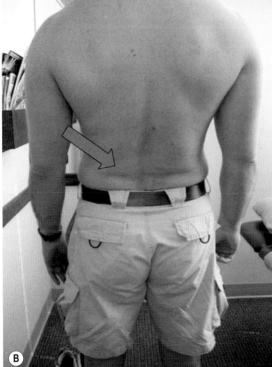

Fig. 4.13 • (A) Note the excessive segmental flexion at L4–5 (arrow). This segment has 'hinged' and translated posteriorly during flexion of the lumbar spine in forward bending. This is non-physiological coupling of motion. (B) Note the horizontal skin crease at L4–5. This segment has 'hinged' and translated anteriorly during extension of the lumbar spine in backward bending. This is also non-physiological coupling of motion.

for the upper three segments rotation is accompanied by contralateral sideflexion. This motion is unidirectional about an oblique axis and also involves slight flexion or extension of the segment (Fig. 4.15). He agrees that at L5–S1 the pattern tends to be ipsilateral (Fig. 4.16) and that L4–L5 is variable. In addition, he notes that individual variation exists and resists any rules for segmental motion patterning.

Vicenzino & Twomey (1993) investigated the conjunct rotation that occurred during lateral bending of the lumbar spine and noted that in 64% of their specimens no conjunct rotation occurred at L5–S1. In the remainder, the direction of rotation was always the same as the direction of sideflexion. This coupling of motion was consistent when the segment was sideflexed from a flexed, neutral, or extended position. Above L5–S1, an interesting pattern emerged. In extension, L1–L2 and L3–L4 rotated opposite to the direction of sideflexion. In flexion, L1–L2 and L3–L4 rotated in the same direction as the sideflexion. Conversely, in extension, L2–L3 and L4–L5 rotated in the same direction as the sideflexion and in flexion L2–L3 and L4–L5 rotated in the opposite direction! The conclusion from this study was that the coupling of motion in the lumbar spine was indeed complex.

The biomechanics of the lumbar spine change with both age and degeneration (Farfan 1973, Gilmore 1986, Grieve 1986, Kirkaldy-Willis et al 1978, Kirkaldy-Willis 1983, Stokes 1986, Taylor & Twomey 1986, White & Panjabi 1978). The instantaneous center of rotation for flexion/extension and/or rotation/sideflexion can be significantly displaced with degeneration, resulting in excessive posteroanterior and/or lateral translation during motions of the trunk (Stokes 1986, White & Panjabi 1978). Consequently, 'on the intersegmental level ... normal loads may in fact be acting about a displaced IAR [instantaneous axis of rotation], thus locally producing abnormal motion' (Gilmore 1986).

In summary, even if the biomechanics of the lumbar spine are confirmed and conclusive, the potential for altered coupling patterns to exist is high, rendering

> clinical observation of a patient [as] the most direct way to assess spine motion clinically, despite its lack of objectivity.
>
> Stokes 1986.

Kinetics – vertical compression of the lumbar segment

Compression of an object results when two forces act towards each other. The main restraint to vertical compression in the lumbar segment is the vertebral body/annulus–nucleus unit, although the zygapophyseal joints have been noted to support up to 20% of

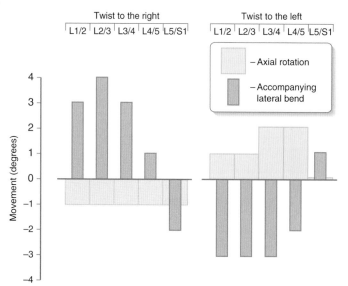

Twist to the right
L1/2 L2/3 L3/4 L4/5 L5/S1

Twist to the left
L1/2 L2/3 L3/4 L4/5 L5/S1

– Axial rotation

– Accompanying lateral bend

Movement (degrees)

Fig. 4.14 • Findings of coupled motion of rotation and lateral bending in the lumbar spine. At the lumbosacral junction, lateral bending occurs in the same direction as the induced rotation. Redrawn from Pearcy & Tibrewal, 1984.

the axial compression load (Fig. 4.17) (Bogduk 1997, Farfan 1973, Gracovetsky et al 1985, Gracovetsky & Farfan 1986, Kirkaldy-Willis 1983). Both the annulus and the nucleus transmit the load equally to the end-plate of the vertebral body. The thin cortical shell of the vertebral body provides the bulk of the compression strength, being simultaneously supported by a hydraulic mechanism within the cancellous core, the contribution of which is dependent upon the rate of loading. When vertical compression is applied slowly (static loading), the nuclear pressure rises distributing its force onto the annulus and the end-

plates. The annulus bulges circumferentially and the end-plates bow towards the vertebral bodies. Fluid is squeezed out of the cancellous core via the veins; however, when the rate of compression is increased, the small vessel size may retard the rate of outflow such that the internal pressure of the vertebral body rises, thus increasing the compressive strength of the unit. In this manner, the vertebral body supports and protects the intervertebral disc against compression overload (McGill 2002). The anatomical structure that initially yields to high loads of compression is the hyaline cartilage of the

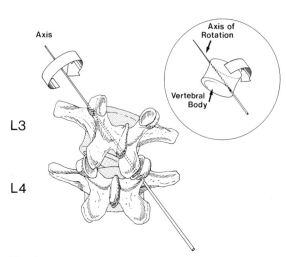

Fig. 4.15 • Left rotation of the L3–4 joint complex couples with contralateral sideflexion.

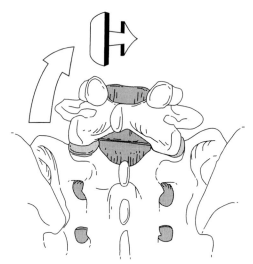

Fig. 4.16 • During right rotation, the L5 vertebra rotates/sideflexes to the right.

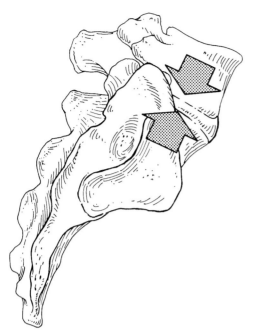

Fig. 4.17 • Compression of the lumbosacral junction.

end-plate, suggesting that this structure is weaker than the peripheral parts of the end-plate (Bogduk 1997). The fracture appears radiographically as a Schmorl's node (Fig. 4.18) (Kirkaldy-Willis et al 1978, Kirkaldy-Willis 1983). This lesion is commonly seen at the higher lumbar levels. The vertebral bony elements fail at the higher load rates, whereas

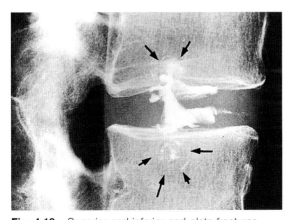

Fig. 4.18 • Superior and inferior end-plate fractures (Schmorl's nodes) detected via a discogram. Note the penetration of the dye into both the superior and inferior vertebral bodies through the end-plate (arrows). Reproduced with permission from Farfan and the publisher Lea & Febiger, 1973.

the end-plate fails first at low rates (McGill 2002). The zygapophyseal joints do not contribute to weight bearing when the lumbar spine is in the neutral position, given that their sagittal and coronal components are oriented vertically. When the lumbar segment is extended, the inferior articular process of the superior vertebra glides inferiorly and impacts the pars interarticularis. When vertical compression is applied in this lordotic position, load can be transferred through the inferior articular process to the lamina (Bogduk 1997).

Kinetics – axial torsion of the lumbar segment

When a force is applied to an object at any location other than the center of rotation, it will cause the object to rotate about an axis through this pivot point. The magnitude of the torque force can be calculated by multiplying the quantity of the force by the distance the force acts from the pivot. Axial torsion of the lumbar vertebra occurs when the bone rotates about a vertical axis through the center of the body (see Fig. 4.16) and is resisted by anatomical factors located within the vertebral arch (65%) as well as by the structures of the vertebral body/intervertebral disc unit (35%) (Bogduk 1997, Gracovetsky & Farfan 1986).

At the lumbosacral junction, the superior articular process of the sacrum (see Figs 3.7, 3.8) is squat and strong in comparison to the inferior articular process of the L5 vertebra, which is much longer and receives less support from the pedicle. Consequently, the inferior process is more easily deflected when the zygapophyseal joint is loaded at 90° to its articular surface. This process can deflect 8–9° medially during axial torsion beyond which trabecular fractures and residual strain deformation will occur (Bogduk 1997, Farfan 1973).

The structure and orientation of the annular fibers are critical to the ability of the intervertebral disc to resist axial torsion. 'The concentric arrangement of the collagenous layers of the annulus ensures that when the disk is placed in tension, shear or rotation, the individual fibers are always in tension' (Kirkaldy-Willis 1983). Under static loading conditions, injuries occur with as little as 2° and certainly by 3.5° of axial rotation (Gracovetsky & Farfan 1986). The ventral band of the iliolumbar ligament (see Fig. 3.16) plays an important role in minimizing torque forces at the lumbosacral junction (Pool-Goudzwaard et al 2003). The longer the transverse process of the L5 vertebra, and consequently the shorter the iliolumbar ligament, the stronger is the resistance of the segment to torsion (Farfan 1973).

Vertical compression also increases the segment's ability to resist torsion by 35% (Gracovetsky & Farfan 1986). During forward flexion of the lumbar spine, the instantaneous center of rotation moves forward (see Fig. 4.11B), thus increasing vertical compression and consequently the ability of the joint to resist torsion (Farfan 1973, Gracovetsky & Farfan 1986).

Kinetics – horizontal translation of the lumbar segment

Translation occurs when an applied force produces sliding between two planes. Posteroanterior translation occurs at a lumbar segment when a force attempts to displace the superior vertebra anterior to the one below (Fig. 4.19). The anatomical factors that resist posteroanterior shear/translation at the lumbosacral junction are primarily the impaction of the inferior articular processes of L5 against the superior articular processes of the sacrum and the iliolumbar ligaments (Bogduk 1997). Secondary factors include the intervertebral disc, the anterior longitudinal ligament, the posterior longitudinal ligament, and the midline posterior ligamentous system (Twomey & Taylor 1985). The passive restraints to anteroposterior translation of a lumbar segment are primarily the longitudinal ligaments, the intervertebral disc, and the capsule of the zygapophyseal joints.

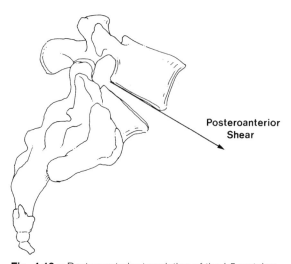

Posteroanterior Shear

Fig. 4.19 • Posteroanterior translation of the L5 vertebra on the sacrum requires control during forward bending of the trunk and in upright postures.

Form closure – the pelvic girdle

Mobility of the sacroiliac joint (SIJ) has been recognized since the 17th century. Since the middle of the 19th century, both postmortem and in vivo studies have been done in an attempt to clarify the movements of the SIJs and the pubic symphysis (PS) and the axes about which these movements occur (Albee 1909, Colachis et al 1963, Egund et al 1978, Goldthwait & Osgood 1905, Hungerford et al 2004, Jacob & Kissling 1995, Lavignolle et al 1983, Lund et al 1996, Meyer 1878, Miller et al 1987, Sashin 1930, Sturesson 1999, Sturesson et al 1989, 2000, Vleeming et al 1990a,b, Walheim & Selvik 1984, Weisl 1954, 1955, Wilder et al 1980).

The investigative methods used include:

1. manual manipulation of the SIJ both at surgery and in a cadaver (Chamberlain 1930, Jarcho 1929, Lavignolle et al 1983);

2. X-ray analysis in various postures of the trunk and lower extremity (Albee 1909, Brooke 1924);

3. roentgen stereophotogrammetric and stereoradiographic imaging after the insertion of tantalum balls into the innominate and sacrum (Egund et al 1978, Sturesson et al 1989, 2000, Walheim & Selvik 1984) and after the attachment of surface markers to the femur, sacrum, and innominate (Hungerford et al 2004);

4. inclinometer measurements in various postures of the trunk and lower extremity, after the insertion of Kirschner wires into the innominate and sacrum (Colachis et al 1963, Jacob & Kissling 1995, Pitkin & Pheasant 1936);

5. computerized analysis using a Metrecom skeletal analysis system (Smidt 1995), and ultrasound evaluation during manual maneuvers (Lund et al 1996).

What do we know from this research?

Kinematics – the pelvic girdle

Motion of the pelvic girdle can occur in all three body planes; anterior and posterior pelvic tilt occurs in the sagittal plane (Fig. 4.20A,B), lateral tilt in the coronal plane (Fig. 4.20C), and axial rotation in the transverse plane (Fig. 4.20D). A combination of all of these motions occurs during gait (Greenman 1990, 1997, Vleeming & Stoeckart 2007). In addition, motion occurs *within* the pelvis; this is known as intrapelvic motion.

Kinematics – intrapelvic motion

Although mobility of the SIJ and PS is small, movement has been shown to occur throughout life (Hungerford et al 2004, Jacob & Kissling 1995, Lund et al 1996, Miller et al 1987, Vleeming et al 1992c, Walheim & Selvik 1984). The quantity of motion available at the SIJ has been debated with several studies reporting differing amplitudes of available motion in both painfree and painful populations (Colachis et al 1963, Jacob & Kissling 1995, Lavignolle et al 1983, Sturesson et al 1989, Weisl 1954, 1955). These studies are difficult to compare as different methods of analysis were used and several have doubtful validity in that surface markers were used. It is difficult, and likely non-ethical, to get approval to use invasive methods for measuring intrapelvic motion in healthy subjects; the only study to do this was Jacob & Kissling's (1995). Sturesson et al's studies (1989, 2000) were invasive in that tantalum balls were inserted into the innominate and sacrum and motion between the markers was analyzed during a variety of functional tasks. These studies (Sturesson et al 1989, 2000) are often quoted to support statements regarding the amplitude of normal SIJ motion; however, it is important to note that the subjects in these studies were women with pelvic girdle pain. Can we rely on studies using subjects in pain to obtain normal biomechanical data?

Jacob & Kissling (1995) inserted Kirschner wires into the innominate and sacrum of healthy, painfree subjects (between 20 and 50 years of age) and analyzed the amplitude of SIJ motion with a three-dimensional stereophotogrammetric method. The position of the innominate and sacrum in the erect standing position was compared to that at the end of forward bending, backward bending, right and left one leg standing. Both the angular and translatoric displacements of the Kirschner wires were noted. The values for rotation and translation were low: 0.4–4.3° of rotation coupled with no more than 0.7mm of translation.

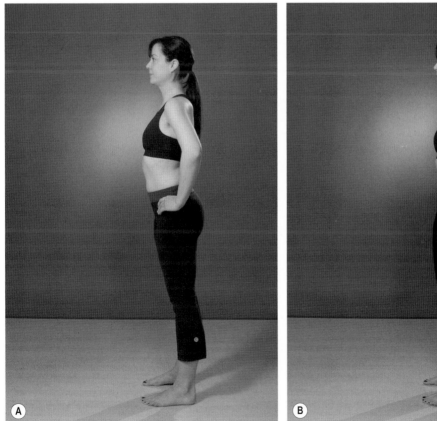
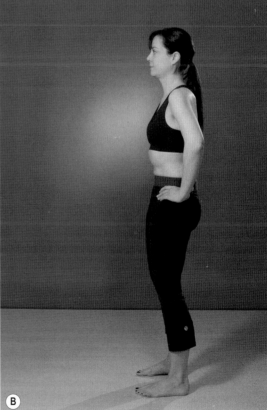

Fig. 4.20 • (A) Anterior pelvic tilt in the sagittal plane. (B) Posterior pelvic tilt in the sagittal plane.

Continued

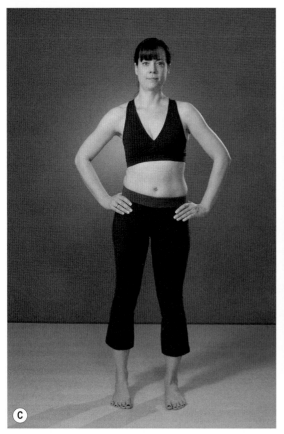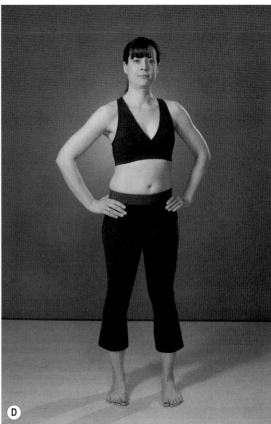

Fig. 4.20—cont'd • (C) Lateral pelvic tilt in the coronal plane. (D) Axial rotation of the pelvic girdle in the transverse plane.

No statistical differences were noted for either age or gender. They postulated that more than 6° of rotation and 2mm of translation were pathological (Jacob & Kissling 1995). It is important to note that, in this study, the motion of the SIJ was measured only when the pelvic girdle was in a vertically loaded position. No comparisons were made between mobility of the relatively unloaded (supine) non-weight bearing SIJ and the loaded (vertical) weight bearing SIJ. Lund et al (1996) used ultrasound imaging to measure displacement of the sacrum relative to the innominate during a rapid posteroanterior 'spring' maneuver applied to the dorsal aspect of the contralateral inferior lateral angle of the sacrum (inducing an oblique axis rotation). Eighty-two percent of the 22 subjects demonstrated greater than 2mm of SIJ movement, suggesting that this joint may be capable of greater passive range of motion than revealed in studies that investigated only active movements.

Buyruk et al (1995a,b, 1999, 2002) used a Doppler imaging system combined with vibration (DIV method) to measure stiffness of the SIJs. This research was repeated and confirmed by Damen et al (2002c). Both groups were able to demonstrate that stiffness of the SIJ is variable between subjects, and therefore the range of motion is potentially variable. This research also suggests that in healthy subjects stiffness of the SIJ is symmetrical, whereas in subjects with unilateral pelvic girdle pain SIJ stiffness is asymmetrical.

In conclusion, it is known that in weight bearing the SIJs are capable of a small amount of both angular and translatoric motion, that the amplitude of this motion is variable between subjects, and that within one subject the motion should be symmetrical between sides. It appears that the amplitude of SIJ motion is greater in non-weight bearing positions (Lund et al 1996).

Few studies have considered the mobility of the PS. Walheim & Selvik (1984) inserted tantalum balls into the left and right superior pubic rami and ischial tuberosities of two healthy subjects, one male and one female. Roentgen stereophotogrammetric analysis was used to measure displacements of the markers during two passive tasks:

1. supine unilateral hip abduction at 90° of flexion; and

2. supine bilateral hip abduction at 90° of flexion;

and three active tasks:

1. active straight leg raise from the supine position;

2. left and right one leg standing; and

3. moving from supine lying to standing.

They found that in both subjects the PS translated less than 2mm vertically and rotated less than 3° about a coronal axis.

Kinematics – intrapelvic motion – terminology

When the sacrum moves symmetrically and bilaterally relative to the innominates at the left and right SIJs, the osteokinematic motion is called nutation and counter-nutation. Nutation of the sacrum occurs when the sacral promontory moves forward into the pelvis about a coronal axis through the interosseous ligament (it nods) (Fig. 4.21). Conversely, counter-nutation of the sacrum occurs when the sacral promontory moves backward about this coronal axis (Fig. 4.22). These terms should be reserved to describe motion of the sacrum relative to the

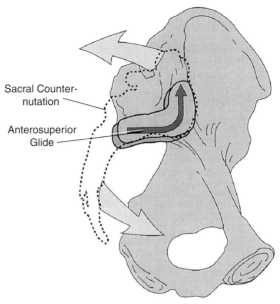

Fig. 4.22 • When the sacrum counter-nutates the promontory moves backwards and the articular surface of the sacrum is thought to glide anterosuperiorly relative to the innominate.

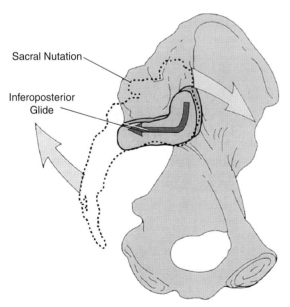

Fig. 4.21 • When the sacrum nutates the promontory moves forward into the pelvis and the articular surface of the sacrum is thought to glide inferoposteriorly relative to the innominate.

innominate regardless of how the pelvic girdle is moving relative to the lumbar spine and femora. In other words, during backward bending, the pelvic girdle should tilt posteriorly and the sacrum should nutate between the posteriorly rotating innominates. If attention was paid only to the motion of the sacrum during this task, one may think it was counter-nutating. When does the sacrum nutate and when does it counter-nutate?

In health, the sacrum is counter-nutated when lying supine and moves into slight nutation in sitting or standing. In other words, whenever an individual is vertical, the sacrum is nutated relative to the innominates. The amount of sacral nutation depends on *how* the individual is sitting or standing. In an optimal, neutral lumbopelvic posture (either sitting or standing) (Fig. 4.23A,B), the sacrum should be slightly nutated between the innominates, but not fully as full nutation is the close-packed, or self-braced, position for the SIJs (see below). During the initial stages of forward or backward bending, the sacrum should completely nutate between the innominates and remain there throughout the full range of motion. On returning to the erect standing posture, the sacrum should move out of the close-packed, fully nutated, position back to slight nutation. When an individual stands in a collapsed posture

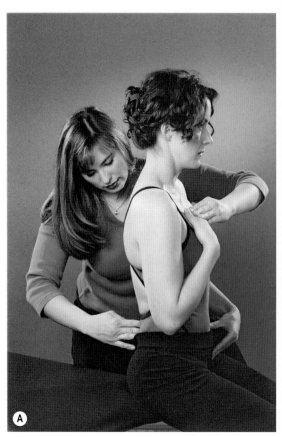
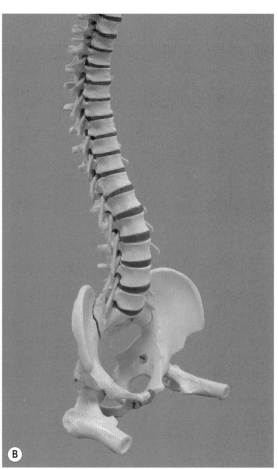

Fig. 4.23 • (A) When the strategy for sitting is optimal the pelvic girdle will be in a neutral posture, as will the lumbar spine. (B) The skeleton in an optimal neutral sitting posture.

(e.g. excessive kypholordosis or anterior pelvic sway posture) (Fig. 4.24), the sacrum is often completely nutated between the innominates. It is not uncommon for this individual to complain of aching in the low back or sacral regions during tasks that involve prolonged standing. No further nutation will occur during forward or backward bending as the total available range of motion has been exhausted. Alternately, when an individual sits in a slumped posture with their center of mass posterior to the SIJs (slouched) (Fig. 4.25A,B), the sacrum is often completely counter-nutated (forced by weight bearing through the coccyx). It is not uncommon for this individual to complain of coccydynia and/or pain specifically just below the PSIS; this is often associated with a painful long dorsal ligament.

Arthrokinematically, when the sacrum nutates relative to the innominate, a linear motion or translation between the two joint surfaces occurs. To date, there have been no studies to validate the following arthrokinematics proposed to occur when the sacrum nutates bilaterally relative to the innominates. During nutation, the proposal is that the sacrum glides inferiorly down the short arm (S1) and posteriorly along the long arm (S2, S3) of the articular surface (see Fig. 4.21). The amplitude of this translation is extremely small, yet can be palpated when the pelvis is in the supine position. Nutation of the sacrum is resisted by its wedge shape, the ridges and depressions of the articular surface, the friction coefficient of the joint surface, and the integrity of the interosseous, sacrospinous, and sacrotuberous ligaments (Vleeming et al 1990a,b) (Fig. 4.26). This is the close-packed, or self-braced, position of the SIJ – a secure position for transferring intermittent high loads.

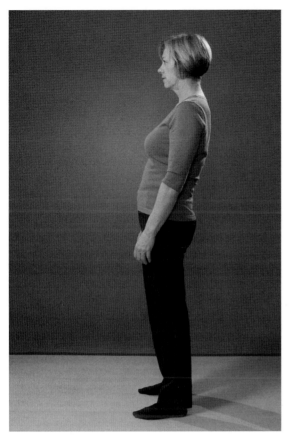

Fig. 4.24 • An anterior pelvic sway posture causes the sacrum to fully nutate between the innominate; this posture is often achieved with a strategy that can create general sacral aching during prolonged standing.

Arthrokinematically, when the sacrum counternutates relative to the innominate, it is proposed that the sacrum glides anteriorly along the long arm and superiorly up the short arm (see Fig. 4.22). This motion is resisted by the long dorsal sacroiliac ligament (Fig. 4.27) (Vleeming et al 1996) and is considered to be a non-optimal position to transfer loads.

The sacrococcygeal joint flexes and extends in response to contraction and relaxation of the pelvic floor (Bø et al 2001). Normally a mobile joint, its motion is primarily restrained by the ventral, dorsal, and lateral sacrococcygeal ligaments.

Rotation of the innominate, relative to the sacrum, occurs about a paracoronal axis through the interosseous ligament of the SIJ and is thought to occur during a variety of functional tasks. Using reflective surface markers on 15 bony landmarks of the femur, innominate, and sacrum, and a motion analysis imaging system, Hungerford et al (2004) investigated the osteokinematic motion of the innominate, relative to the sacrum, during single leg standing with contralateral hip flexion to 90° in both non-painful and pelvic girdle pain populations. They found that when a healthy subject stood on one leg and flexed the contralateral hip (Fig. 4.28), the supporting innominate (weight bearing side) either posteriorly rotated or remained posteriorly rotated relative to the ipsilateral sacrum (the sacrum was, therefore, relatively nutated). In this position, the SIJ is close-packed and able to transfer loads. The non-weight bearing innominate (side of hip flexion) also posteriorly rotated relative to the ipsilateral sacrum during this motion. An associated, and variable, sideflexion/rotation of the innominate was also noted during this task and likely reflects that the axis of motion is not in the pure coronal plane.

Hungerford et al (2004) also investigated the arthrokinematic translation that occurred between the articular surfaces of the innominate and sacrum during posterior rotation of the innominate on both the non-weight bearing and weight bearing sides. They were able to confirm part of what was originally proposed in the second edition of this text (Lee 1999); that is, during posterior rotation of the *non-weight bearing* innominate (side of hip flexion), the innominate glides anterosuperiorly relative to the sacrum (Fig. 4.29). On the weight bearing side, the relative arthrokinematic translation was *posterior* and superior relative to the sacrum (Fig. 4.30). Concurrently, a medial translation was noted, which may reflect increased articular compression during loading. In other words, when the pelvic girdle is self-braced and compressed by the passive and active systems (optimal form and force closure), the direction of the arthrokinematic translation is *not* as predicted in the second edition of this text (Lee 1999). Posterior and superior translation of the articular surface of the innominate relative to the sacrum would effectively 'lock in' the SIJ similar to the mechanism of a bicycle's sprocket and chain. Control of motion, both rotation and shear, would be facilitated during the transference of loads when the articular surfaces engaged in this manner.

Anterior rotation of the innominate is an osteokinematic term used to describe motion of the innominate relative to the sacrum (Fig. 4.31) *or* of the left and right innominates relative to each other. The latter occurs whenever the pelvic girdle is rotated *as a unit* to the left or right (transverse plane rotation) and produces an intrapelvic torsion (IPT). Osteokinematically, an intrapelvic torsion to the left (IPTL)

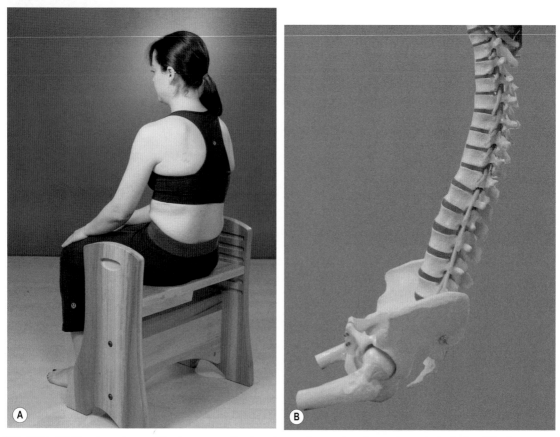

Fig. 4.25 • (A) Slouch or slump sitting is a non-optimal posture as the center of mass is posterior to the SIJs, the sacrum is often forced by gravity into a counter-nutated position, and the direct pressure on the coccyx often leads to coccydynia. (B) The skeleton in slouched/slump sitting.

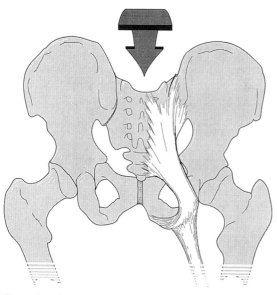

Fig. 4.26 • Sacral nutation is resisted by the interosseous, sacrospinous, and sacrotuberous ligaments. Redrawn from Vleeming et al, 1997.

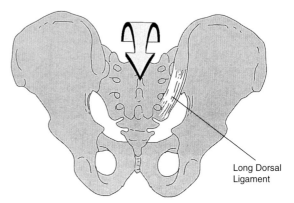

Long Dorsal Ligament

Fig. 4.27 • Counter-nutation of the sacrum tightens the long dorsal ligament. Redrawn from Vleeming et al, 1996.

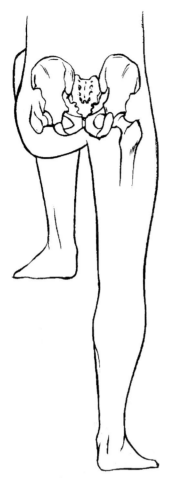

Fig. 4.28 • During one leg standing with flexion of the contralateral hip the non-weight bearing innominate posteriorly rotates relative to the sacrum. In addition, the weight bearing innominate remains posteriorly rotated relative to the sacrum (or posteriorly rotates slightly more).

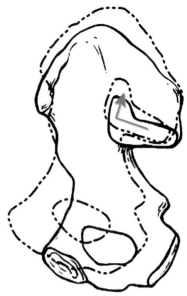

Fig. 4.29 • When an individual transfers weight through one leg and flexes the contralateral hip, the innominate on the non-weight bearing side rotates posteriorly (dotted lines) relative to the sacrum (osteokinematics). The innominate glides anterosuperiorly relative to the sacrum (arrow) (arthrokinematics) (Hungerford et al 2004). The amplitude of the osteokinematic and arthrokinematic motion has been exaggerated in this illustration for visual purposes. In reality, the amplitude of osteokinematic motion is less than 6° coupled with 2–3mm of translation in weight bearing (Jacob & Kissling 1995).

produces anterior rotation of the right innominate relative to the left innominate and left rotation of the sacrum. Both the left and right sides of the sacrum nutate relative to the respective innominate with the right side nutating further than the left (thus the bone rotates to the left). An intrapelvic torsion to the right (IPTR) produces exactly the opposite osteokinematics; the left innominate rotates anteriorly relative to the right innominate and the sacrum rotates to the right with both the left and right sides of the sacrum nutating relative to the respective innominate. These are physiological patterns of osteokinematic motion for intrapelvic motion and occur during gait (when the pelvis rotates in the transverse plane) and during all rotation/lateral bending tasks.

Anterior rotation of the weight bearing innominate *relative to the sacrum* does occur; however, it is thought to be non-optimal if it occurs when the pelvis is loaded as this is the loose-packed, or unlocked, position for the joints of the pelvis. Anterior rotation of the weight bearing innominate occurred in the subjects with unilateral pelvic girdle pain (Hungerford et al 2004). Arthrokinematically, it is felt that when the innominate anteriorly rotates relative to the sacrum, it glides inferiorly down the short arm and posteriorly along the long arm of the SIJ. It is likely that some decompression of the joint surfaces occurs as well. The arthrokinematics of non-weight bearing anterior rotation of the innominate have not been investigated and remain a clinical hypothesis.

In conclusion, it is known that in non-weight bearing the innominate can posteriorly rotate relative to the sacrum and that an arthrokinematic glide between the innominate and the sacrum occurs and is physiological (i.e. follows the articular surfaces). It is also

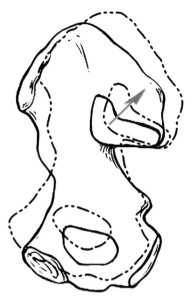

Fig. 4.30 • When an individual transfers weight through one leg and flexes the contralateral hip, the innominate on the weight bearing side either remains posteriorly rotated or posteriorly rotates (dotted line) relative to the sacrum (osteokinematics). The innominate glides *posteriorly* and superiorly relative to the sacrum (arrow) (Hungerford et al 2004). The amplitude of the osteokinematic and arthrokinematic motion has again been exaggerated in this illustration for visual purposes.

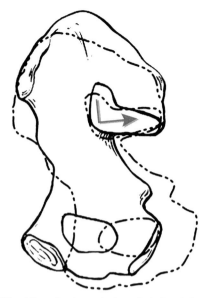

Fig. 4.31 • When the innominate anteriorly rotates (dotted line), it glides inferiorly down the short arm and posteriorly along the long arm of the sacroiliac joint (arrow). The amplitude of the osteokinematic and arthrokinematic motion has been exaggerated in this illustration for visual purposes.

known that in weight bearing, the sacrum should nutate (relative posterior rotation of the innominate) to close-pack, or self-brace, the SIJ and that the arthrokinematic glide during this motion does not follow the articular surfaces, but rather is posterior, superior, and medial. The rest is still clinical hypothesis at this time. It is thought that:

1. sacral nutation occurs during tasks that increase load through the pelvic girdle; and
2. intrapelvic torsion (to the left and/or right) occurs during gait or tasks that induce transverse plane rotation or lateral bending of the trunk and lower extremities.

Counter-nutation of the sacrum relative to the innominate, as well as anterior rotation of the innominate relative to the sacrum, should not occur during any tasks that increase load through the pelvic girdle.

Kinetics – intrapelvic restraints to shear/translation

How does the form of the pelvic girdle contribute to its ability to resist shear or translation of the SIJs

and/or PS during functional tasks? The SIJs transfer large loads and their shape is adapted to this task. The articular surfaces are relatively flat and this helps to transfer compression forces and bending moments (Snijders et al 1993a,b, Vleeming et al 1990a,b). However, a relatively flat joint is theoretically more vulnerable to shear forces. The SIJ is anatomically protected from shear in three ways. First, the sacrum is wedge-shaped in both the anteroposterior and vertical planes and thus is supported by the innominates (see Figs 3.7, 3.8). The articular surface of the SIJ is comprised of two to three sacral segments and each is oriented differently such that when the joint is compressed shear is prevented (see Fig. 3.12) (Solonen 1957). Second, in contrast to other synovial joints, the articular cartilage of the SIJ is not smooth, but irregular, especially on the ilium, and when the joint is compressed this irregularity increases the friction coefficient of the joint (Bowen & Cassidy 1981, Sashin 1930) (see Plates 1–5). Third, cartilage-covered bony extensions (ridges and grooves, see Fig. 3.11) protrude into the joint (Vleeming et al 1990a). All three factors resist translation of the articular surfaces when compression (force closure) is applied to the pelvis. Both form and force closure are required to balance the moment of a large external load.

The PS has less ability to resist shear/translation than the SIJ in that the joint surfaces are relatively flat; the PS has less form closure. The joint surfaces are bound by a fibrocartilaginous disc that is supported externally by superior, inferior, anterior, and posterior ligaments. The PS is vulnerable to shear forces in both the vertical and horizontal plane and relies on 'extra forces' or force closure (compression in the coronal plane), in addition to its passive restraints, for control of vertical shear (Cowan et al 2004).

Form closure – the hip

The femur articulates with the innominate via a ball-and-socket joint, the hip, which is capable of circumductive motion. The hip is classified as an unmodified ovoid joint and in mechanical terms is capable of 12 degrees of freedom of motion along and about three perpendicular axes (Fig. 4.32). This classification does not account for the anatomical or neurophysiological factors that influence and restrain the coupling of motion that actually occurs at the joint.

Kinematics – the hip

Osteokinematically, flexion/extension occurs when the femur rotates about a paracoronal axis through the center of the femoral head and neck; the femoral head should remain centered within the acetabulum through the full excursion of motion. Although variable, approximately 100° of femoral flexion is possible, following which motion of the SIJ and lumbar spine occurs to allow the anterior thigh to approximate the chest (Williams 1995). Approximately 20° of femoral extension is possible (Kapandji 1970). When rotation of the femoral head occurs purely about this axis (i.e. without conjoined abduction/adduction or medial/lateral rotation), the motion is arthrokinematically described as a pure spin. No translation of the femoral head relative to the acetabulum should occur when the joint spins purely.

Osteokinematically, abduction/adduction occurs when the femur rotates about a parasagittal axis through the center of the femoral head. Approximately 45° of femoral abduction and 30° of femoral adduction are possible, following which the pelvic

Fig. 4.32 • The osteokinematic motion of the femur. In mechanical terms, the femur is capable of 12 degrees of freedom along and about three perpendicular axes.

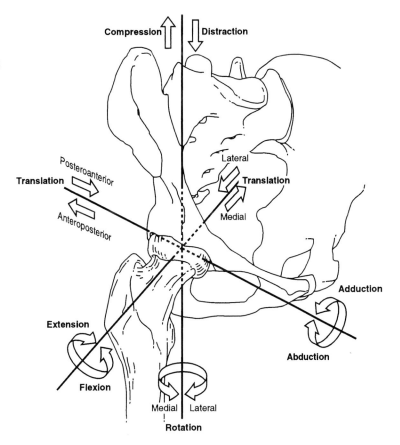

girdle laterally tilts on the lumbar spine (Kapandji 1970). When the femur rotates purely about this parasagittal axis, the head of the femur arthrokinematically transcribes a superoinferior chord within the acetabulum (i.e. the shortest distance between two points); therefore, this motion is described as a pure swing.

Osteokinematically, medial/lateral rotation occurs when the femur rotates about a longitudinal axis. The location of this axis depends on whether the foot is fixed on the ground. When the pelvic girdle rotates about a firmly planted foot, the longitudinal axis of rotation runs from the center of the femoral head through to the lateral femoral condyle. When the foot is off the ground, the femur can rotate about a variety of longitudinal axes, all of which pass through the femoral head and the foot (Williams 1995). Approximately 30–40° of medial rotation and 60° of lateral rotation are possible (Kapandji 1970). Pure femoral rotation about this axis causes the femoral head arthrokinematically to transcribe an anteroposterior chord within the acetabulum and this motion is described as a pure swing (MacConaill & Basmajian 1977).

Functionally, movement of the femur relative to the innominate does not produce pure arthrokinematic motion. Rather, combinations of movement are the norm. The habitual pattern of motion for the non-weight bearing lower extremity is a combination of flexion, abduction, and lateral rotation and extension, adduction, and medial rotation. Arthrokinematically, both motions are impure swings (MacConaill & Basmajian 1977). The close-pack position of the hip is extension, abduction, and internal rotation.

Kinetics – the hip

The hip is subjected to forces equal to multiples of body weight during tasks of everyday living. The anatomical configuration of the joint as well as the orientation of the trabeculae and the orientation of the capsule and the ligaments contribute to its ability to transfer loads without buckling (giving way) or translating during habitual movements. During erect standing in optimal posture, the superincumbent body weight should be distributed equally through the pelvic girdle to the femoral heads and necks. Each hip joint supports approximately 33% of the body weight that subsequently produces a bending moment between the neck of the femur and its shaft (Singleton & LeVeau 1975). A complex system of bony trabeculae exists within the femoral head

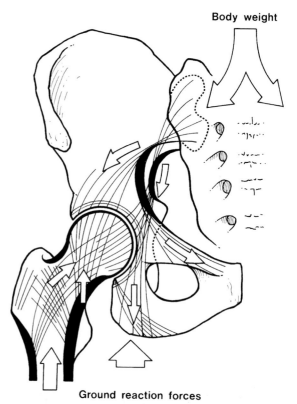

Body weight

Ground reaction forces

Fig. 4.33 • The orientation of the bony trabeculae within the pelvic girdle corresponds to the lines of force met during load transfer through the pelvic girdle. Redrawn from Kapandji, 1970.

and neck to prevent superoinferior shearing of the femoral head during erect standing (Fig. 4.33) (Kapandji 1970). The hip joint is an unmodified ovoid joint, a deep ball-and-socket, and its shape precludes significant shearing in any direction, yet facilitates motion. In spite of this, non-optimal translation (commonly anterior) with or without rotation of the femur often occurs during loading tasks, or open-kinetic chain movements of the hip, leading to uneven distribution of loads between the acetabulum and femoral head, and over time can lead to significant pain and impairment (Lee & Lee 2004a, Sahrmann 2001).

Form closure – the ligaments

For every joint, there is a position called the close-packed, self-braced, or self-locked position where there is maximum congruence of the articular surfaces and maximum tension of the major ligaments.

In this position, the joint is under significant compression and the ability to resist shear, or translation, is enhanced by the tension of the passive structures and increased friction between the articular surfaces (Snijders et al 1993a,b, Vleeming et al 1990b). The close-packed position for the lumbar zygapophyseal joints is end range extension (Bogduk 1997), for the SIJs it is full nutation of the sacrum, or posterior rotation of the innominate (van Wingerden et al 1993, Vleeming et al 1989a,b), and for the hip joint it is extension combined with abduction and internal rotation (Hewitt et al 2002).

Sacral nutation, or posterior rotation of the innominate, increases tension in the sacrotuberous, sacrospinous, and interosseus ligaments (Vleeming et al 1989a,b) (see Fig. 4.26). Counter-nutation of the sacrum, or anterior rotation of the innominate, decreases tension in these major ligaments although the long dorsal ligament becomes taut during this motion (Vleeming et al 1996) (see Fig. 4.27).

The ligaments of the hip joint (see Figs 3.16, 3.37, 3.38) contribute to its form closure as follows (Table 4.1). Extension of the femur winds all of the extra-articular ligaments around the femoral neck and renders them taut. The inferior band of the iliofemoral ligament is under the greatest tension in extension. During lateral rotation of the femur, the iliotrochanteric band of the iliofemoral ligament and the pubofemoral ligament become taut, whereas the ischiofemoral ligament becomes slack. Conversely, during medial rotation of the femur, the anterior ligaments become slack whereas the ischiofemoral ligament becomes taut (Hewitt et al 2002). Abduction of the femur tenses the pubofemoral ligament, and the inferior band of the iliofemoral ligament as well as the ischiofemoral ligament. At the end of abduction, the neck of the femur impacts onto the acetabular rim, thus distorting and everting the labrum (Kapandji 1970). In this manner, the acetabular labrum deepens the articular cavity (improving form closure), thus increasing translatoric motion control without limiting mobility. Adduction results in tension of the iliotrochanteric band of the iliofemoral ligament, whereas the other ligaments remain relatively slack. Adduction of the flexed hip tightens the ischiofemoral ligament (Hewitt et al 2002). The ligamentum teres is under moderate tension in erect standing as well as during medial and lateral rotation of the femur. Flexion of the femur unwinds the ligaments and, when combined with slight adduction, predisposes the femoral head to posterior dislocation if sufficient force is applied to the distal end of the

femur (e.g. dashboard impact); this is a position of least form closure with respect to the ligamentous system.

Force closure theory

According to the original definition, force closure (see Fig. 4.8) pertains to when 'extra forces are needed to keep the object in place' (Snijders et al 1993a). The extra forces increase articular compression, and thus friction between the joint surfaces (Vleeming et al 1990a,b) and also increase the joint's stiffness (stiffness = force/resultant displacement or distance). The 'extra forces' are applied to the joint:

- directly by the resting tone in, and co-contraction of, the muscles that cross the joint; or
- indirectly by the resting tone in, and co-contraction of, the muscles that do not cross the joint but increase tension in the fascia, which does.

Table 4.1 Form closure is augmented when tension increases in the ligaments of the hip joint during motion of the femur

Femoral motion	Ligament	Tension
Extension	All extra-articular ligaments	Taut
Flexion/adduction	All ligaments	Slack
Lateral rotation	Iliotrochanteric	Taut
	Pubofemoral	Taut
	Ischiofemoral	Slack
Medial rotation	Iliofemoral	Slack
	Pubofemoral	Slack
	Ischiofemoral	Taut
Abduction	Pubofemoral	Taut
	Inferior band*	Taut
	Ischiofemoral	Taut
	Iliotrochanteric	Slack
Adduction	Iliotrochanteric	Taut
	Inferior band*	Slack
	Ischiofemoral	Slack
	Pubofemoral	Slack

*Inferior band of iliofemoral ligament.

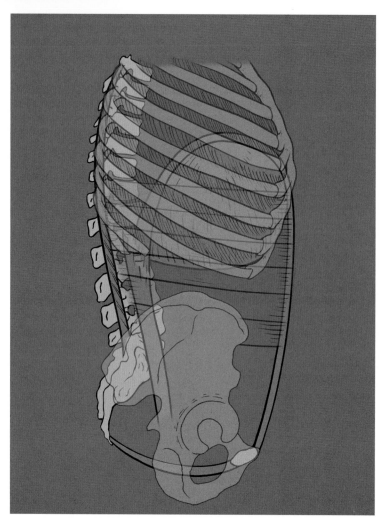

Fig. 4.34 • The abdominal canister is comprised of the lower six thoracic rings (vertebrae and associated ribs), the five lumbar vertebrae, and the pelvic girdle as well as all the muscles and viscera the canister contains. The diaphragm forms the roof of the canister, the pelvic floor forms the floor, and the muscles and fascia of the deep abdomen form the walls.

Translation, or shear, of the joints of the LPH complex is, therefore, prevented by a combination of factors:

• the architecture of the joint (form closure as noted above); as well as

• the compression generated by certain ligaments, muscles, and fascia (force closure).

The muscles and fascia

Function would be significantly compromised if a joint's motion could not be controlled through its full range (see Fig. 4.9). In the joint's neutral zone, the passive system (the capsule and ligaments) cannot contribute to motion control. How the nervous system controls the synergistic function of muscles required to control the 85 joints in the abdominal canister (Fig. 4.34), while allowing necessary movement to occur, during a multitude of tasks of varying loads, predictability, and perceived risk, has been the focus of much research since the last edition of this text. In this section, the muscles and fascial systems (slings) that have the potential to increase force closure through the joints of the LPH complex will be considered. An explanation of the underlying control mechanisms (motor control) will follow.

Using the Doppler imaging and vibration method (DIV method), Richardson et al (2002) showed that co-contraction of the deep muscles of the lumbo-pelvis increases stiffness of the SIJ. The muscles included, but were not necessarily limited to, transversus abdominis, multifidus, and the pelvic floor, and co-contraction was initiated with an abdominal drawing-in, or hollowing, cue. In the same study, stiffness of the SIJ was also augmented by co-contraction of the superficial muscles of the lumbopelvis. The muscles included, but were not necessarily limited to, the external oblique, internal oblique, rectus abdominis, and erector spinae, and co-contraction was initiated with an abdominal bracing cue. They noted that the drawing-in, or hollowing, cue had a bigger effect on stiffness of the SIJ. van Wingerden et al (2004) also used the DIV method to investigate the impact of several other muscles on stiffness of the SIJ, including the biceps femoris, gluteus maximus, erector spinae, and contralateral latissimus dorsi. They found that stiffness of the SIJ increased when 'individual muscles were activated,' although they did note that significant co-contraction of other muscles occurred.

There is a problem with the conclusions from these studies in that individual muscle recruitment is highly unlikely and, therefore, the conclusions should be that an abdominal drawing-in, hollowing and/or bracing cue, as well as a command to contract the biceps femoris, gluteus maximus, or erector spinae, results in increased stiffness of the SIJ. It appears that co-contraction of many muscles can increase force closure of this joint. No conclusion can be made about how much force closure is needed for specific tasks and which co-contraction pattern is the most optimal for different tasks.

In a cadaveric study using springs to simulate the forces produced by co-contraction of the muscles of the pelvic floor, Pool-Goudzwaard et al (2004) showed that, in females, a significant increase in stiffness of the SIJ occurs when the muscles of the pelvic floor contract as a group. There was no significant effect on SIJ stiffness when contraction of an *individual* muscle of the pelvic floor was simulated; in fact, a significant *decrease* in stiffness of the SIJ occurred during a simulated contraction of only iliococcygeus. They also noted that co-contraction of the entire pelvic floor and/or the coccygeus muscle (ischiococcygeus) produced counter-nutation of the sacrum. There was no change in the stiffness of the male SIJs and they hypothesize that this was due to gender differences in joint mobility and in the shape of the pelvis (the female subjects were twice as mobile as the male). The limitation of these studies is that muscle activity is simulated by springs on cadavers, and not in vivo contractions. The role of the pelvic floor muscles in providing 'extra forces' to close the urethra and the role of these muscles in the continence mechanism is considered in Chapter 6.

Using a three-dimensional simulation model, Pel et al (2008) showed that shear forces through the SIJ could be significantly reduced by simulated activation of transversus abdominis and the pelvic floor. They also found that, although gluteus medius, minimus, and piriformis increased compression between the innominates and the sacrum, these muscles were less able to control shear of the SIJ because the total force through the joint still acted primarily in a vertical direction (non-optimal net vector for controlling vertical shear).

Several studies have investigated the contribution of

1. various muscles (Cholewicki et al 1997, Cholewicki & van Vliet 2002, Hodges 2003, McGill et al 2003);
2. the thoracolumbar fascia (Barker et al 2006, Hodges 2003b, Hodges et al 2003a, Vleeming et al 1995a); and
3. intra-abdominal pressure (Cresswell 1993, Cresswell et al 1992, Hodges & Gandevia 2000a,b, Hodges et al 2001a, 2005, Hodges 2003);

to control of motion in the lumbar spine. A number of different methods have been used with the conclusion being that many muscles contribute to force closure of the lumbar spine (i.e. provide 'extra forces to keep the object in place') through mechanisms that compress the spine, tense its fascia, or increase the intra-abdominal pressure and, importantly, that static stability (via increased stiffness) and maintenance of a neutral spine posture can be achieved with minimal levels of co-contraction of the muscles of the trunk (see Fig. 4.3A) (Andersson et al 2002, Cholewicki et al 1997, Cholewicki & van Vliet 2002, Hodges 2003). But knowing which muscles have the capacity to increase force closure of the LPH complex is not enough; we need to understand how the CNS controls and directs the synergistic activity of these muscles to reach the goals of function.

An orchestra is a useful analogy for explaining to patients how the neuromuscular system functions in health. Imagine that each muscle is like an instrument in the orchestra. It is important for the musician to know how to play their instrument well and if you listen closely during the warm up, you will hear beautiful music from this instrument. This is the equivalent to knowing how to contract/relax a specific muscle; in other words, play the muscle. However, during the orchestra's warm-up time, the resultant collective noise from all of the musicians is not harmonious, and certainly not beautiful.

Someone, or something, has to tell the musicians what, and how, to play together to make beautiful music. The 'someone' is, of course, the conductor (the controller, or the CNS) and the 'something' is the piece of music they choose to perform (the task) and the musician (the specific muscle) has to know how to read his/her own part in the score. When the muscles perform in synergy (optimal motor control), beautiful movements occur. What do we know about the controller (CNS), the conductor of the orchestra?

Motor control theory

Much of the research on motor control of the LPH complex has focused on understanding how the CNS controls stability of the spine. As discussed in the introduction, research in the field of spinal stability has continued to evolve and a broader definition of spinal stability that moves beyond static models to encompass the dynamic nature of the spine has emerged. If only *static situations* are considered, using co-contraction of the trunk muscles to stiffen the spine is predicted to be the best strategy for control of the spine; however, in *dynamic situations*, the CNS can choose strategies that use movement to dampen and control perturbations in addition to a stiffness strategy (Hodges & Cholewicki 2007). It is clear that the CNS can switch between different strategies as the task, environment, and goals change.

> The musculoskeletal system is highly redundant, implying that each motor task can be performed in many ways; motor control is constrained by weighted and potentially conflicting criteria, such as achieving the task goal, while avoiding excessive energy consumption. Weights of constraints are contingent upon environmental circumstances, task requirements, and changes in the musculoskeletal system, as well as psychological factors such as motivation and attention.
>
> van Dieen 2007.

When the research is considered together within a larger framework, it is evident that current models do not fully explain this complex system. Hodges & Cholewicki (2007) note that 'investigation of the dynamic control of lumbopelvic stability is the next major challenge facing our understanding of functional control of the spine and pelvis.'

What is the current understanding of this complex system? The following is an interpretation and summary from the current trends in evidence pertaining to motor control and the lumbopelvic region. The reader is encouraged to read the papers and summary chapters cited in this section for more detail on the specifics of the research/evidence.

Stability strategies for the LPH complex – an overview

How does the CNS choose an appropriate strategy to prepare the LPH complex for loads while ensuring that any necessary mobility is allowed, respiration is supported, continence is preserved, and balance or equilibrium is maintained? The challenge for the CNS (the controller or conductor) is to analyze all of the requirements for a specific task, interpret the current status of all systems, and plan the best strategy. The best strategies for stability of the LPH complex will achieve multiple outcomes (Fig. 4.35). They will:

1. control both angular and translatoric motions of the joints, and therefore maintain optimal joint axes and distribute loads appropriately, while allowing the necessary mobility required for the task;
2. control spinal posture/orientation within and between the regions;
3. maintain postural equilibrium; and
4. simultaneously support respiration and continence in potentially changing environments during multiple predictable and unpredictable tasks of varying loads and risk.

When the challenge is unpredictable (sudden change in load, predictability, equilibrium), the CNS must react quickly in response to the perturbation to ensure stability is maintained (return to the intended path of trajectory). Given the considerable redundancy in the motor system, the CNS has multiple muscles and many different strategy options to choose from for any given task (e.g. co-contraction stiffening, alternating muscle activity, use of inertia and dampening, etc.). All strategies will involve multiple muscles, both deep and superficial. The impact on the body of a particular strategy lies in:

1. how much compression/torque is generated;
2. how much stiffness is generated/mobility is allowed/restricted and where;
3. how much the intrathoracic and intra-abdominal pressure is increased; and
4. how well the body can react to unexpected perturbations (internal or external, physical, cognitive, or emotional) that may occur during the task.

Fig. 4.35 • An optimal strategy for any task will ensure that loads are transferred while controlling both angular and translatoric motion of all joints in the kinetic chain, maintaining optimal alignment between the regions (thorax to pelvis, pelvis to lower extremity), and ensuring balance or equilibrium is maintained in spite of any perturbation that may occur. The strategy will not create excessive stress on any of the joints, will support optimal breathing patterns, and will not excessively increase the intra-abdominal pressure such that continence is preserved.

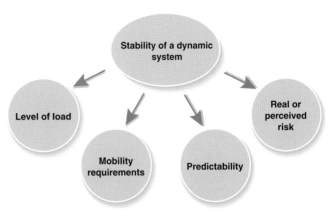

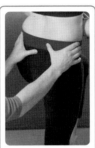
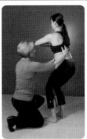
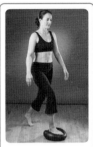

| Control angular and translatoric motion of all joints in the kinetic chain while allowing the necessary range of motion required for the task | Maintain optimal alignment within and between the regions | Ensure that balance is maintained in spite of any perturbation that may occur |

Any strategy can be good or bad; the key is whether the individual is using the 'best,' or most appropriate, strategy for the task at hand given their individual makeup. In order to determine if a given strategy is appropriate for a specific task, the clinician uses information from both the science and a qualitative analysis of movement and performance. The strategy analysis tests for the LPH complex are covered in Chapter 8; Chapters 9 and 12 will discuss the clinical reasoning and aspects of strategy analysis that are currently difficult to measure scientifically and rely on clinical observation. The following sections will focus on what is known from the research.

Stability strategies – the evidence

What influences the strategy chosen by the CNS? The choice depends on the:

1. somatosensory information being relayed to the CNS from the joints, fascia, ligaments, muscles, organs, and skin, as well as how the CNS interprets this information;

2. quantity of the load to be controlled; higher loads require increased activity of more muscles;

3. predictability of the task; can the CNS plan or must it react/respond to perturbations quickly to prevent giving way or buckling and return the system to its intended trajectory?

4. real or perceived risk (threat value); how does the CNS process and influence the information coming from the peripheral system (impact of past experiences, fears, and/or beliefs)?

The CNS must carefully plan the strategy to match the changing demands of the task. For example, walking is a dynamic task and the CNS modulates the activity of the deep and superficial trunk muscles throughout the task such that the greatest activity occurs in conjunction with the peak times of high load (foot strike or times of maximal trunk rotation)

(Saunders et al 2004a, 2005). In addition, it must be prepared to react to any sudden perturbation that throws the subject off its intended trajectory (inadvertently stepping on a rock). How does it do all this? The evidence suggests that given the dynamic nature of the human system the

> trunk muscles do not co-contract to increase stiffness of the spine, which would be a valid strategy for increasing stability in a static sense, but instead they respond in a triphasic manner with alternating flexor and extensor bursts of activity to match the moments imposed on the spine, which is an appropriate strategy to assure stability in a dynamic sense.
>
> Hodges & Cholewicki 2007.

The relative contribution of specific muscles to stability of the LPH complex changes constantly, even during the same task, and is based on the demands of the task *at the moment*, its predictability, and its threat value (real or perceived risk). Stiffening the spine by co-contracting multiple muscles (static/stiffening strategy) is the simplest solution with a lower potential for error (e.g. loss of control of one segment or joint) than a strategy that is dynamic and requires specific activation of muscles synergistically at the right time and in an optimal pattern or sequence. It is proposed that a movement, or control strategy, has greater potential for error (Hodges 2005, Hodges & Cholewicki 2007). When loads are high, predictability low, and an individual perceives a situation or task to be dangerous or highly threatening, the CNS will likely opt to limit the possibility of error and use a co-contraction bracing strategy even though this comes at a cost of higher compression loading, increased energy expenditure, and higher intra-abdominal pressure, and reduces the efficiency of breathing and challenges continence (Fig. 4.36).

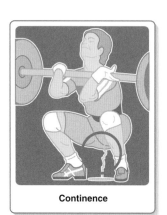
Continence

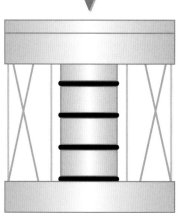

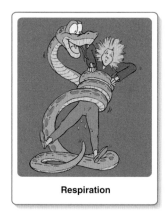
Respiration

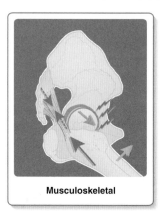
Musculoskeletal

Fig. 4.36 • A co-contraction bracing strategy comes at a cost: (1) higher compression loading of the joints; (2) higher intra-abdominal pressure (more risk of herniation or prolapse); and (3) more restriction to lateral costal expansion of the rib cage thus compromising optimal respiratory patterns.

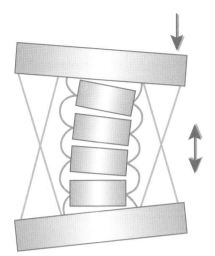

Fig. 4.37 • A dynamic strategy for transferring loads requires a finely tuned neuromuscular system with accurate feedforward and feedback mechanisms that responds to perturbations with predictable movements and not stiffening.

On the other hand, in 'safe' situations or ones of perceived low load/risk, the CNS is more likely to choose a dynamic strategy that allows more mobility, is less compressive to the musculoskeletal system, does not excessively increase the IAP intra-abdominal pressure, and overall is more efficient (requires less energy) (Fig. 4.37). However, there is greater risk for error if the timing of muscle activation is off just a bit, or if the load is not judged accurately, or if an unexpected perturbation is not responded to appropriately. The CNS relies on accurate afferent input from the articular mechanoreceptors, the myofascial receptors, as well as the visual receptors, and considers the load and predictability of the task as well as any past experience and/or beliefs about the task when choosing a strategy (to brace or to move). Some of these motor strategies are preplanned and under automatic control, whereas others can be modulated by voluntary action and training.

Although all muscles are important for effectively transferring loads through the LPH complex, the deep muscles (transversus abdominis, segmental fibers of multifidus, pelvic floor, psoas, deep hip rotators) are better suited to control segmental translation compared to the superficial muscles, as the deep muscles can provide specific segmental compression, whereas the superficial muscles span several segments and compress multiple segments if they are used to control translation. The superficial muscles are better suited to control posture and

motion between regions, as well as static stability. Note that although co-contraction of multiple superficial muscles may be a suitable strategy for intermittently transferring high loads, the problem comes when this strategy is used habitually for all tasks as excessive or sustained compressive loads on the spine can lead to damage or changes in the passive system (Adams et al 1996, Cholewicki & McGill 1996). Furthermore, co-contraction of the superficial multisegmental muscles affects the ability of the spine to move, impacts its ability to absorb and dissipate forces (loss of flexible column), as well as potentially interferes with motion through space (an intended trajectory). Therefore, strategies that create excessive co-contraction bracing may negatively impact functions such as walking, which requires thoracopelvic rotation, and breathing, which requires lateral costal expansion and spinal motion, as well as the capacity for dynamic stability.

An experimental paradigm that provides insights into dynamic control of the spine is the use of fast voluntary arm movements, as moving the arm rapidly creates perturbations of the trunk, and challenges multiple components of spinal stability (postural orientation, postural equilibrium, segmental control) (Belenkii et al 1967, Bouisset & Zattara 1981, Hodges 1997). Anticipatory postural adjustments of the trunk in response to rapid arm movements have been used extensively in research and provide an understanding of how the deep and superficial muscle systems of the trunk contribute to stability of the abdominal canister. The evidence suggests that the strategy used by the CNS to prepare the body for the expected perturbation involves preparatory motion (Belenkii et al 1967, Bouisset & Zattara 1981, Hodges 1997, 2003, Hodges et al 1997, 1999, 2000, 2001b, Hodges & Gandevia 2000a,b, Lee et al 2009, Moseley et al 2002, 2003, Smith et al 2007b). The osteokinematic preparatory movements, the resultant movements, as well as the muscle responses that occur when predictably moving the arm(s) rapidly through flexion and extension, are outlined in Table 4.2.

In short, when either one or both arms are moved rapidly, reactive moments are imposed on the trunk. There is a predictable preparatory movement of the trunk and predictable preparatory muscle activity prior to movement/muscle activity of the arm, as well as a resultant movement of the trunk and a resultant muscle response after movement of the arm. The CNS prepares the trunk for the perturbation with movement, not stiffness, and does so in a

Table 4.2 Anticipatory postural adjustments of the trunk and the associated muscle activity during rapid arm movements

Arm movement	Preparatory trunk movement	Preparatory muscle activity		Resultant trunk movement	Resultant muscle activity
		Deep muscles	Superficial muscles		
Bilateral flexion	Extension (Ext)	TrA,	ES, IO	Flexion	RA, EO
Bilateral extension	Flexion (Fl)	TrA,	EO, RA	Extension	ES, IO
Unilateral L flexion	Ext, RSF RROT	TrA, PFM, diaphragm, deep multifidus	ES, IO, superficial multifidus	Fl, LSF, LROT	RA, EO
Unilateral L extension	Fl, RSF, LROT	TrA, PFM, diaphragm	EO	Ext, LSF, RROT	ES, deep and superficial multifidus

EO, external oblique; ES, erector spinae; IO, internal oblique; LROT, left rotation; LSF, left sideflexion; PFM, pelvic floor muscles; RA, rectus abdominis; RSF, right sideflexion; RROT, right rotation; TrA, transversus abdominis.

Note that the preparatory and resultant responses and movements are relative to the onset of deltoid. Hodges et al 1999, 2000, 2003, 2007, Hodges & Gandevia 2000a,b, MacDonald et al 2009, Smith et al 2007a. Intra-abdominal pressure increases before activation of the deltoid (Hodges et al 2007, 1997, 1999).

predictable manner. All of the superficial trunk muscles (erector spinae, rectus abdominis, external oblique, internal oblique, superficial multifidus) are involved in the postural adjustments and the pattern of activation is specific to the direction of trunk movement (directional specificity). The onset of the superficial trunk muscle activity precedes the preparatory movement.

The deep muscles of the LPH complex

With respect to the deep muscles of the LPH complex, in all of the studies investigating anticipatory postural adjustments in response to rapid arm movements, transversus abdominis responded prior to any other muscle in the trunk or upper extremity regardless of the direction of the perturbation, preparatory and/or resultant trunk movement (non-direction specific), as did the pelvic floor and the diaphragm (Hodges 1997, 2003, Hodges et al 1997, 1999, 2007, Hodges & Gandevia 2000a,b, Sjodahl et al 2009, Smith et al 2007b). When the task was sustained (repetitive rapid arm flexion and extension) there was a sustained, or tonic, response in the activity of the transversus abdominis, pelvic floor, and diaphragm even though activity of all three muscles continued to be phasically modulated for respiration. It has also been shown that the deep and superficial fibers of multifidus are differentially activated during rapid arm movements (MacDonald et al 2009, Moseley et al 2002, 2003). The deepest, most segmental, fibers of multifidus increased activity prior to the superficial fibers during both flexion and extension of one arm. However, the onset of both was earlier than deltoid only with flexion of the arm. In other words, both the deep and superficial fibers of multifidus demonstrate some direction specificity (MacDonald et al 2009). Masani et al (2009) also noted direction-specific, phasic activation in multiple superficial trunk muscles (internal oblique, external oblique, rectus abdominis, and erector spinae) during postural perturbations of the trunk in sitting.

Studies of other dynamic tasks also support that the CNS differentially controls the deep and superficial muscles. During one leg standing with contralateral hip and knee flexion, the onset of the low horizontal fibers of transversus abdominis and internal oblique, as well as multifidus, precedes a weight shift in healthy individuals (Hungerford et al 2003). Surface electromyography (EMG) was used to measure onset times and therefore any difference in the onset timing of transversus abdominis and internal oblique could not be determined in this study. During the active straight leg raise test (lifting one leg off the table while lying supine), the onset of EMG activity of transversus abdominis preceded that of rectus femoris (Cowan et al 2004). Fine-wire EMG was used to measure onset times in this study. Feedforward, or early, activation of transversus abdominis was previously noted during standing lower limb movement (Hodges & Richardson 1997).

It is important to remember that the findings of differential activation for the deep muscles may not be exactly the same for tasks that have different requirements. For example, during walking,

Saunders et al (2004a) found tonic activity of transversus abdominis for 100% of the gait cycle at speeds less than 3ms^{-1}, yet phasic at speeds greater than 3ms^{-1}. There was a brief period of EMG silence in TrA during the airborne phase of the run. In addition, the deep fibers of multifidus were *not* tonically active at any speed and showed phasic bursts of activity that corresponded to times of increased vertical loading (ipsilateral and contralateral heel strike) (Fig. 4.38). Care must be taken not to assume that

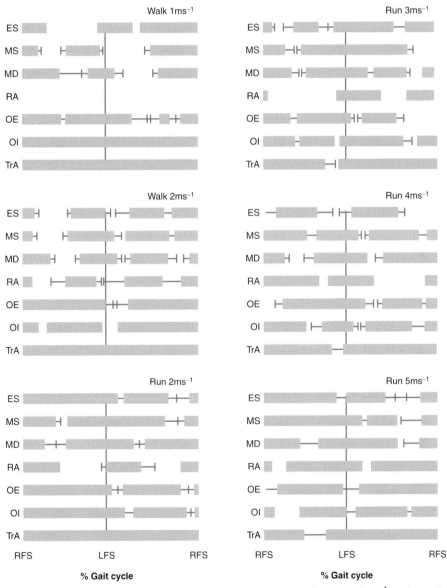

Fig. 4.38 • Onset timing of all muscles measured during walking at speeds less than 3ms^{-1} and speeds greater than 3ms^{-1}. Note the phasic response of the multifidus and the intermittent response of TrA at greater walking/running speeds. Redrawn from Saunders et al, 2004a.

the way the CNS controls the muscles during one task is the same for other tasks.

What is becoming increasingly clear is that, although both the deep and superficial muscle systems are required for stabilization during all tasks, the deep muscles behave differently than the superficial muscles. The evidence suggests that the deep muscles work synergistically (they coactivate) to prepare the body for loads by:

1. increasing the intra-abdominal pressure; and
2. fine-tuning the segmental stiffness of the intervertebral, intrapelvic, and likely the hip joints, prior to the activation of the superficial system;

such that the large moments exerted by the powerful superficial muscles result in:

1. evenly distributed transference of load;
2. maintenance of optimal axes of rotation for each joint in the kinetic chain; and a
3. uniform motion of the entire spine (Hodges & Cholewicki 2007).

Although some authors have argued that the potential contribution of TrA to spinal stability is limited (Grenier & McGill 2007, Kavcic et al 2004), it is important to realize that these studies use models that only consider the control of static rotational buckling, or model TrA as a trunk flexor or lateral flexor; that is, they are looking at one part of stability or asking a research question about one potential role of TrA. Hodges (2003) suggests that activity of transversus abdominis is not related or linked to trunk movement but rather to changes in intra-abdominal pressure. Given all that we have discussed thus far, it is clear that when all of the available evidence is considered, TrA and the deep trunk muscles play an important role in spinal stability, but their role differs from that of the superficial muscles.

In addition to playing a specific role in stability strategies for control of the LPH complex, the deep muscles of the abdominal canister play key roles in respiration and continence. The diaphragm (see Fig. 3.63A,B,C) is the primary respiratory muscle and is known also to contribute to trunk control (Hodges & Gandevia 2000a,b). This muscle is able to 'multitask' in that:

1. its resting tone increases prior to any recorded movement/activity of the arm during rapid arm movement;

2. it remains tonically active during sustained repetitions of flexion/extension of the arm, while simultaneously

3. modulating its activity for respiration (increasing with inspiration and decreasing with expiration).

The activity of the diaphragm is linked to activity of transversus abdominis; however, the opposite pattern of activity modulation is found. Both the diaphragm and TrA are active throughout the respiratory cycle and, although the EMG amplitude of TrA is greater during expiration, the EMG amplitude of the diaphragm is greater during inspiration.

The pelvic floor muscles (see Fig. 3.55A,B) play a key role in dynamic stability of the trunk, which includes controlling motion of the joints of the pelvic girdle and spine in addition to their role in respiration and continence (Pel et al 2008, Pool-Goudzwaard et al 2004). They are tonically active in standing, non-direction specific during rapid arm movements that perturb the trunk, and increase their activation during quiet and resisted expiration (Deindl et al 1993, 1994, Hodges et al 2007, Neumann & Gill 2002, Smith et al 2007b). The increased activation of the pelvic floor has been linked to activation of transversus abdominis (Hodges et al 2007). Coactivation of the pelvic floor with transversus abdominis has also been noted during cues to lift, or contract, the pelvic floor and to hollow, or draw-in, the lower abdomen (Hodges et al 2007, Neumann & Gill 2002, Sapsford & Hodges 2001, Sapsford et al 2001, Smith et al 2007b, Thompson et al 2006). This coactivation results in increased intra-abdominal pressure and therefore increased tension in the thoracolumbar fascia and likely the anterior abdominal fascia/linea alba (Barker et al 2006, Brown & McGill 2009). The muscles of the pelvic floor are also known to increase their activity in an anticipatory, or feedforward, manner during a cough and thus support the endopelvic fascia (suburethral layer) (see Figs 3.59, 3.60), a critical structure for urethral support (Ashton-Miller et al 2001, Ashton-Miller & DeLancey 2007, Barbic et al 2003, Bø and Stien 1994, Constantinou & Govan 1982, Deindl et al 1994, DeLancey 1994, Peng et al 2006). Bø and Stien (1994) have also found coactivation between the muscles of the pelvic floor and the muscles of the urethral wall; this likely facilitates force closure of the urethra and the maintenance of continence during tasks that increase the intra-abdominal pressure.

In summary, the evidence suggests that the deep muscles of the LPH complex work synergistically (not separately) to prepare the body for loads through mechanisms that increase the intra-abdominal pressure, tense the relative fascia (thoracolumbar, endopelvic, and perhaps the anterior abdominal), and specifically increase compression of the joints of the LPH complex to maintain an optimal joint position prior to the activation of the superficial muscle system. This synergy of muscle action (within and between the deep and superficial muscles) is controlled by the CNS and results in the even transference of loads through the LPH complex such that:

1. mobility is maintained while keeping to the intended trajectory, or path of motion;
2. respiration is supported;
3. continence is maintained; and
4. the ability to control expected or unexpected perturbations (internal or external) is ensured.

Compared to the muscles of the lumbopelvic region, few studies have analyzed the onset timing of the deep muscles of the hip during functional tasks (e.g. pectineus, piriformis, superior and inferior gemelli, obturator internus and externus). Andersson et al (1995) investigated the activation patterns of psoas and iliacus using fine-wire EMG and ultrasound guidance during a variety of tasks in standing, sitting, and lying, in healthy subjects. They found coactivation of both muscles during tasks requiring hip flexion (contralateral hip flexion in standing, supine, bilateral or unilateral (ipsilateral) leg raises, sitting in hyperlordosis or angled back at 30°) and no activation of either psoas or iliacus in quiet standing or when the trunk was inclined 30° forward. Selective activity in iliacus occurred only during contralateral hip extension in standing (non-weight bearing), whereas selective psoas activity only occurred in some subjects during contralateral slow lateral bending of the trunk while standing. They conclude that neither psoas nor iliacus plays a role in postural support in standing and that selective activation of iliacus pertains to tasks involving control of hip extension (eccentric) and psoas, in some, pertains to tasks involving control of contralateral lateral bending of the trunk (eccentric). All other tasks involving hip flexion resulted in coactivation of both iliacus and psoas.

No studies could be found that investigated the onset timing, or role, of obturator internus, externus, superior or inferior gemelli, or quadratus femoris, the deepest muscles of the hip and the ones likely involved in the maintenance of the joint's axes of motion.

The superficial muscles – the myofascial slings

As noted above, the superficial muscles play an integral role in strategies used by the CNS for control of the spine and pelvis; superficial muscle activity patterns are related to task characteristics and should occur in synergy with the deep muscles (e.g. Table 4.2). Vleeming & Snijders have described four slings of myofascia that assist in control of the pelvis between the thorax and the legs (Snijders et al 1993a, Vleeming et al 1995a,b). The posterior oblique sling (Fig. 4.39A) connects the latissimus dorsi and the gluteus maximus through the thoracolumbar fascia; the anterior oblique sling (Fig. 4.39B) connects the external oblique, the anterior abdominal fascia, and the contralateral adductors of the thigh; the longitudinal sling connects the peroneii, the biceps femoris, the sacrotuberous ligament, the deep lamina of the thoracolumbar fascia, and the erector spinae; and the lateral sling connects the gluteus medius/minimus, tensor fascia latae, and the lateral stabilizers of the thoracopelvic region. Myers (2001) has described several interconnected deep and superficial slings of muscles and fascia, or, in his words, trains – a novel metaphor for the many myofascial sling systems (Fig. 4.40).

It is likely that there are multiple myofascial slings, deep and superficial, which belong to full body kinetic chains that connect well beyond the LPH complex and link the lower extremity to the pelvis, the thorax to the pelvis, and, through the thorax, the shoulder, head, and neck to the pelvis. The four slings initially described by Vleeming and Snijders sought to explain how specific muscles linked together for load transfer through the pelvis. It is now recognized that, although individual muscles are important for stabilization as well as for mobility, it is critical to understand how they connect and function together (work in synergy). A muscle contraction produces a force that spreads beyond the origin and insertion of the active muscle. This force is transmitted to other muscles, tendons, fasciae, ligaments, capsules, and bones that lie both in series and in parallel to the active muscle (Brown & McGill 2009). In this manner, forces can be produced quite distant from the origin of the initial muscle contraction; this is referred to as a force vector. These muscles connect through the fascia to produce vectors of force that assist in the transfer of load and, when all of the vectors are balanced, they provide optimal alignment of the bones and joints for any task (Fig. 4.41).

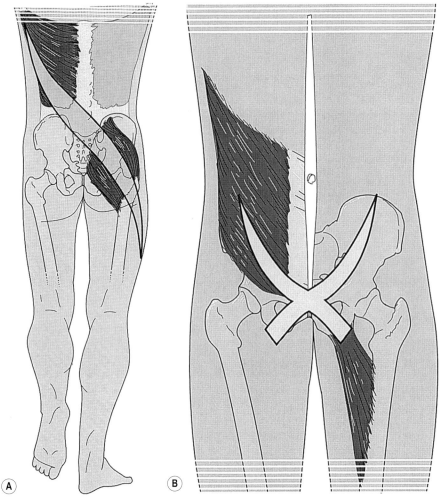

Fig. 4.39 • (A) The posterior oblique sling and (B) the anterior oblique sling, as described by Vleeming et al (1995a).

According to Wikipedia, tensegrity is a portmanteau of the words 'tensional' and 'integrity' and refers to structures, or systems, whose integrity is based on a synergy between balanced tension and compression (Fig. 4.42) (Levin 1997). When the deep and superficial muscle systems work synergistically in any task, there is dynamic tensegrity in that the force vectors come and go according to the demands of the task. This applies to fairly static tasks, such as sitting or standing, as well as complex tasks such as running, swimming, walking, jumping, etc. The vectors of force are constantly changing as the needs of the task are met.

Imbalanced force vectors resulting from non-optimal strategies associated with altered tension in the deep and superficial muscle systems and the myofascial slings (Fig. 4.43) can create malalignment and potentially contribute to loss of stability during single or multiple tasks. A muscle, or part of a muscle, may participate in more than one sling and the slings may overlap and interconnect depending on the task. The hypothesis is that the slings have no beginning or end but rather connect, and are recruited, to assist in the transference of forces. It is possible that the individual slings are part of one interconnected myofascial system with different tasks requiring the selective activation of parts of the whole sling or system. Dysfunction of specific muscles, or specific fascicles within one muscle, often creates non-optimal vectors of force and needs to be identified, and addressed, if restoration of all components of motion control (segmental, regional, and postural equilibrium) is to occur.

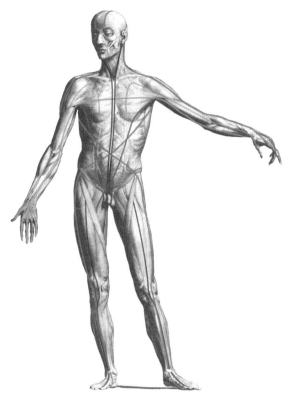

Fig. 4.40 • The 'Anatomy Trains' of myofascial slings according to Myers. Reproduced with permission from Myers and the publisher Churchill Livingstone, 2001.

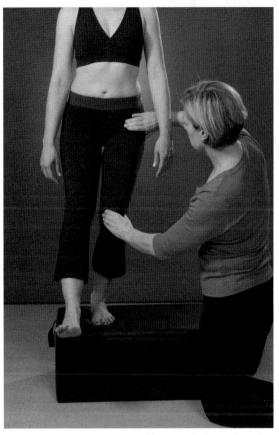

Fig. 4.41 • When the vectors of force are balanced, motion occurs effortlessly and alignment of the skeleton and stability of the joints are maintained.

Moving beyond stability – requirements for beautiful movement

It is evident that there is an increasingly broader view of optimal motor control for spinal stability. The best strategies for stabilization of the LPH complex, and the rest of the spine, will provide control of segmental motion and multisegmental alignment in both static and dynamic situations, while supporting movement, optimal respiration, continence, and control of postural equilibrium (balance). As highlighted above, *which* stability strategy is best to use depends on multiple factors related to the task characteristics and makeup of the individual. Increasing spinal stiffness is only one possible strategy for dynamic tasks; it is often not appropriate and indeed can be detrimental. This is consistent with the clinical observation that increasing spinal stiffness is not appropriate for patients who are already using strategies that make them too stiff. Furthermore, increased stiffness, in some situations, may impair the ability to 'maintain the desired trajectory' in a given task, and thus actually make the spine unstable.

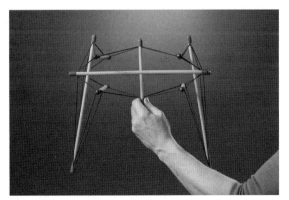

Fig. 4.42 • A tensegrity model of the pelvis (built by Tom Flemons of www.intensiondesigns.com) with balanced tension forces maintaining optimal alignment of the structure.

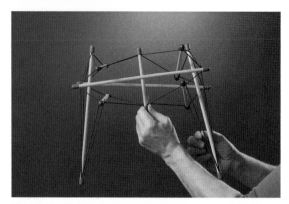

Fig. 4.43 • This is the same tensegrity model of the pelvis with an increased vector of force simulating the pull of rectus femoris. Note the change in alignment of the structure (pelvis).

Still an even broader perspective is one that considers the questions, 'If the spine is stable, does this guarantee optimal performance and function?' or, 'If the spine is stable, does it guarantee that the patient's goals are met in regards to outcomes for the desired task?' It would seem that many have made the assumption that yes, if the spine is stable then optimal function is guaranteed. However, stability is only one requirement for beautiful movement and optimal performance. Anyone who has watched the combination of grace, power, and beauty in the movements of elite athletes intuitively knows that stability is only one characteristic of a system that enables optimal function and performance. Reeves et al (2007), in their review article clarifying terms around spinal stability, note that

> once stability of a system is established, the interest shifts to its performance. Unless the system is stable, there is no reason to discuss its performance. All unstable systems perform poorly.
>
> Reeves et al 2007.

Of interest, Reeves et al (2007) also note that a common mistake is to assign a *level* of stability to a system; in other words, to say that one system is more stable than another.

> A system is either stable or it is not – there should be no index or level of stability ... it is more appropriate to say the system is more robust than more stable ... To discuss stability of a system, whether it is in equilibrium (static) or changing with time (dynamic), we must give a small perturbation and observe the new behavior. If the new behavior is approximately the same as the old, qualitatively speaking, the system is 'stable' ... if the disturbed behavior differs significantly from the old behavior, the system is unstable.

Note that this definition of stability is consistent with that of Hodges & Cholewicki (2007) discussed in the introduction of this chapter; that is, 'if the new behavior is approximately the same as the old' then the system has the ability to 'maintain the desired trajectory despite disturbances' (Hodges & Cholewicki 2007).

Reeves et al define robustness as

> how well [the system] can cope with uncertainties and disturbances [and state that] systems that can significantly change their parameters (i.e. stiffness) without loss of stability are also said to be robust.
>
> Reeves et al 2007.

Therefore, situations can arise where two patients use different strategies, but both strategies provide stability to the spine/pelvis during a specific task. So, in terms of stability, the strategies can be considered equivalent. However, the two strategies may differ in the level of robustness they provide, in that one patient may be able to cope with only a low level of uncertainty (e.g. walking on uneven terrain), whereas the other may be able to cope with greater degrees of uncertainty (e.g. walking on uneven terrain in the dark).

Therefore, evaluation of motor control involves consideration of multiple factors that are required to attain the goal of optimal movement, without injury and pain. Stability of the spine/pelvis is one necessary component. More robust systems are likely to be less susceptible to injury over a wider variety of tasks and contexts, and thus higher levels of robustness are more optimal, and thus more desirable. And ultimately, performance is related to how the spine/pelvis functions in relation to the rest of the body, *how well* the task is completed, and whether or not the outcome matches the patient's task-related goals. We want the whole body to *perform well*. According to Reeves et al (2007),

> performance reflects how closely and rapidly the disturbed position of the system tends to return to the undisturbed position. Accuracy and speed are two main attributes of any control system.

While this definition provides distinct, measurable entities to quantify 'performance,' we suggest that optimal performance is broader than these parameters. Optimal performance must include parameters that reflect quality of movement, which allow an observer to state that one performance looks 'better' than another, and yet both may be achieved with the same speed and accuracy. We can intuitively know that one motor control strategy has more 'flow' or 'ease' or 'grace,' or that it evokes a different emotion when we observe it, but science is not yet able to measure these qualitative aspects of optimal function and performance that allow us to call it 'beautiful movement.'

In summary, for every task, and specific to each individual, there exists an optimal strategy for function and performance (see Chapter 7, *The Integrated Systems Model for Disability and Pain* and *The Clinical Puzzle*, Fig. 7.11). This *strategy for function and performance* is a whole body strategy and reflects a strategy for stability of the LPH complex, as well as measurable parameters, such as speed, accuracy, and robustness, and subjectively determined qualities of movement. An optimal stability strategy is necessary for optimal performance, but does not guarantee it because optimal performance is also related to patient goals and qualitative features. Thus, if non-optimal strategies for stability of the LPH complex are present, these need to be addressed before focusing on parameters such as speed, agility, and endurance. Finally, the optimal strategy for function and performance of a given task will also minimize metabolic costs and thus maximize efficiency and synergy of all systems.

In the second part of this book, assessment tests, clinical reasoning, and movement training techniques are presented that together are aimed at evaluating current strategies for function and performance during specific tasks and understanding the relationship of this strategy to:

- stability of the LPH complex (functional control);
- underlying impairments;
- the pain experience and current problem.

A clinical reasoning process, based in the current science and integrated with clinical expertise, then provides the vehicle for designing treatment programs for the patient with LPH disability and/or pain that aims to facilitate and restore a more optimal strategy for performance of meaningful tasks and move the patient towards an experience of beautiful movement.

Emotional states

It is interesting to consider two people each performing the same task and both using strategies that ensure stability of the spine and pelvis with the same accuracy, speed, and level of robustness, but while in a different emotional state. Do different emotional states affect overall strategy for function and task performance? Studies suggest that emotional states do play a significant role in human function, and are often reflected in the musculoskeletal system (Hodges & Moseley 2003, Moseley & Hodges 2005). In addition to their functional complaints, many patients with pain present with symptoms similar to those seen in individuals who have experienced traumatic events. Negative emotional states such as fear, anxiety, and insecurity can express themselves in maladaptive defensive, or aggressive, postures that correlate with altered muscle activity and further strain on the musculoskeletal system.

Clinically, it appears that if an individual does not have the coping mechanisms necessary to confront their symptoms, they learn to avoid activities that result in pain (Vlaeyen & Linton 2000). This avoidance can persist due to their fear of re-injury or an underlying belief that they are unable to perform because of their condition (fear-avoidance). The muscles of the region can reflect this fear and can become hypertonic, thereby increasing force closure that subsequently results in sustained excessive compression of the LPH complex. This can perpetuate pain. Furthermore, emotional states can contribute to peripheral and/or central sensitization of the nervous system (Butler 2000, Butler & Moseley 2003, Moseley & Hodges 2005), which in turn can create substantial barriers to rehabilitation.

It is important to understand the patient's emotional state, and their belief systems, as affecting the emotional state is often the only way to change the resultant detrimental motor patterns. Sometimes, it can be as simple as restoring hope through education (Butler & Moseley 2003, Moseley 2003a,b, Moseley & Hodges 2005), awareness of the underlying mechanical problem, provision of a clear understandable diagnosis, and a logical course of action. Other times, professional cognitive behavioral therapy is required to retrain more positive thought patterns.

The integrated biomechanics of the lumbopelvic–hip complex

The primary function of the lower quadrant is to move and to simultaneously provide a stable base from which the upper extremity can function (transfer load). Together, the trunk and the lower extremities have the potential for multidirectional movement with a minimum of energy expenditure (Abitbol

1995, 1997, McNeill 1997). Neuromusculoskeletal harmony is essential for optimal function of the LPH complex. In 1911, Meisenbach stated that:

> When the trunk is moved to one side quickly there are direct opposing forces of the lumbar and spinal muscles against the pelvic and leg muscles. Normally these work in harmony and are resisted by the strong pelvic ligaments and fascia to a certain extent. If the harmony of these muscles is disturbed from some cause or another, or if the ligamentous support is weakened, other points of fixation must necessarily yield.

It is traditional to study both anatomy and biomechanics in a regional manner. For example, the lumbar spine is often considered separately from the pelvic girdle, which in turn is investigated separately from the hip. This approach yields information as to how the parts function, but not as to how the parts work together. Although it is necessary to consider the function of the individual parts, rehabilitation is often unsuccessful without consideration of how these parts achieve the harmonious action, as noted by Meisenbach almost a century ago. The regional biomechanics of the lumbar spine, pelvic girdle, and hip have been described under the relevant kinematics section/form closure, previously in this chapter. What follows now is a description of the integrated biomechanics of the LPH complex during the functional tasks that are commonly used in assessment (see Chapter 8).

Forward bending

Forward bending of the body results in posterior displacement of the pelvic girdle. This motion shifts the center of mass behind the pedal base such that slight plantarflexion of the talocrural joints occurs (Fig. 4.44). The pelvic girdle anteriorly tilts on the femoral heads about a transverse axis through the hip joints; the hip joints flex and the femoral heads remain centered in the acetabulum. The thoracic and lumbar spines flex and the sequence of flexion can be varied (cranial to caudal vs caudal to cranial). No lateral bending or rotation should occur in the thoracolumbar column during forward bending.

Within the pelvic girdle itself, there is no relative anterior or posterior rotation between the innominates during forward bending. Both innominates should travel an equal distance as the pelvic girdle anteriorly tilts on the femoral heads. During the initial stages of forward bending, the sacrum completely nutates between the innominates and should remain nutated throughout the full range of motion. On

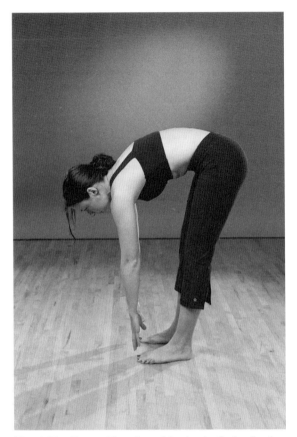

Fig. 4.44 • Forward bending of the body. Optimally, the apex of the forward bending curve should be in the mid-buttock. This model demonstrates a lack of anterior tilt of the pelvic girdle on the femoral heads due to insufficient lengthening of the hamstrings (note the flexion of her knees).

returning to standing, the sacrum remains nutated between the innominates until the erect posture is reached. At this point, the sacrum counter-nutates slightly (remaining relatively nutated) to become suspended once again between the two innominates. At no time during this task should the joints of the pelvis (SIJ or PS) unlock; the innominates should remain posteriorly rotated relative to the sacrum and the femoral heads should remain centered in the acetabula at all times.

The deep and superficial muscle systems work in synergy to allow the smooth transfer of loads through the bones and joints of the LPH complex. There should be no non-optimal translation, or giving way, of any joint in the kinetic chain, or lack of multisegmental motion; these findings reflect a non-optimal strategy for the task.

Backward bending

Backward bending of the body results in anterior displacement of the pelvic girdle. This motion shifts the center of mass anterior to the pedal base such that slight dorsiflexion of the talocrural joints occurs (Fig. 4.45). The pelvic girdle posteriorly tilts on the femoral heads about a transverse axis through the hip joints; the hip joints extend and the femoral heads remain centered in the acetabulum. The thoracic and lumbar spines extend and the sequence of extension can be varied (cranial to caudal vs caudal to cranial).

Within the pelvic girdle itself, there is no relative anterior or posterior rotation between the innominates during backward bending. Both innominates should travel an equal distance as the pelvic girdle posteriorly tilts on the femoral heads. The sacrum

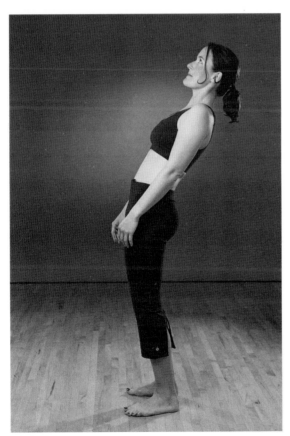

Fig. 4.45 • Backward bending of the body. The pelvic girdle should posteriorly tilt (hip joints extend) such that the apex of the backward bending curve is at the level of the iliofemoral ligament of the hip joint.

should remain nutated relative to the innominates. At no time during this task should the joints of the pelvis (SIJ or PS) unlock; the innominates should remain posteriorly rotated relative to the sacrum and the femoral heads should remain centered in the acetabula at all times.

The deep and superficial muscle systems work in synergy to allow the smooth transfer of loads through the bones and joints of the LPH complex. There should be no non-optimal translation, or giving way, of any joint in the kinetic chain, or lack of multisegmental motion; these findings reflect a non-optimal strategy for the task.

Lateral bending

Right lateral bending of the body is initiated by displacing the upper legs/pelvis to the left, thus maintaining the center of mass within the pedal base (Fig. 4.46). The apex of this lateral bending curve should be at the level of the greater trochanter. The pelvic girdle laterally tilts to the right such that the right femur abducts and the left femur adducts. A left intrapelvic torsion occurs such that the left innominate posteriorly rotates relative to the right innominate, and the sacrum rotates to the left. The lumbar spine laterally bends to the right and, although the lumbar segmental conjunct rotation is variable, a gentle, even curve should result with each segment contributing to the total range of motion. Clinically, L5 appears to rotate/sideflex congruently with the sacrum.

The deep and superficial muscle systems work in synergy to allow the smooth transfer of loads through the bones and joints of the LPH complex. There should be no non-optimal translation, or giving way, of any joint in the kinetic chain, or lack of multisegmental motion; these findings reflect a non-optimal strategy for the task.

Squat

During a functional squat, which is essential for moving from standing to sitting or sitting to standing, the body is lowered/raised in a controlled manner (Fig. 4.47). The hips and knees should flex, the ankles should dorsiflex, and the feet should pronate as the pelvic girdle anteriorly tilts on the femoral heads. The thoracopelvic orientation should not change as the body is lowered/raised, which requires forward movement of the trunk, relative to the base

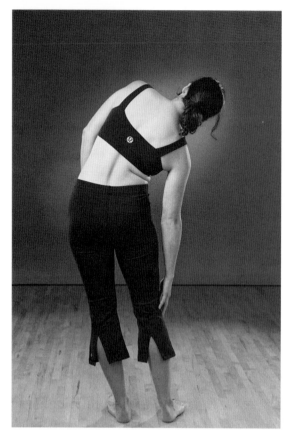

Fig. 4.46 • Lateral bending of the body. Optimally, the apex of the lateral bending curve should be at the level of the greater trochanter.

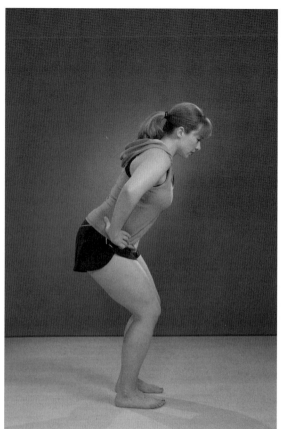

Fig. 4.47 • In a functional squat the manubriosternal junction remains aligned with the pubic symphysis and the mass of the body centered between the feet.

of support, as the hips and pelvis move posteriorly. The center of mass should remain centered over the pedal base of support. Each leg should remain vertically aligned over the center of each foot. The knee joint should not hinge into valgus or varus, or rotate non-physiologically, and the joints of the pelvis should not unlock. In addition, the lumbar spine should retain its neutral orientation and not hinge, or buckle, into segmental or multisegmental extension, flexion, lateral flexion/rotation, or lateral shift. These findings reflect a non-optimal strategy for this task.

Walking

Walking is an excellent example of the Integrated Model of Function in motion. When function is optimal, and one's mood is light and confident, walking is effortless and the individual glides through space with only minimal displacement of the center of gravity. This section will review the osteokinematics of the LPH complex during one cycle of gait. Walking requires motion, and therefore control, of the entire spine, pelvis, and lower extremities and, while the amplitude and pattern of regional motion are individual, an optimal strategy will result in the following kinematics (Gracovetsky 1997, Greenman 1997, Vleeming & Stoeckart 2007).

Femoral motion

During the swing phase of the right lower extremity (from toe-off to heel strike), the right femur moves from an extended to a flexed position. The femoral motion is not an arthrokinematic chordal spin (pure) at the hip joint, but rather an arcuate swing (impure), and therefore associated osteokinematic motions occur. At toe-off, the femur is extended and medially rotated relative to the innominate (the degree of abduction/adduction is variable), and some of the ligaments of the hip joint are taut. As the femur flexes and the pelvic girdle rotates to the left in the transverse plane, lateral rotation of the femur relative to the innominate occurs. The path of femoral motion should remain in the pure sagittal plane.

During the stance phase of the right lower extremity (from heel strike to toe-off), the right femur moves from a flexed to an extended position. Again, this motion is not a pure spin at the hip joint, but rather an arcuate, or impure, swing. The associated motion includes medial rotation although, as mentioned above, the medial femoral rotation is due to transverse plane rotation of the pelvic girdle to the right and therefore the path of femoral motion should remain in the pure sagittal plane. Adduction/abduction during this motion is variable. The ligaments are progressively wound around the femoral neck as the body weight passes anterior to the hip joint. Through the mid-stance position, the winding of the ligaments of the hip joint, together with the myofascial forces, increases compression of the femoral head into the acetabular fossa in a manner that distributes load equally across the articular surface of the femoral head. This increase in tension augments the form closure of the hip joint as the load transfer requirements increase. Adequate stride length requires optimal mobility of the hip joint, which requires a centered femoral head (displaced neither anteriorly nor posteriorly) during all motion. Effective load transfer requires synergistic action of the deep and superficial muscles of the entire LPH complex (optimal force closure and motor control).

Pelvic girdle motion

At right toe-off, the pelvic girdle is rotated in the transverse plane to the right. Through the right swing phase, the pelvic girdle rotates transversely to the left such that at right heel strike the pelvic girdle is rotated in the transverse plane to the left. At left toe-off, the pelvic girdle is rotated in the transverse plane to the left, and through the right stance phase it rotates transversely to the right. As the pelvis rotates to the left and right in the transverse plane, a small amount of alternating intrapelvic torsion occurs (IPTL, with transverse plane rotation to the left; IPTR, with transverse plane rotation to the right).

Lumbar motion

The lower lumbar vertebrae sideflex/rotate in alternate directions as the pelvis rotates in the transverse plane during gait. The direction of lumbar rotation is congruent with the direction of rotation of the pelvis.

When an optimal strategy is used for walking, the center of gravity should travel along a smooth sinusoidal curve both vertically and laterally and the displacement in both planes should be no more than 5cm (Inman et al 1981). This displacement is exaggerated when the walking strategy is non-optimal and there are multiple reasons for this.

Lifting

The forces necessary to support 27kg (59.5lb) during a squat lift can induce a compressive load on the spine of over 7000N (1568 lb) (McGill 2002). Therefore, optimal strategies for transferring load during lifting tasks are essential for injury prevention. Sudden, unexpected perturbations during lifting (trips, slips, poorly calculated load), as well as twisting while lifting, are known to be key mechanical circumstances related to low back injuries (Cholewicki & McGill 1996, Magnussen et al 1996). Similar to all other tasks, when the strategy used for lifting is optimal, the movement is smooth and appears effortless, all joints move congruently (no segmental or multisegmental hinges, kinks, or buckles, no unlocking of the pelvis, or loss of centering of the hip), and the intrathoracic/intra-abdominal pressures are appropriate to the loads such that the musculoskeletal system is controlled/protected, respiration is supported, and continence is preserved.

Summary

Like a well-trained orchestra, beautiful movement (music) requires optimal function of all the joints and muscles (instruments and musicians), the control of which is directed by the CNS (conductor), which plans the movements and activation of specific myofascial slings (comprised of both deep and superficial muscle systems) according to the needs of the intended task (score of music to be played). The CNS adjusts the individual muscle and joint responses (musicians and instruments) as the task progresses from moment to moment (play now, do not play, crescendo, diminuendo, fade). The 'adjustments' occur in response to the feedback the CNS receives from the body's multiple receptors relayed throughout the task (i.e. what does the resultant music sound like?). The CNS must also respond to

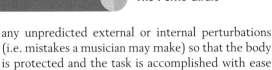

any unpredicted external or internal perturbations (i.e. mistakes a musician may make) so that the body is protected and the task is accomplished with ease (the music resonates as one sound).

While all of this may seem very complex, and indeed to understand how it all works is very complicated, for clinicians it comes down to analyzing the strategy the individual is using for any task being evaluated. The chosen strategy is either appropriate or not, the system is stable or it is not, performance goals are being met or not. The specific tests needed for determining whether or not a strategy is functional and/or optimal for the task being evaluated will be covered in Chapter 8 as well as the subsequent tests and clinical reasoning necessary to determine why the individual is using a non-optimal strategy (Chapter 9). However, before we can present the clinical aspects of this text, consideration needs to be given to what is known about pain and impairments of the LPH complex – on to Chapter 5!

The impaired lumbopelvic–hip complex

Diane Lee   Linda Joy-Lee

5

CHAPTER CONTENTS

Introduction 91
The lumbar spine – form closure deficits . . . 91
The pelvic girdle – form closure deficits 98
The hip/groin – form closure deficits 99
Summary 100
Pain, force closure, motor control, and the
lumbopelvic–hip complex 100
Some common clinical presentations –
lumbar spine 104
Some common clinical presentations –
pelvic girdle 114
Some common clinical presentations –
the hip 121
Emotional states 127
Summary 128

Introduction

The primary function of the lumbopelvic–hip (LPH) complex is to transfer loads safely while addressing the movement requirements of any task in a way that ensures the musculoskeletal components are not injured (either in the short or long term) and the organs are supported/protected. Chapter 4 outlined what is known about the functional LPH complex using the framework of the Integrated Model of Function (Lee & Vleeming 1998, 2004, 2007). This chapter will highlight what is known about the impaired LPH complex, the one that fails to transfer loads effectively and ultimately leads to disability, pain, organ prolapse, or incontinence. Some common clinical features of impairments of the lumbar spine,

pelvic girdle, and hip will be described. Note that, in clinical practice, it is most common to find combinations of impairments in all three regions (lumbar spine, pelvic girdle, and hip). However, in order to determine which impairments are:

1. related to the patient's pain experience;
2. related to compensatory adaptations; and which impairments are
3. the underlying drivers of the key problems;

it is necessary to understand the key patterns and features of common impairments for each region separately. This base understanding of 'clinical patterns' facilitates further understanding of how the regions relate/integrate, and how to perform more complex clinical reasoning (covered in the second part of this text).

The lumbar spine – form closure deficits

While systemic diseases, such as

- genomic spine disorder;
- vertebral osteochondritis or Scheurmann's disease; and
- infection;

as well as metabolic conditions, such as

- osteopenia;
- rheumatoid arthritis;
- ankylosing spondylitis;
- Paget's disease; and
- diffuse idiopathic skeletal hyperostosis (DISH);

are known to cause structural changes in the lumbar spine (Box 5.1), the most common cause of structural changes in the passive system of the lumbar spine occurs secondary to sudden macrotrauma (Taylor et al 1990, Twomey et al 1989) or minor repetitive trauma over time (Farfan 1973, 1978, Kirkaldy-Willis et al 1978, Kirkaldy-Willis & Hill 1979, Kirkaldy-Willis 1983, Taylor & Twomey 1986) (Fig. 5.1). The repetitive use of non-optimal strategies for transferring loads through the LPH complex often creates uneven load sharing and eventually tissue breakdown and pain.

As a reminder from Chapter 4, optimal strategies (see Fig. 4.35):

1. control both angular and translatoric motions of the joints while allowing the necessary mobility required for the task;

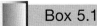

Box 5.1

Pathological soft tissue and bony disorders of the lumbar spine (MacNab 1977)

These are non-mechanical potential sources of peripherally mediated pain arising from the lumbar spine. A multidisciplinary approach including medical management is required for these disorders.

Scheuermann's disease – vertebral osteochondritis.

Infective – pyogenic vertebral osteomyelitis.

Systemic inflammatory – rheumatoid arthritis, ankylosing spondylitis.

Metabolic – osteoporosis, Paget's disease, tuberculosis, Calve's disease, diffuse idiopathic skeletal hyperostosis (DISH).

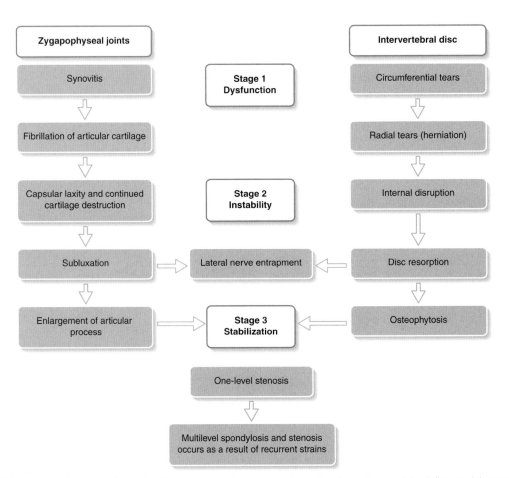

Fig. 5.1 • The spectrum of pathoanatomical changes in the zygapophyseal joints and intervertebral disc, and the potential consequences of these changes on function according to Kirkaldy-Willis (1983).

2. control spinal posture/orientation within and between the regions;

3. maintain postural equilibrium; and

4. simultaneously support respiration and continence in potentially changing environments during multiple predictable and unpredictable tasks of varying loads and risk.

In the lumbar spine, non-optimal strategies fail to control angular and translatoric motion (see Fig. 4.13) and have been classified by O'Sullivan (2000, 2005) as either movement or motion control impairments. According to O'Sullivan, both of the subjects in Figure 4.13 would be classified as motion control impairments as that translation is poorly controlled at L4–5 during forward bending (Fig. 4.13A) and backward bending (Fig. 4.13B). However, it is not uncommon to find both movement and motion control impairments in the same lumbar spine in the same patient (Fig. 5.2A,B). It is even more common to find an impairment in movement in one part of the LPH complex and in control in another (Fig. 5.2C, Video 5.1).

Non-optimal strategies for transferring load often create excessive stress on the joints of the LPH complex and, over time, can lead to structural changes, particularly in the lumbar spine. These changes are often attributed to age (Kirkaldy-Willis & Hill 1979, Kirkaldy-Willis 1983, Taylor & Twomey 1986, 1992) and Bogduk (1997) suggests they are 'natural consequences of the stresses applied to the spine throughout life.' According to Kirkaldy-Willis (1983), structural changes occur secondary to events that result in:

1. synovitis of the posterior zygapophyseal joints (Grade 1–2 sprain);

2. minor circumferential tears of the outer layers of the annulus and the associated anterior and posterior longitudinal ligaments (Fig. 5.3A,B);

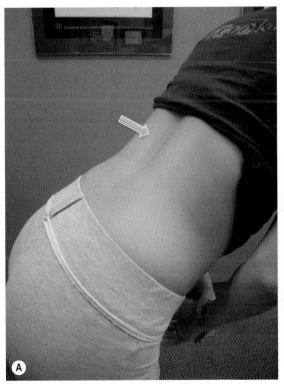
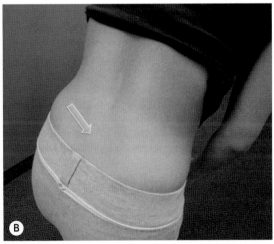

Fig. 5.2 • Movement and motion control impairments. (A) The forward bending strategy of a young woman (18 years) with persistent low back pain. Note how restricted flexion is in the thoracic and upper lumbar spine. She struggled to relax/release the erector spine (arrow) during forward bending and this was the most flexion she could actively achieve as she bent forward. (B) In addition, note that L5–S1 is fully flexed; all of her flexion motion in the lumbar spine was occurring at this segment. L5–S1 provocation tests reproduced her pain. This young woman has both a motion control impairment at L5–S1 and a movement impairment from approximately T6 to L5.

Continued

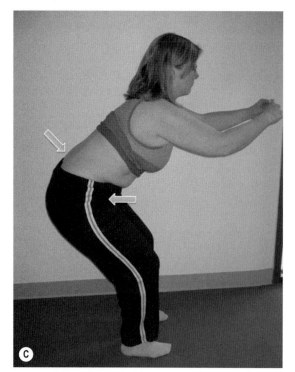

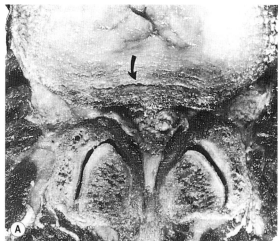

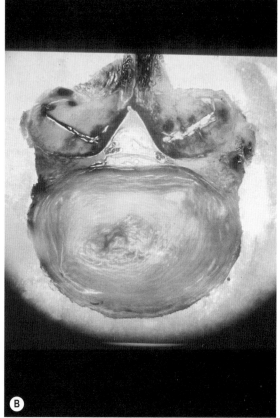

Fig. 5.2 — cont'd • (C) In the squat task, this woman has a movement impairment of her hips (they are not flexing enough for this task) and a motion control impairment at L4–5. She excessively flexes her lumbar spine and L4–5 hinges excessively into flexion and posterior translation.

3. tears of the capsule and ligamentum flavum (Fig. 5.4A,B) as well as subchondral fractures of the superior articular process in more severe injuries (Fig. 5.5). These injuries are not always evident on X-ray (Taylor et al 1990).

These changes are consistent with stage 1 dysfunction (see Fig. 5.1) according to Kirkaldy-Willis (1983). Continued use of non-optimal strategies, combined with intermittent acute (recurrent) flare-ups of back pain, can result in progressive pathoanatomical changes ultimately leading to significant form closure deficits and potentially segmental instability (Fig. 5.6) (Bogduk 1997, Kirkaldy-Willis et al 1978, Kirkaldy-Willis & Hill 1979, Kirkaldy-Willis 1983, Panjabi 1992a,b, Taylor & Twomey 1986, Taylor et al 1990, Twomey et al 1989). Note that in the Kirkaldy-Willis model, 'instability' is defined as the loss of passive system integrity with an increased neutral zone; see Chapter 4 for a discussion of different

Fig. 5.3 • Pathoanatomical changes in the lumbar joints thought to occur during stage 1 dysfunction (Kirkaldy-Willis 1983). (A) Transverse circumferential tears in the annulus fibrosus (arrow). (B) Circumferential tears in the annulus as well as moderate degeneration of the zygapophyseal joints. Dr. Twomey gave this beautiful dissection to Diane after both were keynote speakers in Hong Kong in 1992. The dissection comes from the 1980s research published by Drs Taylor and Twomey while investigating age-related changes in the lumbar spine and is reproduced with permission.

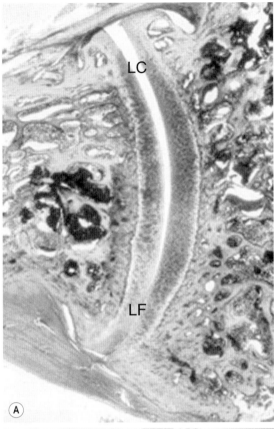

LC

LF

(A)

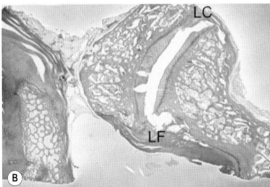

LC

LF

(B)

Fig. 5.4 • Pathoanatomical changes in the lumbar joints thought to occur during stage 1 dysfunction (Kirkaldy-Willis 1983). (A) A healthy zygapophyseal joint courtesy of Drs Twomey & Taylor. Note the smooth, intact articular cartilage and the integrity of the lateral capsule (LC) and the ligamentum flavum (LF) (B) An unhealthy zygaphophyseal joint. Note the difference in the articular cartilage and the tears within the lateral capsule and detachment of the ligamentum flavum. This figure is courtesy of Drs Twomey & Taylor and is reproduced with permission.

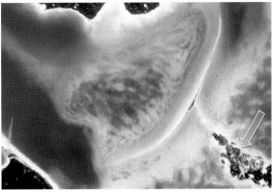

Fig. 5.5 • An unsuspected fracture (not evident on X-ray) of the superior articular process (arrow) in an otherwise healthy zygapophyseal joint in an individual who died in a motor vehicle accident. This figure is courtesy of Drs Taylor and Twomey and is reproduced with permission.

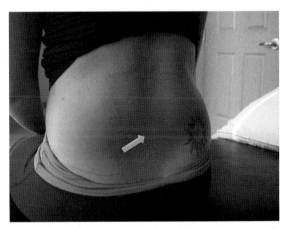

Fig. 5.6 • Note the posterior translation and segmental flexion at L5–S1.

definitions of 'stability' and 'instability.' The progressive pathoanatomical changes include (Fig. 5.7A–D):

1. fibrillation and subsequent loss of the articular cartilage of the zygapophyseal joint(s);

2. laxity of the articular capsule(s) and attenuation of the segmental ligaments;

3. fracture of the articular process with resultant strain deformation of the neural arch;

4. coalescence of the circumferential annular tears into a radial fissure with/without subsequent herniation of the nucleus pulposus, ultimately progressing to marked internal disruption of the disc, loss of disc height, circumferential bulging, and resorption; and/or

5. sclerosis of the adjacent vertebral bodies.

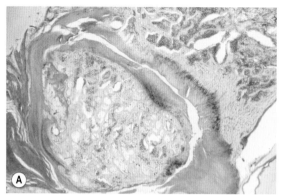

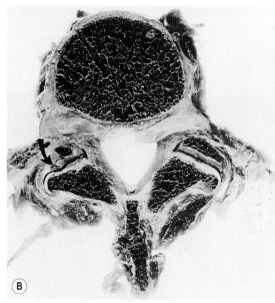

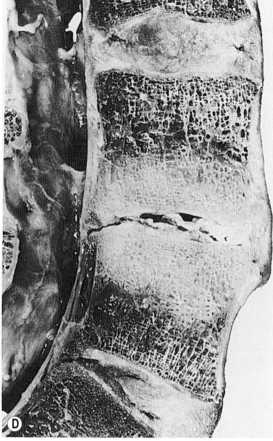

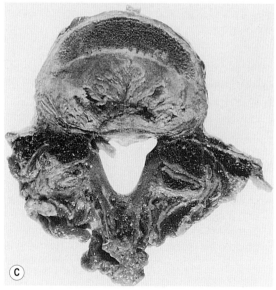

Fig. 5.7 • Pathoanatomical changes in the lumbar joints thought to occur during stage 2 instability (Kirkaldy-Willis 1983). (A) Note the progressive degeneration of the articular cartilage and further loss of integrity of the articular capsule and ligamentum flavum (form closure deficits). This figure is courtesy of Drs Taylor and Twomey and is reproduced with permission. (B) Macroscopic transverse section of the L5–S1 segment. Note the marked degeneration of the left zygapophyseal joint (arrow). Reproduced with permission from Kirkaldy-Willis and the publisher Churchill Livingstone, 1983. (C) Macroscopic transverse section of the L4–L5 segment. Note the coalescence of several radial fissures and the early stages of internal disruption. Reproduced with permission from Kirkaldy-Willis and the publisher Churchill Livingstone, 1983. (D) Macroscopic sagittal section of the lumbar spine. Note the sclerosis of the vertebral bodies above and below the central intervertebral disc, which is markedly resorbed. Reproduced with permission from Kirkaldy-Willis et al and the publisher Spine, 1978.

Collectively, these anatomical changes allow the superior articular process of the inferior vertebra to sublux upwards and forwards during axial rotation of the trunk (Fig. 5.8). This motion consequently narrows the lateral recess, potentially affecting the function of the structures within the intervertebral foramen (Butler 2000, Shacklock 2005, Sunderland 1978).

The posterior zygapophyseal joints can enlarge to develop osteophytes, the intervertebral disc can become fibrotic, and traction spurs may develop on the anterior and/or posterior aspect of the vertebral body, occasionally leading to spontaneous fusion (Fig. 5.9A,B). According to Kirkaldy-Willis (1983), these changes occur during the third stage of the degenerative process (stabilization) (see Fig. 5.1),

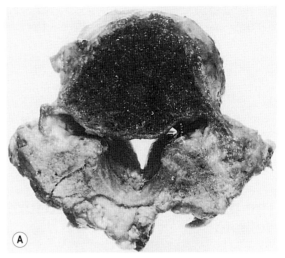

(A)

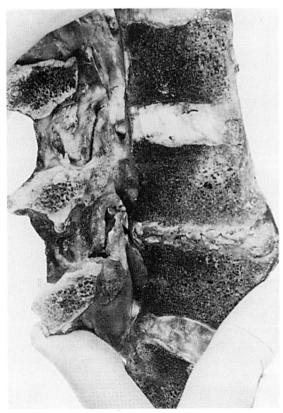

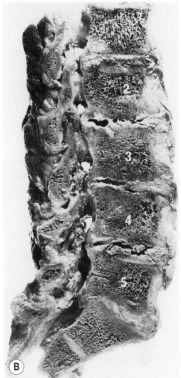

(B)

Fig. 5.8 • Dynamic stenosis of the lateral recess of the lumbosacral junction associated with instability. In this specimen the spinous process of the L5 vertebra has been rotated towards the observer. The zygapophyseal joint has opened (arrow), and the superior articular process has approximated the posterior aspect of the intervertebral disc, subsequently narrowing the lateral recess. Reproduced with permission from Reilly et al and the publisher J B Lippincott, 1978.

Fig. 5.9 • Pathoanatomical changes in the lumbar joints thought to occur during stage 3 stabilization (Kirkaldy-Willis 1983). (A) Macroscopic transverse section of the L5–S1 segment illustrating fixed central and lateral stenosis. The central and lateral canals are markedly narrowed by osteophytosis. Reproduced with permission from Kirkaldy-Willis and the publisher Churchill Livingstone, 1983. (B) Macroscopic sagittal section of the lumbar spine illustrating multilevel spinal stenosis. Reproduced with permission from Kirkaldy-Willis and the publisher Churchill Livingstone, 1983.

and the patient is now often painfree, hypomobile, and no longer unstable. The risk at this stage is the development of fixed central and/or lateral recess stenosis due to osseous trespass on the spinal canal and/or lateral recess with attendant peripheral symptoms of neurogenic vascular claudication. Note that, although the affected segments may no longer be a source of peripheral nociception, the biomechanical effects of these pathoanatomical changes usually create altered stresses on other regions in the kinetic chain and therefore can be a cause of new sources of pain.

The pelvic girdle – form closure deficits

There are also a number of systemic, inflammatory, infective, and metabolic conditions known to cause structural changes in the joints of the pelvic girdle. The majority of these are listed in Table 5.1 and the reader is referred to Bellamy et al (1983) and Gamble et al (1986) for further description of each. Figure 8.97A–D illustrates the structural changes of the sacroiliac joint (SIJ) seen via computed tomography (CT) in patients with Reiter's disease and ankylosing spondylitis.

At the turn of this century, practitioners believed that the SIJ was the major source of sciatica, admitting that, as well as sciatica, 'lumbago [and] backache . . . were frequently caused by an abnormal amount of motion in the pelvic joints, especially the sacroiliac synchondrosis' (Meisenbach 1911). Aside from trauma, non-optimal postural strategies were recognized as being integral to the etiology of dysfunction.

> The etiology of the pelvic girdle dysfunction is not always clear, but there are many features of definite importance. At times, the lesion apparently represents simply an excess of a normal physiological process. At other times, trauma is a definite factor, 'sitting down hard,' or the 'giving way' under severe strains, such as lifting, being the two most common forms of injury. Attitudes or postures are also of importance in causing or predisposing to joint weakness or displacement.
>
> Goldthwait & Osgood 1905.

Structural changes in both the SIJ and the pubic symphysis (PS) have been noted to occur with age and are described in Chapter 3. Kampen & Tillman (1998) note that the morphological changes associated with aging are more pronounced in the articular cartilage lining the ilium, whereas the articular cartilage lining the sacrum often remains unaltered

Table 5.1 Non-mechanical potential sources of peripherally mediated pain arising from the sacroiliac joint (Bellamy et al 1983) and pubic symphysis (Gamble et al 1986). A multidisciplinary approach including medical management is required for these disorders

Sacroiliac joint	Pubic symphysis
Inflammatory disorders	**Congenital anomalies**
Ankylosing spondylitis	Exstrophy of the bladder
Reiter's syndrome	Cleidocranial dysostosis
Inflammatory bowel disease	Dyggve–Melchior–Clausen
Psoriatic spondylitis	syndrome
Rheumatoid arthritis	
Juvenile rheumatoid arthritis	
Pustulotic arthro-osteitis	
Familial Mediterranean fever	
Behçet's syndrome	
Relapsing polychondritis	
Whipple's disease	
Joint infection	**Joint infection**
Pyogenic	Pyogenic
Brucellosis	Tuberculosis
Tuberculosis	Pseudomonas
Metabolic disorders	**Inflammatory disorders**
Gout	'Osteitis pubis'
Calcium pyrophosphate deposition disease	Ankylosing spondylitis
Hyperparathyroidism	Reiter's syndrome
Miscellaneous	**Metabolic disorders**
Osteitis condensans ilii	Renal osteodystrophy
Paget's disease	Hyperparathyroidism
Acro-osteolysis in polyvinyl chloride workers	Chondrocalcinosis
Alkaptonuria	Hemochromatosis
Gaucher's disease	Ochronosis
Tuberous sclerosis	

until old age. The sacral subchondral bone plate is usually thin, whereas the subchondral bone plate of the ilium is thick. Recently, single photon emission computed tomography combined with CT (SPECT-CT) have shown sclerotic changes on both the sacral and iliac surfaces (Figs 5.10, 5.11) in individuals without active systemic disease. These changes are thought to be secondary to repetitive shear forces

Fig. 5.10 • Single photon emission computed tomography combined with CT (SPECT-CT) showing sclerosis secondary to loss of motion control of the sacroiliac joint (SIJ). This is a 34-year-old woman with left lower back pain worsening after delivery of her first child. This SPECT-CT scan shows increased uptake in upper left SIJ and sclerosis of the joint as indicated by the arrowheads. These images are provided courtesy of Dr. M. Cusi and Dr. H. Van der Wall, Sydney, Australia.

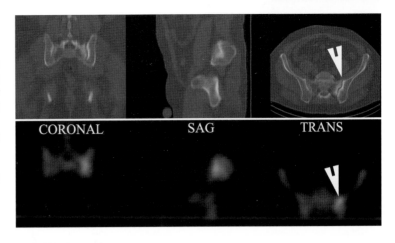

Fig. 5.11 • Single photon emission computed tomography combined with CT (SPECT-CT) showing sclerosis secondary to loss of motion control of the sacroiliac joint (SIJ). This is a 42-year-old man involved in a motor vehicle accident who has a 2-year history of increased right lower back pain. Imaging findings are of increased uptake and sclerosis of the SIJ as indicated by the arrowheads. These images are provided courtesy of Dr. M. Cusi and Dr. H. Van der Wall, Sydney, Australia.

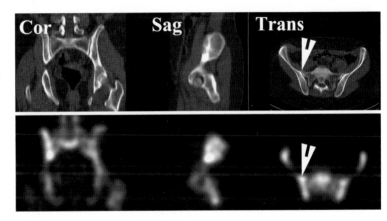

caused by the use of non-optimal strategies for load transfer (based on clinical examination). Similar changes have been noted at the PS, again in individuals with non-optimal strategies for transferring loads and no other disease. Osteitis pubis (pubalgia or athletic pubalgia) used to be considered a 'disease' (note its inclusion in Table 5.1) and is now thought to be the result of 'chronic overload or impaction trauma' (Gilmore 1998, Kunduracioglu et al 2007, Verrall et al 2001), secondary to repetitive jumping, twisting, or turning motions during sprinting, cutting, and kicking tasks. This chronic overload is thought to be due to an imbalance between the abdominal and adductor muscles (Robinson et al 2004, Rodriguez et al 2001). The irregularities of the bony margins of the PS and sclerosis of the pubic ramus are evident via magnetic resonance imaging (MRI) and SPECT-CT.

Structural changes in the joints of the pelvis also occur subsequent to massive trauma that results in fracture or fracture/dislocation of the joint.

Diastases, straddle fractures, intra-articular fractures, and overlapping dislocations of the PS are often associated with ruptured sacroiliac ligaments and/or iliac and sacral fractures (Gamble et al 1986). These massive injuries are often also associated with trauma to the internal pelvic structures and surgical intervention is frequently required.

The hip/groin – form closure deficits

The hip joint can also be afflicted with systemic, inflammatory, infective, and metabolic disorders (Box 5.2, Fig. 5.12). Of a more mechanic nature, tears of the acetabular labrum are increasingly recognized as a source of hip pain and dysfunction (Hunt et al 2007, Torry et al 2006) and are thought to occur with repetitive pivoting motions on the weight

Non-mechanical potential sources of peripherally mediated pain arising from the hip joint (Adams 1973, Cyriax 1954, Shindle et al 2006). A multidisciplinary approach including medical management is required for these disorders

Congenital dislocation of the hip
Perthes' disease
Tuberculosis
Transitory arthritis
Slipped femoral epiphysis
Osteochondritis dissecans
Ankylosing spondylitis
Pyogenic arthritis
Rheumatoid arthritis
Tuberculous arthritis
Osteoarthritis
Ankylosing spondylitis
Paget's disease
Psoriatic arthritis
Septic arthritis
Osteomyelitis
Metastatic bone disease

bearing femur. Dysplasias of the hip and femoroacetabular impingement (both cam and pincher type (Kassarjian et al 2007)) are thought to contribute to acetabular labral tears and osteoarthritis (Ganz et al 2003, McCarthy et al 2003, Tanzer & Noiseux 2004, Tonnis & Heinecke 1999). Some researchers believe that labral 'fraying' or tearing represents the natural history of the aging hip joint as these abnormalities are found in asymptomatic subjects, with the incidence increasing with age (Abe et al 2000).

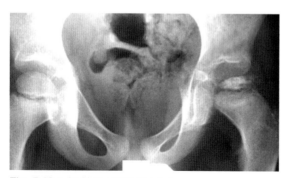

Fig. 5.12 • An X-ray of Perthes' disease.

Chondral tears and capsular injuries of the hip can occur with seemingly minimal trauma (Shindle et al 2006). In addition, 'atraumatic instability of the hip' has been reported as a common complaint in athletes who participate in sports involving repetitive hip rotation with loading (Shindle et al 2006). Although sports such as soccer, hockey, golf, and ballet have been associated with injuries to the passive structures of the hip (Mason 2001, McCarthy et al 2003), most have been reported to be insidious in onset without a specific traumatic event, suggesting that non-optimal strategies for transferring loads through the hip may be a key factor.

Summary

It is evident from this brief literature review that structural changes occur in the joints of the LPH complex over a lifetime, some as a consequence of major trauma and most (more likely, although there is little science yet to support this) as a consequence of non-optimal strategies for transferring loads through the region. As a clinician, it is easy to gain the impression that structural changes in the LPH complex are always accompanied by symptoms; however, it is known that the incidence of spondylosis and osteoarthrosis is just as great in patients with symptoms as in patients without symptoms (Bogduk 1997, Lawrence et al 1966, Magora & Schwartz 1976, Torgerson & Dotter 1976). In addition, it is common for the joints or regions adjacent to the painless one with the structural change to become symptomatic. Regardless of which joint or region is producing pain, it is known that pain can have an impact on the function of the LPH complex.

Pain, force closure, motor control, and the lumbopelvic–hip complex

Several studies have investigated the responses of the deep and superficial muscle systems of the trunk and some of the muscles of the lower extremity during a variety of tasks in subjects with low back, pelvic girdle, and/or groin pain (Cowan et al 2004, Hodges 1996–2009, Hungerford et al 2003, Kaigle et al 1998, O'Sullivan et al 2002, Radebold et al 2000, 2001, van Dieen et al 2003a,b) and urinary incontinence (Chapter 6). There are two excellent chapters that review a lot of this research evidence:

1. Hodges & Cholewicki (2007), chapter 33, Functional control of the spine. In: Vleeming et al (eds) Movement, Stability & Lumbopelvic Pain; and

2. Hodges et al (2009), chapter 11, Lumbar spine: treatment of instability and disorders of movement control. In: Magee et al (eds), Pathology and Intervention in Musculoskeletal Rehabilitation.

They are highly recommended chapters for further reading on the research evidence. A summary of this extensive body of evidence follows.

From the evidence, it is known that the changes in motor control that occur with actual, perceived, and/or experimentally induced lumbopelvic pain are multiple and highly variable. In other words, subjects with pain in similar regions are not homogeneous; their control system (CNS) responds differently to pain (including current pain, past history of pain, and experimentally induced pain). This is highly consistent with what is observed in clinical practice. In research experiments and clinical practice, subjects/patients with low back, pelvic girdle, and/or groin pain of a similar distribution may present with neuromuscular patterns that have increased activation of:

1. both the flexors and extensors of the trunk (co-contraction bracing or trunk-gripping);

2. the flexors of the trunk only (chest-gripping);

3. the extensors of the trunk (back-gripping);

4. the deep and superficial muscles of the hip in a variety of patterns (butt-gripping, hip-gripping); and/or

5. asymmetrical combinations of the above (1–4).

van Dieen (2007) notes that it is not possible to predict the actual neuromuscular consequence of musculoskeletal disorders. The starting point of his 'theory of contingent adaptation' is the 'indeterminacy of behavioral responses to pathology.'

> This framework is based on the recognition that the musculoskeletal system is highly redundant, implying that each motor task can be performed in many ways, and that motor control is constrained by weighted and potentially conflicting criteria, such as achieving the task goal, while avoiding excessive energy consumption. Weights of constraints are contingent upon environmental circumstances, task requirements and changes in the musculoskeletal system, as well as psychological factors such as motivation and attention.
>
> van Dieen 2007.

Simply put, the research evidence suggests that 'there is no consistent adaptation of muscle control during pain' (Hodges & Cholewicki 2007). Both of these statements concur with what is observed in clinical practice.

There are, however, some common features among subjects with low back/pelvic girdle and/or groin pain. Several studies investigating the response of the deep and superficial muscle systems in subjects with lumbopelvic pain during a variety of tasks report increased activation of the superficial trunk muscles compared to patients without pain, either in terms of earlier recruitment or increased amplitude of activity, including:

1. co-contraction of flexor and extensor trunk muscles with sudden unloading of the trunk compared to alternate activity between flexors and extensors in healthy controls (Radebold et al 2000). In the data presented by Radebold et al, activity was increased in at least one superficial trunk muscle; however, the specific muscle varied between individuals, and there was greater variability in their individual muscle reaction times (an indeterminate response);

2. increased activity of the erector spinae (ES) muscles during gait (Arendt-Nielsen et al 1996) and during a sit-up (Soderberg & Barr 1983);

3. increased activation of the external oblique during an active straight leg raise (ASLR) task (de Groot et al 2008);

4. failure of the superficial back muscles (ES) to relax during trunk flexion (Kaigle et al 1998);

5. increased internal oblique (IO), external oblique (EO), and rectus abdominis (RA) activity during gait (Saunders 2004b) and earlier onset of biceps femoris in the swing phase of gait (Vogt et al 2003).

Other studies investigating the timing and activity of the deep and superficial muscle systems report a variety of non-optimal responses including:

1. delayed activity of transversus abdominis (TrA) during rapid arm and leg movements in subjects with low back pain (Hodges 2001, Hodges & Richardson 1996, 1997), delayed or reduced activity of TrA with experimentally induced lumbar pain (Hodges et al 2003b), and delayed TrA activity during a supine ASLR task in subjects with groin pain (Cowan et al 2004);

2. delayed activation of deep fibers of multifidus (dMF) during rapid arm movements in subjects

with recurrent unilateral low back pain but no pain at time of testing (MacDonald et al 2009);

3. loss of differential activation of deep and superficial fibers of multifidus during rapid arm movements in subjects with recurrent unilateral low back pain (painfree at time of testing) (MacDonald et al 2009);

4. loss of tonic activity of TrA during gait (activity was phasic) (Saunders 2004b);

5. delayed activation of TrA/IO and dMF during a single leg loading task in subjects with pelvic girdle pain (Hungerford et al 2003);

6. early onset of biceps femoris and delayed onset of gluteus maximus during a single leg loading task in subjects with pelvic girdle pain (Hungerford et al 2003); and

7. inhibition of multifidus after the zygapophyseal joint is injected with lidocaine (Indahl et al 1995) or saline (Indahl et al 1997).

The structure of the lumbar multifidus (active system changes) has been investigated in subjects with both acute and chronic low back pain and the following findings are consistently noted. There is evidence of:

1. decreased cross-sectional area in segmental multifidus immediately after an acute low back injury (Hides et al 1994) that does not spontaneously resolve (Hides et al 1996);

2. decreased cross-sectional area in segmental multifidus in subjects with chronic low back pain (Danneels et al 2000);

3. rapid atrophy of multifidus after an experimental injury to either the intervertebral disc and/or nerve root (in pigs) (Hodges et al 2006); and

4. fatty infiltration (Kang et al 2007, Kjaer et al 2007) of the multifidus.

Changes have also been noted in the cross-sectional area of psoas in subjects with unilateral sciatica caused by herniation of the intervertebral disc (Dangaria & Naesh 1998).

In summary, in subjects/patients with low back/pelvic girdle and/or groin pain, it is common to find alterations in neuromuscular behavior, which ultimately impact the force closure mechanism during a number of different tasks. In general, it seems the deep muscles are affected in a more consistent way than the superficial muscles. Taken together, alterations in CNS control of the trunk muscles, along with structural changes in the muscles, likely

lead to the changes that have been noted in the articular biomechanics during functional tasks such as:

1. altered segmental kinematics of the lumbar spine (some joints do not move, others are poorly controlled) (Kaigle et al 1998, O'Sullivan 2000, 2005);

2. altered intrapelvic kinematics associated with the loss of the self-bracing or self-locking mechanism (anterior rotation of the innominate during increased loading tasks) (Hungerford et al 2004); and

3. altered hip joint kinematics, such as the loss of centering of the femoral head and unequal distribution of loads across the articular surface (Lee & Lee 2004a, Sahrmann 2001, Torry et al 2006).

Theories abound as to why these neuromuscular and structural changes occur; it has been suggested that the CNS responds/adapts to pain by increasing spinal stiffness through co-contraction bracing of the trunk muscles to prevent movements that provoke pain and to increase stability. Others suggest that the non-optimal neuromuscular patterns are pre-existing and the cause of pain. In patients with recurrent problems, it is likely a combination of reasons. What is evident from both the science and the clinic is that the healthy individual has a wide spectrum of optimal strategies to choose from for multiple tasks (Chapter 4) and can use his/her muscle system in a variety of ways. In subjects with low back pain, the spectrum becomes reduced to predominately one strategy that is used for all tasks. Performing all tasks with the same strategy (trunk-grip, chest-grip, back-grip, butt-grip, etc.) will eventually overload the passive and active system structures that are then consistently and repetitively stressed (Fig. 5.13A–C), which could be a factor in the cause of recurrent LPH pain. Note that non-optimal strategies may themselves be a cause of pain without causing significant pathoanatomical changes.

Panjabi (2006) proposed that co-contraction bracing occurred to compensate for osseoligamentous deficits in the spine (impairments of form closure); however, studies have shown that the same types of neuromuscular response are noted in subjects with no osseoligamentous deficits when pain was experimentally induced (Hodges et al 2003b) and in subjects who perceived a risk of pain (Moseley & Hodges 2005). Hodges et al (2009) present several possible factors to explain the relationship between

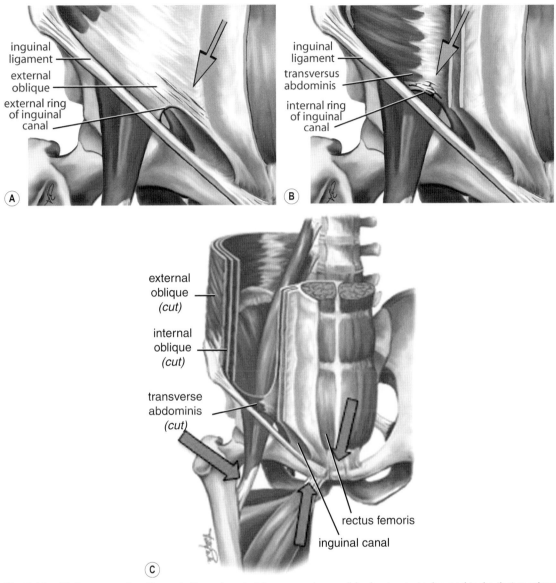

inguinal
ligament

external
oblique

external ring
of inguinal
canal

A

inguinal
ligament

transversus
abdominis

internal ring
of inguinal
canal

B

external
oblique
(cut)

internal
oblique
(cut)

transverse
abdominis
(cut)

rectus femoris

inguinal canal

C

Fig. 5.13 • (A) Common site of tears in the external oblique muscle possibly due to strategies and tasks that overload the tissue. (B) Common site of tears in transversus abdominis possibly due to strategies and tasks that overload the tissue. (C) Common sites of tendinopathy in the 'groin triangle,' again possibly due to strategies and tasks that overload the tissue. Falvey et al (2009) and Brukner & Khan (2007) provide excellent reviews of potential causes of pathoanatomical changes in the 'groin triangle' and the reader is referred to them for further discussion. Reproduced with permission from Brukner & Khan and the publisher McGraw Hill, 2007.

impaired activity of the deep system and increased activity of the superficial system (Fig. 5.14). As noted above, this is an excellent review chapter of the evidence pertaining to motor control and the functional and impaired lumbopelvis.

It is common to see alterations in motor control creating non-optimal strategies for transferring loads through the lumbopelvis. Over time, the repetitive use of poor strategies likely leads to structural changes in the passive system (form closure deficits)

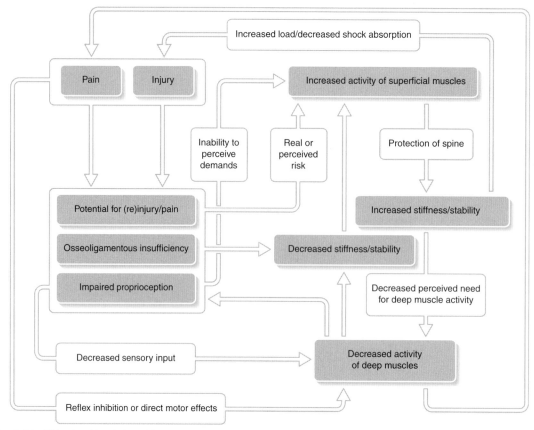

Fig. 5.14 • This algorithm is from Hodges et al (2009) and presents the possible factors that may explain the relationship between impaired activity of the deep muscles and increased activity of the superficial muscles. Pain and injury may lead to opposite changes in the deep and superficial muscles. Redrawn and reproduced with permission from Hodges et al and the publisher Saunders Elsevier, 2009.

and the active system. The non-resolved question is: which came first, the non-optimal strategy and poor load sharing, or an acute traumatic event that produced pain and subsequently altered the neuromuscular strategy? After 30 years of clinical experience, it appears that the answer is both – it takes a chicken and an egg to keep the cycle going!

Some common clinical presentations – lumbar spine

What follows is a brief description of common clinical presentations of patients presenting in a variety of stages of structural change according to the classification schema of Kirkaldy-Willis (1983). Recall that in the Kirkaldy-Willis schema 'instability' is defined as the loss of integrity of the passive system (form

closure mechanism) and does not relate to dynamic stability as discussed in Chapter 4. The clinical presentations in this chapter are hypothetical and based on clinical experience derived from multiple patients. The focus in this chapter is on the mechanical component of the clinical presentation. In reality, all patients present with sensorial (derived in part from mechanical impairments), cognitive, and emotional dimensions that collectively create a unique experience and affect the overall presentation. Pain mechanisms and other features of the clinical presentation are discussed in detail in Chapter 7. In Chapter 9, several case reports of actual patients with combined impairments are presented according to the schema of The Integrated Systems Model (Lee & Lee 2007, Lee et al 2008a,b) and each of these cases considers all three dimensions of the patient's experience (sensorial, cognitive, and emotional).

Lumbar dysfunction with acute pain – stages 1 and/or 2

The history

This individual is usually young (18–35 years of age) and the mode of onset of pain is commonly insidious (postural) or sudden (trauma). They may report that this is an initial episode of low back pain or it may be a recurrent episode. After an initial acute episode of low back pain, there is a suggestion that subsequent acute episodes of low back pain be termed *recurrent episodes* of a *chronic* problem, as the underlying mechanisms contributing to recurrent low back pain are likely to be different from those of a first-time traumatic episode, and recurrence of pain after an acute episode is a common problem (Carey et al 1999, Pengel et al 2003).

The pain may be unilateral or bilateral and is usually localized to the low back (region between T12/12th rib and the iliac crest) and can radiate distally as far as the foot. Dysesthesia is not often reported unless there is an injury to the intervertebral disc that has prolapsed or herniated into the spinal canal/lateral recess. The aggravating activities include the extremes of range of motion (forward/backward bending, rotation), prolonged standing or sitting, and lifting. Rest in the supine lying position (knees over a bolster) usually affords relief.

In the first few days after a traumatic injury (acute inflammatory phase, see Table 7.2), the patient often has marked difficulty walking and getting out of a chair as both tasks require motion of the lumbar spine and are often provocative.

Standing posture

A wide variety of postures and neuromuscular activation patterns will be noted and depend on the CNS's response to pain (remember that the response is indeterminate). Some common patterns include:

1. Overactivation of the erector spinae (the back gripper) → posture: extension of the thorax and lumbar spine (Fig. 5.15A).
2. Overactivation of the external and internal oblique (the chest-gripper) → tendency to flex the thorax relative to the lumbar spine (Fig. 5.15B).
3. Overactivation of both the erector spinae and the superficial oblique abdominals (co-contraction brace, the trunk-gripper) → a neutral posture may be present with this response; trunk alignment depends on the net balance of activity between trunk flexors and extensors (Fig. 5.15C).

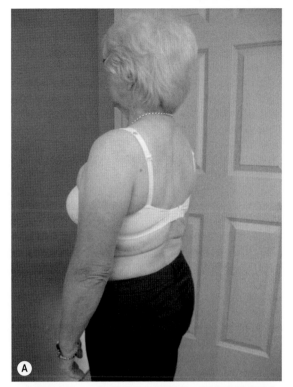

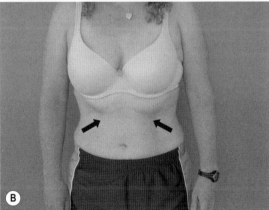

Fig. 5.15 • The central nervous system responds with a wide variety of responses to pain; consequently different strategies for standing posture will be found. (A) The posture of a back-gripper. Note the posterior thoracic tilt and extension of the thoracic and lumbar spines. (B) The posture of a chest-gripper. Note the narrowing of the infrasternal angle and the classical vertical crease (arrows) of the lateral abdominal wall. This neuromuscular response tends to result in an anterior thoracic tilt (flexion of the thoracic spine) and the resultant lumbar posture depends on how the individual adapts to the resultant flexion force.

Continued

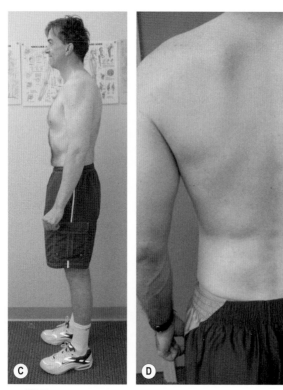

Fig. 5.15 — cont'd • (C) The posture of a trunk-gripper. Both the flexors and extensors of the trunk are overactive in this posture, and although it appears to be neutral it is extremely compressive. (D) Unilateral back-gripper. Note the increased tone in the right erector spinae (arrow).

4. Unilateral overactivation of either of the above muscle groups (Fig. 5.15D) or combined asymmetrical overactivation (one side external and internal oblique, opposite erector spinae or components of the erector spinae).

Load transfer tests

In the first few days after an injury to a lumbar joint (zygapophyseal or intervertebral disc), the patient with acute symptoms will present with marked restriction of all ranges of motion secondary to the neuromuscular protective response. The range of motion is bilaterally limited when the injury is bilateral, and unilaterally limited when the pathology is unilateral. As the intensity of the pain subsides (4–6 days), the pattern of segmental restriction becomes more evident and localized to the traumatized joint.

If the superficial back muscles are overactive, they may restrict motion of L4–L5 or L5–S1 during the one leg standing test (contralateral hip flexion in single leg standing – see Chapter 8). This will affect motion of the ipsilateral innominate as L4 and L5 must be free to rotate to the side of the non-weight bearing lower extremity (side of hip flexion) during this test (Chapter 8, see case report Mike, Chapter 9 Video MQ3 🖱). If the pain has significantly altered motor control, unlocking of the ipsilateral hemipelvis and/or buckling/giving way of the impaired lumbar segment may occur.

Form closure, force closure, and motor control

Initially, severe pain restricts a detailed examination of segmental mobility, integrity of the passive system (form closure mechanism), and the active and motor control systems (force closure mechanism). As the pain subsides and the overactive superficial muscle system is released (Chapter 10), the tests for mobility and motion control can be done. A variable response will be found and depends on the extent of the structural changes.

If in the later phases of this event (remodeling/maturation phase from 4 weeks to 12 months; see

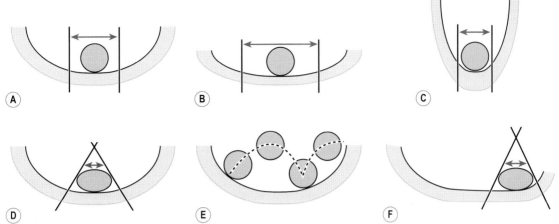

Fig. 5.16 • The neutral zone of motion can be affected by anything that alters compression across the joint. (A) A graphic illustration of the neutral zone of motion in a healthy joint. (B) A joint that is insufficiently compressed due to the loss of form or force closure and/or deficits in motor control will have a relative increase in the neutral zone of motion. (C) A joint that is excessively compressed due to fibrosis will have a relative decrease in the neutral zone of motion. (D) A joint that is excessively compressed due to increased activation of certain muscles will also have a relative decrease in the neutral zone of motion. (E) The bouncing ball reflects an *intermittent* loss of compression/control during a task. (F) A joint that is fixated (subluxed) is excessively compressed and no neutral zone of motion can be palpated (complete joint block).

Table 7.2) restrictive capsular adhesions have created a fibrotic stiff joint, the neutral zone of motion will be reduced and the elastic zone will reveal a very firm end feel (Fig. 5.16C). The tests for the integrity of the passive restraints (Chapter 8) will be normal. If, however, there has been an attenuation of the ligaments/capsule or loss of tensile strength or height of the intervertebral disc, the tests for the integrity of the passive restraints may be positive and this finding puts the impairment into Kirkaldy-Willis' stage 2 – instability (see Fig. 5.1).

The results of the tests for the active and control systems are variable and almost always positive. In other words, there are deficits in the neuromuscular behavior of the deep and superficial muscle systems, and possible structural changes in the active systems, the patterns of which are indeterminate and require specific assessment (Chapter 8).

Treatment

This section describes the specific therapy indicated for restoring mobility of a lumbar motion segment (including the zygapophyseal joints and the intervertebral discs) following a traumatic sprain of the joint as it is this injury that often leads to a stiff, fibrotic segment if not properly managed. Rarely is rest indicated

for the acutely sprained back. Patients are encouraged to remain as active/mobile as possible. However, if there is a suspected fracture of the zygapophyseal joint (see Fig. 5.5) there will be associated inhibition of the deep fibers of multifidus and healing of the bone must precede training of this muscle. The resting position for the painful low back is supine with the hips and knees semi-flexed and supported over a wedge. Once the soft tissue healing has progressed to the stage where load is tolerated, gentle range of motion exercises should be encouraged (pelvic tilting in either the supine and specific segmental mobilization techniques are used to maintain/regain full functional range of motion) (Chapter 10).

When the back pain persists and the individual's strategy for transferring loads has been non-optimal for some time, rendering the low back stiff and rigid, the joints can also become stiff and rigid. This is not apparent until the multi-segmental, superficial muscles of the back are released with techniques described in Chapter 10. In treatment, the goal is to restore segmental mobility to the lumbar spine such that loads are equally distributed. This will require the stiff or compressed segments to be mobilized or released (Chapter 10) and the patient taught ideal strategies for postures and movements necessary for their activities of daily living (Chapters 11, 12).

Lumbar dysfunction with acute pain – stage 2, acute locked back

The intra-articular meniscoid (see Fig. 10.48 A–C) of a moderately degenerated zygapophyseal joint can become trapped during a flexion/rotation load (lift and twist) when the movement and load are poorly controlled. The resulting response of the neuromuscular system (increased activation of the superficial muscles of the trunk) stabilizes/fixates the lumbar segment in what appears to be a 'locked' posture and the findings are as follows.

The history

The mode of onset is usually sudden and the patient vividly recalls the precipitating event. The pain is often unilateral and segmentally specific and intensely aggravated by any motion that inferiorly glides the impaired zygapophyseal joint. The joint most commonly affected is L4–5. The pain may radiate distally down the buttock and posterolateral thigh. Resting in a flexed, laterally translated posture (away from the side of pain) often affords some relief. This is a key finding and differentiates this condition from a prolapsed intervertebral disc, which is usually intolerant to flexion postures.

Standing posture

The patient presents with a classical flexed and laterally translated posture and cannot achieve a neutral lumbar spine posture in any position. Segmentally, the impaired joint is flexed and rotated away from the impaired side. The pelvis is posteriorly tilted and the hip joints are often flexed.

Load transfer tests

Any attempt to correct the postural deformity meets with marked increase in pain. All movements are painful and limited. The protective neuromuscular response restricts all motion at L4–5 and L5–S1. If the pain has significantly altered motor control, unlocking of the ipsilateral hemipelvis and/or buckling/giving way of the impaired lumbar segment may occur.

Form closure, force closure, and motor control

Positionally, the impaired joint is held in flexion and contralateral rotation (away from the side of pain). The neutral zone of motion is completely blocked and the end feel is springy (Fig. 5.16F). Marked inhibition of the deep muscle system is usually present.

Treatment

This condition requires a specific high acceleration, low amplitude thrust technique that is described in Chapter 10. Subsequently, the patient will require instruction on ideal strategies (for posture and movement) and may need specific training to restore function of the deep muscles in order to protect this segment from future episodes of 'locking,' since the underlying form closure deficit remains (Chapters 11, 12).

Lumbar dysfunction with chronic or persistent pain – stages 1 and 2

Clinically, patients with chronic or persistent pain and late stage 1 or stage 2 lumbar dysfunction may or may not have significant structural changes (form closure deficits) (see Figs 5.6, 5.7A–D) and consistently present with motor control and/or active system deficits that impact the force closure mechanism for single or multiple joints within the lumbar spine.

The history

This individual is usually middle aged (35–50 years of age) and has a long history of intermittent low back pain with repeated episodes of exacerbation and resolution. Alternately, this may be the first episode that is not resolving in expected timeframes. The low back pain may be unilateral or bilateral and can refer as far as the distal extent of the segmental dermatome. Dysesthesia is common, though not universal, due to the potential for neurovascular impedance at the intervertebral foramen and/or presence of sensitization of the peripheral or central nervous systems and altered CNS processing (Chapter 7). The aggravating activities frequently include sustained end-range postures (flexion and/or extension of the lumbar spine with or without rotation) and those activities that induce them (prolonged standing or sitting out of neutral spine, prolonged forward or backward bending of the trunk). Rest in the supine lying position with the knees supported over a bolster usually affords relief. The findings of four different segmental impairments will be described.

Lumbar dysfunction – stage 2 flexion control impairment

An individual with a *flexion* control impairment often presents with a segmental kyphosis (Fig. 5.17A), which is exaggerated in flexion (forward bending) (Video 5.1 🖱). The segmental kyphosis is also evident in sitting (Fig. 5.17B). The individual tends to stand and sit with the pelvis posteriorly rotated, the impaired segment flexed and posteriorly translated and the upper lumbar and lower thoracic spine extended. The mode of onset is often flexion/rotation activities, sudden or repetitive. The back pain is usually aggravated by sustained or repetitive flexion tasks (shoveling, gardening, rowing, etc.). The tests for the integrity of the passive system (passive restraints) (Chapter 8) are positive; there is increased anteroposterior translation in the neutral zone and a softer end feel in the elastic zone. The tests for the active and control systems for the impaired segment are positive in flexion loading (i.e. loads requiring control of flexion such as resisted arm extension at 90° shoulder flexion) and the

specific motor control and active system deficits are variable (response is indeterminate). When there is loss of segmental control, the deep fibers of multifidus at that segment are usually impaired in function bilaterally and, if the condition is persistent, there are also structural changes in the muscle (atrophy and fatty infiltration) bilaterally (Fig. 5.18). The responses of TrA and the pelvic floor are variable (absent, delayed, asymmetrical) and often not coactivated with the impaired dMF. The superficial muscle system response is variable with at least one muscle (EO, IO, RA, sMF, ES, etc.) being hyperactive.

Lumbar dysfunction – stage 2 extension control impairment

An individual with an *extension* control impairment presents with an excessive segmental lordosis that is exaggerated in extension (backward bending) (Fig. 5.19A,B) (Video 5.2 🖱). The pelvis can be either anteriorly tilted (see Fig. 10.22A,B) or posteriorly tilted (Fig. 5.19B) and can remain there during backward bending. The upper lumbar spine and

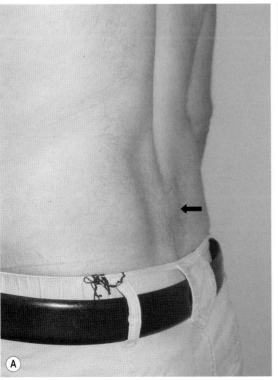 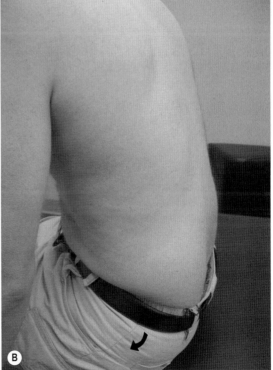

Fig. 5.17 • A patient with a segmental flexion/posterior translation instability at L5–S1. Note the segmental kyphosis at L5–S1 in standing (arrow) (A) and its accentuation in sitting (B). In addition, note the posterior pelvic tilt (arrow) and loss of the lumbar lordosis in sitting.

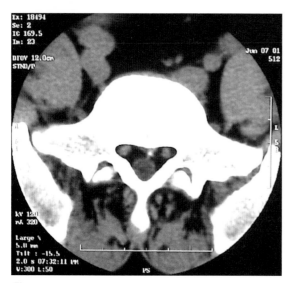

Fig. 5.18 • A magnetic resonance image (MRI) of the lumbosacral junction. Note the dark 'holes' in the deep fibers of multifidus. This is likely due to atrophy and fatty infiltration of the muscle.

lower thoracic spine often remain flexed during backward bending such that the motion hinges around the 'unstable' (defined à la Kirkaldy-Willis) segment (Video 5.3). The mode of onset is often extension and/or rotation activities, sudden or repetitive, and the back pain is usually aggravated by sustained or repetitive extension or rotation tasks (prolonged standing, running, swimming, etc.).

The tests for the integrity of the passive system (passive restraints) (Chapter 8) are positive; there is increased posteroanterior translation in the neutral zone and a softer end feel in the elastic zone. The tests for the active and control systems for the impaired segment are positive in extension loading (i.e. loads that require control of extension such as resisted arm elevation) and the specific motor control and active system deficits are variable (response is indeterminate). When there is loss of segmental control, the deep fibers of multifidus at that segment are usually impaired in function bilaterally and, if the condition is persistent, there are also structural changes in the

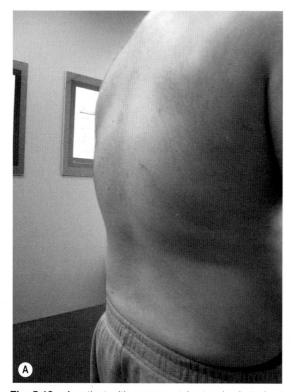

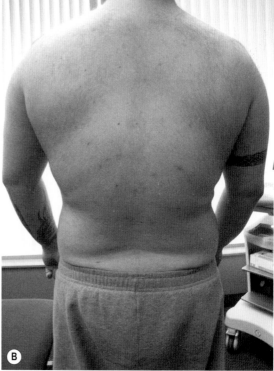

Fig. 5.19 • A patient with a segmental extension/anterior translation instability at L5–S1. (A) In standing, the segmental hinge is not apparent; however, in backward bending (B) the classical 'skin crease' and hinge at L5–S1 is easily seen. Note also the lack of segmental extension in the upper lumbar spine. This is another example of a motion control and a movement impairment occurring at different levels in the same lumbar spine. Watch Video 5.3 to see this individual backward bend with two different strategies.

muscle (atrophy and fatty infiltration) bilaterally (see Fig. 5.18). The responses of TrA and the pelvic floor are variable (absent, delayed, asymmetrical) and often not coactivated with the impaired dMF. The superficial muscle system response is variable with at least one muscle (EO, IO, RA, sMF, ES) being hyperactive.

Lumbar dysfunction – stage 2 rotation control impairment

An individual with a rotation control impairment may present in acute pain with a segmental lateral shift. If the condition is persistent, the pain is less intense and the shift less obvious. In this case, the segment is often flexed and rotated. This loss of segmental lordosis is exaggerated in sitting, the pelvis is often posteriorly tilted, and an intrapelvic torsion (IPT) is common. The mode of onset is often a rotation injury, usually in flexion (lift and twist), and recurrences of pain and impairment are common. The back pain is aggravated by all tasks that require rotation of the lumbar spine (walking, running, twisting, etc.). The tests for the integrity of the passive restraints (Chapter 8) are positive unilaterally; there is increased unilateral posteroanterior or anteroposterior translation in the neutral zone and a softer end feel in the elastic zone. The tests for the active and control systems for the impaired segment are positive in tests requiring rotational control (bilateral or unilateral) and the specific motor control and active system deficits are variable (response is indeterminate). When there is loss of segmental rotation control, the deep fibers of multifidus at that segment are usually impaired in function unilaterally and, if the condition is persistent, there are also structural changes in the muscle (atrophy and fatty infiltration) unilaterally. The responses of TrA and the pelvic floor are variable although most often asymmetrical in response to a verbal cue. In addition, there is loss of coactivation of TrA with the dMF often in a contralateral pattern (left dMF and right TrA). The superficial muscle system response is variable with at least one muscle (EO, IO, RA, sMF, ES) being hyperactive.

Treatment

In treatment, the goal is to restore segmental mobility to the lumbar spine such that the load is equally distributed. This will require that the patient be taught ideal strategies for postures and movements necessary for their activities of daily living (Chapters 11, 12). The impaired joint is commonly compressed (see Fig. 5.16D) by overactivation of the superficial muscle system, which will require release

(Chapter 10) prior to retraining segmental control via retraining coordination of the deep and superficial muscle systems (Chapter 11) followed by integration into functional tasks (Chapter 12). Note the difference in the extension hinge at L5–S1 during backward bending before and after treatment (Fig. 5.20A–D, Video 5.3).

Lumbar dysfunction – stage 2 multidirectional control impairment

The segment that lacks control in multiple directions is severely impaired. This individual has often had multiple episodes of acute back pain with increasing levels of disability after each event. The back pain is aggravated by all loading tasks in every direction and there is minimal range of functional (controlled) motion. It is difficult to assess the integrity of the passive system (passive restraints) (Chapter 8), as there is usually marked co-contraction bracing of the superficial muscle system preventing accurate motion analysis of the deeper structures. The tests for the active and control systems for the impaired segment are positive and the specific motor control and active system deficits are variable (response is indeterminate) and often involve multiple muscle groups. The deep fibers of multifidus are usually impaired in function bilaterally at the impaired segment and there are consistent structural changes in the muscle (atrophy and fatty infiltration) bilaterally (see Fig. 5.18). The response of TrA is often absent and coactivation of the superficial muscle system common (EO, IO, RA, sMF, ES).

Treatment

The individual with a segmental multidirectional control impairment is very difficult to treat conservatively. Although the approach is the same as for the unidirectional control impairment (Chapters 10–12), the response to treatment is often not ideal. These individuals may require a consultation for surgical stabilization; however, prolotherapy should be tried first (Chapter 11).

Neurological conduction status

Impedance of neurological function (motor, sensory, reflex) and neural mobility can occur with stage 2 impairments ('instability') as the increased segmental translation that occurs during loading can interfere with the dimensions of the lateral recess (see Fig. 5.8).

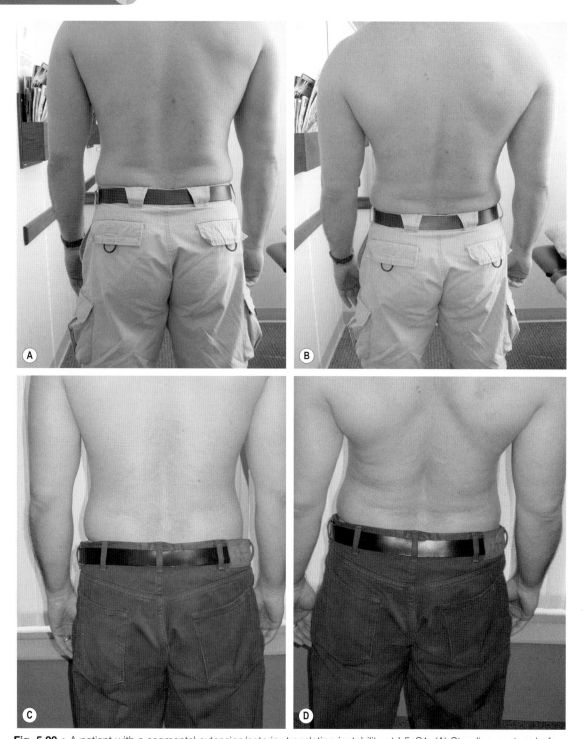

Fig. 5.20 • A patient with a segmental extension/anterior translation instability at L5–S1. (A) Standing posture before treatment. (B) Backward bending strategy before treatment. (C) Standing posture after treatment. (D) Backward bending strategy after treatment. Note how the load in backward bending is now distributed throughout the lumbar spine, and there is significantly less hinging at L5–S1 despite even greater backward bending range of motion compared to the pre-treatment movement.

The relevant neurodynamic test(s) would then be positive. The spectrum of neurological impedance is variable and depends on the degree of pathology. The patient may present with minimal motor weakness or sensory dysesthesia in the early stages, and later with a complete motor nerve block and sensory anesthesia. Careful objective evaluation is mandatory to detect the early neurological decompensation. Sensitization of the peripheral and central nervous systems can cause a wide variety of both sensorial and motor perceptions, and it is crucial to differentiate this from the true loss of neural conduction.

Lumbar dysfunction with chronic or persistent pain – stage 3

Continued use of non-optimal strategies combined with intermittent acute flare-ups of back pain can result in progressive pathoanatomical changes, ultimately leading to significant form closure deficits. In stage 3 (stabilization) the osteophytes on the posterior zygapophyseal joints and intevertebral disc can create spontaneous fusion (see Fig. 5.9A). According to Kirkaldy-Willis (1983), when these changes occur the patient is painfree. The risk at this stage is the development of fixed central and/or lateral stenosis due to osseous trespass on the spinal canal and/or lateral recess with attendant peripheral symptoms of neurogenic vascular claudication. The primary complaint is dysesthesia and pain in the lower extremities often induced by tasks that require extension and rotation of the lumbar spine such as walking. Forward bending and sitting in flexion affords temporary relief, as does intermittent lumbar traction. The lumbar lordosis is often reduced and mobility extremely restricted in this stage (Fig. 5.21A–C). Motor control training to balance activation of the superficial and deep muscle systems (release any hypertonicity in the superficial muscle system and train better strategies for load transfer using more activation of the deep muscle system) are sometimes beneficial; however, if the structural changes are excessive, surgical intervention may be required. Optimizing mobility and control in adjacent joints in the kinetic chain (e.g. thorax, hips) as well as changing strategies for function can help unload the affected segments by creating better load sharing during functional tasks, and can improve functional status as well as prevent further deterioration of the pathoanatomical changes.

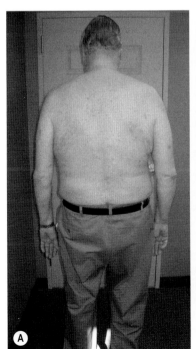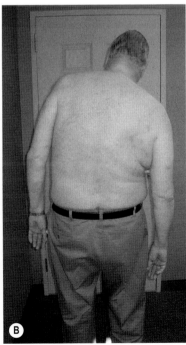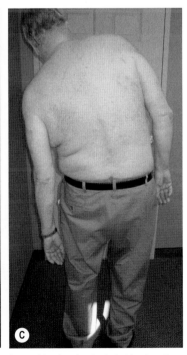

Fig. 5.21 • A patient with marked central canal stenosis from L1 to L5. (A) Note the loss of lumbar lordosis in his standing posture and the marked limitation of (B) left and (C) right sideflexion. This is a very stable, non-painful lumbar spine. His primary complaint was bilateral numbness in his legs and feet that occurred while walking.

Some common clinical presentations – pelvic girdle

All conditions pertaining to the pelvic girdle result in either excessive compression and, therefore, restriction of the SIJ/PS, or insufficient compression, and poor control, of the SIJ/PS regardless of whether the etiology is non-mechanical (see Table 5.1) or mechanical. What follows is a brief description of some common clinical presentations of patients with either excessive or insufficient compression of the SIJ and/or PS secondary to deficits in either the form or force closure/motor control mechanisms. Remember that it is very common to find asymmetrical imbalances in compression of the pelvis; that is, excessive compression on one side of the pelvis (SIJ/PS) and insufficient compression/control on the other side.

Excessive compression of the SIJ

Excessive compression of the SIJ can result from systemic articular pathology, such as ankylosing spondylitis (fusion), mechanical articular pathology that causes fibrosis of the capsule (fibrotic stiff joint) (see Fig. 5.16C), or mechanical neuromuscular pathology that causes compression secondary to overactivation of certain muscles (Fig. 5.16D). There are three muscles that, when hypertonic, can compress and limit both passive and active mobility of the SIJ. Each muscle (together with the forces produced by the fascial system) appears to compress a specific part of the SIJ.

1. Ischiococcygeus (see Fig. 3.62A,B) compresses the inferior part of the joint, prevents a parallel glide between the innominate and sacrum, and induces posterior rotation of the innominate when gentle anteroposterior pressure is applied to the innominate (Chapter 8);
2. Piriformis (Fig. 3.62A,B) compresses all three parts of the SIJ preventing a parallel glide at all parts of the joint (superior, middle, and inferior); and the
3. Superficial fibers of multifidus (see Fig. 3.55A) compress the superior part of the joint, prevent a parallel glide between the innominate and sacrum, and induce an anterior rotation of the innominate when gentle pressure is applied to the innominate (Chapter 8).

The history

The mode of onset for the SIJ that is excessively compressed by fibrosis (stiff) is either systemic/inflammatory, resulting in an intra-articular synovitis, or traumatic. The joint stiffens in response to the joint inflammation/sprain and the patient usually presents several months later complaining of pain in the opposite SIJ, lumbar spine, or groin. The fibrotic joint is rarely the current source of pain, although patients may report that their symptoms began there.

The mode of onset for the SIJ compressed by overactivation of muscles (hypertonicity) is often insidious and may occur as a consequence of pregnancy and delivery or secondary to the use of strategies in sports/life that repetitively induce external rotation of the hip (e.g. ballet, soccer, hockey) or repetitive asymmetrical vertical loading combined with power (kicking, cutting motions, rotational drives as in golf). The location of the pain is variable and depends on the tissues that are being stressed or overused in the altered biomechanics produced by this compression. If the SIJ is the source of nociception, the pain will likely be between the iliac crest and the gluteal fold and may radiate down the posterolateral thigh to the knee. Activities that aggravate a compressed SIJ often include tasks that require IPT (walking, full body rotation tasks). It is important to note that a compressed SIJ (due to muscle hypertonicity) can occur secondary to an underlying passive system impairment (form closure deficit), where the muscle hypertonicity is an attempt to compensate for the underlying passive instability. The patient's history determines whether an underlying insufficiency of the passive system is a likely hypothesis.

Standing posture

The fibrotic, stiff SIJ is not evident in postural analysis; however, the SIJ that is myofascially compressed secondary to overactivation of the external rotators of the hip has a classical appearance (Fig. 5.22B). Normally, the lumbopelvic region should resemble the shape of a pyramid (Fig. 5.22A) with a wide pelvic base narrowing superiorly at the waist. When an individual develops a strategy for transferring load that uses predominantly the deep external rotators of the hip joint as well as the ischiococcygeus, the constant activation of these muscles compresses the inferior aspect of the SIJ. This is called a buttgripping strategy (Fig. 5.22B). The bilateral buttgripper has a buttock that resembles an inverted pyramid and, in standing, a large divot posterior to

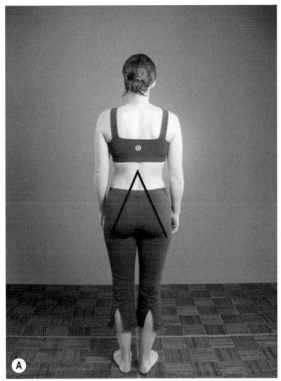

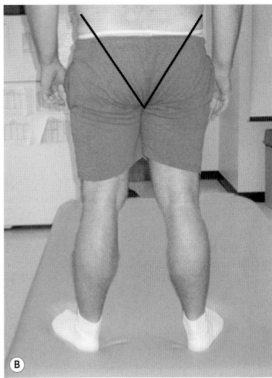

Fig. 5.22 • (A) The shape of an optimal lumbopelvic–hip pyramid. (B) The shape of a butt-gripper; the pyramid is inverted. Note the externally rotated position of both lower extremities.

the greater trochanter can be seen and palpated. The bilateral butt-gripper tends to stand with the pelvic girdle posteriorly tilted, the L4–5 and L5–S1 joints flexed, and the lower extremities externally rotated. If the leg does not appear to be externally rotated at the foot, then a compensatory rotation occurs at the knee and through the foot. The unilateral butt-gripper often stands with the pelvis rotated in the transverse plane and an IPT.

Load transfer tests

In both forward and backward bending, the fibrotic, stiff SIJ will create an IPT and the asymmetry will be consistent each time the individual moves in the sagittal plane. Axial rotation will be limited towards the side of the restriction and lateral bending will be limited away from the side of the restriction. A SIJ that is myofascially compressed unilaterally by the external rotators of the hip joint will create similar findings, although the direction of the lateral bending restriction can be variable. In addition, an IPT will be produced and the direction depends on the specific muscles involved; some may create

an altered axis of motion for the hip. The apex of the forward bending curve is often in the thorax (Fig. 5.23, Video 5.4 🖱).

During the one leg standing test, the individual with the fibrotic, stiff SIJ will have reduced motion during flexion of the ipsilateral hip (compared to the opposite SIJ) and will have no difficulty transferring load (no unlocking during single leg loading). The myofascially compressed joint may move symmetrically during flexion of the ipsilateral hip or may not, depending on the strategy used for the task, and it frequently 'unlocks' during single leg loading. The ASLR test is often negative when the SIJ is fibrotic or stiff. There is a notable difference in the effort required to lift one leg off the table, and adding more compression to the pelvic girdle does not reduce the effort required to perform this task; in fact, compression may make it more difficult to lift the leg. This finding suggests that the pelvis is already excessively compressed (Video 5.5 🖱). The myofascially compressed SIJ will have variable responses to compression during the ASLR, depending on which muscles are overactive (creating different vectors), and to what degree they are overactive. Generally, it is more difficult to lift one

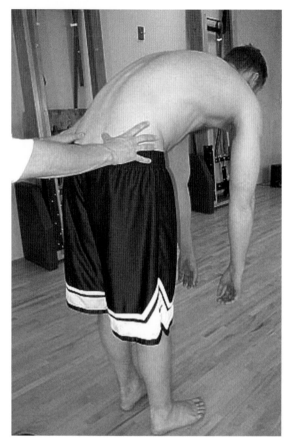

Fig. 5.23 • This is the pattern of forward bending commonly seen in an individual who cannot release the hip joints to allow the pelvic girdle to tilt anteriorly relative to the femoral heads (butt-gripping). Note the open hip angle (minimal hip joint flexion) and the excessive thoracolumbar flexion.

leg off the table, but only certain patterns of compression across the pelvis (Chapter 8) will reduce the effort to perform the task; other patterns of compression will make the task harder. In the extremely compressed SIJ (where all parts of the joint are held by hypertonic muscles), any compression pattern makes the leg harder to lift.

Form closure, force closure, and motor control

The fibrotic, stiff SIJ has a reduced neutral zone of motion at all three parts of the SIJ (superior, middle, and inferior), whereas the myofascially compressed SIJ commonly has one part of the joint restricted and the location depends on which muscle is hypertonic. The elastic zone of the fibrotic, stiff joint has a

consistently hard end feel, whereas the myofascially compressed joint has a muscular resistance quality. In both cases, the form closure mechanism is intact (normal passive restraints). The results of the tests for the active and control systems (force closure and motor control) are variable and almost always positive. In other words, there are deficits in the neuromuscular behavior and/or integrity of the deep and superficial muscle systems, the pattern of which is indeterminate and requires specific assessment (Chapter 8).

Treatment

This section describes the specific therapy indicated for restoring mobility of the SIJ following a traumatic sprain of the joint as it is this injury that often leads to a stiff, fibrotic SIJ if not properly managed. If the injury results in an intra-articular synovitis, several pain provocation tests will be positive (Chapter 8) and the goal of treatment at this time is to reduce the load through the joint such that healing can occur. The SIJ is a difficult joint to rest as most postures/ positions compress the joint. Clinically, it appears that the best resting position for the painful SIJ is sidelying with the painful side uppermost and the hip and knee supported on a pillow between the legs. Weight bearing activities such as walking, standing, and sitting should be minimized during the first few days. A cane can help to reduce the loading through the pelvis when vertical. Sacroiliac belts increase compression of the joint and often increase pain during this stage of healing.

As the pain and inflammation settles, passive and active range of motion of the joint should be encouraged (Chapter 10). If the patient presents several weeks or months after the initial injury, it is possible that the SIJ has become stiff and fibrotic. A specific mobilization technique is the treatment of choice (Chapter 10). In treatment, the goal is to restore symmetrical mobility between the left and right SIJ such that loads are equally shared and rotation forces are not distributed to the low back or hip. This will require that the patient be taught ideal strategies for postures and movements necessary for their activities of daily living (Chapters 11, 12) after the stiff SIJ is mobilized.

The myofascially compressed SIJ is treated with specific release techniques directed towards the specific muscles responsible for the excessive compression (Chapter 10). Subsequently, retraining of intrapelvic control via activation and coordination of the deep and superficial muscle systems (Chapter 11) followed by integration into functional tasks (Chapter 12) is provided.

Insufficient compression of the SIJ and PS

Repetitive or single trauma to the pelvic girdle as a consequence of pregnancy and delivery, sport, work or motor vehicle accidents can cause changes in neuromuscular function and control, and pain that further impacts the behavior of the neuromuscular system and results in non-optimal strategies for transferring loads through the pelvic girdle. Significant trauma, or microtrauma over prolonged periods of time, can lead to pathoanatomical changes and passive instability of the SIJs and/or PS. Unlike the lumbar spine, very little research has been done to document any structural changes that occur as a consequence of insufficient articular compression of the pelvic joints. Recent research using SPECT-CT shows promise in being able to identify individuals with mechanical instability of the SIJs and PS (see Figs 5.10, 5.11).

The history

This individual is usually young (17–35 years of age at the time of the initial event) with either a short (if this is an initial episode) or long history of pelvic girdle pain (if this is a recurrent episode). The pain is often, though not always, either unilateral over the SIJ and buttock or over the PS and groin. The aggravating activities frequently include unilateral weight bearing (walking, climbing stairs), bending forward or lifting, lying supine and rolling over from this position. The most comfortable position for the painful pelvis is sidelying in the semi-Fowler's position with the painful side uppermost. Comfort is enhanced with a body pillow that allows the flexed hip and knee to be supported. The findings of three different motion control impairments will be described.

SIJ – vertical control impairment

An individual with a vertical control impairment of the SIJ often presents with difficulty walking and limps into the treatment room. They are often reluctant to bear full weight through the impaired side of the pelvis in either sitting or standing, and compensate with a variety of strategies (Fig. 5.24). The mode of onset is often sudden or repetitive vertical loading through the lower extremity or ischial tuberosity

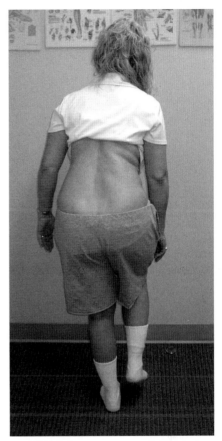

Fig. 5.24 • This woman is unable to transfer load through the left hemipelvis in this one leg standing task. One cause may be a vertical control impairment of the sacroiliac joint; further analysis of the articular, neural, myofascial, and visceral systems is required for differentiation.

(a fall landing hard on the leg or buttock). Consistent with the findings of Hungerford et al (2004), unlocking of the impaired side of the pelvis occurs when the individual attempts to bear weight and single leg load. However, there is a range of presentations in regard to the point during the task at which loss of control of the hemipelvis (SIJ/PS) occurs. Some individuals cannot even shift their weight to the impaired side, whereas others are able to fully load into single leg stance and only lose intrapelvic control (unlock) when they attempt a higher load task, such as a one-leg squat. The ASLR test is often positive with a notable difference in the effort required to lift one leg off the table. Adding more compression to the pelvic girdle just below the anterior superior iliac spines (ASISs) reduces the effort required to perform this task. Damen et al (2002a,b) note that compression of the pelvic girdle just below the ASIS increases the stiffness/compression of the SIJ, whereas compression of the pelvic girdle just above the greater trochanter increases the stiffness/compression of the PS. Clinically, often only certain patterns of compression across the pelvis (bilateral anterior, bilateral posterior, unilateral anterior combined with unilateral posterior – see Chapter 8) will reduce the effort required to perform the task (Lee & Lee 2004a). A positive ASLR test (effort decreases with specific and appropriate compression) suggests that the pelvis is insufficiently compressed (force closed) during the performance of this task.

In the absence of a fixation of the SIJ (see below), the positional findings are often unremarkable unless the compensatory strategies used to control the hemipelvis result in an IPT. The passive mobility tests for the SIJ reveal asymmetry of neutral zone motion with more motion in both the anteroposterior and craniocaudal planes on the affected side. The end feel of the elastic zone is 'softer' and pain is often provoked during this test. If there are significant structural changes in the passive restraints, the tests for the integrity of the passive restraints and the form closure mechanism (Chapter 8) will be positive; that is, when the joint is passively positioned into the close-packed position there will still be movement available. If the passive restraints are functional, any structural changes are not significant enough to impact passive stability of the SIJ. The tests for the active and control systems for the pelvic girdle are positive and the specific motor control and active system deficits are variable (response is indeterminate) and often involve multiple muscles (deep and superficial). The deep fibers of the lumbosacral multifidus are usually impaired in function unilaterally and there are consistent structural changes in the muscle (atrophy and fatty infiltration) (see Fig. 5.18). The responses of TrA and the pelvic floor are variable, although most often asymmetrical, in response to a verbal cue. In addition, there is loss of coactivation of TrA with the dMF in either a contralateral (left dMF and right TrA) or ipsilateral (left dMF and left TrA) pattern. The superficial muscle system response is variable with at least one muscle (EO, IO, RA, sMF, ES) being hyperactive.

Treatment

In treatment, the goal is to restore motion control of the SIJ during a variety of vertical loading tasks (both static and dynamic). This will require that the deep

and superficial muscle systems are released if necessary (Chapter 10) and then trained, coordinated (Chapter 11), and subsequently integrated into functional tasks (Chapter 12). If there is a form closure deficit and restoring optimal recruitment patterning of the deep and superficial muscle systems fails to provide control during vertical loading tasks, prolotherapy is indicated (Chapter 11).

SIJ – horizontal control impairment

An individual with a horizontal control impairment of the SIJ often presents with difficulty performing forward bending tasks (Fig. 5.25). The mode of onset is often traumatic and it is common to find that a lifting/twisting injury precipitated the initial event. These patients can be mistakenly thought to have a lumbar disc injury due to the mechanism of injury;

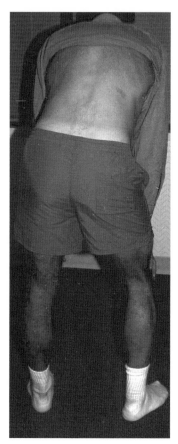

Fig. 5.25 • A patient with a horizontal translation control impairment of the right sacroiliac joint has marked difficulty forward bending and often supports the trunk by walking the hands down the thighs.

if a thorough assessment of the pelvis is not included in the examination, then the horizontal control impairment of the SIJ can be missed. In forward bending, inconsistent findings prevail and depend on the strategy chosen. An intermittent and variable IPT is commonly seen and the pelvis frequently unlocks unilaterally (innominate anteriorly rotates relative to the ipsilateral sacrum) during the forward bend. The findings from the one leg standing test are variable and inconsistent, the pelvis may or may not unlock during single leg loading, and asymmetry of intrapelvic motion is commonly found. The ASLR test is often positive with a notable difference in the effort required to lift one leg off the table. Adding more compression to the pelvic girdle at the level of the ASISs reduces the effort required to perform this task. Clinically, often only certain patterns of compression across the pelvis (bilateral anterior, bilateral posterior, unilateral anterior combined with unilateral posterior – see Chapter 8) will reduce the effort to perform the task (Lee & Lee 2004a). This finding suggests that the pelvis is insufficiently compressed (force closed) during the performance of this task.

In the absence of a fixation of the SIJ (see below), the positional findings are often unremarkable unless the compensatory strategies used to control the hemipelvis result in an IPT. The passive mobility tests for the SIJ reveal asymmetry of neutral zone motion with more motion in the anteroposterior plane on the affected side. The end feel of the elastic zone is often 'softer' and pain is often provoked during this test. If there are significant structural changes in the passive restraints, the tests for the integrity of the passive restraints (Chapter 8) will be positive; when the joint is passively positioned into the close-packed position there will still be movement available in the anteroposterior plane. If the form closure mechanism is intact (no neutral zone motion available when the joint is close-packed), any structural changes in the passive restraints are not significant enough to impact passive stability of the SIJ. The tests for the active and control systems of the pelvic girdle are positive and the specific motor control and active system deficits are variable (response is indeterminate) and often involve multiple muscle groups. The deep fibers of the lumbosacral multifidus are usually impaired in function unilaterally and there are consistent structural changes in the muscle (atrophy and fatty infiltration). The responses of TrA and the pelvic floor are variable, although most often asymmetrical in response to a verbal cue. In addition, there is loss of coactivation

of TrA with the dMF in either a contralateral (left dMF and right TrA) or ipsilateral (left dMF and left TrA) pattern. The superficial muscle system response is variable with at least one muscle (EO, IO, RA, sMF, ES) being hyperactive.

Treatment

In treatment, the goal is to restore motion control of the SIJ during a variety of horizontal loading tasks. This will require that the deep and superficial muscle systems are released if necessary (Chapter 10) and then trained, coordinated (Chapter 11), and subsequently integrated into functional tasks (Chapter 12). If there is a form closure deficit and restoring optimal recruitment patterning of the deep and superficial muscle systems fails to provide control during vertical loading tasks, prolotherapy is indicated (Chapter 11).

PS – vertical control impairment

An individual with a vertical control impairment of the PS presents complaining of midline anterior pelvis and/or unilateral groin pain that is aggravated by vertical loading tasks, especially those that involve abduction of the lower extremity. The mode of onset is either sudden and traumatic (forceps delivery, straddle impact loading of the pelvis) or repetitive excessive loading using poor strategies. The SIJ usually (though not always) unlocks during vertical loading tasks, and increased craniocaudal translation is evident at the PS when the leg hangs unsupported from the pelvis (see Fig. 8.61C), and during other tasks that require control of vertical loading through the PS (Fig. 8.61A,B). The ASLR test is often positive with a notable difference in effort required when lifting one leg off the table. Adding more compression to the pelvic girdle at the level of the greater trochanter focused anteriorly to generate a force vector across the PS reduces the effort required to perform this task. This finding suggests that the pelvis is insufficiently compressed (force closed) during the performance of this task.

In the supine position, one pubic tubercle may be higher than the other, and an IPT may or may not be present depending on the compensatory strategies being used to control the hemipelvis. The tests for the active and control systems for the PS are positive (current recruitment pattern/force generated by the muscle systems is insufficient to control translation of the PS) and the specific motor control and active system deficits are variable (response is indeterminate) and often involve both the deep and superficial muscle systems. Hypertonicity of the short adductors (on the inferiorly sheared side), the opposite rectus abdominis, and the oblique abdominals is common, as are deficits in the recruitment patterning of the pelvic floor and TrA. Depending on whether or not the patient has concurrent low back pain, there may or may not be changes in the lumbar multifidus. If the tests for the integrity of the passive restraints are positive, this suggests that there are structural changes in the joint associated with this impairment.

Treatment

In treatment, the goal is to restore motion control of the PS during a variety of loading tasks. This will require that the deep and superficial muscle systems of the trunk are released if necessary (Chapter 10) and then trained, coordinated (Chapter 11), and subsequently integrated into functional tasks (Chapter 12). Once a symmetrical co-contraction of the deep muscles is attained, the integrity of the active and control systems should be retested. In addition, the function of the hip joint should be assessed and treated (see below) and any hypertonicity of the muscles attaching to the pubic rami released and balanced.

Insufficient force closure of the pelvic girdle can also occur as a consequence of loss of structural integrity of the linea alba (diastasis rectus abdominis) and/or endopelvic fascia. These conditions are discussed in Chapter 6 as they commonly, although not exclusively, occur as a consequence of pregnancy and delivery.

The acute locked SIJ

The mechanism underlying this condition is poorly understood (see Chapter 10 for a detailed discussion of this topic); yet, every time I begin to believe that the condition does not exist, it never fails that someone arrives in the clinic with what appears to be an acute locked SIJ. Note that this is not the most common condition to see in a general outpatient orthopedic clinical practice.

The history

The mode of onset is always traumatic and usually involves a significant fall on the buttocks (excessive vertical load), a lifting twisting event (excessive horizontal load), or a sudden force up the lower extremity while seated (motor vehicle accident). There is immediate pain over the fixated SIJ and inability to load through the pelvic girdle. After a vertical loading injury, the aggravating activities include any weight bearing through the affected side (standing, walking, sitting). After a horizontal loading injury, the aggravating activities include forward bending or rotation. The patient often states that no position gives them relief from pain. It is common for them to state that they have 'put their hip or pelvis out.' This impairment significantly impacts the ability to walk and the patient often arrives ambulating with crutches or a cane. The patient who has sustained a horizontal loading injury and has an acute locked SIJ walks in a forward bent, laterally shifted manner. It is readily apparent to even a casual observer that something is very wrong.

Standing posture

The pelvis is postured in a non-physiological alignment. As a reminder from Chapter 4, osteokinematically, an IPT to the left (IPTL) produces anterior rotation of the right innominate relative to the left innominate and left rotation of the sacrum. Both the left and right sides of the sacrum nutate relative to the respective innominate with the right side nutating further than the left (thus the bone rotates to the left). An IPTR (IPT to the right) produces exactly the opposite osteokinematics; the left innominate rotates anteriorly relative to the right innominate and the sacrum rotates to the right with both the left and right sides of the sacrum nutating relative to the respective innominate. These are physiological patterns of osteokinematic motion for intrapelvic motion and occur during gait and all rotation/lateral bending tasks. All other positional findings of the three bones of the pelvis are non-physiological; this is what is seen with an acute locked SIJ.

Load transfer tests

The fixated SIJ appears to totally block all movement such that the positional findings noted in standing persist in forward/backward bending, sitting, and lying supine or prone. No intrapelvic motion occurs during single leg loading and contralateral hip flexion, and the fixated SIJ does not unlock when loaded in any task. The ASLR test is negative in that, although there is a notable difference in the effort required to lift one leg off the table, adding more compression to the pelvic girdle actually increases the effort required to perform this task (see case report Julie, Chapter 9, Video JG3).

Form closure, force closure, and motor control

There is no palpable motion in the neutral zone of the fixated SIJ; it is extremely compressed and, therefore, it is not possible to test for the integrity of the form closure mechanism at this time. The joint requires immediate decompression via a high acceleration, low amplitude thrust technique (Chapter 10) following which an increased amplitude of neutral zone motion becomes immediately apparent. The tests for the integrity of the form closure mechanism will now identify if there has been a structural change in the passive restraints as a consequence of the injury. The tests for the integrity of the active and control systems (force closure and motor control) for the pelvic girdle are positive and the specific motor control and active system deficits are variable (response is indeterminate) and often involve multiple muscle groups. The deep fibers of the lumbosacral multifidus are usually impaired in function unilaterally. The responses of TrA and the pelvic floor are variable, although most often asymmetrical in response to a verbal cue. In addition, there is loss of coactivation of TrA with the dMF in either a contralateral (left dMF and right TrA) or ipsilateral (left dMF and left TrA) pattern. The superficial muscle system response is variable with at least one muscle (EO, IO, RA, sMF, ES) being hyperactive.

Subsequent treatment

Subsequent to the release of the SIJ, the goal is to restore motion control of the SIJ during a variety of loading tasks. An external support (SI belt) is usually required until the deep and superficial muscle systems of the trunk are trained, coordinated (Chapter 11), and integrated into functional tasks (Chapter 12). If there is a form closure deficit (articular instability due to structural changes in the passive restraints) and restoring optimal recruitment and patterning of the deep and superficial muscle systems fails to provide control of the joint during loading tasks, prolotherapy is indicated (Chapter 11).

Some common clinical presentations – the hip

Structural changes of the hip occur secondary to:

1. non-mechanical conditions such as those listed in Box 5.2 and Figure 5.12;

2. major trauma such as a fracture through the joint or a fracture of the neck of femur resulting in a change in position of the femoral head; or

3. repetitive trauma to the articular structures (capsule, ligaments, labrum) that occurs as a consequence of non-optimal strategies for transferring load.

Non-optimal strategies for loading through the hip joint are often produced by neuromuscular imbalances such as altered recruitment and patterning of the deep and superficial muscles of the hip, with or without associated hypertonicity (altered resting tone) (Janda 1978, 1986). Non-optimal strategies create non-optimal postures and movement control of the femoral head during loading (Lee & Lee 2004a, Sahrmann 2001). A butt-gripping (Fig. 5.22b) or hip-gripping strategy (overactivation of the short adductors combined with the external rotators) (Fig. 5.26) creates a net force vector that often results in anterior or anteromedial translation of the femoral

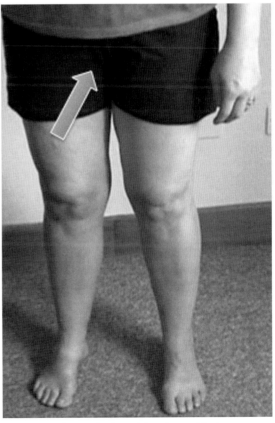

Fig. 5.26 • Overactivation of the short adductors combined with the deep external rotators often forces the femoral head anterior; this is the hip-gripping strategy.

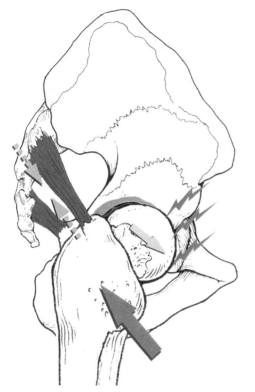

Fig. 5.27 • Overactivation of the deep external rotators of the hip pulls the greater trochanter posteriorly (large arrow) and forces the femoral head anteriorly.

head in the acetabulum (Fig. 5.27). Many muscles can collectively produce a postural displacement of the femoral head (see case reports in Chapter 9). If persistent, unbalanced vectors from hypertonic muscles and/or altered muscle recruitment patterns can be a precursor to early degeneration of the articular surfaces of the hip as well as structural changes in the acetabular labrum (labral fraying and tears). Consequently, patients can present with patterns of pain referred from multiple structures around the groin/hip and movement restrictions that are often combined with intermittent loss of motion control (commonly associated with 'clicking,' 'popping,' or 'giving way' in certain ranges of motion) that are due to:

1. excessive compression and malalignment of the joint secondary to muscle imbalances;
2. structural changes in the articular labrum (labral tears and fraying) and femoral acetabular impingement (FAI); and
3. structural changes in the articular cartilage (osteoarthritis).

The clinical presentation of each will be described below.

Excessive compression and malalignment of the hip secondary to muscle imbalance

Non-optimal strategies for transferring load through the hip joint are often produced by altered recruitment patterns of the deep and superficial hip muscles. Some common patterns include:

1. delayed or absent activation of psoas and early activation of rectus femoris, tensor fascia lata, and/or sartorius;
2. delayed or absent activation of psoas and early activation of the short adductors and piriformis; or
3. co-contraction bracing of gluteus medius/minimus and short/long adductors.

The functional range of motion of the hip (the range available with the femoral head staying centered in the acetabulum) becomes limited if the femoral head is translated anteriorly or anteromedially as a consequence of these non-optimal patterns (in resting tone or activity during movement).

The history

This individual can be young, middle aged, or old and the mode of onset is commonly insidious. It is not uncommon for the pain to be felt initially in other areas of the body that are compensating for the restricted hip (pelvis, low back, knee).

The joints of the low back and/or pelvic girdle can be overly stressed and ultimately painful when the hip fails to share the load during a task that requires more functional motion than it has. For example, consider Figure 5.2C. As this woman squats, her hips fail to flex and her lumbar spine flexes excessively to compensate; this is her usual strategy for a squat. Her primary complaint is low back pain that is aggravated by prolonged sitting. She is completely unaware that this is due to the strategy she is using to perform the squat and that her non-painful hips are creating this impairment. Other patients may be aware of tender trigger points in the superficial muscles of the hip and have attempted to 'stretch them out' without success. They find temporary release from muscle release techniques such as massage, but, because they do not change their movement strategies, the 'tightness' in their hip(s) returns.

Table 5.2 Frequency of pain referral to the buttock, thigh, groin, leg, knee, and foot

Anatomical Region	Percentage of Patients with Pain
Buttock	71
Thigh	57
Anterior	27
Lateral	27
Posterior	24
Medial	16
Groin	55
Leg	16
Lateral	8
Posterior	8
Anterior	4
Medial	2
Foot	6
Knee	2

Over time, the posterior buttock and/or groin may become painful and the movement restriction of the hip more evident. When the hip joint itself becomes symptomatic, the location of pain can be variable (Table 5.2, see Fig. 7.6).

Standing posture

Several non-optimal postural alignments and strategies can create malalignment of the femoral head secondary to muscle imbalance of the deep and superficial hip muscles; a common one is the anterior pelvic sway posture (unilateral or bilateral) (Fig. 5.28). Malalignment may also be due to altered control (or neural drive) of the muscles of the lumbopelvic canister, such as:

1. a butt-gripping strategy (see Fig. 5.22B) (increased activation of the external rotators of the hip); and
2. a hip-gripping strategy (see Fig. 5.26) (increased activation of the short adductors and posterior abductors of the hip).

Load transfer tests

When the hip joint is restricted in flexion and/or extension unilaterally, full forward and/or backward bending of the trunk will produce a transverse plane rotation of the pelvic girdle as well as an IPT. A compensatory, multisegmental rotoscoliosis of the lower lumbar spine also occurs. When abduction or adduction of the hip is limited, lateral bending of the trunk will be restricted as the pelvic girdle

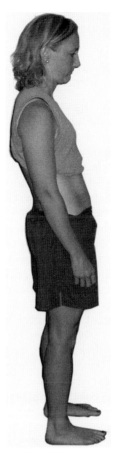

Fig. 5.28 • The anterior pelvic sway posture/strategy can lead to malalignment of the femoral head, as can the butt-gripping strategy (Fig. 5.22B) and the hip-gripping strategy (Fig. 5.26).

cannot translate in the coronal plane without deviation. Axial rotation of the trunk is limited in both directions when the femoral head is anteriorly translated in the acetabulum.

During single leg loading with contralateral hip flexion (one leg standing test (Chapter 8)), the restriction in functional motion is only apparent if the muscle imbalance significantly limits mobility of the hip to less than 60° of flexion. On the weight bearing side, the femoral head may rest anteriorly/anteromedially and stay there throughout the task or shift further anteriorly/rotate internally/externally during the task (Chapter 8). The loss of femoral head centering can also be felt during many other tasks including forward/backward bending, lateral bending, rotation, and/or a squat. In supine, the femoral head often continues to rest anterior relative to the acetabulum and remain, anterior or shifts anterior during horizontal loading tasks. All of these findings reflect poor motor control for optimal function of the hip.

Form closure, force closure, and motor control

Hypertonicity of the superficial and deep hip muscles prevents testing of the integrity of the passive restraints of the hip (form closure mechanism). Once the muscles are released (Chapter 10) full functional range of motion with the femoral head maintained centrally in the acetabulum often occurs and the form closure tests reveal healthy, intact ligaments, labrum, and capsule. If, however, the hip posture has been anterior or non-centered for some time, the underlying articular structures can become restricted and a true articular deficit (stiff joint) becomes apparent. This joint now requires a specific articular mobilization technique to restore full functional range of motion (Chapter 8). Alternately, articular deficits such as labral tears may become apparent when testing the form closure after releasing the hypertonic muscles (see below). The results of the tests for the motor control and active systems (force closure) are variable and almost always positive. In other words, there are deficits in the neuromuscular behavior of the deep and superficial muscles of the hip, the pattern of which is indeterminate and requires specific assessment (Chapter 8).

Treatment

This section describes the specific therapy indicated for restoring mobility of the hip joint that is compressed and malaligned secondary to an imbalance of the deep and superficial muscles of the hip. The hypertonic muscles are treated with specific release techniques (positional release, *release with awareness* (Lee & Lee 2004a), dry needling) directed towards the specific muscles responsible for the excessive compression and malalignment (Chapter 10). Subsequently, retraining of hip mobility and control via activation and coordination of the deep and superficial hip muscles (Chapter 11) followed by integration into functional tasks (Chapter 12) is provided.

Structural changes of the hip joint

It is commonly reported that non-optimal biomechanics of the hip joint can lead to structural changes in the joint including labral tears and cartilage

compression (chondral lesions) (Austin et al 2008, Brukner & Khan 2007, Hunt et al 2007, Shindle et al 2006, Torry et al 2006). Torry et al (2006) note that 'maintaining an appropriate femoral head position within the joint capsule and labral complex is paramount to normal hip function and failure in this mechanism can lead to debilitating labral and cartilage compression in active individuals.' In other words, non-optimal strategies for transferring loads through the hip can lead to structural changes; a labral tear is one structural change (Fig. 5.29A,B), articular degeneration of the joint is another (Fig. 5.30A,B). Subluxation and dislocation of the joint can occur as a consequence of sports and motor vehicle accidents and these injuries are also known to lead to articular instability (Shindle et al 2006), labral tears, and joint degeneration. More often, however, atraumatic 'instability' with associated labral tears and hip joint degeneration is reported and thought to be due to the overuse of repetitive motion, especially weight bearing rotation and extension (Shindle et al 2006).

Acetabular labral tears

Acetabular labral tears were first described in 1957 (Paterson 1957) and have received considerable investigation and interest in the last decade.

The history. Most individuals with an acetabular labral tear are young to middle-aged women (more than men) who have been involved in athletic activities, particularly those that involve repetitive pivoting motions on the weight bearing femur (soccer, golf, ballet). The onset of pain is usually insidious and primarily located in the anterior hip or groin (90% according to Burnett et al 2006). The pain is often constant and dull with intermittent episodes of sharp pain and is aggravated by weight bearing activities (walking, pivoting, sitting). Fifty-three percent also report popping or clicking in the joint and 41% report true locking (Burnett et al 2006). Concomitant pain in the pelvic floor has also been associated with this condition (Hunt et al 2007).

Standing posture. The postures noted above (see **Excessive compression and malalignment of the hip secondary to muscle imbalance**) are the same ones noted in individuals with acetabular labral tears as the non-optimal strategy produced by the muscle imbalance is often responsible for creating the condition. The femoral head almost always rests anterior or anteromedial in the acetabulum in all positions – standing, sitting, and prone lying.

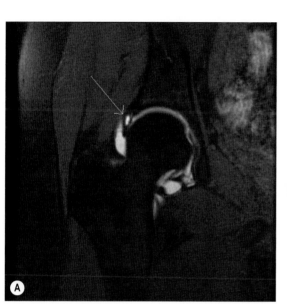

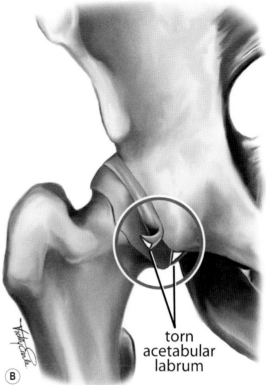

torn
acetabular
labrum

Fig. 5.29 • Actebular labral tear. (A) Arthrogram. (B) Graphic representation of a torn acetabular labrum. Reproduced with permission from Brukner & Khan and the publisher McGraw Hill, 2007.

Load transfer tests. Persistent anterior/anteromedial translation of the femoral head limits the ability of the pelvis to anteriorly tilt during forward bending of the trunk and, if the condition is unilateral, results in a transverse plane rotation of the pelvis and an IPT. Backward bending is also limited and asymmetrical as the anterior structures of the hip are already stretched at the beginning of the motion and restrict further posterior tilt of the pelvis (extension of the hip). During single leg loading, if the femur begins in an anteriorly translated position, an anterior shift will not be felt as the joint is loaded, as the shift has already occurred. If the femoral head is centered in standing, it often shifts anterior/anteromedial as weight is taken through the impaired hip joint. Note that these are the same findings as outlined above; the structural changes commonly occur as a consequence of these same non-optimal strategies.

Form closure, force closure, and motor control. Hypertonicity of the posterior hip abductors (gluteus medius and minimus) and deep hip external rotators combined with hypertonicity of the tensor fascia latae (TFL), rectus femoris (RF), sartorius, and short adductor muscles is common. Notable restriction of flexion/adduction and internal rotation of the hip is present (positive inner quadrant or scour test) and may be associated with a click. Until the hypertonic muscles are released, it is not possible to differentiate the articular cause for this motion restriction (labral tear) from a neuromuscular cause (hypertonicity of muscles preventing full range of motion). Indeed Austin et al (2008) note that there is limited evidence 'supporting various physical examination techniques to identify intra-articular pathology of the hip, particularly acetabular labral tears.' Most authors suggest that consideration of multiple test findings, especially those tests that reproduce the patient's pain and clicking, is necessary to reach a clinical diagnosis. This concurs with our experience. Many times patients will present with magnetic resonance arthrogram (MRA) findings identifying a labral tear, yet their physical presentation is remarkably similar to

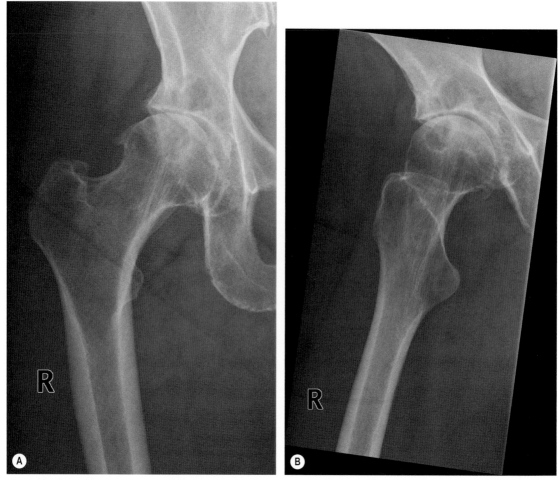

Fig. 5.30 • These (A) anteroposterior and (B) frogleg lateral radiographs of the hip demonstrate superolateral joint space narrowing and sclerosis, large subchondral cysts, and osteophytes consistent with osteoarthritis.

that of someone with an excessively compressed hip joint secondary to muscle imbalances without an associated labral tear.

Diagnostic imaging. The increasing use of diagnostic imaging has led to more frequent diagnoses of acetabular labral tears (Brukner & Khan 2007), yet it is important to note that this finding is likely a structural consequence of the repetitive use of non-optimal strategies for transferring load through the hip. The next structural change with the continued use of non-optimal strategies is progressive degeneration of the hip joint itself (see below).

Treatment. Treatment begins by releasing the hypertonic muscles that are responsible for creating the non-optimal strategy for transferring load through the hip (Chapter 10). Subsequently, training for hip mobility and control, including activation and

coordination of the deep and superficial hip muscles (Chapter 11) followed by integration into functional tasks (Chapter 12), is provided. If pain, clicking, or locking persists and acute flare-ups of pain increase in frequency, consideration should be given for surgical intervention to arthroscopically debride the torn part of the labrum (Hunt et al 2007). Image-guided injections with or without corticosteroid have also been recommended for persistent synovitis of the joint (Hunt et al 2007).

Articular cartilage degeneration

The history. Severe trauma or repetitive microtrauma over prolonged periods of time can lead to structural changes in the articular cartilage and osteoarthritis (Fig. 5.30A,B). When the changes are moderate, the hip can produce pain in a variety of patterns (see Table 5.2) and this pain is often aggravated by activities that load the joint including walking, stair climbing/descent, and squatting. The pain may be worse in the morning or after activity. This individual is often middle aged or older unless there is a history of hip dysplasia. Hip dysplasia and femoroacetabular impingement are widely accepted as major initiators of early hip degeneration (Hunt et al 2007), including labral tears.

Standing posture. When degeneration of the articular surfaces of the hip is moderate to severe, the patient is often reluctant to load through the joint and tends to avoid symmetrical standing postures. The hip may be postured in slight flexion and external rotation on the impaired side.

Load transfer tests. The hip joint that is moderately to severely degenerated will produce rotation and torsions of the pelvis very early in the task. The ability of the individual to single leg load through the impaired hip depends on the intensity of the hip pain and the impact of the painful joint on the neuromuscular control. As the degeneration gets more severe, the level of ability to load the joint decreases.

Form closure, force closure, and motor control. There may be associated muscle imbalances and after the hypertonic muscles are released the true articular deficit becomes apparent.

Degeneration of the hip joint progresses over time such that, in the presence of early pathology, the only objective finding may be a slight limitation of medial rotation, flexion and adduction in 90° of femoral flexion. As the pathology progresses, the range of motion becomes progressively restricted and the pattern is variable. The end feel of an arthritic joint is very hard. The results of the tests for the force closure mechanism are variable and almost always positive. In other words, there are deficits in the neuromuscular behavior and/or integrity of the deep and superficial muscles of the hip, the pattern of which is indeterminate and requires specific assessment (Chapter 8).

Treatment. This section describes the specific therapy indicated for restoring mobility of the hip joint following a traumatic sprain of the joint as this injury can lead to a stiff, fibrotic joint if not properly managed. If the injury results in an intra-articular synovitis, weight bearing will be difficult and the goal of treatment at this time is to reduce the load through the joint such that healing can occur. Clinically, it appears that the best resting position for the painful hip is supine with the painful hip and knee supported on

a bolster. The amplitude of hip flexion depends on where in the range of motion the femoral head is able to center in the acetabulum; this is the goal. Weight bearing activities such as walking, standing, and sitting should be minimized during the first few days. A cane (used with the opposite upper extremity) can help to reduce the loading through the hip joint when vertical.

As the pain and inflammation settles, passive and active range of motion of the joint should be encouraged (Chapter 10). If the patient presents several weeks or months after the initial injury, it is possible that the hip joint has become stiff and fibrotic. A specific mobilization technique is the treatment of choice (Chapter 10). In treatment, the goal is to restore full mobility of the hip with the femoral head centered in the acetabulum such that loads are equally shared between the low back, pelvis, and hip. This will require the patient to be taught ideal strategies for postures and movements necessary for their activities of daily living (Chapters 11, 12) after the stiff hip is mobilized.

Emotional states

As a reminder from Chapter 4, emotional states are influenced by past experiences, beliefs, fears, and attitudes and can significantly impact motor control and consequently affect strategies for function (Hodges & Moseley 2003, Moseley 2007a,b, Moseley & Hodges 2004, Vlaeyen & Linton 2000, Vlaeyen & Vancleef 2007, Waddell 2004).

Negative emotional states such as fear, anxiety, and insecurity can express themselves in maladaptive defensive or aggressive postures, which correlate with altered muscle activity and further strain on the musculoskeletal system.

Clinically, it appears that, if an individual does not have the coping mechanisms necessary to confront their symptoms, they learn to avoid activities that result in pain (Vlaeyen & Linton 2000). This avoidance can persist due to their fear of re-injury or an underlying belief that they are unable to perform because of their condition (fear-avoidance). The neural drive to the muscles of the region can reflect this fear and the muscles can become hypertonic, thereby resulting in excessive compression of the LPH complex, either symmetrically or asymmetrically. This can perpetuate pain and cause peripheral and/or central sensitization of the nervous system (Butler 2000, Butler & Moseley 2003, Moseley & Hodges 2005),

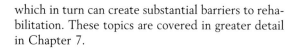

which in turn can create substantial barriers to rehabilitation. These topics are covered in greater detail in Chapter 7.

Summary

In clinical practice, patients present with a combination of the impairments noted in this chapter in a multitude of patterns that may involve all regions (lumbar spine, pelvis, and hip(s)). Clinical reasoning and logic are essential for the development of prescriptive treatment plans and this is covered in detail in the second part of this text. Through a series of case reports, we will revisit most of the above impairments in 'real stories' and demonstrate how the research evidence is considered along with clinical expertise to develop sound hypotheses from which prescriptive treatment plans are derived. Before we get to the clinical part of this text there is one more group of patients to discuss, those who experience persistent impairments and disability as a consequence of pregnancy and delivery; this topic is covered in Chapter 6.

Pregnancy and its potential complications

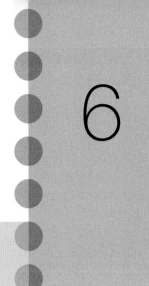

6

Diane Lee

CHAPTER CONTENTS

Prevalence of pelvic girdle pain
and urinary incontinence 129

The impact of pregnancy and delivery
on the pelvis 130

Urinary continence and incontinence 139

Postpartum health for moms – restoring
form and function after pregnancy 144

Summary 144

Every year millions of women deliver babies and go on to lead painfree functional lives; however, there are many who do not. What do we know about the prevalence (percentage in the total population) of pregnancy-related pelvic girdle pain (PRPGP) and the potential postpartum complications, namely the loss of pelvic organ support and urinary incontinence (UI)? This chapter will discuss the prevalence of PRPGP and UI, describe the impact of pregnancy and delivery on multiple systems (passive, active, and control (Panjabi 1992b)), and then discuss UI in greater detail.

Prevalence of pelvic girdle pain and urinary incontinence

Pregnancy-related pelvic girdle pain – prevalence

The prevalence of PRPGP can be difficult to determine from the literature. According to Ostgaard (2007), the true prevalence of pelvic girdle pain (PGP) in the general population is not known; however, in the pregnant population both his studies (Ostgaard et al 1991), as well as those of Albert et al (2002), found a prevalence of approximately 20%. A systematic review (Wu et al 2004) of PRPGP estimates the prevalence of both pelvic girdle and low back pain to be 45% during pregnancy and 25% postpartum. When only 'serious' pain is considered, this number drops to 25%, which is closer to the prevalence reported by Ostgaard et al (1991) and Albert et al (2002). Ostgaard (2007) notes that fortunately the majority of women recover within 3 months of delivery; however, 5–7% do not (Ostgaard & Andersson 1992).

Can we predict who is going to continue having pain postpartum? According to Damen et al (2001), if a woman has greater than 7/10 on a visual analogue pain scale (VAS) and asymmetrical laxity of the sacroiliac joints (SIJs), there is a greater chance that their PRPGP will not resolve. Gutke et al (2007) note that a combination of low back *and* pelvic girdle pain, dissatisfaction at work, and an older maternal age are predictors for non-resolution after delivery. Where is the pain most often felt? Rost et al (2004) studied the pain distribution of 870 postpartum patients and reported that 76% have pain around the SIJ and 57.2% around the pubic symphysis (PS). They found that the pain is not constant and is aggravated by vertical loading tasks such as walking, standing, sitting, and changing positions.

Urinary incontinence – prevalence

What do we know about the prevalence of UI in postpartum women? Wilson et al (2002) followed 7,882 women for up to 7 years after delivery and tracked

DOI: 10.1016/B978-0-443-06963-5.00006-7

the prevalence of UI. At 5–7 years after delivery, 44.6% of the women had some degree of UI. An interesting finding was that, over the 6-year course of this study, 27% of the incontinent women became continent and 31% of continent women became incontinent. This suggests that some women were able to optimize their strategies for load transfer postpartum whereas others were not; their non-optimal strategies led to UI over time. In this study, the biggest predictor for developing and sustaining incontinence postpartum was prepartum incontinence. Again, this suggests that the women used non-optimal strategies for transferring loads through their pelvis prior to becoming pregnant and the experience did not help to restore optimal function.

Pregnancy-related pelvic girdle pain and urinary incontinence – combined prevalence

Is there a relationship between PRPGP and UI? Smith et al (2008) reviewed the data collected in 14,779 younger (age 18–25 years) and 14,099 mid-age (45–50 years) women surveyed in the Australian Longitudinal Study on Women's Health to determine the prevalence of back pain among parous compared to nulliparous women. In addition, they investigated the association between incontinence and back pain among nulliparous, pregnant, and postpartum women. With respect to low back pain (not specifically PGP but both low back and PGP), the pregnant women experienced more back pain than the postpartum or nulliparous women in the younger age group, whereas the middle-aged women did not show any difference in the prevalence for back pain. With respect to incontinence, the findings were the same for both age groups. However, there was a descending order in the prevalence of incontinence with the pregnant group demonstrating the greatest level of incontinence, followed by the non-pregnant parous group, and finally the nulliparous group. Of note, although this is a very large study, there is a significant age group missing as women between the ages of 25 and 45 were not surveyed.

Pool-Goudzwaard et al (2005) conducted a multi-center study in Holland to investigate, in part, the association between, and the prevalence of, pregnancy-related low back/pelvic girdle pain and pelvic floor disorders in women aged 30–50. In this small study of 66 patients, 52% reported a combination of low back and/or pelvic girdle pain along with pelvic floor dysfunction, which included voiding dysfunction, UI, sexual dysfunction, and/or constipation. Of these 52%, 82% stated that their symptoms began with either low back or pelvic girdle pain.

Summary

Pregnancy and delivery appear to increase the risk of developing incontinence in some women of all ages and, in addition, a small number will continue to have pelvic girdle pain after the 3-month postpartum period.

The impact of pregnancy and delivery on the pelvis

Considering the anatomical changes that occur in the abdominal canister during the 9 months of pregnancy and the forces and potential trauma to the passive, active, and control systems of the lumbopelvis, it is understandable that long-term changes in both anatomy and function occur, and it is amazing that the prevalence is not higher. What happens to each of the systems during pregnancy and delivery and how do these changes impact on the function of the pelvis and its organs for postpartum women?

The passive system

During pregnancy, the joints of the pelvic girdle become lax secondary to relaxation of the ligaments of the SIJs and the PS (Brooke 1930, Buyruk et al 1999, Damen et al 2001, Hagen 1974, Kristiansson 1997, Young 1940). This process begins during the fourth month and continues until the seventh month of pregnancy, following which only a slight increase in mobility occurs. Great variation in the degree of both transverse and superoinferior widening of the PS has been noted radiologically (Brooke 1930, Hagen 1974), with the average increase being 5mm. Although widening of the PS is universally found in postpartum women (Wurdinger et al 2002), a correlation between this widening and pelvic pain either during pregnancy or in the postpartum phase has not been found (Ostgaard 1997, 2007, Wurdinger et al 2002). Similarly, Damen et al (2002b) have shown no statistical correlation between increased laxity of the SIJs and pelvic pain in pregnancy. There is a correlation, however, between asymmetrical laxity of the SIJ and pelvic pain in pregnancy (Damen et al 2001).

According to Hagen (1974), relaxation of the pelvic girdle in pregnancy is due to the presence of a specific high-molecular-weight hormone, relaxin, which together with estrogen causes

> depolymerization of hyaluronic acid ... Compressive, shearing and tensile forces constitute a chronic trauma increasing the concentration of hyaluronidase ... This interferes with the humoral conditions needed for pelvic stability and very likely also plays a certain role as a pathogenetic factor in pelvic relaxation.

Marnach et al (2003) did not find a correlation between any of the pregnancy-related hormone levels (including relaxin) and the presence of joint laxity; therefore the evidence is conflicting as to what causes relaxation of the joints of the pelvis during pregnancy. It is commonly thought that articular mobility is increased during this time secondary to increasing weight of the trunk and rising intra-abdominal pressure. The anatomical changes associated with pregnancy are universal and often occur without symptoms (Damen et al 2001, 2002b).

The active system

The fascia of the abdominal wall, low back, and pelvic floor plays a crucial role in the transference of loads through the trunk (Barker et al 2006, Barker & Briggs 2007, DeLancey et al 2003, Dietz & Steensma 2006, Hodges et al 2007, Pool-Goudzwaard et al 2004). The anterior abdominal fascia, in particular the linea alba, and the endopelvic fascia are at risk for excessive stretching and/or tearing during pregnancy and delivery. Although the endopelvic fascia has received considerable investigation (see below), the linea alba has not.

Linea alba and diastasis rectus abdominis

Universally, the most obvious visible change during pregnancy is the expansion of the abdominal wall. Some abdomens accommodate this stretch very well with no residual damage to either the skin or the underlying fascia, including the linea alba. In others, the damage appears extensive (Fig. 6.1). One structure particularly affected by the expansion of the abdomen is the linea alba, the complex connective

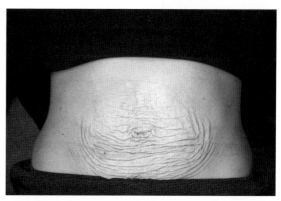

Fig. 6.1 • This postpartum woman has extensive damage to the skin, superficial and deep abdominal fascia, and the linea alba as a consequence of her two pregnancies.

tissue that connects the left and right abdominal muscles (Figs 3.45, 3.46, 3.47). The width of the linea alba is known as the inter-recti distance and varies along the length from the xyphoid to the PS. According to Rath et al (1996), in women below the age of 45, the inter-recti distance at a point half-way between the umbilicus and the xyphoid (UX point) should measure no more than 1.0cm (Fig. 6.2A), 2.7cm at a point just above the umbilicus (U point) (Fig. 6.2B) and 0.9cm at a point half-way between the PS and umbilicus (PU point) (Fig. 6.2C). After the age of 45, these measures increase to 1.5cm (UX), 1.7cm (U), and 1.4 cm (PU), respectively. A diastasis of the rectus abdominis (DRA) (separation of the left and right rectus abdominis muscles and widening of the linea alba) is diagnosed when the width exceeds this amount (Fig. 6.3A–C).

There is little research on this condition; Boissonnault & Blaschak (1988) found that 27% of women have a DRA in the second trimester and 66% in the third trimester of pregnancy. Fifty-three percent of these women continued to have a DRA immediately postpartum and 36% remained abnormally wide at 5–7 weeks' postpartum. Coldron et al (2008) measured the inter-recti distance from 1 day to 1 year postpartum and noted that the distance decreased markedly from day 1 to 8 weeks, and that without any intervention (e.g. exercise training or other physiotherapy) there was no further closure at the end of the first year. In the urogynecological population, 52% of patients were found to have a DRA (Spitznagle et al 2007). Sixty-six percent of these women had at least one support-related pelvic floor dysfunction (stress urinary incontinence (SUI), fecal incontinence, and/or pelvic organ prolapse).

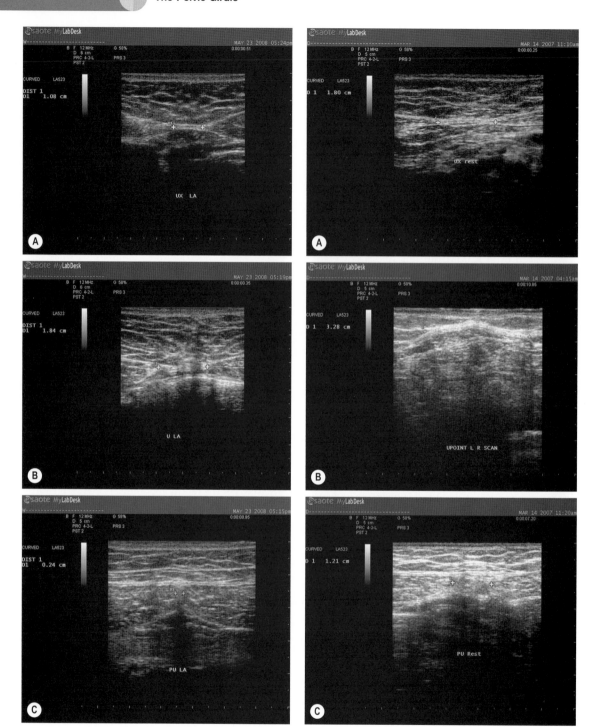

Fig. 6.2 • These are three ultrasound images of a normal linea alba in a nulliparous woman. (A) Supraumbilical region between the umbilicus and the xyphoid. (B) Just above the umbilicus. (C) Infraumbilical region between the pubic symphysis and the umbilicus below the transition zone (Chapter 3).

Fig. 6.3 • These are three ultrasound images of diastasis rectus abdominis in a multiparous woman. (A) Supraumbilical region between the umbilicus and the xyphoid. (B) Just above the umbilicus. (C) Infraumbilical region between the pubic symphysis and the umbilicus below the transition zone (Chapter 3).

Summary

Separation of the abdominal wall occurs in many women in the third trimester of pregnancy and, without intervention, many do not return to normal width by 1 year. There appears to be a correlation between support-related pelvic floor dysfunction and DRA in over 50% of the urogynecological population. Could this be the impact of using non-optimal strategies for transferring loads?

There are no studies yet to guide clinicians towards the best treatment for postpartum women with DRA. Clinically, it appears that some women with DRA are able to generate sufficient force closure of the low back and pelvis and fully recover function even though the inter-recti distance remains wider than normal (see case report Melissa, Chapter 9 🖰). Others, with the same increase in inter-recti width, fail to regain function; in other words, all strategies fail to provide stability for the low back/pelvis during multiple loading tasks (see case report Christy, Chapter 9 🖰). The differentiating factor does not appear to be the width of the linea alba and research is planned that will allow us to accurately predict who will require surgery and who will not. Currently, it appears that as long as

1. forces can be transmitted through the linea alba (i.e. tension can be generated between the left and right rectus abdominis, Video 8.7 🖰); and
2. the forces are sufficient to stabilize the joints of the low thorax, lumbar spine, and pelvis, function can be restored *regardless* of the inter-recti distance. In other words, the goal is not to close the diastasis but rather to generate tension through it.

Video 6.1 🖰 is a video clip of a postpartum woman with DRA who participated in our Postpartum Health for Moms program (www.discoverphysio.ca). There is a significant change in the tension of the linea alba noted both on palpation and ultrasound imaging (increased echogenicity) from 8 weeks to 1 year postpartum. Although the inter-recti distance did not change significantly with this training, her function certainly improved. Watch Video 6.2 🖰 to observe a session with a woman with DRA who is 8 days' postpartum. The sooner an optimal strategy for transferring loads between the thorax and the pelvis is restored, the better. Video 6.3 🖰 is a session with the same woman 4

months later. Her linea alba is still significantly separated just above, at, and below the umbilicus and this structural deficit appears to be compromising her ability to stabilize the L3–4 segment during flexion and rotation loading tasks. Although tension can be felt in the linea alba during:

(a) a curl-up task; and even more strongly during
(b) a pre-contraction of the deep system prior to a curl-up task;

it does not take much force through her elevated arms to overcome her ability to stabilize her thorax on her pelvis. The force closure mechanism for control at L3–4 has been compromised by the structural deficit in the active system (DRA). The assessment tests demonstrated in these video clips, and the interpretation of the ultrasound imaging, are described in Chapter 8 and the postural training in standing in Chapter 12.

Surgical abdominoplasty has been noted to reduce back pain in patients with DRA (Toranto 1988), although the mechanism is unknown. Marin Valladolid et al (2004) found that the intra-abdominal pressure (IAP) increased by 31% in healthy women who underwent an abdominoplasty for cosmetic reasons (no DRA). In women with DRA, this increase in IAP may facilitate stabilization of the lumbopelvis by increasing tension in the anterior and posterior fascial systems.

It is important to note that an abdominoplasty to correct a DRA can also create problems if consideration is not given to how much the abdominal wall is tightened. Watch Video 8.5a 🖰 to view the behavior of a healthy linea alba (at the U point) during a curl-up task and then watch Video 6.4 🖰, an ultrasound image of the midline anterior abdominal wall and linea alba during a curl-up task in a woman who had an abdominoplasty to repair her DRA and consequently developed difficulty breathing and increased midthoracic pain. Note how her left and right rectus abdominis overlap at all three points – UX, U, and PU – and there is essentially no linea alba. There was insufficient 'flexibility' in the abdominal wall to allow lateral costal expansion of her rib cage or rotation of her thorax.

The endopelvic fascia – paravaginal and rectovaginal defects

There is more research on the fascia of the pelvic floor (endopelvic fascia), which is a very complex and important structure for pelvic floor function and pelvic organ support (see Chapter 3 for an anatomical review). The majority of injuries to the endopelvic fascia are thought to occur during a vaginal delivery, although defects have also been found in nulliparous women.

Ashton-Miller & DeLancey (2009) note that the pubovisceral muscle undergoes a stretch ratio of 3.26 at the end of the second stage of labor; in other words, this muscle stretches over three times its resting length. Dietz & Lanzarone (2005) studied the prevalence of major trauma to the pubovisceral muscles (see Fig. 3.56B) with 3D perineal ultrasound in primiparous women 1–4 weeks before delivery and then 2–6 months' postpartum. Thirty-six percent of the women who delivered vaginally had an avulsion of the pubovisceral muscle and their postpartum stress urinary incontinence was thought to be directly related to this avulsion. Specifically, they found the avulsion to occur at the inferomedial aspect of the pubovisceral muscle where it inserts into the arcus tendineus fascia pelvis (Figs 6.4, 6.5). This deficit can lead to a prolapse of the bladder (cystocele, Fig. 6.6A–C).

What impact does this avulsion have on the strength of the pubovisceral muscle? Dietz & Shek (2007) investigated the relationship between levator avulsion (diagnosed with both clinical palpation and 3D ultrasound) and clinical grading of levator ani muscle strength (Oxford grading scale) in 1,112 postpartum women. The prevalence of avulsion was 23% in this group and was associated with a highly significant reduction in the overall Oxford grading; in other words, the muscle tested weak.

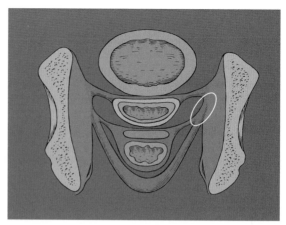

Fig. 6.5 • The circle on this illustration denotes the location of disruption of the rectovaginal fascia and the puborectalis muscle. Redrawn from Retzky & Rogers, 1995.

They also found that older women were more at risk for this avulsion (Dietz & Simpson 2007).

The impact of a vaginal delivery on the rectovaginal fascia (see Figs 3.58, 3.59) has also been investigated via perineal ultrasound. The lateral insertion of the rectovaginal fascia may be torn off the puborectalis muscle (see Fig. 6.5) and transverse tears can open up in the fascia during the crowning of the baby's head (Fig. 6.7) (Dietz & Steensma 2005). Alternately, the rectovaginal fascia may detach from the perineal body. This detachment destabilizes the perineal body as the continuity between the cardinal and uterosacral ligaments, the rectovaginal septum, and the perineal body is lost (Cundiff & Fenner 2004). The perineal body is no longer suspended from the sacrum (Chapter 3) and hypermobility of the perineal body can result. On perineal ultrasound, a true defect of the rectovaginal fascia can be seen in the mid-sagittal plane as herniation of the rectal wall and rectal contents (if any) into the vagina at the level of the anorectal junction (Fig. 6.8).

To further analyze the role of a vaginal delivery in producing these rectovaginal fascial defects, Dietz & Steensma (2006) used perineal ultrasound imaging to assess the state of the levator ani and its related fascia during a maximum Valsalva maneuver (Fig. 6.9) in primiparous women 1–4 weeks before a vaginal delivery and 2–6 months afterwards. Prior to delivery of their first child, two women (of 68 in total) were found to have a rectovaginal fascial defect and a true rectocele and this number increased to eight women after childbirth. In a small percentage (6/68) a new

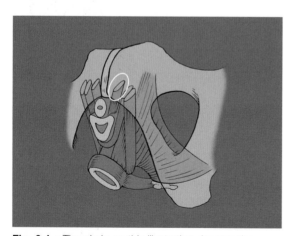

Fig. 6.4 • The circle on this illustration denotes the location where Dietz & Lanzarone (2005) found a high prevalence of avulsion of the pubovisceral muscle after vaginal delivery. Redrawn from Ashton-Miller and DeLancey, 2007.

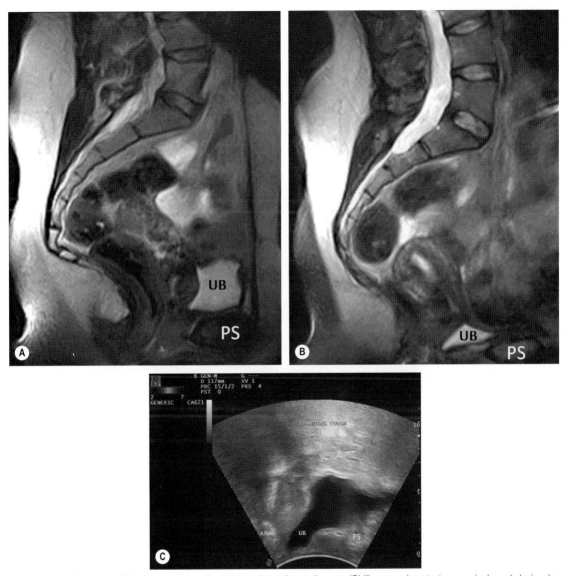

Fig. 6.6 • (A) This is a MRI of a woman with stress urinary incontinence (SUI) secondary to trauma induced during her vaginal delivery. This image is a sagittal slice of her pelvis in the midline taken when she is lying supine. Note that the bladder (UB) rests on the pubic symphysis (PS) as it should. (B) This MRI is of the same woman in standing. Note how her bladder has 'slid' off the pubic symphysis and is well below the level of the levator ani and PS. (C) This is an ultrasound image (perineal view) of the same woman in standing. The image is captured during the peak of her cough. A large deficit of the posterior bladder and urethral support is evident.

rectocele was caused by the vaginal delivery. The authors concluded from this study that rectocele can exist in nulliparous women (a previous study had found a prevalence of 12% in this group (Dietz & Clarke 2005)) but did not know why. Possibly, longstanding non-optimal strategies for load transfer could create fascial laxity and/or tearing. Alternately, myofascial trauma incurred through sport, such as falling straddle on a balance beam in gymnastics or across a bicycle bar, could be responsible.

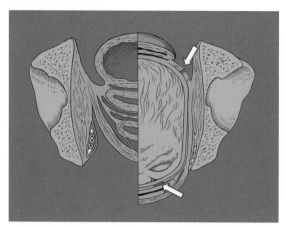

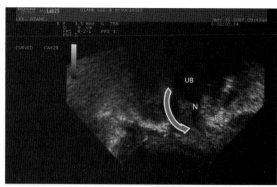

Fig. 6.7 • Excessive stretching of the birth canal during a vaginal delivery potentially causes tears in the endopelvic fascia anteriorly and rectovaginal fascia posteriorly (arrows), as well as compression of the pudendal vessels and nerve. Redrawn from Retzky & Rogers, 1995.

Fig. 6.9 • This is a perineal ultrasound image of the pelvic structures during a Valsalva maneuver in a multiparous woman with a rectocele. Note the descent of the rectal and posterior vaginal structures during this maneuver. See videos of perineal ultrasound imaging in Chapters 8 and 9 for a comparison of normal versus abnormal responses. N, bladder neck; PS, pubic symphysis; UB, urinary bladder.

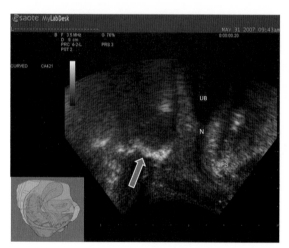

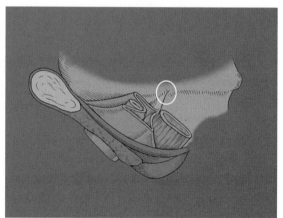

Fig. 6.8 • This is a perineal ultrasound image of the pelvic structures at rest (see Fig. 8.92A for a review of the normal pelvic structures seen via perineal ultrasound imaging). Note the hyperechogenicity of the rectal fascia (arrow) suggesting increased tension in this structure. This is commonly seen when there is a rectocele. N, bladder neck; PS, pubic symphysis; UB, urinary bladder.

Fig. 6.10 • The circle on this illustration indicates the location of disruption of the rectovaginal fascia from the arcus tendineus fascia pelvis (ATFP). Redrawn from Leffler et al, 2001.

While investigating the structural integrity of the urethral and anterior vaginal wall support system during surgery for cystourethrocele and SUI, DeLancey (2002) found paravaginal defects of the arcus tendineus fascia pelvis in only 3% of 71 women (as opposed to 36% and 23% found in Dietz's studies).

However, in 97.6% of these women, detachments of the arcus tendineus fascia pelvis (ATFP) were found posteriorly from the *ischial spine* (Fig. 6.10). He concluded that the ATFP usually detaches from the ischial spine and not from the pubis, and that the detachment tends to occur bilaterally. In this study, slightly more than 50% of the 71 women also had visible abnormalities in the pubococcygeal muscles including generalized atrophy and occasionally 'strips of muscles that were missing.' In several women, the loss of muscle was so great that the superior aspect of the perineal membrane could be seen from the space of Retzius. DeLancey found that a dorsal detachment of the arcus from the ischial spine was associated with anterior vaginal wall descent, and he felt that the paravaginal defect most often arises because the connection between the ATFP and the ischial spine becomes detached allowing the vagina to swing caudally (Fig. 6.11A,B). Detachment would subsequently compromise the stiffness of the suburethral tissues, and this would have a significant impact on continence (more on DeLancey's hammock hypothesis of continence to follow).

Regardless of what has let go or avulsed, any significant loss of the fascial support can have consequences to the function of the pelvic floor complex, both in terms of postural support/control of the pelvis and low back as well as organ support and continence. The symptoms that are most strongly associated with a true rectocele diagnosed via perineal ultrasound imaging are:

- incomplete emptying of the bowel;
- assisted evacuation with digitation (Dietz & Korda 2005);
- pelvic pressure;
- the need to splint the perineum to defecate; or
- impaired sexual relations, difficult defecation, and fecal incontinence (Cundiff & Fenner 2004).

Summary

Defects of the endopelvic fascia and its associated muscles both anteriorly and posteriorly have been noted in a significant number of postpartum women. The loss of the myofascial integrity will have consequences for organ support, continence, and postural support/control.

As a clinician, what is the best way to diagnose these defects so that they may be appropriately referred for surgical correction if necessary? Dietz et al (2006, Dietz & Shek 2008) compared intravaginal palpation to 4D perineal ultrasound imaging to see if clinical palpation could detect the fascial abnormalities of the inferomedial aspect of the pubovisceral muscle. Unfortunately, there was a poor correlation in that the anatomical abnormalities were missed (2006) or not agreed on (2008) by vaginal palpation. Two-dimensional perineal ultrasound is a more affordable option for clinical physiotherapists and is showing promise (Peng et al 2006, 2007) for a more specific diagnosis of pelvic floor muscle function; however, more research is needed using this tool in comparison to the 4D imaging studies. Perineal imaging for pelvic floor function is discussed in Chapter 8, a skill well worth investigating if you work with the postpartum population, especially those with pelvic floor dysfunction.

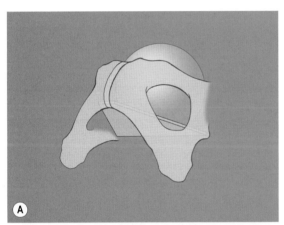

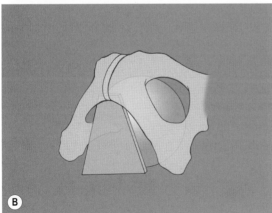

Fig. 6.11 • (A) When the endopelvic fascia is intact the organs of the pelvis are well supported. (B) When the lateral suspension between the vagina, rectum, and the arcus tendineus fascia pelvis (ATFP) is lost (dorsal detachment of the arcus from the ischial spine) the vagina and rectum swing caudally. Redrawn from DeLancey, 2002.

The control system

A constant low level of electromyography (EMG) activity in the levator ani has been noted in standing (Hodges et al 2007). In a postural perturbation study using a repetitive arm movement paradigm (Bouisset

& Zattara 1981), *increased* activity of the pelvic floor muscles was noted (via anal and vaginal EMG) *before* any activity was recorded in the deltoid (Smith et al 2007a,b). With respect to the *direction* of arm movement, there was no difference noted in the EMG activity of the levator ani; in other words, the activation of the levator ani was non-direction dependent. The increase in the intra-abdominal pressure occurred *after* the increase in anal pressure, which suggests that the anal pressure is *not* due to transmission of pressure from the abdominal cavity but more likely due to the contraction of the levator ani. In quiet breathing, the modulation of the pelvic floor EMG was linked to activity of transversus abdominis and was greatest during expiration.

There have been no studies investigating the behavior of either transversus abdominis or the pelvic floor in pregnancy. Clinically, in a healthy pregnancy, these deep muscles appear to continue to function in synergy (Fig. 6.12A,B, Video 6.5 , see case report Christy, Chapter 9, Videos CD12, CD13). Several studies have investigated the control system (behavior of the pelvic floor and abdominal wall) in subjects with either pelvic girdle pain and/or incontinence and will be discussed below.

The viscera

The pelvic viscera include the primary organs of the pelvic girdle namely the sigmoid colon, uterus (together with the ovaries and fallopian tubes), and bladder, as well as all the ligaments and fascial connections that support them. Impairments of this system include:

- altered pelvic organ position due to:
  - ○ ligamentous or fascial laxity, tears, or altered tensions in the suspensory system. Pregnancy results in all the uterine ligaments being distended sometimes up to four times their normal length (Barral 1993);
  - ○ hormonal changes (progesterone levels);
  - ○ turgor effect of abdominal organs (predominantly gas);
  - ○ turgor effect of pelvic organs (predominantly fluid);
  - ○ altered pressure gradients between pulmonary, abdominal, and pelvic cavities (Barral 1993);
- altered organ mobility due to:
  - ○ adhesions or restrictions secondary to;
  - ○ infection;
  - ○ surgery;
  - ○ trauma (vaginal delivery, pelvic fractures, blunt trauma);
  - ○ visceral spasm (increased tone in smooth muscle fibers of colon or bladder);
- altered organ function including but not limited to:
  - ○ inflammatory organ conditions such as cystitis, enteritis, or prostatitis;
  - ○ infective conditions (urinary tract);
  - ○ endometriosis;
  - ○ fibroids/tumors/cysts.

The Barral Institute (www.barralinstitute.com) offers a full series of courses in visceral anatomy, assessment,

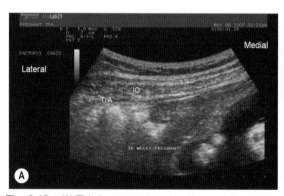
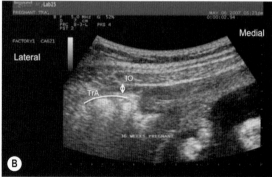

Fig. 6.12 • (A) This is a transabdominal view of the right anterolateral abdominal wall of a woman 36 weeks' pregnant prior to a command to contract the transversus abdominis (TrA) muscle. (B) This is the same view of the same abdomen in response to a verbal cue to contract the TrA muscle. Note the lateral slide, the corseting (line), and the broadening of TrA (double-headed arrow) in response to the contraction – an ideal response. See this optimal response in Video 6.5 .

and treatment in an osteopathic approach, which address organ position, mobility, and function. The specifics of this approach are beyond the scope of this book, yet highly recommended by the author.

Urinary continence and incontinence

Urinary incontinence (UI) is defined as the involuntary leakage of urine (Abrams et al 2002). Stress urinary incontinence (SUI) (leakage that occurs during physical exertion) is the most common type. Urge urinary incontinence (UUI) is defined as leakage that is precipitated by a sudden strong urge or desire to void and often occurs along with SUI (mixed or MUI). Cundiff (2004) presents an interesting historical perspective on how the various theories of causation of UI have evolved as well as the subsequent surgical treatment.

The prevalence of UI in the postpartum population has been presented above (44.6%). Nygaard et al (1994) note that this condition is not limited to women bearing children and that in a study of 144 nulliparous female athletes aged 18–21 years, 28% suffered from SUI. Bø & Borgen (2001) found that 41% of elite female athletes experience SUI. Fantl et al (1996) state that incontinence affects four out of 10 women, about one out of 10 men, and about 17% of children below the age of 15. Clearly, this is a significant problem for both nulliparous and parous women, and some men; given the findings of Pool-Goudzwaard et al (2005) and Smith et al (2006), this problem should not be considered separately from the lumbopelvic pain population.

In two excellent review articles, Ashton-Miller et al (2001, 2007) explain the mechanism by which continence is achieved during functional tasks. Essentially, continence relies on optimal function of two systems – the urethral support system and the urethral sphincter closure system.

Urinary continence – the urethral support system

The structures that provide support for the urethra include:

1. the passive system: this includes the endopelvic fascia, which is a dense fibromuscular layer that includes fibroblasts, α-smooth muscle cells, and elastin as well as type III collagen, which are all loosely organized to provide an elastic fibromuscular layer (Cundiff & Fenner 2004). This layer surrounds the vagina and attaches it to the arcus tendineus fascia pelvis laterally. At the top of the vagina, this layer blends with the cardinal and uterosacral ligaments, which attach posteriorly and cranially to the presacral fascia, thus suspending the vagina over the levator ani. The endopelvic fascia posterior to the vagina (between it and the rectum) is called the rectovaginal septum and extends to the perineal body caudally and to the arcus tendineus fascia pelvis and arcus tendineus levator ani laterally through the arcus tendineus fascia rectovaginalis (see Figs 6.5, 6.10). In the horizontal plane, the arcus tendineus fascia pelvis and the arcus tendineus fascia levator ani are suspended and anchored between the pubic bone anteriorly and the ischial spine posteriorly. This three-dimensional honeycomb web supports and suspends the urethra, vagina, and rectum, and the integrity of this fascial web is essential for continence and pelvic organ position;

2. the active system: this system supports and reduces tension in this three-dimensional fascial hammock and includes the levator ani (pubovisceralis, pubococcygeus, puborectalis, iliococcygeus) and the ischiococcygeus muscles. These muscles contain primarily type 1 (slow twitch) fibers and exhibit constant resting tone (Hodges et al 2007). There are a few type 2 fibers that allow an appropriate response of the pelvic floor to sudden increases in intra-abdominal pressure during a cough, sneeze, or sudden lift;

3. the control system: this system includes the pudendal nerve and direct branches from S3 and S4, which innervate the levator ani, as well as the central control mechanism, which coordinates the feedforward/feedback responses between the viscera and the musculoskeletal system.

Together, the passive, active, and control systems form a dynamic hammock of support for the urethra (Fig. 6.13), and the integrity and function of these systems is essential if continence is to be preserved during tasks that increase intra-abdominal pressure. If the fibromuscular layer gives way easily because of an active system deficit or if the layer is not stiffened at the right time or with the right amount of force secondary to a control system deficit (delayed timing of pelvic floor muscle (PFM) contraction or

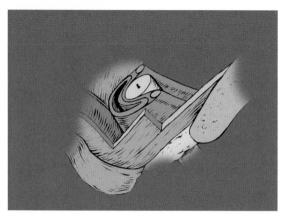

Fig. 6.13 • The hammock of support for the urethra depends on the integrity of the endopelvic fascia and its lateral extensions to the arcus tendineus fascia pelvis (ATFP) as well as the proper activation of the levator ani that supports it. Redrawn from DeLancey, 1994.

weakness), the hammock will fail to provide an adequate backstop against which the urethra can be compressed. Ashton-Miller et al (2001) provide an analogy that is very useful for educating incontinent patients. Imagine a garden hose (the urethra) with water (urine) running through it lying on a trampoline bed (the pelvic floor). Stepping on the hose will block the flow of water if the bed is very stiff and provides an equal and opposite counterforce (functional pelvic floor). If the bed is very flexible (i.e. there is loss of myofascial support), the downward pressure on the hose will cause the bed; to stretch and allow the hose to indent the bed, meanwhile the flow of water will continue uninterrupted. The flexibility of the bed is determined by the contraction of the muscles of the pelvic floor as well as the stiffness of the fascia to which the muscles attach. If the muscles are weak, or do not contract at the right time, or if the fascia is lax or torn, the bed will not become stiff enough in time to prevent the water from running through the hose (DeLancey 2002, DeLancey et al 2007).

Urinary continence – the urethral sphincter closure system

In addition to extrinsic compression of the urethra due to contraction of the levator ani and intra-abdominal pressure, the urethra is intrinsically closed by a system of muscles both intrinsic and extrinsic to the urethra itself. The urethra contains a complex system of both striated and smooth muscle, and together with the vascular elements within the sub-mucosa these muscles contribute to resting urethra closure pressure. The striated sphincter muscles, namely the extrinsic compressor urethra and urethro-vaginal sphincter, are also composed of type 1 fibers and are well suited to maintain constant tone. Resting urethral closure pressures are higher in continent women than incontinent, and the resting closure pressures are affected by age (Hilton & Stanton 1983).

Constantinou & Govan (1982) measured the intraurethral and intrabladder pressures in healthy continent women during both a Valsalva maneuver and a cough and found that, during a cough, the intraurethral pressure increases approximately 250ms before any pressure increase is detected in the bladder. This did not occur during a Valsalva (bearing down or straining). This suggests an anticipatory reflex between the pelvic floor and urethra. Thind et al (1991) confirmed this anticipatory closure of the urethra. They also noted that the urethral pressure remained elevated for a short time after the pressure normalized in the bladder.

Bø & Stein (1994) used needle EMG to measure activity in the wall of the urethra during a cough and Valsalva, as well as during activation of the hip adductors, abdominals, and gluteal muscles. They found that the urethral wall contracted synergistically with the pelvic floor, hip adductors, and gluteals and also during a cough. They concluded that strengthening the pelvic floor will also strengthen the urethral wall; but will it restore the anticipatory reflex mechanism?

Sapsford et al (2001) investigated the coactivation pattern of the pelvic floor and abdominals via fine-wire EMG for the abdominal wall and surface EMG for the pelvic floor, and found that the abdominals contract in response to a pelvic floor contraction command and that the pelvic floor contracts in both a 'hollowing' and 'bracing' abdominal command. They also found that a submaximal command of pubococcygeus elicited the *greatest* response in transversus abdominis. The results from this research suggest that the pelvic floor can be facilitated by coactivating the deep abdominals and vice versa. However, it is wrong to assume that all patients will be able to contract the muscles of the pelvic floor through verbal commands alone, through either abdomen or the pelvic floor. Bump et al (1991) found that only 50% of women could actually perform a pelvic floor muscle contraction with just a verbal instruction. Careful analysis is required to ensure that the reflex connection between the transversus abdominis and the pelvic floor is intact before this strategy is used.

Stress urinary incontinence

Stress urinary incontinence can result when there is loss of the integrity, or function, of the pelvic floor (muscles and fascia) secondary to a major trauma or microtrauma over prolonged periods of time. Non-optimal strategies for transferring load through the pelvis can lead to incontinence, particularly those which excessively increase the intra-abdominal pressure (Smith et al 2007a,b, Thompson et al 2006) and result in the bladder being repetitively compressed inferiorly. Non-optimal strategies include:

- abdominal bulging and breath-holding (see Fig. 8.42);
- excessive oblique abdominal activation with thoracolumbar flexion and posterior pelvic tilt (see Fig. 8.41B,C);
- excessive erector spinae activation with thoracolumbar extension and anterior pelvic tilt (see Fig. 8.40).

When the bladder is observed with transabdominal ultrasound imaging, these strategies appear to cause excessive bladder motion. In a group of pelvic girdle pain patients, O'Sullivan et al (2002) noticed through transabdominal ultrasound imaging that the bladder descended during an ASLR test. When compression was applied to the pelvic girdle, this descent was minimized.

How much descent of the bladder is optimal, or normal, during functional activities? Peschers et al (2001) measured the mobility of the bladder neck via perineal ultrasound during a Valsalva and cough in 39 healthy nulliparous women (Videos 8.11, 8.12). They found that the bladder neck descended a variable amount (2–32mm) in both a Valsalva and cough, and questioned the long-held view that SUI was associated with urethral mobility. Like the SIJ (Buyruk et al 1995b), there appears to be a wide variation in the amount of motion possible and continence relies more on control and urethral closure rather than amplitude of motion of the urethra.

Howard et al (2000) investigated descent of the bladder neck during a cough and Valsalva in three groups of women: nulliparous continent (17 subjects), primiparous continent (18 subjects), and primiparous incontinent (23 subjects). There was no statistical difference in the amount of bladder neck mobility between the groups, again suggesting that movement of the urethra is not what determines one's continence status. When they compared the amount of bladder neck movement during a cough and Valsalva, they noted that in the two continent groups there was less movement during a cough. The incontinent group conversely demonstrated no difference in the amount of movement during either task. Clearly, something was happening during a cough in the continent women that was not happening in the incontinent group. All three groups generated the same amount of cough pressures; however, the stiffness value (pressure change divided by bladder neck mobility) was greatest in the nulliparous continent group, second highest in the primiparous continent group, and lowest in the primiparous incontinent group. Howard et al (2000) hypothesize that the reason for these differences is a functional pelvic floor in the continent women. They showed that stiffness of the pelvic floor was much less in incontinent women than in continent women. They propose that the compliant pelvic floor in the incontinent women provides less resistance to deformation during the transient increases in intra-abdominal pressure (the trampoline bed goes down) such that urethral closure cannot be ensured and stress incontinence becomes possible. Thind et al (1991) noted that the amplitude of the anticipatory pressure rise in the urethra was less in women with SUI and suggest that this is due to *weakness* of the pelvic floor, but perhaps a compliant or more flexible floor could also be the cause.

Allen et al (1990) investigated 96 nulliparous women both prenatally and postpartum to determine if childbirth caused damage to the pelvic floor muscles and/or its nerve supply. They showed that a vaginal delivery impairs the strength of the pelvic floor and noted that recovery had not occurred at 2 months postpartum. They also demonstrated via needle EMG that vaginal delivery caused a partial denervation of the pelvic floor in 80% of these women. Women who had a long, active second stage of labor showed the most EMG evidence of denervation. Ashton-Miller et al (2001, 2007) feel that if the nerve to the levator ani is damaged the denervated muscles will atrophy, thus placing more stress on the passive supporting structures (endopelvic fascia), which over time will stretch and result in organ prolapse. Alternately, as noted above, a paravaginal defect can occur, which causes a separation in the endopelvic fascia. This effectively reduces the stiffness of the fascial layer that supports the urethra and can occur unilaterally or bilaterally. When this occurs, the pelvic floor must take over to support the organ position and provide active closure to the urethra. However, they note 'if the muscle is completely detached from the fascial tissues, then it may be able to contract; but that contraction may not be effective in elevating the urethra or stabilizing its position' (Ashton-Miller et al 2001).

Bø et al (1990) demonstrated in a randomized clinical trial that retraining the function of the pelvic floor (awareness training coupled with strength and endurance training) is effective for some women (60%) in the treatment of SUI. However, it is important to note that 40% of the women in this study did not improve with just exercises for strengthening the pelvic floor muscles.

Deindl et al (1994) compared the activity pattern of pubococcygeus in nulliparous continent and parous stress urinary incontinent women. They found two differences in the incontinent group:

1. a voluntary 'squeeze' of the pubococcygeus showed an endurance deficit (shorter holding times); and
2. an asymmetrical and uncoordinated pattern of activation (left versus right) commonly occurred. Sometimes the response was only unilateral.

Barbic et al (2003) also investigated the pattern and timing of muscle activation of the levator ani in both continent and incontinent women. They found that both the left and right levator ani contracted prior to any pressure increase in the bladder and that the timing of this activation was delayed in the incontinent group. They concluded that an important aspect of a

> stable bladder neck is the timely activation of the levator ani muscle. The activation, which precedes the contraction of other muscles . . . , might enable a pretension of the endopelvic fascia tissue, which becomes less compliant for stretching by downward forces of increased abdominal pressure.

Is there a difference in the timing of activation of the pelvic floor in incontinent women? Smith et al (2007b) repeated the trunk perturbation study of Hodges et al (2007) using the repetitive arm movement paradigm in 16 women with SUI and compared the results to a group of normal continent controls. During shoulder flexion and extension, the EMG activity of the pelvic floor increased before the onset of anterior deltoid in the continent women (confirming the findings of Hodges et al (2007)); however, the EMG activity of the pelvic floor increased *after* the onset of deltoid in women with SUI. There was a timing delay in the activation of the levator ani in response to the postural perturbation. These findings confirm those of the earlier study of Barbic et al (2003).

In the same study, Smith et al (2007a) had both groups repeat the task with a full bladder and found there were no differences in the two groups. The EMG activity of the pelvic floor *decreased* in both the continent and incontinent group when the bladder was moderately full. Interestingly, the EMG activity of the superficial abdominals and the erector spinae increased. This would certainly make it a challenge to remain continent. Of note, they found that the raw EMG activity of the pelvic floor was greater in women with SUI, even though it has been found that in women with SUI these muscles are 'weak' (Bø 2003, Deindl et al 1994, Mørkved et al 2004).

In the previous study (Smith et al 2007a), the applied postural perturbations were predictable. The subjects moved their arm rapidly in response to a randomly changing light color (different color of light was assigned a different direction of movement). In part of a subsequent study (Smith et al 2007b), the predictability of the task was removed. The subjects were blindfolded and a 1-kg weight was dropped 30cm unpredictably into a bucket held in their outstretched arms. The EMG activity of several muscles was recorded during this task and the following was found. The raw EMG of the pelvic floor was increased in both the mildly and severely incontinent group of women. The raw EMG of the external oblique muscle was also greater in the women with severe SUI. In response to a sudden load, the severely incontinent group chose a strategy that increased the activation of the external oblique and the pelvic floor. This combination of increased pelvic floor EMG and external oblique EMG would increase intra-abdominal and intravesical pressure and certainly pose a greater challenge for continence. The EMG responses were greater for both the continent and the incontinent subjects and Smith et al (2007b) suggest that the nervous system overestimates the required activity when the perturbation is unexpected.

These findings certainly challenge the premise that incontinence is only associated with reduced or weak pelvic floor muscles and suggest that non-optimal strategies for load transfer through the entire abdominal canister may be important in the treatment of SUI. This is supported by Thompson et al (2006) who studied the EMG activity of multiple muscles in a subgroup of women with SUI who were known to consistently depress the pelvic floor when attempting a lifting PFM contraction (identified via real-time ultrasound imaging (Thompson et al 2005)). The muscle activation patterns were measured via superficial EMG during a PFM contraction and Valsalva. Increased EMG activity was noted in the pelvic floor muscles, internal oblique, erector spinae, and rectus abdominis (i.e. a coactivation bracing strategy) during an attempt to contract the pelvic floor. They were unable to isolate a contraction of the deep system only (Fig. 6.14). They also noted an increase in EMG

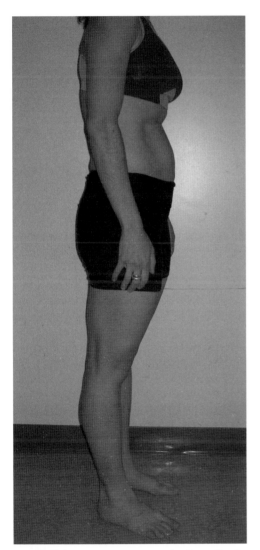

Fig. 6.14 • This postpartum woman is attempting to contract her transversus abdominis by thinking of drawing her navel to her spine, a common cue used for training the deep muscles of the abdominal wall. All that is hollowing is her upper chest as she overactivates the external oblique muscles bilaterally. This pattern of abdominal activation is commonly seen in women with stress urinary incontinence.

activity in all muscles measured during a Valsalva. When measured at rest, they also noted increased EMG activity in the pelvic floor and the external oblique, a finding consistent with those of Smith et al (2007b).

Conversely, Sapsford et al (2008) investigated the activity of the pelvic floor muscles in various sitting postures (slump supported, upright unsupported, and very tall upright sitting) and found that, compared to a continent group of women, the incontinent women had lower resting tone in the pelvic floor in all three sitting postures. The amount of activation of the pelvic floor varied between postures (least in slump supported sitting versus upright supported sitting) in both groups; however, according to this study, pelvic floor activation in sitting is less in women with incontinence. Smith et al (2007b) found that pelvic floor activation in standing is more in women with incontinence – different task, different strategy.

Using 2D perineal ultrasound imaging, Peng et al (2007) developed a method for analyzing displacement, trajectory, velocity, and acceleration of the anorectal angle (ARA) during a PFM contraction, Valsava, and cough in both continent and incontinent women. The results of this study have resolved the question arising from the study of Howard et al (2000): what is the difference in the cough mechanism in continent versus incontinent women? In the continent group, a contraction of the pelvic floor resulted in a cranioventral lift of the ARA, towards the urethra (see Fig. 8.89B, Video 8.10), a Valsalva caused the ARA to move caudodorsally (Fig. 8.89C, Video 8.11), and a cough resulted in a small cranioventral lift followed by a dorsocaudal movement that went past the initial starting position followed by a final return in the cranioventral direction to the initial position (Fig. 8.89D, Video 8.12). In the incontinent group, the trajectory of the ARA during a PFM contraction was variable and often the lift was not directed towards the urethra (Video 8.13). In this group, the ARA *only moved caudodorsal* in both a Valsalva (Video 8.14) and cough (Video 8.15).

According to Peng et al (2006):

> It appears that the functional PFM in continent women provide support to the urogenital structures before and during a cough, acting like a brake to resist or limit the dorsal-caudal movement that occurs as IAP inevitably rises during a cough. In women with SUI, this PFM "brake" appears to have been applied late, or is diminished, demonstrated by the increased displacement of the ARA.

An increasing body of evidence suggests that delays in the timing of PFM activation can impact on function. Continence of urine during the transference of loads through the pelvic girdle requires optimal bladder position and control and this depends, in part, on the individual's ability to effectively contract and sustain a tonic co-contraction of the deep muscles in a properly timed manner. Even with an intact endopelvic fascia, delayed activation of the pelvic floor will reduce the suburethral support. Ashton-Miller & DeLancey (2007) note 'an individual with muscles that do not function properly has a problem that is not surgically correctable.'

DeLancey (2005) reports:

> Each year, pelvic floor dysfunction affects between 300 000 and 400 000 American women so severely that they require surgery. Approximately 30% of the operations performed are re-operations. The high prevalence of this problem indicates the need for preventive strategies, and the common occurrence of re-operation indicates the need for treatment improvement. Efforts at prevention and treatment improvement will only be possible if research clarifies causative mechanism and scientifically valid studies discover why operations fail. By reaching a goal of 25% prevention we could save 90 000 women from experiencing pelvic floor dysfunction and with 25% treatment improvement we could avoid 30 000 women from needing a second operation.

These are powerful and thought-provoking numbers. The high re-operation rate suggests that the non-optimal strategies for load transfer that contributed to the loss of function persisted postoperatively. Is the cause always only a failure of anatomy due to trauma? This is not likely given the evidence. DeLancey then says, 'to achieve these goals we must discover specific events or behaviors in a woman's life that lead to these problems and that are amenable to preventive strategies.'

Summary

The evidence suggests that the pelvic floor plays a significant role in closure of the urethra. In health, the pelvic floor muscles have a constant low level of activity and have feedforward activation in response to perturbation of the trunk (i.e. increase their activation in anticipation of load). The pelvic floor muscles should coactivate with transversus abdominis and this synergistic activation facilitates lumbopelvic function and urethral closure when the fascial system is intact and the control system is working well.

Postpartum health for moms – restoring form and function after pregnancy

The Postpartum Health for Moms program was first introduced in 2001 (Lee 2001) and updated in 2006 (Lee & Lee 2006) in an attempt to educate the moms of the world and encourage them to proactively restore their form and function after pregnancy even if they do not have back pain or incontinence.

The pitch is this:

> The goal of this program is to provide you with the knowledge and skills you need to restore optimum function of your low back and pelvis. The program specifically addresses the consequences that occur through the experience of pregnancy and delivery. The information, as well as the exercises, will help to restore optimal loading strategies for your low back and pelvic girdle. Optimal movement and loading strategies can potentially reduce the risk of future low back and pelvic pain, as well as prevent problems such as uterine prolapse and bladder dysfunction.

Personal trainers, exercise instructors, and physiotherapists have been keen to adopt this program into their facilities as more and more women become proactive and understand the importance of preventive health care. The Postpartum Health for Moms program provides the trainer/therapist with the educational tools (slides in Microsoft Powerpoint format and an extensive client workbook) necessary to deliver the relevant information contained in this book in a group class. It is hoped that we will see more of these education/exercise classes worldwide and that, by restoring form and function after pregnancy, the prevalence of PRPGP, organ prolapse, and incontinence will lessen. A shift is occurring in the attitudes of moms and we find that, unlike 20 years ago, most women are less inclined to accept that having children means sacrifices to their postural support/control and/or continence. More information on this program can be found online at www.discoverphysio.ca

Summary

The research, as well as clinical experience, suggests that orthopedic physiotherapists must include assessment and treatment of the pelvic floor in both their pelvic girdle pain patients as well as their patients with stress urinary incontinence. Similarly, pelvic

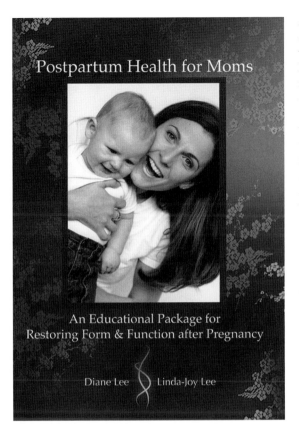

Postpartum Health for Moms

An Educational Package for
Restoring Form & Function after Pregnancy

Diane Lee   Linda-Joy Lee

floor therapists who primarily treat perineal pain, incontinence, and organ prolapse must include

assessment and treatment of the entire abdominal canister (Lee & Lee 2004b, 2007). Both are treating the same condition, non-optimal strategies that have led to failed load transfer through the lumbopelvic region, manifested either through a loss of motion control of the joints of the low back and/or pelvis, a loss of closure of the urethra or a loss of organ position. The research supports our understanding of the function and dysfunction of the *whole* abdominal canister and not just its parts. Treatment of the impaired lumbopelvic–hip complex must focus on an integrated approach, one that considers the restoration of optimal strategies and addresses impairments in multiple systems. Optimal strategies for function and performance will ensure controlled mobility, preservation of continence and organ support, and respiration. Pregnancy and delivery can significantly alter the strategies women use for transferring loads both through the musculoskeletal components of the pelvis and its organs. By restoring optimal strategies for function and performance in both the symptomatic and asymptomatic population, it is hoped that we will impact the prevalence of PRPGP, organ prolapse, and incontinence.

This completes the theoretical part of this text. By now, you are hopefully asking, 'How do I release this muscle or mobilize that joint and how do I facilitate the restoration of synergy and coordination between the deep and superficial muscles systems?' 'When do I do what?' That is what part 2 of this text is all about!

Clinical practice – the reality for clinicians

Linda-Joy Lee   Diane Lee

7

CHAPTER CONTENTS

Knowledge – what every practitioner
needs to know for clinical practice 147

Evidence-based practice – where did it
come from? Where is it going? 148

Understanding pain – what do we need
to know? 152

Classification and clinical prediction rules –
are we searching for the Holy Grail? 158

It's about more than pain – integrated
systems for optimal health 163

The Integrated Systems Model for Disability
and Pain – a framework for understanding
the whole person and their problem 165

Summary 171

Knowledge – what every practitioner needs to know for clinical practice

All health practitioners spend a considerable number of years gaining the knowledge necessary for their chosen career. What types of knowledge are there and what do practitioners need on a daily basis? Knowledge can be categorized as:

1. propositional, theoretical, or scientific knowledge (Higgs & Titchen 1995), also known as declarative knowledge (Jensen et al 2007); and

2. non-propositional or professional craft knowledge (knowing how to do something) (Higgs & Titchen 1995) or procedural (Jensen et al 2007). Non-propositional knowledge also includes personal knowledge or knowing oneself as a person and in relationship with others.

Propositional, or declarative, knowledge refers to the content knowledge that one's profession is based on and includes factual information derived from formal research trials (Chapters 4, 5). In addition, this category includes theoretical knowledge developed from existing empirical protocols and principles derived from dialogue with professionals in the same discipline and logic (Higgs 2004).

Non-propositional, or procedural, knowledge pertains to knowing how to do things pertaining to one's profession (craft and personal knowledge), such as how to mobilize a joint, release a hypertonic muscle, rewire a neural network, train a movement pattern, and/or motivate an individual to change. This knowledge is gained through reflection on both professional and personal experiences (what worked, what did not work, and how could it have been 'done' or handled differently to achieve a different outcome). Historically, non-propositional knowledge formed the basis for both medicine and physiotherapy. All therapy is influenced by a practitioner's perspective, their personal knowledge, values, and beliefs. This factor contributes to the outcome of an intervention and is often not considered in clinical trials studying the efficacy of a particular treatment (i.e. a trial that aims to identify whether manipulation or exercise is more effective for the treatment of low back pain).

Most practitioners continue to take postgraduate courses or attend professional conferences to improve their knowledge pertaining to clinical theory and research (propositional) as well as their technical skills (non-propositional or craft); however, Rivett & Jones (2004) note that there is a tendency in both courses

DOI: 10.1016/B978-0-443-06963-5.00007-9

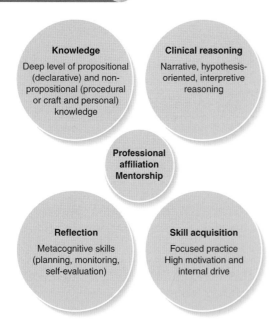

Fig. 7.1 • Five components for the development of clinical expertise. Adapted from Jensen et al, 2007.

and conferences to neglect an essential component of daily clinical practice – *clinical reasoning*. How should the practitioner integrate into clinical practice the newly learned scientific and theoretical knowledge? Who is it appropriate for and when is the new skill appropriate to use? Clinical practice is, and always will be, a blend of science and 'art' with a healthy dose of logic and reasoning. Clinical expertise comes from reasoning, reflection, skill acquisition, and the continual life-long pursuit of knowledge (propositional (declarative) and non-propositional (procedural and personal)) (Fig. 7.1) (Jensen et al 2007). This takes time, discipline, and often mentorship and professional affiliation both with individuals and groups.

Recently, for best practice, there is increasing pressure for practitioners to become evidence-based when making all clinical decisions. However, it appears that this term, evidence-based practice, means different things to different people. What is evidence-based practice and what is its history?

Evidence-based practice – where did it come from? Where is it going?

In 1989, when the first edition of this text was published, the term evidence-based practice had yet to be coined. Gaining access to anything published

(clinical opinion or scientific research) meant a trip to the university library, scrolling through the Index Medicus looking for any relevant article, and then heading to the stacks where the journal was filed, hoping it was there. The next step was to wait in a long line for the photocopier with a fistful of nickels in hand. In 1989, the internet was used only by the Department of Defense; it was released for public use in 1992.

In the 1970s and 1980s, peer-appointed leaders in physiotherapy taught a variety of clinical theories, protocols, and techniques largely based on their experience and expertise. Therapists seeking more knowledge for their clinical practice attended their short-term courses and often became advocates for their models. At that time, it was common to be asked what kind of therapist you were and which model you followed (i.e. Maitland, Cyriax, Kaltenborn, or McKenzie (Fig. 7.2)). Fortunately, the founders of the Canadian Academy of Manipulative Therapy (Cliff Fowler, David Lamb, and John Oldham) decided against embracing just one of these approaches and against personalizing an approach for themselves and subsequently developed an integrated curriculum that provided information on all models. Canadian manual therapists have been exposed to an integrated approach since the inception of postgraduate training in orthopedic manual therapy in 1975, and have consistently used reasoning and critical thinking to understand both impairments and the mechanisms driving the patient's pain experience.

The term 'evidence-based' was first used in 1990 by David Eddy and 'evidence-based medicine' in 1992 by Guyatt et al. The methodologies used to determine 'best evidence' were largely established by the Canadian McMaster University research group led by David Sackett and Gordon Guyatt. Professor Archie Cochrane (Fig. 7.3), a Scottish epidemiologist, has been credited with increasing the acceptance of the principles behind evidence-based practice (Cochrane 1972). Cochrane's work was honored through the naming of centers of evidence-based medical research, Cochrane Centers, and an international organization, the Cochrane Collaboration. Since the early 1990s there has been an explosion of research evidence, and accessibility to this evidence has been facilitated for those involved in research or formal study through easy internet access to full-text articles in indexed journals. Unfortunately, access to full-text articles is still limited, or expensive, for clinicians not affiliated with research centers or universities.

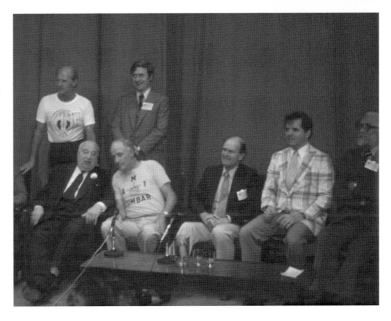

Fig. 7.2 • The keynote speakers from the IFOMT meeting in Christchurch, New Zealand in 1980. From left to right: Front Row – Dr. James Cyriax, Mr. Robin McKenzie, Mr. Geoff Mailtland, Dr. Sandy Burkart, Dr. Alan Stoddard. Back Row – Secretary of IFOMT Mr. Ian Searle and speaker Dr. Stanley Paris.

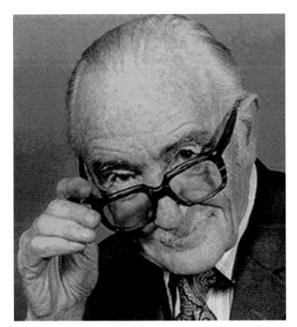

Fig. 7.3 • Professor Archie Cochrane for whom the Cochrane Collaboration is named.

Evidence-based medicine categorizes and ranks the different types of clinical evidence. The terms 'levels of evidence' or 'strength of evidence' refer to the protocols for ranking the evidence based on the strength of the study to be free from various biases. The highest level of evidence for therapeutic interventions is a systematic review, or meta-analysis, including only randomized, double-blind, placebo-controlled trials that involve a homogeneous patient population and condition. Expert opinion has little value as evidence and is ranked the lowest due to the placebo effect, the biases inherent in both the observation and reporting of the cases, and difficulties in discerning who is really an expert. Table 7.1 outlines the Oxford Centre for Evidence-based Medicine Levels of Evidence and was produced by Bob Phillips, Chris Ball, Dave Sackett, Doug Badenoch, Sharon Straus, Brian Haynes, and Martin Dawes.

Evidence-based practice (EBP) embraces all disciplines of health care (not just medicine) and has become synonymous with best practice, but what does the term really mean? To some, it appears that EBP means that a clinician can only use assessment tests and treatment techniques/ protocols that have been validated through the scientific process with high ranking studies as valued by the 'levels of evidence.' This is difficult to adhere to for many reasons, one being that there is not enough evidence at this time. Indeed, could there ever be enough scientific evidence for every situation met in clinical practice? Sackett et al (2000) define EBP as 'the integration of best research evidence, with clinical expertise and patient values' (Fig. 7.4). They note that,

Table 7.1 Oxford Centre for Evidence-based Medicine Levels of Evidence (May 2001)

Level	Therapy/ Prevention, Aetiology/Harm	Prognosis	Diagnosis	Differential diagnosis/ Symptom prevalence study	Economic and decision analyses
1a	SR (with homogeneity*) of RCTs	SR (with homogeneity*) of inception cohort studies; CDR[†] validated in different populations	SR (with homogeneity*) of Level 1 diagnostic studies; CDR[†] with 1b studies from different clinical centers	SR (with homogeneity*) of prospective cohort studies	SR (with homogeneity*) of Level 1 economic studies
1b	Individual RCT (with narrow confidence interval[‡])	Individual inception cohort study with >80% follow-up; CDR[†] validated in a single population	Validating** cohort study with good[†††] reference standards; or CDR† tested within one clinical centre	Prospective cohort study with good follow-up****	Analysis based on clinically sensible costs or alternatives; systematic review(s) of the evidence; and including multi-way sensitivity analyses
1c	All or none[§]	All or none case-series	Absolute SpPins and SnNouts[††]	All or none case-series	Absolute better-value or worse-value analyses[††††]
2a	SR (with homogeneity*) of cohort studies	SR (with homogeneity*) of either retrospective cohort studies or untreated control groups in RCTs	SR (with homogeneity*) of Level >2 diagnostic studies	SR (with homogeneity*) of 2b and better studies	SR (with homogeneity*) of Level >2 economic studies
2b	Individual cohort study (including low quality RCT; e.g. <80% follow-up)	Retrospective cohort study or follow-up of untreated control patients in an RCT; Derivation of CDR[†] or validated on split-sample[§§§] only	Exploratory** cohort study with good[†††] reference standards; CDR[†] after derivation, or validated only on split-sample[§§§] or databases	Retrospective cohort study, or poor follow-up	Analysis based on clinically sensible costs or alternatives; limited review(s) of the evidence, or single studies; and including multi-way sensitivity analyses
2c	'Outcomes' research; Ecological studies	'Outcomes' research		Ecological studies	Audit or outcomes research
3a	SR (with homogeneity*) of case–control studies		SR (with homogeneity*) of 3b and better studies	SR (with homogeneity*) of 3b and better studies	SR (with homogeneity*) of 3b and better studies
3b	Individual case–control study		Non-consecutive study; or without consistently applied reference standards	Non-consecutive cohort study, or very limited population	Analysis based on limited alternatives or costs, poor quality estimates of data, but including sensitivity analyses incorporating clinically sensible variations

Table 7.1 Oxford Centre for Evidence-based Medicine Levels of Evidence (May 2001) – cont'd

Level	Therapy/ Prevention, Aetiology/Harm	Prognosis	Diagnosis	Differential diagnosis/ Symptom prevalence study	Economic and decision analyses
4	Case-series (and poor quality cohort and case–control studies§§)	Case-series (and poor quality prognostic cohort studies***)	Case–control study, poor or non-independent reference standard	Case-series or superseded reference standards	Analysis with no sensitivity analysis
5	Expert opinion without explicit critical appraisal, or based on physiology, bench research or 'first principles'	Expert opinion without explicit critical appraisal, or based on physiology, bench research or 'first principles'	Expert opinion without explicit critical appraisal, or based on physiology, bench research or 'first principles'	Expert opinion without explicit critical appraisal, or based on physiology, bench research or 'first principles'	Expert opinion without explicit critical appraisal, or based on economic theory or 'first principles'

Produced by Bob Phillips, Chris Ball, Dave Sackett, Doug Badenoch, Sharon Straus, Brian Haynes, Martin Dawes since November 1998.

Users can add a minus-sign to denote the level of that which fails to provide a conclusive answer because of: EITHER a single result with a wide confidence interval (such that, for example, an ARR in an RCT is not statistically significant but whose confidence intervals fail to exclude clinically important benefit or harm); OR a systematic review with troublesome (and statistically significant) heterogeneity. Such evidence is inconclusive, and therefore can only generate Grade D recommendations.

Grades of Recommendation: A, consistent Level 1 studies; B, consistent Level 2 or 3 studies or extrapolations from Level 1 studies; C, Level 4 studies or extrapolations from Level 2 or 3 studies; D, Level 5 evidence or troublingly inconsistent or inconclusive studies of any level.

'Extrapolations' are where data is used in a situation which has potentially clinically important differences than the original study situation.

*By homogeneity we mean a systematic review that is free of worrisome variations (heterogeneity) in the directions and degrees of results between individual studies. Not all systematic reviews with statistically significant heterogeneity need be worrisome, and not all worrisome heterogeneity need be statistically significant. As noted above, studies displaying worrisome heterogeneity should be tagged with a '–' at the end of their designated level.

†Clinical Decision Rule. (These are algorithms or scoring systems that lead to a prognostic estimation or a diagnostic category.)

‡See note above for advice on how to understand, rate and use trials or other studies with wide confidence intervals.

§Met when all patients died before the Rx became available, but some now survive on it; or when some patients died before the Rx became available, but none now die on it.

§§By poor quality cohort study we mean one that failed to clearly define comparison groups and/or failed to measure exposures and outcomes in the same (preferably blinded), objective way in both exposed and non-exposed individuals and/or failed to identify or appropriately control known confounders and/or failed to carry out a sufficiently long and complete follow-up of patients. By poor quality case–control study we mean one that failed to clearly define comparison groups and/or failed to measure exposures and outcomes in the same (preferably blinded), objective way in both cases and controls and/or failed to identify or appropriately control known confounders.

§§§Split-sample validation is achieved by collecting all the information in a single tranche, then artificially dividing this into 'derivation' and 'validation' samples.

††An 'Absolute SpPin' is a diagnostic finding whose specificity is so high that a positive result rules-in the diagnosis. An 'Absolute SnNout' is a diagnostic finding whose sensitivity is so high that a negative result rules-out the diagnosis.

†††Good reference standards are independent of the test, and applied blindly or objectively to applied to all patients. Poor reference standards are haphazardly applied, but still independent of the test. Use of a non-independent reference standard (where the 'test' is included in the 'reference', or where the 'testing' affects the 'reference') implies a Level 4 study.

††††Better-value treatments are clearly as good but cheaper, or better at the same or reduced cost. Worse-value treatments are as good and more expensive, or worse and equally or more expensive.

**Validating studies test the quality of a specific diagnostic test, based on prior evidence. An exploratory study collects information and trawls the data (e.g. using a regression analysis) to find which factors are 'significant'.

***By poor quality prognostic cohort study we mean one in which sampling was biased in favor of patients who already had the target outcome, or the measurement of outcomes was accomplished in <80% of study patients, or outcomes were determined in an unblinded, non-objective way, or there was no correction for confounding factors.

****Good follow-up in a differential diagnosis study is >80%, with adequate time for alternative diagnoses to emerge (e.g. 1–6 months acute, 1–5 years chronic).

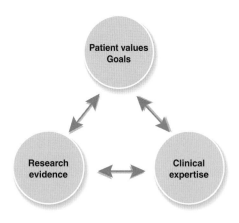

'External clinical evidence can inform, but can never replace individual clinical expertise, and it is this expertise that decides whether the external evidence applies to the patient at all, and if so, how it should be integrated into a clinical decision'
Sackett et al 2000

Fig. 7.4 • The three components of evidence-based practice as defined by Sackett et al (2000).

External clinical evidence can inform, but can never replace individual clinical expertise, and it is this expertise that decides whether the external evidence applies to the patient at all, and if so, how it should be integrated into a clinical decision.

Clinical expertise, as noted above, comprises both propositional (declarative) and non-propositional (procedural, craft, and personal) knowledge; in other words, knowing what, and how, to do the right thing at the right time (clinical reasoning and skill). The type of knowledge gained from scientific studies contributes to building only one kind of knowledge. In EBP according to Sackett et al's definition, clinical expertise plays an equal role alongside the research evidence. A key goal of the second section of this text is to facilitate the development of clinical expertise by exploring multiple types of knowledge. A third component of EBP is the patient's values and goals, which come from the person for whom all of the research and expertise is intended to help.

Recently, the term 'evidence-informed' has surfaced, the intent being to suggest that, as there is not enough research evidence for every situation met in clinical practice, the clinician should be informed of what is known and make their clinical decisions accordingly. However, if we can agree with Sackett et al's definition of EBP, there is no need to modify the term as clinical expertise (reasoning and skill) is considered part of the definition of best practice.

Understanding pain – what do we need to know?

Understanding the neurophysiology of pain mechanisms is essential knowledge for treating patients with lumbopelvic–hip (LPH) pain. Since the proposal of the gate control theory of pain by Melzack and Wall in 1965, significant advances in pain research and therapy have occurred. It is not our intent to provide an in-depth coverage of this topic here, but instead to highlight key features and establish a common language to be used throughout this book. For a more in-depth discussion, historical and sociocultural perspectives, and tools to help educate patients in pain neurophysiology, the reader is referred to extra reading in this topic (see Interest Box 1).

Interest Box 1

Further material for understanding the neurophysiology of pain

Butler D S 2000 The sensitive nervous system. NOI Group Publications, Adelaide, Australia

Butler D S, Moseley G L 2003 Explain pain. NOI Group Publications, Adelaide, Australia

Strong J, Unruh, A M, Wright A, Baxter G E 2002 Pain, a textbook for therapists. Churchill Livingstone, Edinburgh

Main C J, Spanswick C C 2000 Pain management: an interdisciplinary approach. Churchill Livingstone, Edinburgh

Melzack R 2001 Pain and the neuromatrix in the brain. Journal of Dental Education 65(12): 1378–82

Melzack R 2005 Evolution of the neuromatrix theory of pain. The Prithvi Raj Lecture: Presented at the third World Congress of World Institute of Pain, Barcelona, 2004. Pain practice: the official journal of World Institute of Pain 5(2):85–94

Moseley G L 2007 Reconceptualising pain according to modern pain science. Physical Therapy Reviews 12:169–178

Melzack R, Wall P D 1996 The challenge of pain Penguin Global, London (or later edition)

Wall P D 1999 Pain: the science of suffering. Weidenfield & Nicholson, London (or later edition)

What causes pain? Searching for the pain driver

The search for 'the pain driver' in peripheral tissues began when Descartes, in the 17th century, proposed that specific pathways existed from the peripheral tissues to the passive brain to transmit information notifying the brain of tissue injury (Fig. 7.5). The premise that injury of the tissues (ligaments, connective tissue, bones, nerves, organs, etc.) is the cause of pain is the basis of the *pathoanatomical* or *biomedical* model of pain, and has prevailed in the assessment and treatment of pain until quite recently. This model has led to research and increased understanding about nociception, including the stimuli that can cause it (mechanical, thermal, and chemical), which peripheral tissues

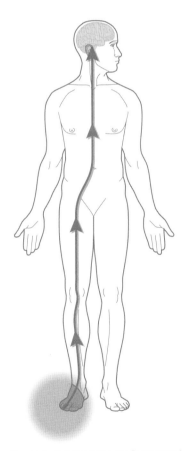

Fig. 7.5 • Descartes' 'L'homme de Descartes' – 1664 and the Specificity Theory of Pain. Descartes believed that there were specific pathways that transmitted information of tissue injury directly to the brain, with the brain being a passive recipient of information from the periphery.

can be painful and the pain patterns they generate (Fig. 7.6). Clinicians believed that if the tissues could heal or be fixed (by whatever means, including by anesthetic injection, anti-inflammatory medication, or removal of the offending tissue) then the nociception would stop, the pain would go away, and the patient would recover function.

However, it is now well recognized that the pathoanatomical model is limited in several ways. Lumbopelvic pain commonly exists in the absence of any findings on diagnostic tests (X-ray, CT scan, blood tests, nerve conduction tests, etc.), and damaged tissues can be identified in people who experience no pain (Nachemson 1999, Waddell 2004) (see Figs 5.3B and 5.7A). Tissues heal and yet the pain experience persists. Furthermore, a focus on only treating 'the painful tissue' neglects to consider that other systems or structures, which may be dysfunctional but *painfree*, could be the underlying cause of excessive mechanical stresses on the painful structures, or the cause of decreased blood flow or nutritional supply. In order to resolve the pain, the *painfree* but *impaired* structures need to be treated for long-term resolution. Identification of what tissue hurts does not provide insight as to *why* it hurts. Finally, significant developments in neuroscience have changed our understanding of what pain is, and have required us to reframe and change our thinking.

We now understand that at any time in one patient there are *many* 'pain drivers' that do not exist solely in the peripheral tissues. Rather than looking for one source of pain, we need to consider that multiple mechanisms are at play in the experience of pain in all our patients. These mechanisms can be broadly separated into *peripherally mediated* (nociception and peripheral neuropathic pain) or *centrally mediated* (related to processing in the central nervous system (CNS)) (Butler 2000) (Fig. 7.7A), and will be discussed in more detail later in this section.

Classifying pain – timelines and mechanism of injury

Patients are commonly classified according to the timeline or duration of their pain experience, and the cause or mechanism of their injury. In general, problems are considered to be *acute* if they are within the first 6 weeks to 3 months (depending on the type of tissue injured) after an initiating incident (Brukner & Khan 2002, Magee et al 2007). Tissue injury results in a known sequence

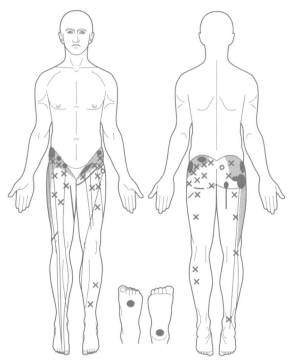

Fig. 7.6 • Pain patterns of patients with hip pathology who experienced at least 90% pain reduction 30 minutes after a fluoroscopically guided intra-articular anesthetic injection into the hip joint. Redrawn from Lesher et al, 2008.

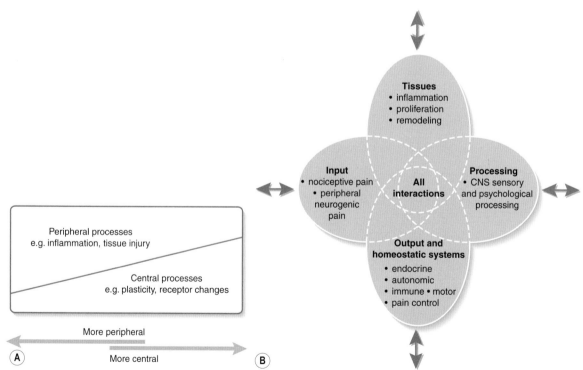

Fig. 7.7 • (A) Overlap of peripheral and central pain mechanisms. Redrawn from Butler, 2000, p. 50.
(B) The pathobiological mechanisms involved in pain states including tissue mechanisms and pain mechanisms.
The arrows represent varying contributions by mechanisms. Note that this figure is redrawn from Butler, 2000 and the International Association for the study of Pain (IASP) has now amended definitions and pain terminology (Loeser & Treede 2008) such that the word 'neuropathic' is preferred to 'neurogenic'.

Table 7.2 The stages of tissue healing. From Brukner & Khan (2007)

Phase	Tissue response
Acute inflammatory phase 0–72 hours	Damaged tissue is filled immediately with erythrocytes and inflammatory cells. Phagocytosis of necrotic cells occurs within 24 hours. Fibroblasts slowly lay down collagen scar
Proliferation/repair phase 2 days–6 weeks	Fibroblasts are the predominant cells, initially resulting in large amounts of scar collagen with excessive cross-links. As stress is applied to the healing tissue, the amount of cross-linking is reduced and the tensile strength of the tissue is increased
Remodeling/maturation phase 4 weeks–12 months	Total collagen content within the tissue is slowly reduced, and the scar tends towards assuming the structure of the pre-injured tissue. The initial severity of the injury will largely influence the time taken for complete remodeling to occur

of events aimed at protecting and repairing the damaged structures. These stages of tissue healing (Table 7.2) occur in three overlapping stages that have been given multiple names but refer to the same processes:

1. acute inflammatory stage;
2. subacute or proliferation stage;
3. chronic or maturation and remodeling stage.

The term *chronic* is often used to indicate the persistence of pain beyond the normal timeline for tissue healing (Bonica 1953, Merskey & Bogduk 1994), as opposed to a stage of the tissue healing process. In the *Classification of Chronic Pain* (Merskey & Bogduk 1994) published by the International Association for the Study of Pain, it is noted that the normal time for healing 'may be less than one month, or more often, more than six months. With nonmalignant pain, three months is the most convenient point of division between acute and chronic pain, but for research purposes six months will often be preferred.' Chronic pain is also further outlined as 'a persistent pain that is not amenable, as a rule, to treatments based upon specific remedies, or to the routine methods of pain control such as non-narcotic analgesics' (Merskey & Bogduk 1994).

More recently, the term *persistent* low back pain has emerged in the literature, to indicate pain that continues past the expected timeframe for tissue healing. Others are suggesting that *acute episodes* of low back pain would be better termed *recurrent episodes* in a *chronic* problem, as the underlying mechanisms contributing to recurrent low back pain are likely to be different from a first-time traumatic episode of low back pain, and recurrence of pain after an acute episode is a common problem (Pengel et al 2003).

Acute pain, especially when related to a specific initiating incident, is commonly perceived as being relatively straightforward in terms of what pain mechanisms are at play. These are generally accepted to be types of peripherally mediated pain (nociceptive or peripheral neuropathic) related to tissue damage and the resultant inflammatory processes are aimed at restoring homeostasis in the body. However, is any pain experience truly simple? Consider the following report:

> A builder aged 29 came to the accident and emergency department having jumped down on to a 15-cm nail. As the smallest movement of the nail was painful he was sedated with fentanyl and midazolam. The nail was then pulled out from below. When his boot was removed a miraculous cure appeared to have taken place. Despite entering proximal to the steel toecap the nail had penetrated between the toes; the foot was entirely uninjured.
>
> BMJ 1995.

The initial logical hypothesis in this case was that acute trauma to the foot was causing severe nociceptive input from the damaged tissues. However, as physical examination revealed completely intact tissues, this cannot explain the patient's pain experience. Clearly other pain mechanisms were at play, despite the timeline (acute onset) and mode of onset (traumatic) of the pain.

Empirical evidence now exists to explain these kinds of stories. A consistent factor that has emerged from the pain sciences is that the *meaning* of the pain experience, and especially the *threat value* of the experience, is significant. In other words, does the pain signify something harmful or not? Although some may continue to function and keep going in spite of pain, others are completely debilitated by the mere thought of the sensation. There is increasing evidence to support that an individual's experience of pain is significantly influenced by the way they think and feel about the situation as a whole,

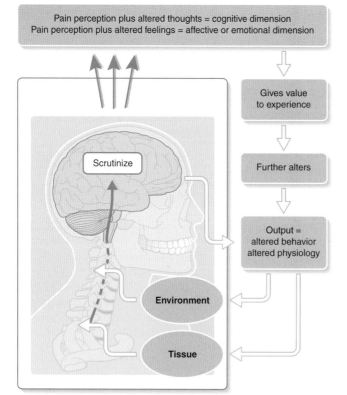

Fig. 7.8 • The Mature Organism Model of Gifford (1998). Adapted from Jones & Rivett, 2004 and Gifford, 1998.

regardless of the severity of tissue injury. The story above illustrates these influences; his pain experience is an example of 100% centrally mediated pain, driven by his beliefs (cognitive dimension) and emotional state (affective dimension) related to the event (having a nail driven through his boot). It is clear that we cannot separate the tissues from the person to which they belong; we are integrated beings and our experience of our body (whether positive or negative) is the result of complex interactions and processes occurring in the brain.

Thus, although it is important to know the mechanism of onset and timeframes related to the pain experience, we must take care that this information does not lead us to assume that certain timelines *necessitate* certain pain mechanisms. Acute pain can be largely driven by central mechanisms. Persistent pain can also be largely driven by peripheral mechanisms. That is, persistent or chronic pain states may have central components, but these are not necessarily the dominant mechanism for every patient simply because the pain experience has persisted for a long period of time. Although evidence supports that 'the relationship between pain and

the state of the tissues becomes less predictable as pain persists' (Moseley 2007b), we need to remember that the pain experience is uniquely individual. Regardless of whether the pain is a newly occurring event or a persistent experience, it is a multidimensional experience, and thus any person presenting with pain should be evaluated with a framework in mind that allows for the consideration of all these factors. As Butler (2000, p. 53) notes,

> Overlap of mechanisms is the key feature because the boundaries are often fuzzy. There will be differing contributions of mechanisms to the injury state over time, person and injury.

Classification by pain mechanisms

So what are the different biological mechanisms that drive the pain experience? Pain mechanisms can be further categorized (Figs 7.7B, 7.8) (Butler 2000, Gifford 1998) as they relate to:

1. input into the nervous system;

2. processing in the nervous system; and

3. output from the nervous and other systems.

The brain receives continuous information from the body and the environment (input mechanisms or all sensory pathways) that is assessed and interpreted (processing at both conscious and unconscious levels) prior to producing a response (output mechanisms). Some of this incoming information is nociceptive. There are many factors that determine an individual's behavior and pain experience (physical, cognitive, emotional) in response to nociceptive input, including:

- contextual factors of the immediate circumstance (i.e. how dangerous is this sensation in the light of environmental and internal factors?); as well as
- past experiences and personal knowledge that collectively contribute to the individual's beliefs, attitudes, emotions, and physical responses.

Input mechanisms as they pertain to pain include all the sensory information reaching the central nervous system (CNS) from the body internally and externally. This includes nociceptive pain from tissues including bones, ligaments, tendons, muscles, connective tissue, viscera, etc. (Butler 2000, Gifford 1998, Wright 2002) and peripheral neuropathic pain from neural tissue outside of the CNS. Processing occurs in the dorsal root ganglion and in the CNS. In the brain, an individual's thoughts and feelings (cognitions + emotions = perception) are integrated and can influence the output mechanisms, which include:

1. somatic or motor (altered posture, altered motor control);
2. autonomic (increased sympathetic response for 'fight or flight');
3. neuroendocrine (increased stress, heightened emotions, hormonal changes); and
4. neuroimmune.

Thinking within the context of stress biology creates a broader framework for understanding pain. Gifford (1998), in proposing the mature organism model (Fig. 7.8), notes that

> ...the sensation of pain is seen as a perceptual component of the stress response whose prime adaptive purpose is to alter our behaviour in order to enhance the processes of recovery and chances of survival. Stress biology and the stress response broadly considers the systems and responses concerned with maintaining homeostasis.

It has been proposed that continued activation of the stress regulation systems and excessive or prolonged cortisol output has a destructive effect on peripheral tissues such as muscle, bone, and nerve tissue, thereby perpetuating a vicious cycle of stress, pain, and tissue injury (Melzack 2005).

In his *Neuromatrix Theory of Pain*, Ronald Melzack (2001, 2005) highlights the need to assess and treat the whole person, not just the painful parts.

> The body is felt as a unity, with different qualities at different times... [Together all outputs] produce a continuous message that represents the whole body [which he also describes] as a flow of awareness.

Melzack's model has four components (2001, 2005):

1. the body-self neuromatrix – an anatomical substrate in the brain of the body-self;
2. cyclical processing and synthesis of nerve impulses, which produces a neurosignature;
3. the flow of neurosignatures is projected back to areas of the brain, the sentient neural hub, which converts them into the flow of awareness; and
4. activation of an action neuromatrix occurs to provide the pattern of movements to bring about the desired goal.

> The neuromatrix, distributed throughout many areas of the brain, comprises a widespread network of neurons which generates patterns, processes information that flows through it, and ultimately produces the pattern that is felt as a whole body. The stream of neurosignature output with constantly varying patterns riding on the main signature pattern produces the feelings of the whole body with constantly changing qualities...The final, integrated neurosignature pattern for the body-self ultimately produces awareness and action.
>
> Melzack 2005.

Figure 7.9 is a modification of Melzack's representation of the body-self neuromatrix to illustrate the sensorial, cognitive, and emotional dimensions of pain. Perhaps the best summary for this section, highlighting the broad view we need to take when considering pain, comes from this leader in the study of pain himself, Ronald Melzack (2001).

> We have traveled a long way from the psychosocial concept that seeks a simple one-to-one relationship between injury and pain. We now have a theoretical framework in which a genetically determined template for the body-self is modulated by the powerful stress system and the cognitive functions of the brain, in addition to the traditional sensory inputs. The neuromatrix theory of pain – which places genetic contributions and the neural–hormonal mechanisms of stress on a level of equal importance with

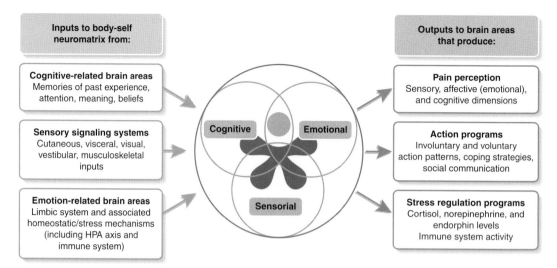

Fig. 7.9 • An adaptation of Melzack's body-self matrix (2001, 2005). HPA axis, hypothalamic–pituitary–adrenal axis.

the neural mechanisms of sensory transmission – has important implications for research and therapy. The expansion of the field of pain to include endocrinology and immunology may lead to insights and new research strategies that will reveal the underlying mechanisms of chronic pain and give rise to new therapies to relieve the tragedy of unrelenting suffering.

It is very clear that as clinicians we need to be aware of all the possible mechanisms that can create pain and to challenge ourselves to have an open mind as we seek to understand each individual's unique pain experience in order to determine which mechanisms are primary for them in all stages of their rehabilitation process.

Classification and clinical prediction rules – are we searching for the Holy Grail?

Given the multidimensional nature of pain, it is not surprising that using pain presentation (location, duration, onset) as the sole means to classify patients and determine best treatment has been ineffective. Fritz and colleagues (2007) report that despite over 1,000 randomized clinical trials investigating the effectiveness of interventions for the management of low back pain, 'the evidence remains contradictory and inconclusive' (Fritz et al 2007). One key reason believed to contribute to this state of the evidence is the lack of classification of low back pain patients into subgroups, not only for studying treatment efficacy, but also for determining

etiological and prognostic factors (Gombatto et al 2007, Leboeuf-Yde et al 1997, Riddle 1998). Sahrmann in the late 1980s noted,

> As we all know, general diagnoses such as low back pain or hip pain do not often relate to the cause or to the underlying nature of the condition.
>
> Sahrmann 1988.

As clinicians have long recognized, it is now widely accepted that patients with low back pain, pelvic girdle pain, and hip pain do not form homogeneous populations, but consist of multiple subgroups with different combinations of underlying impairments (physical and psychosocial), and these subgroups require different treatment approaches for best outcomes. Furthermore, given that multiple factors contribute to lumbopelvic or hip pain, it is also unrealistic to expect that one single type of treatment modality will resolve a patient's presenting pain and functional limitations. Thus, the pursuit of valid ways to identify subgroups of patients with low back and pelvic girdle pain has become an increasingly prominent theme in the literature over the last three decades.

The classification for lumbopelvic pain has evolved since the pathoanatomically based classification of MacNab (1977) with a variety of patient characteristics proposed for use in creating homogeneous subgroups (Bernard & Kirkaldy-Willis 1987, Coste et al 1992, Delitto et al 1995, Fritz et al 2007, Kirkaldy-Willis 1983, McKenzie 1981, O'Sullivan 2005, O'Sullivan & Beales 2007, Reeves et al 2005, Sahrmann 2001) (Table 7.3). O'Sullivan (2005)

Table 7.3 Multiple proposals for the classification of patients

Model/System	Description	Diagnostic/Classification determinants
Pathoanatomical (Nachemson 1999, Kirkaldy-Willis & Hill 1979, Kirkaldy-Willis 1983, MacNab 1977)	Focuses on structural changes that occur as a consequence of inflammation, infection, metabolic disorders, trauma, and/or disease (pathology based)	Radiological diagnosis, blood work
Mechanical diagnosis and therapy (MDT aka the McKenzie Method) (McKenzie 1981)	Directional preference and centralization or peripheralization of pain with repeated movements. Four subgroups: The derangement syndrome The dysfunction syndrome The posture syndrome The other group	Rapidly reversible symptoms with repeated movements in a specific direction
Peripheral pain generator model (Laslett & Williams 1994, Laslett et al 2005)	Attempts to identify the painful peripheral pain-generating structure with the main therapeutic intervention being to block or denervate the nociceptive source	Diagnostic blocks of various peripheral structures seeking to relieve pain
Neurophysiological pain model (Butler 2000)	Generation and maintenance of pain both peripherally and/or centrally mediated (central and/or peripheral sensitization of neural networks)	Subjective examination Confirmed/negated by features of the objective examination
Psychosocial model (Waddell 2004)	Cognitive and emotional factors such as negative thinking, fear avoidance behaviors, and hypervigilance	Subjective examination
Treatment-based classification system (Delitto et al 1995, updated criteria Fritz et al 2007)	Intended for patients with acute/acute exacerbation of LBP. Patients placed into treatment categories based on patterns of signs and symptoms: manipulation specific exercise (flexion, extension, lateral-shift patterns) stabilization traction	Subjective examination, objective examination features based on clinical experience and propositional knowledge. Specific exercise grouping based primarily on centralization/peripheralization principles (McKenzie 1981). Updated criteria include disability questionnaire data and are based on CPRs and scientific research. Traction group removed in updated classification
Movement System Impairment (MSI) System (Sahrmann 2001)	Based on the kinesiopathic model of movement (KPM); musculoskeletal pain develops as a result of repeated movements and postural alignments in the same direction across daily activities, causing repeated loading and microtrauma. LBP subgroups: lumbar flexion lumbar extension lumbar rotation lumbar rotation with flexion lumbar rotation with extension	Subjective and objective examination aimed to identify the direction of movement and alignment that is related to LBP. Symptoms are monitored in response to standardized movement and alignment tests, along with observation of timing of relative motion of body segments, and the response to modification of alignment/movement

CPR, clinical prediction rule; LBP, lower back pain.

noted that a limitation of many classification systems is that only a single dimension (pathoanatomical, psychosocial, neurophysiological, motor control, signs and symptoms, etc.) is often used to create subgroups. Classification systems will be most useful in clinical practice if variables across multiple domains are used to create subgroups.

Features that have been incorporated into different systems include (note this is not intended to be an exhaustive list):

- presence or absence of identifiable underlying pathology (pathoanatomical, peripheral pain generator models);
- pain presentation (central, unilateral, with or without radiation of symptoms to the lower extremity) (signs and symptoms models);
- underlying pain mechanisms/neurophysiology;
- response of pain to movement (centralization or peripheralization) (signs and symptoms models) (movement impairment models);
- physical impairments such as loss or increase of mobility, altered motor control, altered posture/spinal alignment, and the relationship of symptom provocation to these impairments (motor control models, signs and symptoms models, movement impairment models);
- response to specific treatments (manipulation, stabilization exercises, specific exercises, traction); and
- psychosocial and cognitive features such as fear avoidance, coping strategies, and beliefs (biopsychosocial models).

In recent years, the development of clinical prediction rules (CPRs) has emerged as another method to classify patients. CPRs are derived statistically with the aim of identifying the combinations of clinical examination findings that can predict a condition or outcome. Thus, they are proposed to be a useful tool to assist in clinical decision-making by improving the accuracy of diagnosis, prognosis, or prediction of response to specific treatment protocols (Beattie & Nelson 2006, Cook 2008, Fritz 2009). Development of CPRs in physiotherapy has mainly focused on the response to treatment protocols (Fritz 2009) in order to identify subgroups of patients most likely to respond to a specific treatment approach. It is important to note that, at this time, CPRs are still in their infancy of development

and validation, and are not yet at the appropriate stage to be widely applied in clinical practice (Cook 2008).

It has been suggested that CPRs will best impact physiotherapy practice where there is complexity in the clinical decision-making process, and that 'an appeal of CPRs is their potential to make [the] subgrouping process more evidence based and less reliant on unfounded theories and tradition' (Fritz 2009). However, the use of CPRs should be balanced with the knowledge that

> Clinical prediction rules provide probabilities of a given diagnosis or prognosis but do not necessarily recommend decisions. Clinical prediction rules can be of great value to assist clinical decision-making but should not be used indiscriminately. They are not a replacement for clinical judgment and should complement rather than supplant clinical opinion and intuition.
>
> Beattie & Nelson 2006.

Research on specific subgroups and development of classification systems will definitely provide a much better understanding of the specific impairments, mechanisms, and psychosocial features that characterize subgroups and their response to treatment. As Melzack wrote about the evolution of the gate control theory of pain,

> As historians of science have pointed out, good theories are instrumental in producing facts that eventually require a new theory to incorporate them.
>
> Melzack 2001.

However, it is important to recognize that there are limitations on how information gained from classification systems, CPRs, clinical trials, and indeed the findings of any scientific study, can be translated and applied into the reality of clinical practice. Firstly, statistical averages tell us about the average response of the group defined by the characteristics used in design of the study. Individual responses may be to a greater or lesser degree than the average, or even in the opposite direction of the reported response. Indeed, practicing clinicians are well aware of the many patients they have seen who do not fit the data from clinical trials or other studies. These clinical cases provide valuable insight and can generate questions for further research. Secondly, although the data provide relatively unbiased information, the interpretation and conclusions made from the data, and published alongside the data, are subject to bias just as much as clinical opinion is subject to bias. It is also important to recognize that a *lack of* data or science does not invalidate a technique or approach, nor does it mean that approaches that have been studied are necessarily superior. In clinical practice, application of any classification system/CPR requires care to ensure that it does not create a rigid, narrow mindset. Placing the patient 'in a box' could prevent the clinician from considering other options for treatment that may be greatly beneficial. Neglecting to provide these other options could then result in suboptimal outcomes.

Consider the one domain of underlying pain mechanism as a way to create subgroups. Butler (2000) notes that,

> The word 'division' can be instant trouble because these mechanisms all occur in a continuum. All pain states probably involve all mechanisms, however in some, a

dominance of one mechanism may become obvious. Pain mechanisms are not diseases or specific injuries. They simply represent a process or biological state.

In their classification of pelvic girdle pain disorders, O'Sullivan & Beales (2007) categorize non-specific pelvic pain disorders into two groups, one that has centrally mediated pain, and one that has peripherally mediated pain (Fig. 7.10). Although the group of centrally mediated pain is further classified into those with non-dominant psychosocial factors and those with dominant psychosocial factors, the treatment protocol for the subgroup of centrally mediated pelvic girdle pain is medical management (central nervous system modulation), psychological (cognitive behavioral therapy), and functional capacity rehabilitation. Specific interventions directed at identified physical impairments in the periphery are not recommended, and yet it is highly unlikely that

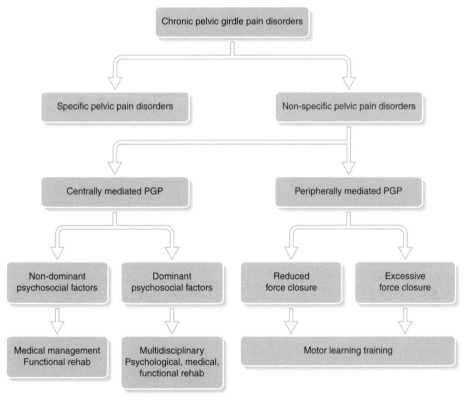

Fig. 7.10 • The mechanism-based classification for chronic pelvic pain (O'Sullivan & Beales 2007) begins by dividing patients according to the specificity of their condition (specific versus non-specific) and then by how their pain is mediated (peripherally or centrally). Where would you put the patient who has reduced force closure of one sacroiliac joint (SIJ) and excessive force closure of the other? Or the patient who has a stiff SIJ that will not respond to motor learning training? How do we classify the patient with multiple impairments that collectively are creating their pain experience and functional problem(s)/disability?

many patients will have 100% centrally mediated pain. In the authors' experience, even in patients with a strong contributor of central sensitization to their pain experience, careful assessment often reveals specific meaningful tasks that relate to a consistent reproduction of symptoms (see case study Julie K, Chapter 9 📖). It is reasonable to suggest that even if peripheral mechanisms contribute only 20% to the complete picture, addressing that 20% in addition to the other approaches will provide the greatest chance for the best outcome. Furthermore, it is likely that, by addressing the physical impairments, psychosocial variables will also be impacted, further advancing the goals of treating drivers of central sensitization.

It is also crucial to recognize that our patients change as a result of their changing life circumstances and our interactions with them (both physical and personal). Thus, during the course of treatment continual re-evaluation is necessary to adapt the treatment program accordingly. Sticking to a rigid plan based on an initial placement into a subgroup may result in the provision of suboptimal care.

Finally, in our quest for better classification schemes and science to support and test our clinical approaches, it is important to remember that at the end of the day, no matter how detailed and well defined our classification schemes, the person presenting to the clinician is a unique *individual* with unique life experiences. There will never be one recipe for treatment that is the best fit for all patients. Furthermore, patient values and beliefs are central to the treatment process, and if they do not want to receive what is considered 'best practice' from the current evidence, we cannot force it on them. Given the same impairment in the tissues, no two individuals will have exactly the same perception and presentation (experience and behavior) because 'how they manifest their pain or illness is shaped in part by who they are' (Jones & Rivett 2004). A reminder: the highest level of evidence for therapeutic interventions is a systematic review, or meta-analysis, of only randomized, double-blind, placebo-controlled trials that involve a homogeneous patient population and condition. Is this possible in the light of what is known about pain? Do homogeneous populations really exist in clinical practice? (See Interest Box 2.)

Science can provide us with an abundance of knowledge to challenge, refine, reshape, and validate our clinical practice, but it cannot provide all of the information needed in any individual patient encounter; it does not paint the whole picture of the patient. In order to treat patients effectively, therapists need to have well-organized knowledge including propositional (knowledge ratified by research trials), non-propositional (professional craft or 'knowing how' knowledge), and personal (knowledge gained from personal experiences (Jones & Rivett 2004)).

> Understanding and successfully managing patient's problems requires a rich organization of all three types of knowledge. Propositional knowledge provides us with theory and levels of substantiation by which the patient's clinical presentation can be considered against research-validated theory and practice. Non-propositional professional craft knowledge allows us the means to use that theory in the clinic while providing additional, often cutting-edge (albeit with unproven generality) clinically derived evidence. Personal knowledge allows a deeper understanding of the clinical problem to be gained within the context of the patient's particular situation and enabling us to practice in a holistic and caring way.
>
> Jones & Rivett 2004.

Personal and craft knowledge cannot be learned from RCTs, mechanistic studies, basic physiology studies, or clinical prediction rules. Ultimately, it is the development of *clinical expertise* that creates optimal patient care. According to Ericsson & Smith (1991), expertise has been defined as 'having the ability to do the right thing at the right time.'

Clinical expertise has two components: skill acquisition (do the right thing) and clinical reasoning (at the right time). Clinical reasoning skills facilitate the organization and integration of knowledge gained both in and out of the clinic, and the wise application of that knowledge for each individual patient. The development of clinical expertise is discussed further in Chapter 9, and is the focus of the second part of this book.

Different classification systems provide us with a variety of perspectives to grow our knowledge base. However, hoping to find '*the* best classification system' to apply in every situation in clinical practice is like searching for the Holy Grail – it cannot be found. We are unique people trying to help other unique people. We need to re-evaluate how we value the 'levels of evidence' and the role of science in directing clinical practice, and develop a more balanced view that values the insight that is uniquely derived from clinical practice. The clinical 'lab' plays a key role in new knowledge generation through the development of innovative techniques for assessment and treatment, which can then be tested by science. Knowledge gained from clinical experience is not more important than science, but it certainly is no less important. Overall, maintaining

Interest Box 2

On 'Evidence-based medicine' and Pharmacology – new directions

An excerpt from, 'Disease Diagnosis and Therapy Customized to Each Person's Genetic Make-up', Prof. Ronald Reid. *UBC Alumni News.*

> *Personalized medicine based on the individuality of the human genome will allow physicians and pharmacists to accurately characterize disease and identify not only the best drug to be administered to a particular patient for a specific disease, but also the correct, safe, and effective drug dose the first time.*

> *Pharmacogenomics uses information from the human genome to diagnose disease and predict the efficacy and toxicity of drug therapy, a concept that has come to be known as 'personalized medicine.' The technology involved is complex, requiring large-scale experimental approaches combined with equally complex statistical and computational analyses. The fundamental strategy in a pharmacogenomics approach is to expand the scope from examining variations in single genes, proteins, and metabolites to studying the interaction of all genes, proteins, and metabolites that are relevant to disease diagnosis and a successful therapeutic outcome.*

> *The application of pharmacogenomics to health care emphasizes that the present paradigm of 'evidence-based medicine,' the techniques of which are derived from randomized and double blind clinical trials, is inconsistent with 'personalized medicine.'*

> *The application of statistical information derived from clinical drug trials on large populations results in a standard dose range for the population, which both overdoses and underdoses a small but significant portion of that population. The failure to recognize patients as individuals is likely a factor in adverse drug and toxic drug–drug interactions that account for 100,000 patient deaths, two million hospitalizations, and $100 billion in health care costs in the United States yearly.*

> *Finally, the realignment of the medical paradigm from 'evidence-based' to 'personalized' via the application of pharmacogenomics should provide a viable solution to optimize disease diagnosis and patient therapy and significantly reduce costs to the health care system.*

There are limitations and dangers of 'failing to recognize patients as individuals.' This supports a questioning of the current value placed in the hierarchy of the 'levels of evidence,' and the value physiotherapy research is currently placing in classification systems and clinical prediction rules. The findings from randomized clinical trials tell us about how to treat populations, but day-to-day clinical practice involves treating individual people. We can learn many things from these studies. But let us critically evaluate what these studies can tell us, and what they *can't*. Over the last 30 years, the pendulum has swung in physiotherapy from blindly following the 'guru of the day' to only doing what the science tells us we should do. It is time to reconsider the valuable insights that clinical expertise brings, and to find a middle ground that uses knowledge gained from *all* sources to find the best multimodal treatment approaches for our patients.

---

an open mind and broad perspective will assist both scientists and clinicians to discover how best to work together and learn from each other in the common goal of providing best care for our patients.

It's about more than pain – integrated systems for optimal health

It has been long recognized that simply relieving a patient's pain does not necessarily result in a full return to all functional activities. Furthermore, there are subgroups of patients, such as high-level athletes, whose functional goals and measures (race time, power delivery in a stroke for example) are just as, if not *more*, meaningful to them than the relief of pain. Indeed, there is an increasing market in helping people *without pain* to optimize performance as well as prevent injury by facilitating strategies for better posture and movement. Pain is not a problem for these people, but an inability to meet their functional goals is. Non-painful impairments are also recognized as a potential contributor to the development of pain, both in sites distal to the impaired area and in the area itself. Furthermore, if we take the broader view that 'pain is an opinion on the organism's state of health rather than a mere reflexive response to injury' (Ramachandran in Doidge 2007), we need to alter our focus and consider what it means to be 'in health' and not only what it means to be 'in pain.' The World Health Assembly has defined health as 'a state of complete physical, mental, and social well-being and not merely the absence of disease or infirmity' (WHO Constitution). Speaking at the 1985 annual conference of the American Medical Association (Seattle, USA), Dr. Paul Brenner defined health even more broadly as 'the full acceptance and appreciation of life.' Restoring health is about more than removing disease; creating optimal strategies for function and performance is about more than removing pain.

What it means to be 'in health' is individually defined. Therefore, changing our focus from removing pain to restoring optimal health and optimal strategies for function and performance is intrinsically linked to the patient's values and goals. Our role as clinicians is to best facilitate and empower patients on their journey to achieve their personal optimal health and function. To do this effectively, we need not only to understand their pain, but also to understand them as a person. Jones & Rivett (2004) refer to this as 'understanding both the problem and the person.'

> To understand and manage patients and their problems successfully, manual therapists must consider not only the physical diagnostic possibilities (including the structures involved and the associated pathobiology) but also the full range of factors that can contribute to a person's health, particularly the effects these problems may have on patients' lives, and the understanding patients (and significant others) have of these problems and their management.

This paradigm requires that clinicians broaden their perspectives and skill sets, and also opens up a wider range of potential and possibility for effecting change.

The Integrated Model of Function (Chapter 4, Fig. 4.5) was developed from anatomical and biomechanical studies of the pelvis, as well as from the clinical experience of treating patients with lumbopelvic pain (Lee 2004, Lee & Vleeming 1998, 2004, 2007). From its inception, The Integrated Model of Function focused on evaluation of the function of the pelvis, and how the pelvis effectively transfers loads across tasks with varying characteristics. The model addresses *why* the pelvis is painful by identifying the underlying impairments in four specific components: form closure, force closure, motor control, and emotions. This is in opposition to pathoanatomical models that seek to identify only pain-generating structures. This model has continued to evolve with the publication of anatomical, biomechanical, and neurophysiological research as well as the clinical expertise gained through collaborative efforts worldwide and remains a useful framework to understand the pelvis in function and in dysfunction.

The Integrated Systems Model for Disability and Pain evolved from working with the Integrated Model of Function and was first introduced in 2007 as the System-Based Classification for Failed Load Transfer (Lee & Lee 2007, 2008a,b, Lee et al 2008a). We have since recognized that using the word 'classification' is limiting for this model because its primary purpose is not to place patients into homogeneous subgroups. In contrast, it is a framework to understand and interpret the unique picture of each individual patient in the clinical context to facilitate decision-making and treatment planning. The model provides a context to organize all the different types of knowledge needed (scientific, theoretic, professional craft, procedural, and personal) and provides for the development and testing of multiple hypotheses as the multidimensional picture of the patient emerges. A multimodal treatment plan can then be designed based on the complete picture of the person and their presenting problem(s).

The Integrated Systems Model for Disability and Pain allows clinicians to characterize all the components that contribute to what Melzack terms the 'message that represents the whole body' as a 'flow of awareness' (Melzack 2005). It is an integrated, evidence-based model that considers disability and pain as defined and directed by the patient's values and goals. The model relates impairments found in systems, underlying pain mechanisms, and the impact of these impairments on their current whole body strategies for function and performance. Thus, the model analyzes the patient's current whole body strategies, determines the underlying reasons for those strategies, and relates these to current knowledge about the necessary state required in all systems to provide optimal strategies for function and performance, and ultimately for health. As a systems-based model, it has inherent flexibility to evaluate and integrate new evidence from research and innovative clinical approaches as they emerge. As a patient-centered model, it can continually adapt to changing goals and values of the patient. As the model applies to the whole person, rather than to a specific type of pain presentation or body region, it can be used across pain and disease populations and is not only applied to patients with lumbopelvic or pelvic girdle pain. However, for the context of this book, specific examples for patients with problems in the low back, pelvic girdle, and hip regions will be used to illustrate the model. In the context of the LPH complex, the Integrated Model of Function fits within, and is encompassed by, The Integrated Systems Model for

Disability and Pain. The Integrated Model of Function provides a way to subgroup patients with failed load transfer (FLT) in the LPH complex – those with a primary form closure, force closure, motor control, or emotional deficit (Chapter 5).

The broader Integrated Systems Model for Disability and Pain also considers how a patient could be subgrouped according to the primary system impairment of patients and also considers the role of the *rest of the body and mind* to the observed FLT in the LPH complex. For example, is the primary impairment causing the FLT intrinsic to the pelvic girdle itself (SIJ laxity creating pelvic-driven pelvic girdle pain – see case report part 1 of Julie G, Chapter 9 🖱]) or extrinsic to the pelvic girdle (foot-driven pelvic girdle pain – see case report Louise 🖱 or thorax-driven pelvic girdle pain – see case reports part 2 of Julie G and part 2 of Louise 🖱]) or due to a negative cognitive/emotional state (see case report Julie K 🖱). The Integrated Systems Model for Disability and Pain also considers the interaction and contribution of multiple systems (articular, myofascial, neural, visceral, hormonal, neuroendocrine, etc.).

Therefore, although The Integrated Systems Model is based on the identification of the multisystem impairments that are the key drivers behind the problems facing the whole person, which could then be used to subgroup patients, the primary purpose of the model is to provide a framework for building a unique tapestry that tells the patient's story. It also facilitates clinical reasoning 'on the fly' as the patient's story unfolds and the clinician begins to understand the significant pieces of their tapestry. When used reflectively, it is our goal that The Integrated Systems Model will facilitate, foster, and promote the development of clinical expertise (see Fig. 9.2).

The Integrated Systems Model for Disability and Pain – a framework for understanding the whole person and their problem

Underlying constructs of the model

Before we can describe the components or systems of The Integrated Systems Model, it is important to define its underlying constructs. These include the definitions of key terms and are as follows:

1. The terms 'body,' 'function/functioning,' 'disability,' 'impairment,' and 'health condition' are taken from the International Classification of Functioning, Disability and Health (ICF) definitions (p. 189–190, 2001):

   Body functions are the physiological functions of body systems, including psychological functions. 'Body' refers to the human organisms as a whole, and thus includes the brain. Hence, mental (or psychological) functions are subsumed under body functions.

   Functioning is an umbrella term for body functions, body structures, activities and participation. It denotes the positive aspects of the interaction between an individual (with a health condition/[perceived problem(s)]) and that individual's contextual factors (environmental and personal factors).

   Disability is an umbrella term for impairments, activity limitations and participation restrictions. It denotes the negative aspects of the interaction between an individual (with a health condition) and that individual's contextual factors (environmental and personal factors).

   Impairment is a loss or abnormality in body structure or physiological function (including mental functions).

   Health condition is an umbrella term for disease, disorder, injury, or trauma. A health condition may also include other circumstances such as pregnancy, ageing, stress, congenital abnormality, or genetic predisposition.

2. In a state of optimal health, an individual will have the option to choose from a wide variety of strategies that provide for optimal function and performance during any meaningful task (movement, activity, or role in a desired context and environment). Determining whether a task is meaningful requires an understanding of the person and their values and goals.

3. By definition, optimal function and performance occurs in a state of health, and will be a state free from undesired pain experiences. Given the definitions of health above, optimal function and performance is individually defined, and attainable in the presence of any health condition, although it may be influenced by specific features of the health condition.

4. Pain is not the only reason that people become disabled. Disability, or the inability to do what the person wants to do, can exist without pain.

5. Optimal function and performance for any task requires the synergistic, integrated operation of

multiple systems in the body. 'Synergy' is defined as a 'combined or cooperative action or force' (Webster's New World College Dictionary), and 'simply defined, it means that the whole is greater than the sum of its parts' (Wikipedia). To 'integrate' is to 'form, coordinate, or blend into functioning or unified whole' (Merriam-Webster's Online Dictionary). Synergy and integration require that each system, and thus the components of each system down to the cellular level, is functioning, and that the many complex feedback and feedforward mechanisms that control each system are working optimally. Then, the systems must work together to produce desired outputs in the body. Congruence of information received from feedback and sensory systems is also important. Not all the underlying mechanisms that produce the integrated, synergistic operation of body systems are fully understood, although science is continuing to reveal the connectedness and interdependence of body systems. Melzack's concept of the body-self neuromatrix (see Fig. 7.9) highlights this need for synergy and integration.

6. Impairment(s) in any one or combination of systems can give rise to undesired outputs in one or more systems. These outputs include painful states, non-optimal posture and movement (inefficient, loss of desired performance or output), loss of function, overactive and/or sustained stress response, and negative emotional states.

7. Designing and implementing the most effective treatment plan for restoring health depends on identifying the relevant impairments in the key systems that are barriers to healing and that need to be addressed in order to restore function and health. The relevance of each impairment is determined through a clinical reasoning process that uses a combination of different types of reasoning (Chapter 9). Each impairment is evaluated in the context of meaningful tasks to determine how much the impairment contributes to the non-optimal strategies for function and performance, and the pain experience. The impairments/systems/regions with high contribution values are

called the key 'driver(s)' in this model. The term 'pain driver' is used to refer to the underlying cause(s) of the pain experience, which could be the pain mechanism itself or a multitude of combined impairments that collectively increase physical and psychological stress and perpetuate the pain experience by exceeding the adaptive/coping mechanisms of specific tissues and the person as a whole. Note that as the human body is dynamic, that is a *changing* entity, the key drivers for disability and/or pain at different points in time can change. Furthermore, the driver(s) of disability may be different from the driver(s) of pain.

8. The Integrated Systems Model is applicable to disability and/or pain of any duration; that is, from acute onset to chronic, persistent, or recurrent problems.

9. Every person is unique genetically, emotionally, cognitively, culturally, and socially; the activities and roles that have meaning for them and their pain experience will be uniquely their own. In this way, the specific combination of impairments and systems that contribute to output experiences will be different for each patient. However, taken together, science and clinical expertise provide us with the necessary information to allow us to identify common patterns and parameters for normal and abnormal functioning of systems, as well as how subgroups of patients with certain common features (determined in research by inclusion and exclusion criteria of the study) respond to different treatment approaches. This information is invaluable and indispensable, and the continued pursuit of furthering our knowledge base (both propositional and non-propositional knowledge) in research and in the clinic creates a continually refined understanding of what allows us to enjoy health. However, knowledge gained from either the clinic or the research lab has limitations. Clinicians must constantly examine their emerging hypotheses for multiple types of bias. Although clinical practice guidelines derived from research can be helpful and provide new insight, they may also be

inappropriate and incorrect for certain patients. Therefore, caution is always necessary when developing general treatment protocols based on 'homogeneous populations' as homogeneous populations are an illusion and do not truly exist outside of research constructs.

10. Each person is a dynamic entity and can change from moment to moment and day to day. Science continues to find more evidence of this. Clinically, this implies that continual reassessment is essential for revising hypotheses about the drivers of the patient's problem.

Components of the model: the Clinical Puzzle – a tool for clinical reasoning and developing clinical expertise

The Clinical Puzzle (Fig. 7.11) is a graphic that conceptualizes the Integrated Systems Model for Disability and Pain. It represents the person and their problem(s), and the systems that support optimal strategies for function and performance. The puzzle is used clinically and in teaching as a tool for clinical reasoning and decision-making. See Chapter 9 – case reports for multiple examples of the Clinical Puzzle in action.

The person in the middle of the puzzle

At the center of the model is the patient, the person in the middle of the clinical puzzle. Seeking to understand the unique makeup of the person (the color, shape, and content of their tapestry), without judgment, is the goal of listening to the patient's story. It is essential that during the subjective examination the therapist creates a supportive, compassionate environment that allows the patient to tell their story freely. Open-ended questions, such as 'What can I do for you today?' or 'Please tell me your story' create an

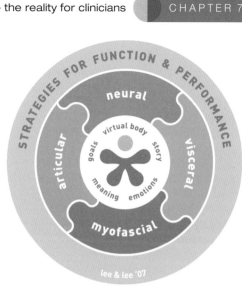

Fig. 7.11 • The Integrated Systems Model – the Clinical Puzzle. The Clinical Puzzle conceptualizes The Integrated Systems Model for Disability and Pain. The outer circle of the puzzle represents the strategies for function and performance that the patient currently uses for meaningful tasks. Meaningful tasks are determined from listening to the patient's story. Impairment in any piece(s) or loss of congruence and synergy between the pieces of the puzzle (the 'systems') within the outer circle can 'drive' non-optimal strategies for function and performance, and non-optimal strategies can also 'drive' impairments in any system(s). The center piece of the puzzle represents several systems that relate to the person and the sensorial (sensations, perceptions), cognitive (beliefs, attitudes, motivations), and emotional (fears, anger, anxiety) dimensions of their current experience. It also includes systemic systems (such as endocrine balance, immune function) and genetic factors. It is the place where primary symptoms, goals, and barriers to recovery are noted. The four other pieces of the puzzle represent the various systems in which impairments are assessed and noted during the clinical examination. During this process, the therapist also considers and reflects upon the relationship of these impairments to the person in the middle of the puzzle (e.g. the meaning these impairments may or may not have, how they relate to health conditions or genetic factors) and the relevance these impairments may have to the non-optimal strategies for function and performance during meaningful tasks. All clinical puzzles are unique as no two individuals have the same life experiences and this graphic is a useful tool for organizing the key information gained through the examination process and for reflection and interpretive reasoning of the findings.

invitation for the patient to share the things about their current experience that are most meaningful and relevant to them, along with their goals and values. This is in contrast to the therapist who has a checklist of questions to obtain answers to, and who strongly directs the subjective examination along a path that the therapist deems (in their wisdom) to be the best. This checklist format of subjective examination is more likely to miss out on essential information from the patient.

Understanding the person in the middle of the Clinical Puzzle also incorporates information about the sensorial, cognitive, and emotional dimensions to their experience of their problem(s). Problems may be disability and/or pain. The sensorial dimension includes the location and behavior of the problem(s), the cognitive dimension includes their beliefs and attitudes about their current experience, and the emotional dimension encompasses both positive and negative feelings about the experience. Problems such as incontinence (stress and/or urge), symptoms of pelvic organ prolapse, difficulty with breathing, and effortful movement, are all examples of problems that the patient may not talk about if they are only asked about their pain, but that are important to identify when present. From these multiple dimensions, the therapist can glean potential barriers to, and potential facilitators of, recovery.

How the patient perceives their body and their current experience of their body constitutes the current state of their *virtual body*. The virtual body is made up of both conscious and unconscious components. As the objective examination proceeds, discrepancies between the actual body and the virtual body will become evident. An example of this would be when a patient perceives that they are standing with equal weight bearing on both feet, but postural examination reveals that the center of mass is shifted to load one extremity to a greater degree than the other.

Meaningful tasks are postures and/or activities that are determined by aggravating activities, relieving activities, activities associated with negative beliefs and emotions (e.g. movements of which the patient is fearful), activities in specific environments or contexts, and the patient's goals (e.g. what would you really like to do that you are not currently able to do due to this problem?). All characteristics of meaningful tasks, including biomechanical requirements, environmental, social,

and emotional context, must be considered during the objective examination in order to most accurately analyze the strategies used by the patient during the meaningful task analysis.

The center of the puzzle (the person in the middle of the Clinical Puzzle) also represents their genetic makeup and systemic health status, including the nutritional, neuroendocrine, autonomic, and homeostatic/stress/immune systems. Past experiences, social background, and other psychosocial features are also a part of the center of the puzzle.

The process of the subjective examination and understanding the patient's story is further discussed in Chapter 8 (assessment) and Chapter 9 (case reports). The experienced clinician will start to link information in the patient's story and form initial hypotheses that direct the priorities of the objective examination to follow.

Strategies for function and performance

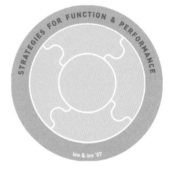

The meaningful tasks identified from the patient's story direct the tasks chosen for analysis of strategies for function and performance, and are noted in the outside ring of the puzzle. These tasks, or the relevant component movements of the task, must be assessed to determine if the patient is using an *optimal* or *non-optimal* strategy for the meaningful task. As the strategies that people use for whole body function are a result of, and depend on, the integrated function of all systems in the body, including all the systems represented by the person in the middle of the puzzle, the 'strategies ring' encircles the entire puzzle. If a non-optimal strategy is observed, the objective findings characterizing how the strategy is non-optimal are written beside the task listed in the outer circle of the puzzle. Strategy analysis is further discussed in Chapters 8, 9, and 12.

Articular, myofascial, neural, visceral systems

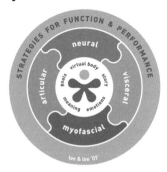

The four other pieces of the puzzle represent the systems that are assessed during the clinical examination. Specific impairments, as well as information gained from diagnostic tests (e.g. X-rays, MRI, etc.) and other sources, are charted within the relevant system in the puzzle. The therapist also considers and reflects upon the relationship of these impairments to the person in the middle of the puzzle (e.g. sensorial, cognitive, and emotional dimensions of the problem(s)) and the relationship these impairments have to the non-optimal strategies for function and performance during meaningful tasks.

As the examination proceeds, the therapist evaluates whether or not the observed non-optimal strategies for function and performance for each meaningful task are *appropriate* or *inappropriate* given all the information available (beliefs about the task, state of tissue healing/integrity of tissue, characteristics of the task and the task context including load requirements, mobility requirements, level of predictability, threat value, availability of accurate proprioceptive input). Note that for some tasks the patient may have appropriate strategies (side bent lumbar spine posture due to acute radicular pain), whereas for other tasks the patient may have inappropriate strategies (fear of moving in any direction in the lumbar spine due to pain that only occurs in one direction of movement). If the therapist has reason to believe that a strategy is inappropriate, determining the reasons why a patient chooses a particular strategy is essential for identifying the driver(s) of the problem and planning the most effective treatment program.

Specific impairments in the *articular, myofascial, neural,* and *visceral* systems for the LPH complex are listed in Tables 7.4a–d. The articular system includes the bones and joints (passive structures) in the musculoskeletal system. The myofascial system includes muscle, and its tendinous and fascial connections, as well as the multiple layers of fascia throughout the body. The neural system includes all components of the central and peripheral nervous system. It also includes the neural drive to muscles, which is reflected in the resting tone and activity or control of the muscle system. The visceral system includes all the viscera of the body.

An impairment in any piece(s) of the puzzle within the outer circle (the 'systems'), or loss of congruence and synergy between the pieces of the puzzle, can 'drive' non-optimal strategies for function and performance. Conversely, non-optimal strategies for function and performance can drive

Table 7.4a The conditions associated with the articular system of the Clinical Puzzle

Articular

Capsular sprain or tear
Ligament sprain or tear (grades I–III)
Labral or intra-articular meniscal tear
Intervertebral disc strain/tear/herniation/prolapse
Fracture
Joint subluxation or dislocation
Periosteal contusion
Stress fracture
Osteitis, periostitis, apophysitis
Osteochondral/chondral fractures, minor osteochondral injury
Chondropathy (softening, fibrillation, fissuring, chondromalacia)
Synovitis
Apophysitis
Fibrosis/osteophytosis of the zygapophyseal and intervertebral joints, sacroiliac joint, hip joint

Table 7.4b The conditions associated with the myofascial system of the Clinical Puzzle

Myofascial

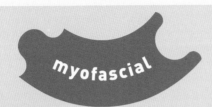

Intramuscular strain/tear (grades I–III)
Muscle contusion
Musculotendinous strain/tear
Complete or partial tendon rupture or tear
Fascial strain/tear
Tendon pathology – tendon rupture, partial tendon tears, tendinopathy (acute or chronic), paratendinopathy, pantendinopathy
Skin lacerations/abrasions/puncture wounds
Bursa – bursitis
Muscular or fascial scarring or adhesions
Loss of fascial integrity of the anterior abdominal wall including diastasis rectus abdominis
Sports hernia (tear of transversalis fascia)
Hockey hernia (tear of the external oblique)
Inguinal hernia
Loss of fascial integrity of the endopelvic fascia leading to cystocele, enterocele, and/or rectocele

Table 7.4c The conditions associated with the neural system of the Clinical Puzzle

Neural

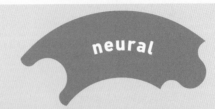

Peripheral nerve trunk or nerve injury (neuropraxia, neurotemesis, axonotemesis)
Central nervous system injury
Altered motor control
Absence of recruitment, inappropriate timing (early or late) of muscle recruitment
Inappropriate amount (increased or decreased) of muscle activity (all relative to demands of task)
Hypertonicity or hypotonicity of muscles at rest
Altered neurodynamics
Sensitization of the peripheral or central nervous system
Altered central nervous system processing

or create impairments within any of the systems inside the puzzle (the person in the middle of the puzzle, the neural, myofascial, articular, and visceral systems). Thus, the entire puzzle is connected, linked, and interdependent and visually represents the integrated systems required for optimal health. All clinical puzzles are unique as no two individuals have the same life experiences.

If one considers all of the possible combinations of impairments and the associated findings that can lead to disability and/or pain, the LPH complex can seem complicated. In reality, when reflective critical thinking and a thorough examination are used, the primary cause and initial treatment plan emerges. The Clinical Puzzle for The Integrated Systems Model is a useful tool for understanding the whole person and their problem(s). It allows for organization of key information gained through the examination process, comparing and contrasting this information to current propositional knowledge and personal knowledge of the clinician, and for

Table 7.4d The conditions associated with the neural system of the Clinical Puzzle

Visceral

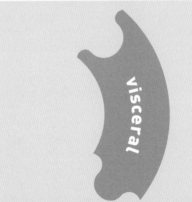

Inflammatory organ disease or pathology (e.g. appendicitis, cystitis, acute ulcerative gastritis, pleuritis, endometriosis)
Infective disorders of the pelvic organs
Organ disease

reflection and interpretive reasoning of the findings. This facilitates the formation of hypotheses to explain the relationships between physical impairments, pain mechanisms, psychosocial features, disability, health conditions, and the patient's values and goals. The goal of the clinical reasoning process, facilitated by the puzzle, is to determine which hypothesis provides the 'most likely and most lovely' explanation of the patient's whole experience, from which an integrated multimodal treatment plan is formulated and implemented. As treatment evolves over several sessions, the focus often changes as the patient journeys towards function and better health.

Summary

Together with the theoretical and scientific information presented in part 1, this chapter has laid the foundation for the rest of this text. Now it is time to put The Integrated Systems Model for Disability and Pain to work and show you how we use it in clinical practice to facilitate the resolution of the patient's unique Clinical Puzzle. There are still a lot of skills to acquire (tools and techniques for assessment (Chapters 8, 12) and treatment techniques (Chapters 10, 11, 12)) and clinical reasoning to learn (Chapters 8, 9, 12) and we hope you find the format of part 2 informative and thought-provoking. The case reports in Chapters 9 and 12 come from our patients and course participants who have volunteered their stories to be shared. Please respect their privacy and do not copy or use their stories or video clips for anything other than your own education.

By now, you should understand that we do not follow recipes or clinical guidelines; we read the research thoroughly and rely on our clinical expertise and sound reasoning skills and logic to guide our clinical practice. We believe that our job is to empower patients to know more about themselves and their state of health so that they can become aware of how their faulty posture, movement, thinking, and/or lifestyle habits can drive their problem(s) and prevent them from attaining the level of function and performance they desire. Ultimately, we hope to motivate them to make the changes necessary to feel better, move better, and be better – it's up to them.

Techniques and tools for assessing the lumbopelvic–hip complex

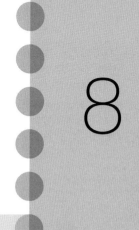

8

Diane Lee   Linda-Joy Lee

CHAPTER CONTENTS

Introduction 173
Subjective examination: understanding the person in the middle of the puzzle 174
Objective examination: developing and testing hypotheses 175
Summary 254

Introduction

Management of patients with lumbopelvic–hip (LPH) disability with or without pain/incontinence using The Integrated Systems Model approach begins with a thorough assessment that includes both a subjective and objective examination. It has been reported that

> Patients with sacroiliac joint (SIJ) pain exhibit no characteristic feature such as aggravation or relief of their pain by sitting, walking, standing, flexion, or extension.
>
> Dreyfuss et al 1996.

This research is not consistent with our clinical experience; however, this finding is not surprising if all patients with sacroiliac joint (SIJ) pain were considered as a homogeneous group (i.e. considered as all having the same impairments and same sensorial, cognitive, and emotional dimensions in their experience). Clinical experience suggests that lumbopelvic and/or hip symptom behavior tends to follow common patterns when patients with similar *impairments* (i.e. deficits in either the articular, neural, myofascial, visceral, and/or systemic systems, and features of 'the person in the middle of the puzzle' (Chapter 7)) are considered. In other words, when patients are subgrouped according to specific impairments, and not by the location/behavior of their pain, characteristic features (similar stories) emerge. Therapists who take the time to reflect on the histories and behavior of symptoms in patients with different LPH impairments will be rewarded later with the ability to recognize similar patterns quickly. Being a reflective practitioner is essential for the development of clinical expertise (Jensen et al 2007). However, it is important to remember that two patients with similar impairments may require different management when consideration is given to the cognitive and emotional dimensions of their experience (Chapter 7). The intent of this chapter is to describe and illustrate the subjective and objective examination for the lumbar spine, pelvic girdle, and hip. The focus of this chapter is on skill acquisition. Although some clinical reasoning will be discussed in this chapter, Chapter 9 will elaborate further on the significance of the findings from both individual and multiple tests through case reports.

© 2011, Elsevier Ltd.
DOI: 10.1016/B978-0-443-06963-5.00008-0

Subjective examination: understanding the person in the middle of the puzzle

The goal of the subjective examination is to hear the patient's story or history, which has ultimately brought them for treatment. Additionally, the examination provides the opportunity for the therapist to learn the significance and meaning, or to gain an understanding, of the experience, as well as the impact it has had on the patient's life, cognitively and emotionally. The way they view and experience their (virtual) body is often revealed through the subjective examination as well as what they hope to achieve from therapy (their goals and meaningful activities). During the interview, any red or yellow flags that may influence treatment decisions are noted. In The Integrated Systems Model the patient's values, beliefs, and goals are at the center of all clinical decision-making, thus the subjective examination is a critical part of the assessment process. The interview begins by introducing yourself and then asking the patient, 'What can I do for you today?' or 'Tell me your story.' This allows the patient to tell their story in their own way and also affirms that they are responsible for setting the goals for therapy. After the examination is completed, the therapist and patient decide together whether or not the goals are realistic.

There are key questions in every subjective examination that include inquiries regarding:

- their age, general health, and medications;
- the mode of onset of symptoms;
- the location and behavior of symptoms, such as aggravating and relieving factors (sensorial dimension of their experience);
- the impact of their pain/symptoms on sleeping;
- the results of any imaging studies;
- their current occupation/leisure/sport activities and desired levels of activities and goals; and
- their thoughts, beliefs, and feelings around their problem (cognitive and emotional dimensions).

Other questions may arise as the interview proceeds.

General health and medications

1. What is the status of the patient's general health? Do they have any conditions that may affect healing (e.g. diabetes). If dry needling is to be included in the treatment plan, it is mandatory to ask if the patient has any infectious diseases that are transmittable through blood such as hepatitis and, HIV, or bleeding disorders.
2. Is the patient currently taking any medication for this or any other condition? If dry needling is to be included in the treatment plan it is mandatory to ask if they are taking any medications that thin the blood such as warfarin (coumadin).

Mode of onset

1. How did the problem begin – suddenly or insidiously?
2. Was there an element of trauma? If so, was there a major traumatic event over a short period of time, such as a fall or motor vehicle accident, or was there a series of minor traumatic events over a prolonged period of time, such as the habitual use of improper lifting/sitting/training technique? With respect to wound repair, is the patient presenting during the substrate, fibroblastic, or maturation phase of healing?
3. Is this the first episode requiring treatment or has there been a similar past history of events? If this is a repeat episode, how long did it take to recover from the previous one and was therapy necessary at that time? If so, what therapy was beneficial, if any?
4. Is the problem a consequence of a pregnancy and/or delivery? If so, when did the symptoms begin, what was the nature of the delivery, and how much trauma occurred to the pelvic floor and/or abdominal wall?

Pain/dysesthesia

1. Exactly where is the pain/dysesthesia? Is it localized or diffuse and can its quality be described?
2. How far down the limb or limbs do the symptoms radiate? Do the symptoms radiate into the abdomen or thorax?

3. Do certain postures or movements change the pain/dysesthesia? If so, which activities (including how much) aggravate the symptoms? It is important to be as specific as possible with aggravating activities. For example, if running exacerbates the pelvic girdle pain, can the patient identify what part of the gait cycle is provocative (heel strike, mid-stance in single leg loading, swing through)? Or, is there a specific context that is more aggravating for a certain task (e.g. racing versus training rides)?

4. If the patient cannot offer any aggravating activities, ask them specifically what effect prolonged sitting, standing, walking, stair-climbing and descent, rolling over in bed, getting in/out of a chair/car, cough and/or sneeze have on their symptoms?

5. Does anything provide relief?

Direct the questions pertaining to the symptom behavior so as to determine whether the symptom is dominantly peripherally mediated or centrally mediated.

Sleep

1. Are the symptoms interfering with sleep? Does rest provide relief?

2. What kind of bed does the patient sleep in and what position is most frequently adopted?

Imaging studies

1. What are the results of any adjunctive diagnostic tests (i.e. X-ray, computed tomography (CT), magnetic resonance imaging (MRI), relevant laboratory tests, etc.)?

Occupation/leisure activities/sport

1. What level of physical activity is required for full function? Specifically, what are the requirements for work, leisure, and sport?

2. What is their current level of activity? Determine the type of activity, frequency, and intensity so that a comparison can be made to the requirements determined from (1).

3. What are the patient's goals from therapy? It is often valuable to ask the patient, 'Are there any things you would like to do but are not doing because of your pain or injury?' and 'What would it take to help you meet your goals?'

Cognitive/emotional considerations

In order to gain insight into the patient's experience (their understanding, beliefs, attitudes, emotions, expectations, and motivations), it is helpful to finish the examination by asking questions such as, 'How do you feel about your current physical status and recovery process?' and 'What do you think is wrong/going on?' and 'What do you think it would take to facilitate your recovery?' Pay attention to the use of the word 'should' as this often reveals their beliefs about what they are meant to do to help their problem and may feel guilty about not doing.

At the end of the subjective examination note the patient's primary complaints and their goals in the center of their Clinical Puzzle (Chapter 7), along with any physical, cognitive, or emotional barriers to the recovery process (features of the meaning perspective). Also note any potential facilitators to recovery, as these can be key positive motivators for embracing the new strategies required for recovery. Make sure to note the tasks (or components of these tasks) that have meaning for the patient in the outer circle of the Clinical Puzzle (strategies for function and performance) as you will want to create ways to reproduce these tasks during the assessment and treatment process (see also Chapter 12). The meaningful task is derived from the patient's goals as well as the activities that aggravate their pain. For example, if the patient's goal is to run 5km and they report that weight bearing on the right leg increases their pain, then single leg loading, or one leg standing, has meaning for them and this task is entered in the outer circle of the puzzle for analysis.

Objective examination: developing and testing hypotheses

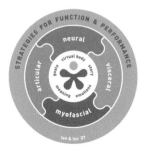

Bogduk (1997) states that biomechanical diagnoses require biomechanical criteria. He notes that 'pain on movement is not that criterion. Movement analysis (including posture/position, mobility, and motion control tests during multiple tasks) is, in part, biomechanical, and yet we have struggled to show reliability for many tests commonly used in clinical practice.

Several studies (Albert et al 2000, Carmichael 1987, Dreyfuss et al 1996, Herzog et al 1989, Laslett & Williams 1994, Laslett et al 2005, Maigne et al 1996, Ostgaard et al 1994, Potter & Rothstein 1985, Robinson et al 2007) have investigated the interexaminer reliability of pain provocation, position, and mobility tests for the pelvic girdle. Although the pain provocation tests have shown reliability individually (Albert et al 2000, Laslett & Williams 1994, Ostgaard et al 1994), the position and mobility tests have not (Dreyfuss et al 1996, Potter & Rothstein 1985, Robinson et al 2007). When test findings are clustered, good percentage agreement and reliability have been found (Arab et al 2009, Laslett et al 2005, Robinson et al 2007). Both novice and expert clinicians rarely rely on the findings of one test alone; the development of hypotheses from multiple test findings (hypothetical deductive reasoning) and reflection on and interpretive reasoning of the test results is a more accurate way of describing and thus investigating clinical practice (Jensen et al 2007, Jones & Rivett 2004, Kerry et al 2008, Kerry 2009) (Chapter 9).

Albert et al (2000) note that the low reliability of position and mobility tests may be due to examiner bias and skill, and propose that instead of abandoning these tests we should seek to improve the skills of the examiners. They emphasize that a higher degree of standardization for all tests is required if interexaminer reliability is to occur.

The tests for LPH function continue to evolve and as we understand more about the factors that influence the test findings (Chapter 2) they will hopefully be able to withstand the scrutiny of scientific research. Some of the tests presented in this chapter have met this scientific challenge and will be identified as such. Other tests are based on clinical expertise and are presented with good intention, recognizing their lack of intertester reliability when considered in isolation. They remain the best we have and, when a clinical reasoning process is applied to multi-test findings, sound hypotheses, logical diagnoses, and treatment plans can be made (Chapter 9).

The objective examination is divided into tests that analyze the strategies chosen for specific tasks (meaningful task analysis), and then specific regional tests that analyze the contribution of each of the systems or puzzle pieces (articular, neural, myofascial, and visceral systems) to the observed non-optimal strategy. This chapter will describe and illustrate how to perform these tests (skill acquisition) and note the optimal and non-optimal test results. The clinical reasoning of multi-test findings will be discussed through a review of several case reports in Chapter 9.

Strategies for function and performance – general principles

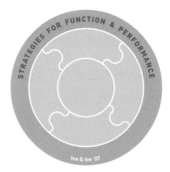

As outlined in Chapter 4, the ability to function optimally across the diverse spectrum of human activity requires that we can access and choose multiple strategies. There is not *one way* in terms of the amount of muscle activity, timing of muscle activity, and coordination or pattern of muscle activation that is optimal across all possible tasks. Futhermore, our central nervous system (CNS) needs to have the ability to match the strategy to the specific demands of the task whether it is sitting at a desk or running a marathon. It is a common clinical observation that patients lose movement options. That is, they have fewer strategies for function and performance to choose from, or they 'get stuck' in one or two strategies that they apply to multiple tasks. In some cases the strategy is appropriate for the task, but in other tasks the same strategy causes pain and loss of function/disability.

For each task, there are multiple characteristics, or factors, that need to be considered to determine which strategy should be used, including:

- What are the loading requirements (how much load needs to be transferred, and how does the amount vary during the task)?
- What are the mobility requirements (how much does each joint in the kinetic chain need to move in order to distribute load, dampen perturbation, and provide range of motion)?
- How predictable is the situation (external or environmental)? How does the person feel about the level of predictablity of the situation (internal)?

- What is the threat value of the situation (real and perceived)?
- Is there accurate proprioceptive and interoceptive information being relayed to the CNS (from the somatosensory system including the joints, ligaments, fascia, skin, vestibular system, and visual system)?
- Is there accurate processing and output of information by the CNS to the musculoskeletal, autonomic and/or endocrine systems (many factors can influence this)?

In addition to these factors, each individual brings a unique structural makeup (due to genetic factors, systemic disease, and injury history, for example), meaning perspective, social context, and environmental context. Given the complexity of, and the challenges in, objectively measuring all these characteristics, how is the therapist to determine if the patient has chosen an optimal strategy for the task being analyzed?

Scientific research can provide ideas to guide our analysis. Differences in motor control between groups with low back pain, pelvic girdle pain, and hip pain compared to healthy controls have been studied for some tasks (Chapters 4, 5). Note that in these studies the definition of 'healthy' was variable. However, scientists can differ in their interpretation of these findings, as some may argue that changes in groups with back pain are necessary and adaptive, whereas others may argue that the changes are non-optimal and maladaptive. It can be said that overall we have a much greater understanding of the underlying mechanisms and principles for motor control of spinal stability, and these principles serve to guide and inform the reflective, critically thinking clinician. Still it is unlikely that science will ever be able to test every possible task and delineate what is 'ideal' or 'normal' motor control for all tasks in all possible contexts and environments for every individual.

How do you decide if the patient is using an optimal strategy for the task being analyzed? We propose an approach that is based on an integration of research in both basic and applied science and extensive clinical experience in movement analysis and training. The basic principles for task analysis draw from multiple disciplines, but have strong influences from the fields of biomechanics, human movement, sports psychology, and neuroscience.

As task analysis involves integrated total body movement, in clinical practice we consider all the joints in the kinetic chain when analyzing strategies. Impairments in any area of the body can create a non-optimal strategy. For the purposes of this book, the focus is on the LPH complex; thus, the principles will be outlined in the context of this region as a base and then expanded upon in later chapters.

Key components of strategy analysis

When the CNS is successful at planning the best, or optimal, strategy (Figs 4.35, 8.1):

1. all joints of the kinetic chain will be controlled in both angular and translatoric motions, while allowing the necessary range of motion required for the task;
2. spinal posture and orientation will be controlled both within and between regions and be appropriate for the task;
3. postural equilibrium will be maintained; and
4. respiration, continence, and internal organ support and function will be maintained.

In addition, there will be enough movement (i.e. give) in the system to dampen and control multiple predictable and unpredictable challenges of varying loads and risk in potentially changing environments (see Chapter 4 for references). Therefore, we can determine whether a strategy is optimal based on the ability of the individual to demonstrate these features (1–4) during any task. Failure to maintain any of the above features is an indication that the patient is using a non-optimal strategy for the task. Once a non-optimal strategy has been determined, the next step is to decide if it is appropriate or not. For example, a non-optimal strategy may be appropriate when there is tissue injury and the state of healing is currently associated with inflammation (acute ankle sprain, muscle tear, inflamed nerve or organ, etc.).

In terms of segmental joint control and spinal posture and orientation, each joint in the kinetic chain is assessed for *the loss of optimal alignment, biomechanics, and/or control required for the task being analyzed*. If there is loss of optimal alignment, biomechanics, and/or control, this is defined as *failed load transfer* (FLT) at that joint. Segmental loss of control often correlates with changes in postural orientation. However, multisegmental malalignment and/or poor control can also occur, and the inability to maintain the required spinal posture or orientation required for the task can then be described by the position of the malalignment and/or direction of loss of control and the levels and regions involved

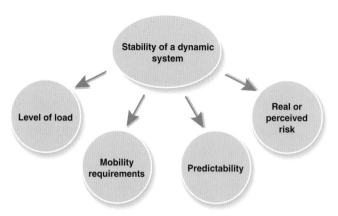

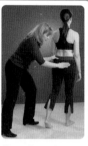

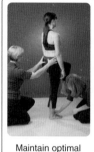

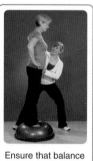

Fig. 8.1 • The requirements of an optimal strategy for any task.

Control angular and translatoric motion of all joints in the kinetic chain while allowing the necessary range of motion required for the task

Maintain optimal alignment within and between the regions

Ensure that balance is maintained (postural equilibrium)

All need to be maintained in spite of any perturbation that may occur, and allow optimal respiration and appropriate IAP increases

(e.g. increased extension from T11–L3). Loss of postural equilibrium during a task is also noted in addition to *when* in the task (timing) this occurs. Respiration, continence, and organ position can be assessed by observation, palpation, and, on occasion, ultrasound imaging. Any non-optimal features are noted, as well as any subjective reports of altered breathing, loss of continence, or sense of pressure in the pelvic floor.

Once the areas of FLT in the kinetic chain are identified, further assessment is required to determine the relative timing of FLT in each area – in other words, which joint fails at the earliest point in the task? For example, if the right side of the pelvis unlocks (right innominate rotates anteriorly relative to the ipsilateral side of the sacrum) and the right hip translates anteriorly (right femoral head shifts anteriorly relative to the acetabulum) during one leg standing, the next step is to determine if the non-optimal

biomechanics of the SIJ and the right hip occur at the same time, or if one occurs before the other. The joint that gives way first is more likely to be the primary impairment. The timing of FLT is charted in the outer ring of the Clinical Puzzle (strategies for function and performance) beside the assessed task.

Subsequently, the impact on the timing of FLT between the various joints is noted when the task is repeated with more optimal biomechanics (Box 8.1). This is achieved through the use of verbal cues and/ or manual support. If it is possible to correct the biomechanics (alignment and control) through verbal cuing and/or manual support, the impact of this correction on:

1. range of motion;
2. strength output on resisted tests;
3. ability to automatically control other joints in the kinetic chain that exhibited FLT;

Box 8.1

Strategy analysis: summary

During any task

- Identify all areas of FLT in the kinetic chain – assess for non-optimal biomechanics
- Establish *relative timing* between areas of FLT; determine which joint(s) exhibit FLT at the earliest point in the task
- Use verbal cues and manual correction to provide better biomechanics at the areas of FLT (one at a time) and assess the impact of correction on:
  (a) ROM;
  (b) resisted tests;
  (c) FLT at other joints in the chain;
  (d) pain;
  (e) effort to move/experience of the patient in ease of movement

Consider

- The relationship of the identified areas of FLT and the pain presentation. Given the patient's story, are the observed non-optimal biomechanics consistent with your hypothesis about the pain-generating structure?
- Given the patient's story and the specific types of FLT (loss of control, loss of mobility, etc.), which systems are *most likely* to be responsible for the FLT observed and therefore the next pieces of the puzzle to assess?

4. the behavior of pain during the task; and the
5. effort required to perform the task can be noted.

The specific tasks analyzed are chosen from the findings of the subjective examination. The key tasks that must be assessed are those that relate to the functional positions and movements that are meaningful to the patient (meaningful task analysis). These are usually the painful or aggravating activities, movements, or positions they find difficult, and those that pertain to their functional goals. For example, if someone notes pain or difficulty during walking then vertical loading tasks associated with single leg loading are indicated. On the other hand, if someone notes that prolonged sitting aggravates their symptoms, then the strategies used for sitting, including squat and stand to sit, are assessed.

The following section includes several tasks that are commonly analyzed in the assessment of pain and impairment of the LPH complex. Included are key screening tests that will reveal impairments of the LPH complex. Note that not all of these tests are necessary for every examination. Hypothesis generation and the clinical reasoning process (Chapter 9)

will direct the clinician in prioritizing which tests are most relevant for each patient, enabling a tailored, time-efficient assessment. In subsequent chapters (Chapters 9, 12), other tasks are chosen for analysis as they were pertinent to the patient's Clinical Puzzle. Multiple video clips of all of these tests both before and after treatment can be viewed online in the case reports in Chapter 9. Advanced task analysis that further simulates meaningful activities is described and illustrated in Chapter 12. The purpose of this section is not to list all of the potential tasks that can be analyzed clinically, but rather to illustrate the principles involved in examining the LPH complex in the context of strategy analysis for any task. These base principles will then be further expanded and elaborated upon in the case reports (Chapter 9) and in principles for training new posture and movement strategies (Chapter 12).

Strategies for function and performance

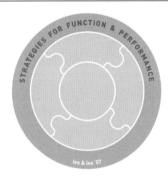

Walking

Careful observation of the patient's strategies used during walking can be informative as walking requires optimal LPH function. Initially, deviation of the top of the head in the vertical and/or coronal planes is noted. When the strategy chosen for walking is optimal, there is minimal deviation of the head in either plane. Failed load transfer through the pelvis and/or hip joint often manifests as a deviation in the coronal plane of the pelvis relative to the lumbar spine and hip (subtle hip drop/Trendelenburg sign (Fig. 8.2A) or compensated Trendelenburg sign (Fig. 8.2B). Asymmetry in stride length and time spent in each phase of the gait cycle can be indicative of impairments within the LPH complex (loss of mobility and/or motion control). Consideration should also be given to the biomechanics of the foot from heel strike through mid-stance to push off, as

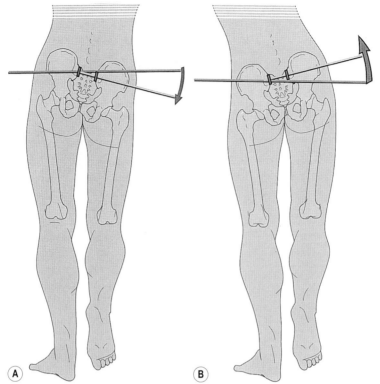

Fig. 8.2 • (A) In a true Trendelenburg gait, the pelvic girdle tilts away laterally from the impaired side in the mid-stance phase of the gait cycle. (B) In a compensated Trendelenburg gait, the pelvic girdle tilts laterally towards the impaired side in the mid-stance phase of the gait cycle.

the foot can be a driver for failed load transfer in the pelvis (see case report Louise, Chapter 9 📁), and to the contralateral thoracopelvic rotation required, which may be absent in cases of thorax-driven failed load transfer in the pelvis.

Standing posture

Malalignment of posture is not necessarily indicative of pelvic girdle impairments (there could be an extrinsic driver for the malalignment); however, impairments within the pelvic girdle (intrinsic drivers) can induce postural malalignment. The *impact* of a specific impairment (intrinsic or extrinsic to the pelvic girdle) is often seen affecting alignment and function of multiple regions.

Optimal postural alignment exists (Fig. 8.3A) when:

- In the sagittal plane, a vertical line passes through the external auditory meatus, the bodies of the cervical vertebrae, the glenohumeral joint, slightly anterior to the bodies of the thoracic vertebrae transecting the vertebrae at the thoracolumbar junction, the bodies of the lumbar vertebrae, the sacral promontory, slightly posterior to the hip joint and slightly anterior to the talocrural joint and naviculo-calcaneo-cuboid joint. The primary spinal curves should be maintained (i.e. gentle even lumbar lordosis, gentle even thoracic kyphosis, and gentle even cervical lordosis).

- There are no kinks, shifts, hinges, or transverse plane rotations in the entire spinal curve.

- The pelvic girdle as a unit should be in neutral in all three planes: coronal, sagittal, and transverse (Fig. 8.3A,B). Figure 8.4A–D illustrates the pelvic girdle in various non-neutral positions and the impact of this on the entire body.

- The innominates should not be rotated relative to one another (Fig. 8.5A) and the sacrum should not be rotated (Fig. 8.5B) (no intrapelvic torsion (IPT)). If an IPT is found, the relative position of each bone determines whether the torsion is physiological or non-physiological. A physiological

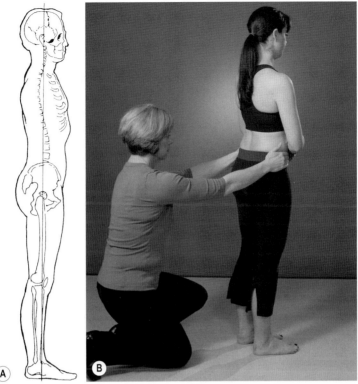

Fig. 8.3 • (A) Optimal posture in standing. (B) Standing posture, palpation. To assess the posture of the pelvic girdle in standing, the therapist positions themselves directly behind the patient. It is important for the therapist to be centered and consistent in their positioning so that kinesthetic sense and reliability are not affected by different starting positions on reassessment. The anterior aspect of the pelvic girdle is palpated bilaterally and its resting position in all three body planes (anteroposterior tilt, lateral tilt, transverse plane rotation) is felt and visualized. Kinesthetic appreciation of position can be taught by having the therapist close their eyes while palpating to remove any visual conflict/bias. During our courses we have found that the therapist's kinesthetic sense is often more reliable than their visual sense.

IPT occurs naturally during tasks that twist the pelvis. A non-physiological IPT exists when the pelvic bones are rotated incongruently with one another (i.e. right anteriorly rotated innominate associated with a left posteriorly rotated innominate and a *right rotated* sacrum).

• The femoral head should be centered in the acetabulum and symmetrical between the left and right sides (Fig. 8.6A–D). The femur should not be internally or externally rotated and the patella should be centered between the medial and lateral femoral condyles. The femoral Q-angle will vary depending on the individual's anatomical structure, but should not cause the patella to tilt (medially/laterally).

• Inferiorly, the talus should rest on top of the calcaneus with the foot neither excessively supinated nor pronated, with no rotation of the tibia and fibula at the knee joint (relative to the femur) (Fig. 8.7A,B). The forefoot should have a gentle dorsal arch (transverse arch), the longitudinal arch should be present medially, and the toes should remain long and flat on the floor.

• The thorax should not be tilted anteriorly, posteriorly (Fig. 8.4A), or laterally (Fig. 8.4D), nor should it be rotated relative to the pelvic girdle. The manubriosternal (MS) junction should be in the same coronal plane as the pubic symphysis (PS) and the anterior superior iliac spines (ASISs) of the innominate. Intrathoracic

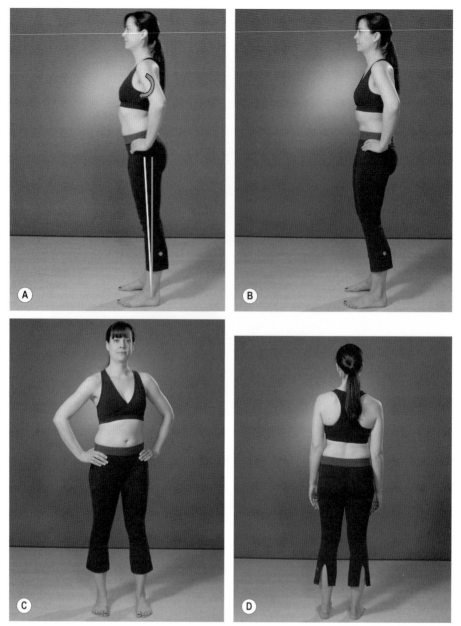

Fig. 8.4 • Standing posture. (A) This model is posturing her pelvis deliberately into an anterior pelvic tilt. Note the associated anterior pelvic sway. The center of mass is displaced anteriorly; note the angle between the vertical line and the anterior line between the greater trochanter and the lateral malleolus. A posterior thoracic tilt has also accompanied this change in pelvic position (arrow). (B) In this illustration the model has deliberately posteriorly tilted her pelvis. She is habitually a back-gripper (overactivates her erector spinae) and this posture is difficult for her to adopt. Note the activation of the superficial abdominal wall and the flexion of her knees required for her to tilt her pelvis posteriorly. This posture and muscle activation pattern can be seen in patients who have been instructed to flatten their low back to reduce an anterior pelvic tilt. It is obviously not optimal. (C) The model is now deliberately rotating her pelvis to the left in the transverse plane and it is quite excessive so that it is visible in this photograph. The rotation has continued through her thorax, but transitions into right rotation in the upper thorax (which is seen by the upper thorax shift to the left), which is a compensatory derotation that continues into her cervical spine. (D) This is a frontal view of this model's normal posture; it is non-optimal. Her pelvic girdle is rotated to the left in the transverse plane, although it is difficult to see in this illustration. Note the left lateral shift of her thorax relative to her pelvis associated with a right rotation and right lateral bend. Her head and neck are left rotated. The right shoulder girdle is lower than the left; however, this could be secondary to the position of her thorax.

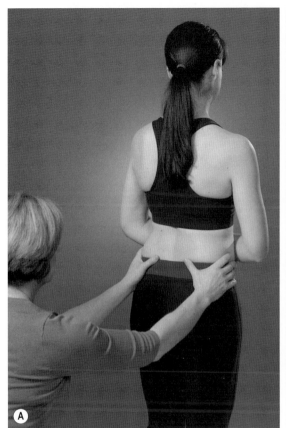
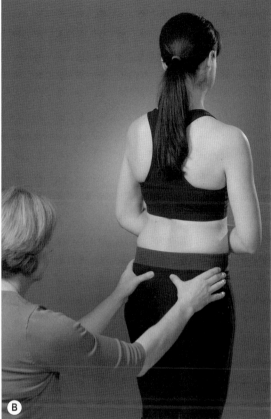

Fig. 8.5 • Standing posture, intrapelvic position. (A) To assess the relative intrapelvic position of the left and right innominates and the sacrum in order to note the presence or absence of a physiological or non-physiological intrapelvic torsion, begin by palpating the innominates. Note the therapist's centered position directly behind the patient. Also note that this test is not just about the level of the posterior superior iliac spines (PSISs). The innominate is a large bone and as much of it should be palpated as possible with the entire hand, not just the thumb and fingertips. The innominates should not be rotated relative to one another. (B) The sacral position is determined by palpating the left and right inferior lateral angles (ILA) and noting the dorsoventral relationship. A dorsal left ILA suggests that the sacrum is rotated to the left. Using the sacral sulcus depth to determine sacral rotation is not valid as the dorsal aspect of the sacrum is covered by multifidus, which has been shown to atrophy with lumbopelvic pain (Hides et al 1994, Hodges et al 2006). Consequently, a deeper sacral sulcus may have nothing to do with sacral position, although it may be indicative of a contributing factor for sacral dysfunction (loss of multifidus function).

positional analysis is beyond the scope of this text; however, it is important to note that the myofascial connections that link the thorax to the pelvis together with poor segmental thoracic control are often responsible for ongoing pelvic girdle pain and dysfunction; this is the thorax-driven pelvic impairment.

• The clavicles and the scapulae should be symmetrical with the clavicles slightly elevated laterally and the scapulae slightly rotated upward with the inferior angle on the chest wall.

• The head and neck should be centered over the thorax with the eyes level; the chin should be parallel to the ground.

Note key findings from the standing posture analysis in the outer ring of the Clinical Puzzle (strategies for function and performance).

Forward bending in standing

Initially, the patient is instructed to bend forward (Fig. 8.8) and the ease with which they do so is noted.

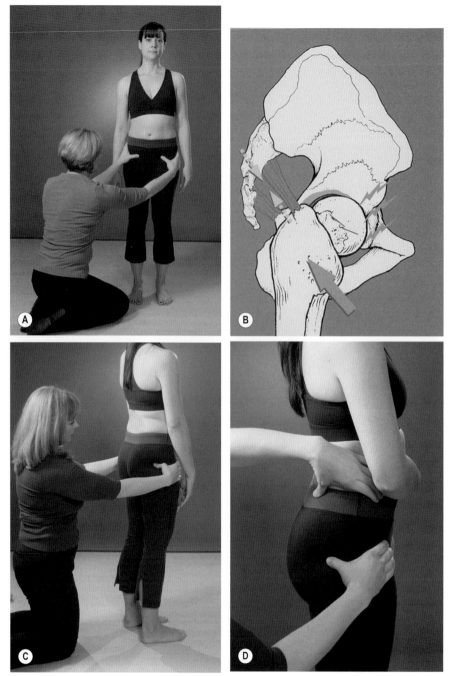

Fig. 8.6 • Standing posture, femoral head position. The femoral heads are palpated midway between the anterior superior iliac spine and the pubic symphysis just below the line of the inguinal ligament. (A) When the femoral head is centered there will be a slight spring/give to the inguinal ligament, and an indent at the hip fold will be felt. When the femoral head is anterior, marked tension in the inguinal ligament (often associated with local tenderness) will be felt, as will the prominence of the femoral head. In this illustration the therapist is off to the patient's right side for photographic purposes only: the therapist should be centered directly in front of the patient. (B) Muscle imbalances around the hip joint can create single or multiple force vectors, which result in anterior displacement of the femoral head. (C) When the femoral head is centered in standing there is equal tension in the front and back of the hip, no 'divot' in the posterolateral buttock, and the greater trochanter projects directly laterally. (D) Note the anterior displacement of the femoral head in this subject. Anterior displacement of the femoral head can be associated with either internal or external rotation of the femur; check the inferior femoral condyle to note the direction of femoral rotation (not shown).

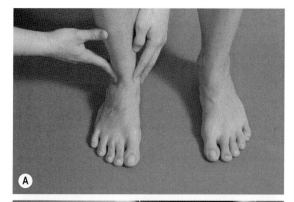

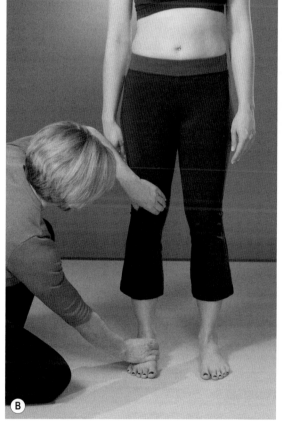

Fig. 8.7 • Standing posture, position of the talus. (A) In a neutral standing posture the head of the talus should rest on the anterior facet of the calcaneus directly beneath the tibia and fibula. The position of the talus is assessed by palpating the medial and lateral aspects of the dome and noting the angle the talus makes with the lower leg (should be directly in line). The lower leg (tibia and fibula) should not be rotated internally or externally. (B) When the talus is in an optimal position relative to both the foot and the lower extremity, the patella and talus will not be rotated relative to one another.

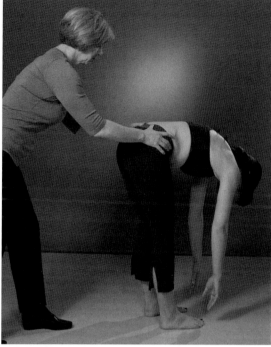

Fig. 8.8 • Forward bending in standing. Initially, the patient is asked to bend forward and the range of available motion, the location of the primary motion/restriction, and the symmetry of motion is noted. Watch for any deviations of the pelvis or thorax from the sagittal plane.

Note the apex of the sagittal curve for the whole body and then specifically note:

1. any rotation of the pelvic girdle or the thorax in the transverse plane (thoracopelvic or pelvicofemoral rotation);
2. the symmetry of the paravertebral fullness between the thorax and the pelvic girdle; it should be equal on both sides of the spinal column;
3. the ability of the femoral heads to center or remain centered in the acetabulum (Fig. 8.9);
4. any intrapelvic torsion; the pelvic girdle should anteriorly tilt symmetrically over the femoral heads (Fig. 8.10) with no torsion;
5. the relative intersegmental mobility of the lumbar spine (segmental kyphosis/lordosis or rotation). The spinal segments should flex symmetrically without shifting or hinging (Fig. 8.11). If a segmental hinge or buckle is present, note the timing of this in relation to any femoral head displacement (or intrapelvic torsion). Often the low back gives way when the hips fail to move;
6. any loss of control of the right or left side of the pelvis (Fig. 8.12). The innominate should remain

185

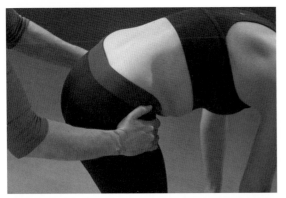

Fig. 8.9 • Forward bending in standing, hip motion control. The femoral heads are palpated anteriorly (remember to stay centered behind the patient) and the presence/absence of femoral head 'seating' or centering is noted as the patient bends forward. If in the standing postural examination one femoral head is noted to be anterior, particular attention is paid to the response of this hip during movement tasks. If the femoral head fails to center, note whether this occurs with a rotation of the pelvis, and which occurs first (i.e. note whether this is a hip-driven pelvic rotation or an intrinsic pelvic rotation with no hip involvement).

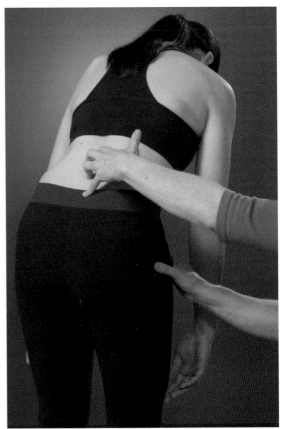

Fig. 8.11 • Forward bending in standing, lumbar motion. The interspinous spaces between the lower lumbar vertebrae are palpated with one hand and the intersegmental mobility is noted and compared between levels as the patient bends forward. All levels should flex symmetrically. If a segmental hinge into flexion is felt (one segment flexes excessively compared to those above and/or below it), the timing of this non-optimal motion should be assessed (early, middle, or late in the overall range of forward bending). Compare the timing of the excessive flexion with the movement analysis of the hip (one hand palpates the femoral head anteriorly and the other palpates the interspinous spaces). It is common to find excessive motion segmentally in the lumbar spine when one or both hip joints fail to move optimally into flexion during forward bending of the trunk (butt-gripping strategy).

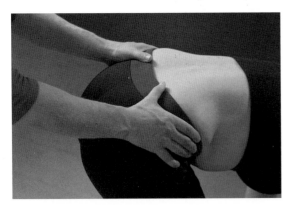

Fig. 8.10 • Forward bending in standing, intrapelvic motion. There should be no relative rotation between the two innominates as the pelvic girdle tilts anteriorly on the femoral heads. Note how the therapist's hands are palpating as much of the innominate as possible and not just the posterior superior iliac spines.

posteriorly rotated relative to the sacrum throughout the forward bend. When the pelvis unlocks, the innominate can be felt to rotate anteriorly relative to the ipsilateral sacrum (Hungerford et al 2004, 2007).

Repeat the forward bend test three or four times to note the consistency/inconsistency of any positive findings and the ease with which the patient is able to bend forward repeatedly. If there are multiple regions of failed load transfer, note the sequential timing of each (i.e. which fails first). Use verbal and manual cues to correct the biomechanics of one region and note the impact of this correction

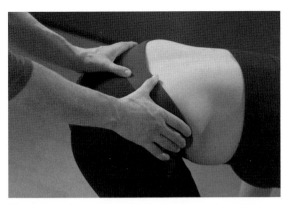

Fig. 8.12 • Forward bending in standing, intrapelvic control. The innominate is palpated with one hand while the sacrum is palpated at either the spinous process of S2 or the ipsilateral inferior lateral angle (ILA). The two bones should move as a unit as the pelvic girdle anteriorly tilts symmetrically over the femoral heads. Watch and feel for early, middle, or late anterior rotation of the innominate relative to the sacrum as the patient bends forward. Remember that the amplitude of motion for the sacroiliac joint is very small while weight bearing (4–6°), and even when the pelvis unlocks completely during this task the movement is very subtle, yet palpable. Examples of an unlocking pelvis can be seen online in the clinical cases in Chapter 9.

on the others. Note the key findings from this task analysis in the outer ring of the Clinical Puzzle (strategies for function and performance).

Backward bending in standing

Initially, the patient is instructed to backward bend and the ease with which they do so is noted. Note the apex of the sagittal curve for the whole body and then specifically note:

1. any rotation of the pelvic girdle (Fig. 8.13) or the thorax in the transverse plane (thoracopelvic or femoral/pelvic rotation);
2. the ability of the femoral heads to remain centered in the acetabulum as the pelvic girdle tilts posteriorly (hips extend);
3. any intrapelvic torsion (Fig. 8.13);
4. the relative intersegmental mobility of the lumbar spine (segmental kyphosis/lordosis or rotation). The spinal segments should extend symmetrically without shifting or hinging. If a segmental hinge or buckle is present, note the timing of this in relation to femoral motion (Fig. 8.14). Often the low back gives way into extension when the pelvic girdle cannot tilt posteriorly on the femoral heads;

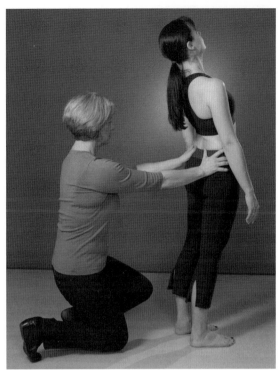

Fig. 8.13 • Backward bending in standing, pelvic girdle motion. There should be no rotation of the pelvic girdle in the transverse plane as the patient backward bends. In addition, there should be no relative rotation between the two innominates as the pelvic girdle posteriorly tilts on the femoral heads. Note how the therapist's hands are palpating as much of the innominates as possible and not just the posterior superior iliac spines. Feel for a small amount of anterior pelvic sway and watch for any segmental hinging (excessive extension) in the lumbar spine.

5. any loss of control of the right or left side of the pelvis (Fig. 8.15). The innominate should remain posteriorly rotated relative to the sacrum as the pelvic girdle tilts posteriorly throughout the backward bend. When the pelvis unlocks, the innominate can be felt to rotate anteriorly relative to the ipsilateral sacrum. Even though the pelvic girdle is tilting posteriorly, it is the relative motion between the innominate and the sacrum that is important to assess.

Repeat the backward bend test three or four times to note the consistency/inconsistency of any positive findings and the ease with which the patient is able to backward bend repeatedly. If there are multiple

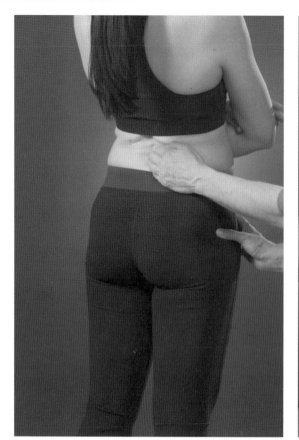

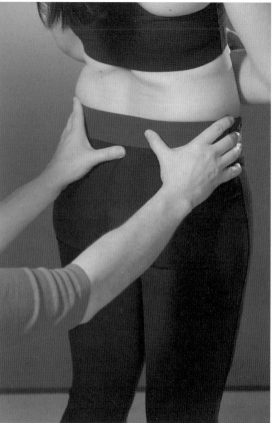

Fig. 8.14 • Backward bending in standing, lumbar motion. The interspinous spaces between the lower lumbar vertebrae are palpated with one hand and the intersegmental mobility is noted and compared between levels as the patient backward bends. All levels should extend symmetrically. If a segmental hinge into extension is felt (one segment extends excessively compared to those above and/or below it), the timing of this non-optimal motion should be assessed (early, middle, or late in the overall range of backward bending). Compare the timing of the excessive extension with the movement analysis of the hip (one hand palpates the femoral head anteriorly while the other palpates the interspinous spaces). It is common to find excessive motion segmentally in the lumbar spine when one or both hip joints fail to move optimally into extension during backward bending of the trunk.

Fig. 8.15 • Backward bending in standing, intrapelvic control. The innominate is palpated with one hand while the sacrum is palpated at either the spinous process of S2 or the ipsilateral inferior lateral angle (ILA). The two bones should move as a unit as the pelvic girdle posteriorly tilts symmetrically over the femoral heads. Watch and feel for early, middle, or late anterior rotation of the innominate relative to the sacrum as the patient backward bends. Remember that the amplitude of motion for the sacroiliac joint is very small in weight bearing (4–6°), and even when the pelvis unlocks completely during this task the movement is very subtle, yet palpable.

Lateral bending in standing

Initially, the patient is instructed to bend laterally while the ease with which they do so is noted. Notice the apex of the coronal curve for the whole body and then specifically pay attention to:

1. any rotation of the pelvic girdle or the thorax in the transverse plane (thoracopelvic or femoropelvic rotation); the body should remain in the coronal plane;

regions of failed load transfer, note the sequential timing of each (i.e. which fails first). Use verbal and manual cues to correct the biomechanics of one region and note the impact of this correction on the others. Note the key findings from this task analysis in the outer ring of the Clinical Puzzle (strategies for function and performance).

2. the ability of the femoral heads to remain centered in the acetabulum as the pelvic girdle tilts laterally (one hip abducts while the other adducts, and the axis of the hip joint should remain centered);

3. any intrapelvic torsion; ideally a small amount of physiological intrapelvic torsion will occur (left lateral bending often induces a slight IPTR);

4. the relative intersegmental mobility of the lumbar spine. The spinal segments should sideflex symmetrically without shifting or kinking. If a segmental or multisegmental restriction is present, note the relationship this has with levels of activity in the paravertebral muscles (Fig. 8.16A,B);

5. any loss of control of the right or left side of the pelvis (Fig. 8.16A,B).

Repeat the lateral bend test three or four times to note the consistency/inconsistency of any positive findings and the ease with which the patient is able to lateral bend repeatedly. Record the key findings from this task analysis in the outer ring of the Clinical Puzzle (strategies for function and performance).

One leg standing

This test is also known as the Gillet test, stork test, or kinetic test and examines the ability of the low back, pelvis, and hip to transfer load unilaterally (motion control test), as well as for the hip to flex, the low

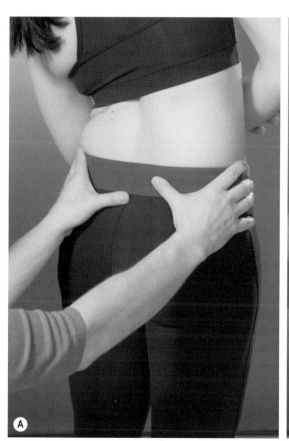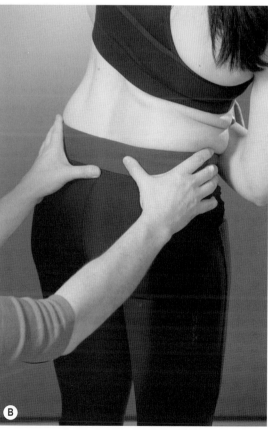

Fig. 8.16 • Lateral bending in standing. (A) Note the lack of left lateral bending at multiple segments in the low lumbar spine (L3–4, L4–5, L5–S1) as well as the lack of right pelvic sway and left lateral pelvic tilt in this model. The therapist's hands in this illustration are noting any unlocking of the right side of the pelvis during this task as well as the lack of optimal motion of the pelvic girdle as a unit. (B) While the pelvic girdle as a unit is moving better relative to the lower extremities, note the multisegmental restriction of right sideflexion of all the lumbar segments and the increased activity of the left paravertebral muscles during right lateral bending.

back to rotate, and the pelvis to allow an intrapelvic torsion (intrapelvic mobility test).

Initially, the patient is instructed to stand on one leg and to flex the contralateral hip and knee towards the waist. Repeat on the opposite side and observe the effort required and the ability to perform this task. The pelvis should not anteriorly/posteriorly/laterally tilt, nor rotate in the transverse plane as the weight is shifted to the supporting limb. Subsequently, note:

1. the ability of the non-weight bearing innominate to rotate posteriorly relative to the ipsilateral sacrum (Fig. 8.17). There should be a small amount of posterior rotation during this task and the quality and amplitude should be symmetrical

between the left and right sides. This test assesses active movement of the innominate relative to the sacrum;

2. the ability of the non-weight bearing femoral head to remain centered as it flexes. If there is an altered axis of motion, note the timing and range in which this occurs;

3. any loss of control of the right or left side of the pelvis during single leg loading (Fig. 8.18). The innominate should remain posteriorly rotated relative to the sacrum throughout the task. When the pelvis unlocks, the innominate can be felt to rotate anteriorly relative to the ipsilateral sacrum.

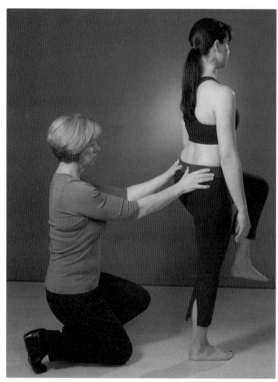

Fig. 8.17 • One leg standing, intrapelvic mobility. The innominate is palpated with one hand while the other palpates the sacrum at either S2 or the ipsilateral inferior lateral angle (ILA). Note the quality and quantity of posterior rotation of the non-weight bearing innominate and compare this movement to the opposite side: it should be symmetrical. Many factors can impede osteokinematic motion of the innominate – the sacroiliac joint (SIJ) is only one of them – therefore this test should not be considered as only a mobility test for the SIJ.

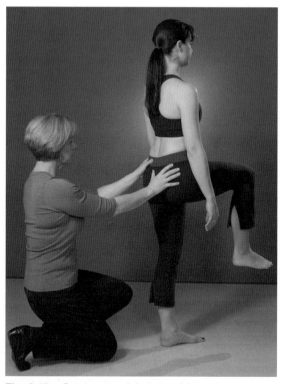

Fig. 8.18 • One leg standing, intrapelvic motion control. The innominate is palpated with one hand while the sacrum is palpated at either the spinous process of S2 or the ipsilateral inferior lateral angle (ILA). The two bones should move as a unit as the pelvic girdle shifts laterally over the weight bearing lower extremity. Watch and feel for early, middle, or late anterior rotation of the innominate relative to the sacrum on the weight bearing side as the patient transfers their weight (this is non-optimal). Remember that the amplitude of motion for the SIJ is very small in weight bearing (4–6°), and even when the pelvis unlocks completely during this task the movement is very subtle, yet palpable.

This test has shown good intertester reliability (Hungerford et al 2007). This task can be made more challenging by having the patient perform a single leg squat. Note the timing (early, middle, or late) of any loss of control (unlocking) during the weight shift, contralateral leg lift, and/or single leg squat;

4. the ability of the femoral head to remain centered in the acetabulum as load is transferred through the hip joint (Fig. 8.19A,B). Pay attention to the timing of any loss of control (femoral head centering) during this task (early, middle, late);

5. note the alignment of the lower extremity, femur to pelvis (Fig. 8.20), femur to tibia, talus to patella (Fig. 8.21), talus to ankle mortise, and changes through the foot as load is transferred through the weight bearing limb.

Repeat the two parts of the one leg standing test three or four times to determine the consistency/inconsistency of any positive findings and the ease with which the patient is able to perform this task repeatedly. If there are multiple regions of failed load transfer, discern the sequential timing of each (i.e. which fails first). Use verbal and manual cues to correct the biomechanics of one region and note the impact of this correction on the others. Record the key findings from this task analysis in the outer ring of the Clinical Puzzle (strategies for function and performance).

Squat

The strategy an individual uses to squat often sets the stage for how they sit (see below). Squat strategy also has implications for how the patient's gym

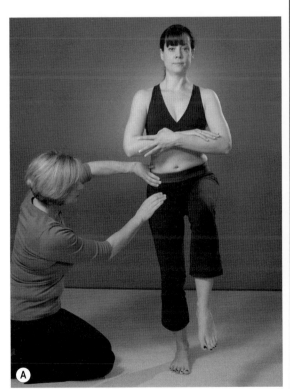
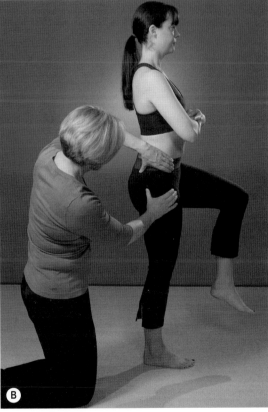

Fig. 8.19 • One leg standing, hip motion control. The innominate is palpated with one hand while the femoral head is palpated anteriorly (A) or the greater trochanter is palpated laterally (B). The femoral head should remain centered in the acetabulum during this task and the femur should not rotate internally or externally. Watch and feel for anterior femoral translation (the femoral head will become more prominent anteriorly and push into your fingers) as well as any femoral rotation (easily palpated via the greater trochanter), and note the timing of this loss of hip control.

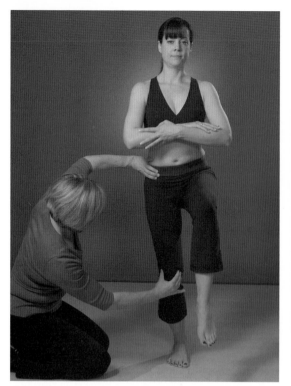

Fig. 8.20 • One leg standing, hip control. Femoral rotation can also be detected by palpating the distal medial and lateral femoral condyles during this task. The femur should remain vertical beneath the pelvic girdle.

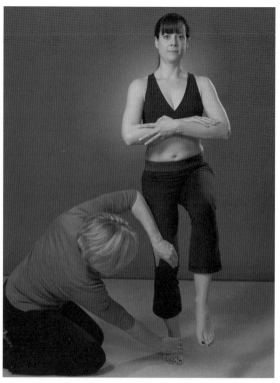

Fig. 8.21 • One leg standing, foot control. It is not uncommon to see a combination of foot, knee, hip, and intrapelvic control problems. In this test, the therapist is palpating the talus to assess any loss of talar position and control during this task. The talus should remain centered on the top of the calcaneus and the loss of talar position during the transference of weight suggests that a more detailed assessment of the foot is in order.

program and technique relates to their pain and dysfunction/disability. Note that the strategy they use to do squats in the gym may be different from how they move into a sitting position, as the task context can affect the strategy. There are many things to consider when evaluating the strategy for a squat and several variations that can be applied to the task. The optimal biomechanics of a squat are described in Chapter 4. Initially, the patient is asked to squat as if they were going to sit into a chair. If the patient reports in their subjective history that 'squats at the gym' are an aggravating activity, then the question should be reframed as, 'Show me how you do your gym squats' so that the task analysis replicates as closely as possible the aggravating task. This should include simulating how they hold any weights (front loaded with a bar, dumbbells in hands at the sides, etc.), as this variable can dramatically change strategy and, unless specifically assessed, key areas of failed load transfer may be missed. When assessing squat tasks, the therapist should note:

1. any loss of control of the right or left side of the pelvis during the squat (Fig. 8.22). The innominate should remain posteriorly rotated relative to the ipsilateral sacrum throughout the task. Note the timing (early, middle, or late) of any loss of control (unlocking);

2. the ability of the femoral heads to remain centered as load is transferred through the hip joints and they flex (Fig. 8.23A,B). Note the timing of any loss of control (loss of femoral head centering) during this task (early, middle, late);

3. the alignment of the thorax to the pelvis and the ability to maintain neutral thoracic and lumbar curves throughout the task. The distance between the MS junction and the PS should not change during an optimal squat (Fig. 8.24A). If the distance increases (Fig. 8.24B) there is extension

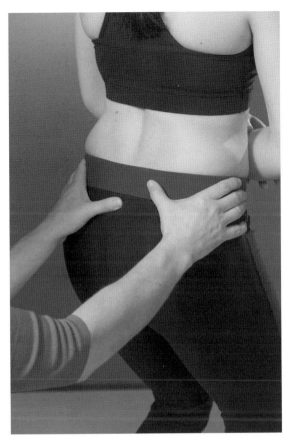

Fig. 8.22 • Squat, intrapelvic control. The innominate is palpated with one hand while the sacrum is palpated at either the spinous process of S2 or the ipsilateral inferior lateral angle (ILA). The two bones should move as a unit as the pelvic girdle tilts anteriorly over the weight bearing lower extremity. Watch and feel for early, middle, or late anterior rotation of the innominate relative to the sacrum. Remember that the amplitude of motion for the sacroiliac joint is very small in weight bearing (4–6°) and even when the pelvis unlocks completely during this task the movement is very subtle, yet palpable.

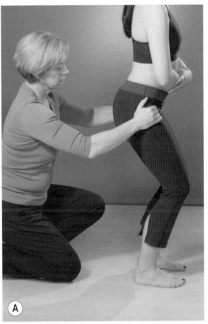

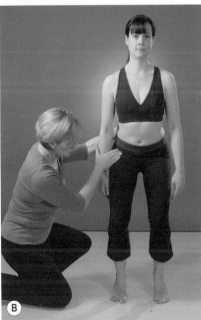

Fig. 8.23 • Squat, hip motion control. The femoral heads are palpated (A) bilaterally (remember to stay centered behind the patient) or (B) unilaterally, and the presence/absence of femoral head 'seating' or centering is noted as the patient initiates and proceeds through a squat. If in the standing postural examination one femoral head is noted to be anterior, particular attention is paid to the response of this hip during movement tasks. If the femoral head fails to center, note whether this induces a rotation of the pelvis as a consequence or causes the pelvic joints to unlock or lose control.

of the spine, multisegmentally and/or segmentally, somewhere in the thoracic and/or lumbar spine; if the distance decreases (Fig. 8.24C) there is flexion of the spine occurring multisegmentally and/or at a segmental hinge somewhere in the thoracic and/or lumbar spine. The spinal segments should not translate or hinge during this task (Fig. 8.24D). If a segmental hinge or buckle is present, note the timing of this in relation to any femoral head displacement (Fig. 8.24E). Often the low back gives way when the hips fail to move and it is not uncommon for

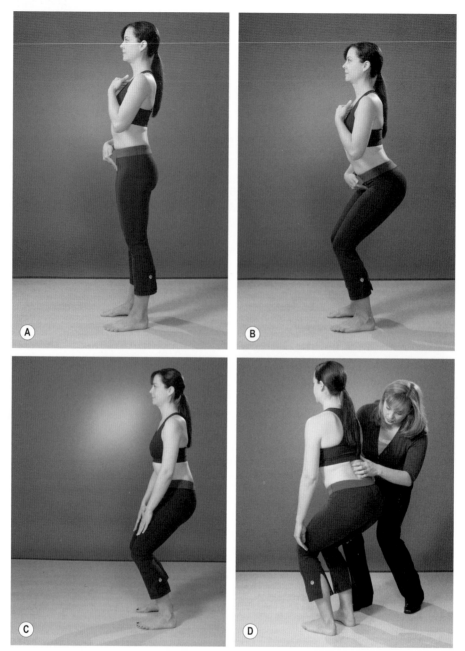

Fig. 8.24 • Squat. (A) Starting position. The patient palpates the manubriosternal junction and the pubic symphysis as a reference point for thoracopelvic orientation during the squat. (B) Thoracopelvic orientation. This patient is using a strategy called back-gripping. This means that she overactivates her erector spinae during this task; note the posterior tilt of her thorax relative to the pelvic girdle and the lengthening of the distance between her manubriosternal junction (MS) and pubic symphysis (PS). (C) This is a butt-gripping strategy for a squat. Note the posterior tilt of the pelvic girdle relative to the femurs and the shortening of the distance from the MS to the PS. As a back-gripper, this is difficult for this model to simulate; note the persistent posterior tilt of the upper thorax. It is common for patients who have been told to 'stay upright' or to 'lift the chest' when squatting in the gym to demonstrate this non-optimal pattern. (D) Squat, lumbar motion control. The interspinous spaces between the lower lumbar vertebrae are palpated with one hand and the intersegmental mobility noted and compared between levels as the patient squats. All levels should remain in the neutral position. If a segmental hinge into flexion or extension is felt (one segment flexes or extends excessively compared to those above and/or below it), the timing of this non-optimal motion should be assessed (early, middle, or late).

Continued

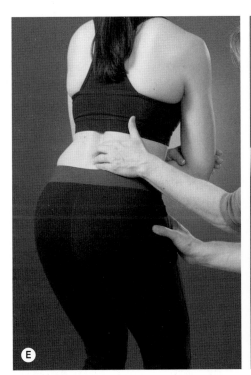
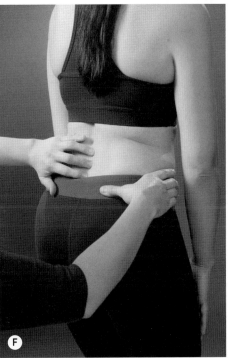

Fig. 8.24 – cont'd • (E) Compare the timing of the loss of control with movement analysis of the hip (one hand palpates the femoral head anteriorly while the other palpates the interspinous spaces). It is common to find excessive motion segmentally in the lumbar spine when one or both hip joints fail to move optimally into flexion during a squat. (F) Combined lumbar spine and pelvic girdle control impairments are not uncommon, with both or either regions contributing to peripheral pain generation. If unlocking of one side of the pelvis has already been determined (by palpating the innominate and sacrum (see Fig. 8.22)), then the timing of unlocking of the pelvis and loss of control of lumbar spine segments can be determined by palpating the innominate with one hand and the lumbar segments with the other.

the level of the segmental hinge to be a pain generator. Also note the timing of the loss of lumbar segmental control relative to pelvic girdle unlocking (Fig. 8.24F), which is important to determine in cases of combined lumbar spine/pelvic girdle impairment and pain;

4. the ability to change this alignment should also be assessed as it gives an indication of the rigidity and commitment to strategy between the pelvis and thorax (Fig. 8.25A,B);

5. the ability of the femurs to rotate externally and internally at the hip joint while in the squat position (Fig. 8.26) as this gives an indication of the commitment to a butt-gripping strategy;

6. the ability of the pelvic girdle to tilt laterally to the left and right while in the squat position (Fig. 8.27).

7. the ability to maintain all of the key components of an optimal squat and then rise up onto the toes (sling squat) (Fig. 8.28).

If there are multiple regions of failed load transfer, pay attention to the sequential timing of each (i.e. which fails first). Use verbal and manual cues to correct the biomechanics of one region and observe the impact of this correction on the others (see case report Louise, Chapter 9, Video LL14 🖰). Record the key findings from this task analysis in the outer ring of the Clinical Puzzle (strategies for function and performance).

Step forward/step backward

Step forward/step backward task analysis is integral to walking and running and thus to many sports as well. If any non-optimal strategies were observed

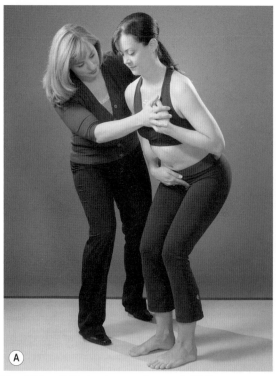 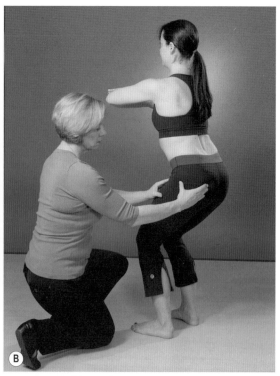

Fig. 8.25 • Ability to change alignment. (A) Response to cues to change. The patient has been given cues to relax the back muscles to allow the thorax to gently tilt anteriorly (not to purposely anteriorly tilt the thorax but rather to relax the muscles that are causing the posterior tilt). Her ability to follow both verbal and tactile cues is noted. This provides some indication of how committed she is to this strategy for squatting. (B) Verbal and tactile cues can also be used to assess commitment to the butt-gripping strategy. Cues to relax the posterior muscles of the deep buttock (let the sitz bones go wide) and allow the femurs to center in the acetabulum are given and the response noted. This model loves to posteriorly tilt her thorax! She was, and still is, a dancer and back-gripping is a common strategy among this group.

during walking, the step forward and/or step backward tasks provide a method of breaking down the gait cycle and palpating various joints in the kinetic chain for failed load transfer. Similar to the squat task analysis, several things should be noted including:

1. any loss of control of the right or left side of the pelvis, especially at the points in the gait cycle that the patient identified as problematic in their story. For example, if a runner reports pain or a sense of 'less stability' on heel strike with the right foot, the right side of the pelvis should be palpated during a step forward with the right foot (Fig. 8.29A), and control of the right SIJ noted during the right leg gait cycle into left step forward. The left side of the pelvis should also be assessed for control in the same task (Fig. 8.29B), at the point of right heel strike, to gain insight as to whether the non-optimal loading of the right leg is due to poor mechanics on push off from the left.

The innominate should remain posteriorly rotated relative to the ipsilateral sacrum throughout the task. Note that the pelvic girdle will rotate in the transverse plane and an IPT left and right will occur during normal gait, but at no point should unlocking occur between the innominate and sacrum. Note the timing (early, middle, or late) of any loss of control (unlocking) during the task;

2. the ability of the femoral head to remain centered in the acetabulum as load is transferred through the hip joint as it flexes and extends at different points in the gait cycle (Fig. 8.30A–C). Note the timing of any loss of control (loss of femoral head centering) during this task (early, middle, late). A patient may have good control of femoral head position on loading (heel strike) but then may lose control as the hip moves into extension (mid-stance to toe-off); it is key for treatment prescription to identify both the joints in the

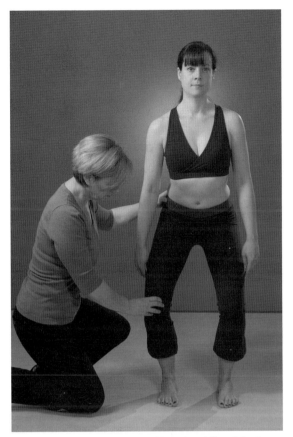

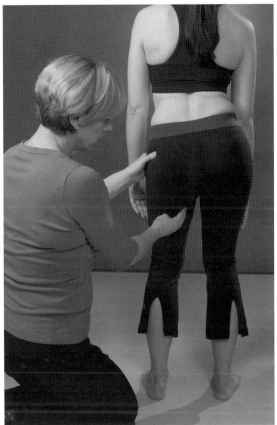

Fig. 8.26 • Squat, hip mobility. Note the ability of the femur to rotate externally and internally while the patient holds a squat. When the strategy for this task is optimal, loads will be transferred without creating articular rigidity. As such, the hip and foot should be free to move even though they are bearing weight.

Fig. 8.27 • Squat, pelvic salsa. Note the ability of the pelvis to tilt laterally to the left and right while the patient maintains a squat position. This task reveals the ability of the hip abductors and adductors to contract eccentrically and concentrically, and many hip imbalances can be seen and felt during this task. In this illustration, the therapist is palpating the adductors during a left lateral tilt of the pelvis to ensure they are able to lengthen eccentrically during this task. Non-optimal vectors of force (vector analysis) are easily palpated during this task.

kinetic chain where control is lost, as well as the direction of loss of control;

3. the maintenance of an appropriate lumbar spine curve throughout the task. Rotation and sidebending should occur as the pelvis rotates in the transverse plane; however, these movements should be evenly distributed througout the lumbar curvature. The spinal segments should not translate or hinge during this task. If a segmental hinge or buckle is present, note the timing of this in relationship to any unlocking of the pelvic girdle, femoral head displacement, or lack of mobility. Often the low back gives way when the hips fail to move, or as a consequence of the loss of control of the pelvic girdle under the lumbar spine;

4. the alignment of the thorax and lower extremity to the pelvis. Non-optimal foot, ankle, knee, and thorax biomechanics can be extrinsic drivers of failed load transfer in the pelvis and their contribution may become more evident in these tasks. For example, the one leg standing (OLS) test may reveal non-optimal biomechanics in the foot, but these will be even more apparent during the transition from foot flat to toe-off during a step forward task (Fig. 8.31A). Counter-rotation between the lower thorax and the pelvis is

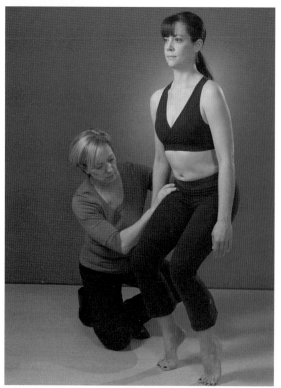

Fig. 8.28 • Sling squat. While the patient maintains the squat position, ask them to rise up onto their toes bilaterally. The task reveals the patient's ability to dissociate movement between the foot and the lower extremity while simultaneously maintaining control at the knee, hip, pelvic girdle, and lumbar spine. The only joints that should move are in the foot and ankle. Note the alignment of the foot, ankle, and knee during this very challenging task.

necessary for optimal walking and running. If the thorax cannot rotate well in one direction, this may contribute to failed load transfer through the hip and pelvis on the leg contralateral to the direction of decreased rotation, especially from mid-stance to toe-off (the thorax-driven pelvis) (Fig. 8.31B).

If there are multiple regions of failed load transfer, pay attention to the sequential timing of each (i.e. which fails first). Use verbal and manual cues to correct the biomechanics of one region and note the impact of this correction on the others (see case report Louise, Chapter 9, Video LL14 🖱). Note the key findings from this task analysis in the outer ring of the Clinical Puzzle (strategies for function and performance).

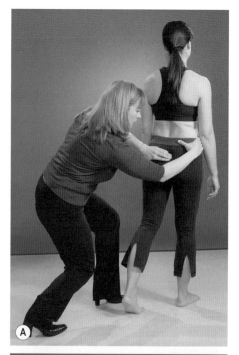

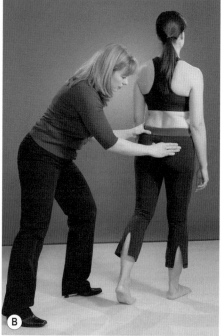

Fig. 8.29 • Step forward – intrapelvic control. Palpate the innominate with one hand and the sacrum with the other. Ask the patient to take a step forward and note any failed load transfer (unlocking or anterior rotation of the innominate relative to the sacrum) on (A) the ipsilateral and then (B) the contralateral side of the forward step. Note the timing of the failed load transfer (early, middle, or late in the task).

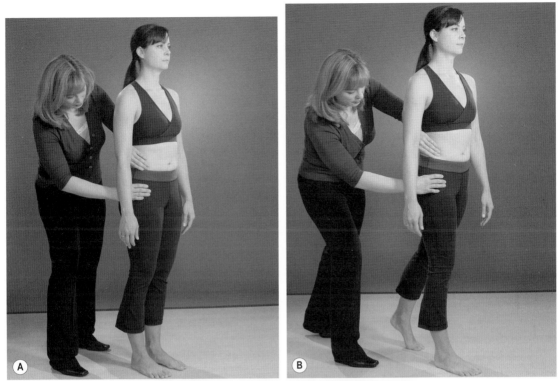

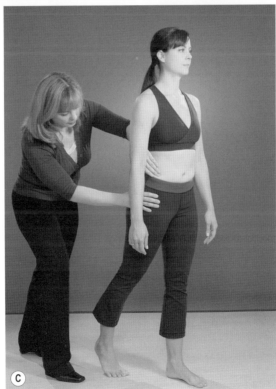

Fig. 8.30 • Step forward – hip motion control. (A) Note the position of the femoral head relative to the innominate in the starting position. Note any loss of femoral head centering as the patient takes a step forward with (B) the ipsilateral leg as well as (C) the contralateral leg. Compare findings to the contralateral hip.

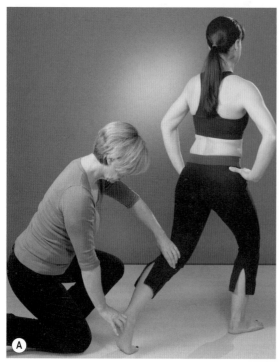
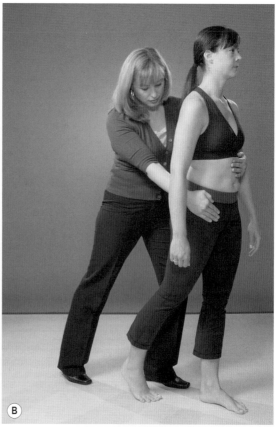

Fig. 8.31 • Step forward – extrinsic factors for LPH control. (A) Non-optimal foot and ankle biomechanics through all phases of gait can be an extrinsic cause of failed load transfer in the LHP complex. In this illustration the therapist is monitoring the alignment of the tibia/fibula and hindfoot and watching the loading strategy of the entire lower extremity and foot during a step forward/lunge. (B) Here the therapist is monitoring thoracopelvic rotation through left mid-stance and right push off. The pelvis should rotate to the right and the thorax to the left at this stage.

Sitting posture

Prolonged sitting is commonly reported as being aggravating for patients with lumbopelvic and/or groin/hip pain. Sitting posture analysis begins with asking the patient to sit 'as they usually do' and then noting the following:

1. Is the pelvis sitting in neutral on the support surface or is it

   (a) posteriorly tilted (Fig. 8.32A); or

   (b) twisted (IPT) (Fig. 8.32B) When there is an IPT this will affect the apparent length of the femurs. Compare the length of the femurs and note which one is longer. This is often associated with the side of pelvis that is 'tucked under,' or gripped.

2. Palpate the position of the hip anteriorly, just below the inguinal ligament midway between the PS and anterior superior iliac spine (ASIS) (Fig. 8.33). The femoral heads should be well seated into the acetabulum and you should feel a 'groove' or folding at the groin. If the axis of the hip is non-optimal (commonly on the side of butt-gripping), you will palpate a fullness in the groin compared to the other side, and a lack of the folding of the hip. This is often associated with the side of the pelvis that is 'tucked under,' and correcting the seating of the femoral head can normalize an IPT.

3. What is the resting posture of the spinal column (neck, thoracic and lumbar spine)? The primary curves should be maintained. Are there any

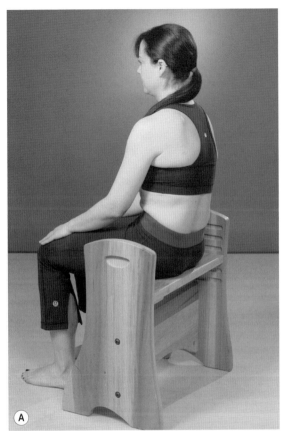

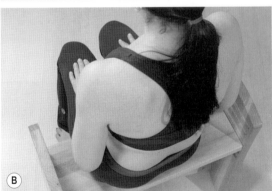

Fig. 8.32 • Sitting posture. This model is sitting in a non-neutral pelvic position. (A) Note the posterior pelvic tilt, the loss of the lumbar lordosis, and her open hip angle. Her head is forward and, although her pony tail obscures the cervical curve, the lordosis is accentuated. (B) The model is now simulating the 'twisted' (IPT) sitting posture that is also non-optimal. Note how her right buttock is 'tucked under,' inducing a thoracopelvic rotation as well as an intrapelvic torsion. This position limits movement between the thorax and pelvis and is a common finding in patients who complain of low back, mid back, and neck pain during sitting tasks.

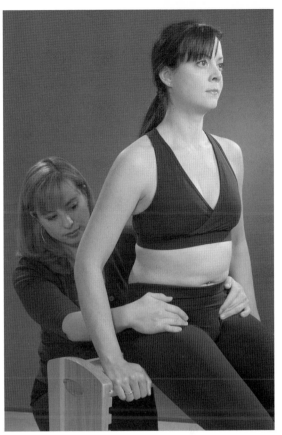

Fig. 8.33 • Sitting posture. An intrapelvic torsion results when the femoral head fails to center during the sitting task. The anteriorly translated femoral head is easily palpated in the groin.

segmental hinges, shifts, or kinks anywhere in the spinal column? How do these curves change if you reposition the pelvis into neutral?

4. Do they still have ability to:

   (a) move their hips (check external and internal rotation of the femurs);

   (b) rotate their thorax (Fig. 8.34); and

   (c) breathe?

An optimal sitting strategy will not stiffen the hip joints or the thorax (this reflects the ability to move in and out of neutral spine, which is important during sustained sitting), and the pelvis will rest in a neutral position on the support surface. Note that careful consideration of the patient's story will help design a more specific and meaningful task assessment. For example, if the patient reports minor difficulties with sitting at work, consider the multiple variables

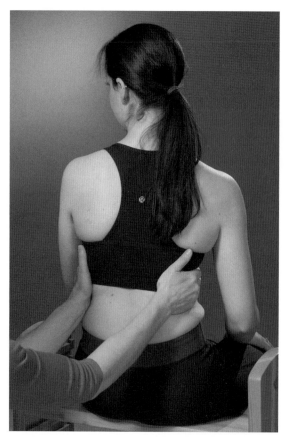

Fig. 8.34 • Sitting posture, available thoracopelvic rotation. Note the ability of the thorax to rotate freely to the left and right and compare the quality (resistance) and quantity of motion between sides. The thorax should be able to rotate freely to the left and right when the strategy for sitting is optimal.

in the work environment. The above simple sitting assessment will need to be modified. In addition to considering ergonomic factors, a 'concentration sitting position' can be simulated by simply asking the patient to imagine that they are working on a project that requires a lot of focus and attention. Observe the impact this 'concentration mode' has on their strategy for sitting. Even if the desk environment in the clinic is not exactly the same as at the patient's work, interesting changes in sitting strategy can occur when the concentration and frame of mind are changed. This variation in strategy will help to reveal any other factors, in addition to the biomechanical factors, that may be associated with symptoms.

Note the key findings from this task analysis in the outer ring of the Clinical Puzzle (strategies for function and performance).

Prone knee bend/hip extension

These tasks allow more specific analysis of extension control for the LPH complex. They were originally developed to assess the role of the pelvis in patients with recurrent hamstring strains and runners with hamstring or ischial symptoms (possible referred pain) during the mid-stance to toe-off phases of gait. Some of these athletes did not necessarily have pain but simply reported decreased power on push off (primary performance complaint, see case report Mike, Chapter 9 🖱). These tests help to determine when the pelvis needs to be addressed in patients with hamstring strains in order for full return to function and decreased risk of recurrence. They also can differentiate lumbar spine drivers from pelvic girdle drivers.

From the prone position, ask the patient to bend one knee to 90° of flexion (a prone knee bend) and then to do the same with the other leg. Note any reproduction of pain and, if pain is present, in which part of the hamstring (medial or lateral, and/or mid-belly). Ask the patient to think about the effort required to *initiate* the movement of the leg off the table as they repeat the movements, and to report if one leg feels harder to bend/lift than the other. Note which leg is heavier and repeat the prone knee bend with this leg while you palpate and identify any:

1. intrapelvic torsion (Fig. 8.35A);
2. segmental hinging into extension or flexion in the lumbar spine (Fig. 8.35B);
3. loss of control of the femoral head in the acetabulum (Fig. 8.35C); and/or
4. loss of control (unlocking) of the ipsilateral or contralateral side of the pelvis (Fig. 8.35D,E).

Optimally, the pelvis should remain neutral, the lumbar spine should not hinge into extension at any segment, the femoral head should remain centered in the acetabulum, and the innominate should not rotate anteriorly relative to the sacrum at either SIJ. The following modifications are then applied if FLT is identified in any of the areas above. Note whether there is a change in effort to perform the task while:

1. the sacrum is nutated passively on the side where unlocking was noted (Fig. 8.36A);

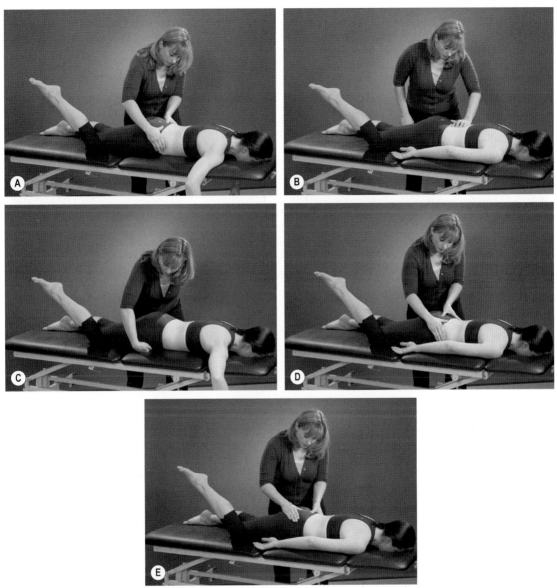

Fig. 8.35 • Prone knee bend. From the prone position ask the patient to bend one knee and note: (A) any intrapelvic torsion – both innominates are palpated and any rotation between them noted as the foot is lifted from the plinth (initiation of movement) and the knee bends; (B) any segmental hinging of the lumbar spine – the interspinous spaces are palpated and any hinging into either flexion or extension is noted as the foot is lifted from the plinth (initiation of movement) and the knee bends; (C) any loss of control of the femoral head in the acetabulum – the anterior aspect of the femoral head is palpated and any loss of centering noted as the foot is lifted from the plinth (initiation of movement) and the knee bends; (D) any loss of control of the ipsilateral sacroiliac joint – the sacrum and the ipsilateral innominate are palpated and any unlocking of the ipsilateral and (E) contralateral side of the pelvis noted as the foot is lifted from the plinth (initiation of movement) and the knee bends.

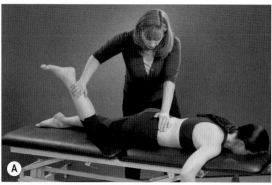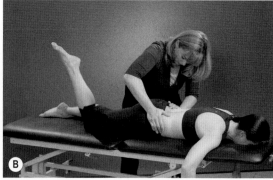

Fig. 8.36 • Prone knee bend. (A) Poor control of the joints of the pelvic girdle is often responsible for apparent hamstring weakness. In this illustration the therapist is comparing the 'strength' response of the hamstrings with the sacrum passively nutated. If increased strength is noted when the sacrum is passively nutated, it is likely that pelvic girdle control is a factor in the original 'weakness' noted. (B) The pelvis can be passively compressed in a variety of locations (this illustration is demonstrating bilateral posterior compression) and the change in effort to perform the prone knee bend task noted.

2. the pelvic girdle is aligned and compressed
   (a) bilaterally across the anterior aspect;
   (b) bilaterally across the posterior aspect (Fig. 8.36B);
   (c) obliquely from left anterior to right posterior; or
   (d) obliquely from right anterior to left posterior; and/or
3. the femoral head position is manually controlled.

The test can be done at a higher load by using isometric resistance (manual muscle test of the hamstrings). Observe any tendency for the tibia to rotate (an effort to bias the medial or lateral hamstrings), any reproduction of pain, as well as any loss of control in the lumbar spine, pelvis, or hip. This resisted test is useful for those patients who cannot feel a difference in effort between the right and left sides in the prone knee bend alone.

Subsequently, ask the patient to extend the hip while keeping the knee extended and note any:

1. intrapelvic torsion;
2. segmental hinging into extension in the lumbar spine;
3. loss of control of the femoral head in the acetabulum;
4. loss of control of the ipsilateral or contralateral SIJ (right or left side of the pelvis); as well as
5. the timing of loss of control of the lumbar spine, SIJ, or hip (Fig. 8.37A,B, Video 12.2a 🖱).

Optimally, the pelvis should remain neutral, the lumbar spine should not hinge into extension at any segment, and the femoral head should remain centered

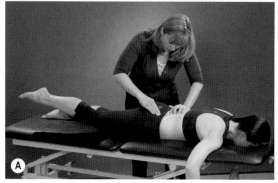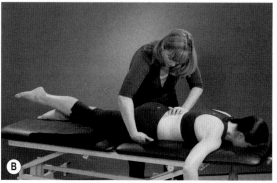

Fig. 8.37 • Prone hip extension. The therapist is noting the timing of loss of control between a lumbar segment and (A) the right sacroiliac joint and (B) the right hip joint. The joint that gives way first is the primary impairment, although attention may need to be directed to both during treatment.

in the acetabulum. Ask the patient to quantify the effort required to lift the extended leg from the prone position (0 = no problem, 5 = unable) and then note the difference in effort when:

1. the sacrum is nutated passively;

2. the pelvic girdle is aligned and compressed

   (a) bilaterally across the anterior aspect;

   (b) bilaterally across the posterior aspect;

   (c) obliquely from left anterior to right posterior; or

   (d) obliquely from right anterior to left posterior; and/or

3. the femoral head position is manually corrected.

A higher load can be added by providing isometric resistance to hip extension. Note the strength on the right and left sides and use the weaker side to continue the test. Repeat the test while passively nutating the sacrum and note any change in hip extension strength (Fig. 8.38). Optimally, the patient will not notice any difference in effort between the right and left legs to perform the prone knee bend/hip extension tests (± resistance), and no differences will be detected with any manual modifications (nutation of the sacrum, pelvic compressions, femoral head centering). However, if areas of failed load transfer were noted initially (SIJ, lumbar spine, or hip), then one or more of the manual modifications may decrease the effort experienced on testing. If this occurs, then a non-optimal strategy for control of the lumbar spine, pelvic girdle, and/or hip can be considered a key contributor to the loss of hip extension power noted both subjectively by the athlete and objectively by the examiner. Further tests are required to determine why the strategy is non-optimal (specific system impairment).

Record the key findings from this prone knee bend/hip extension task analysis in the outer ring of the Clinical Puzzle (strategies for function and performance).

Clinical reasoning. The patient with a true structural deficit in the hamstring muscle (myofascial system impairment) will demonstrate minimal or no changes in perceived effort, pain, or ability/muscle strength output when the prone knee bend/hip extension tests (± resistance) are performed with and without the modifications to augment control of the lumbar spine, pelvis, and hip joints (Video 8.1). In certain patients, poor LPH control may have been a predisposing factor to the hamstring injury. It is our experience that even these patients do not demonstrate marked differences in effort or strength output when the affected hamstring is tested with and without lumbopelvic support, if the main impairment is a structural deficit in the hamstring. A small improvement may be felt but the painful lesion will still test weak and painful, especially in an acute or subacute injury. As the tissue deficit heals, if poor lumbopelvic control is present, these tests will then reveal that it is time to include proximal control and treatment; that is, the test modifications *will* make a change to the effort and/or strength output on the tests. It is our opinion that these findings indicate that the patient will not fully recover from the hamstring injury without treating impairments in the proximal systems.

Patients with referred posterior thigh pain will have significant and marked changes in effort, strength, and pain responses to the modifications to the prone knee bend/hip extension tests (± resistance) applied to the LPH region (see case report Mike, Chapter 9, Video MQ5). Note that if any of the proximal compressions or joint control modifications make the effort or strength output *worse*, this is also supportive of a lumbopelvic driver, and indicates that the system is under too much compression. Manual tests that decrease compression on the relevant components of the lumbopelvic complex (Lee 2004, Lee & Lee 2004a) will then improve the responses to the tests. In either case, the significant change in symptoms, perceived effort, and strength output with alterations to the LPH complex indicate that the 'hamstring pain' has significant proximal drivers and is most likely *not* a true structural deficit of the hamstring muscle.

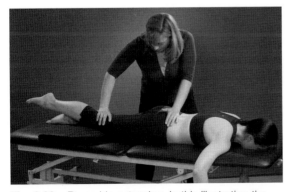

Fig. 8.38 • Prone hip extension. In this illustration the therapist is noting the change in hip extension strength when the sacrum is passively nutated. When hip extension strength improves with passive nutation of the sacrum, an intrapelvic control impairment is suggested.

Active straight leg raise

The supine active straight leg raise (ASLR) test (Mens et al 1999, 2001, 2002) has been validated as a clinical test for assessing load transfer between the trunk and the lower extremity in patients with peripartum pelvic girdle pain. When the LPH complex is functioning optimally, the leg should rise effortlessly from the table (the effort can be graded from 0 to 5) (Mens et al 1999) and the pelvis should not move (flex, extend, laterally bend, or rotate) relative to the thorax and/or lower extremity (Fig. 8.39).

The application of compression to the pelvis has been shown to reduce the effort necessary to lift the leg for peripartum patients with pelvic girdle pain and poor strategies for transferring load (Mens et al 1999). Clinically, it is our experience that this test is useful for multiple patient groups, not only those with impairments secondary to pregnancy and delivery. In addition, we have proposed (Lee 2004, Lee & Lee 2004a) that by varying the location of this compression during the ASLR (see below), further information can be gained that will assist the clinician with hypothesis development and when reasoning the findings from multiple tests.

The supine patient is asked to lift the extended leg 5cm off the table and to note any effort difference between lifting the left and right leg. Does one leg seem heavier or harder to lift? The strategy used to stabilize the thorax, the low back, and the pelvis during this task is observed. The leg should flex at the hip joint and the pelvis should not rotate transversely nor laterally, tilt anteriorly or posteriorly relative to

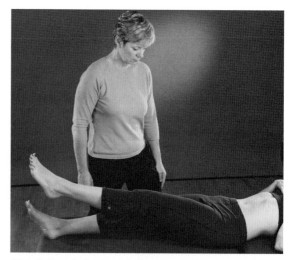

Fig. 8.40 • Active straight leg raise, non-optimal. This model is demonstrating a non-optimal strategy for an active straight leg raise. Note the rotation of her pelvic girdle to the left and the extension of the thoracolumbar spine.

the lumbar spine (Fig. 8.40). The rib cage should not draw in excessively (overactivation of the external oblique muscles) (Fig. 8.41A–C), nor should the lower ribs flare out excessively (overactivation of the internal oblique muscles). Overactivation of the external and internal oblique will result in a braced, rigid ribcage and limit lateral costal expansion on inspiration. The thoracic spine should not extend (overactivation of the erector spinae) (see Fig. 8.40), nor should the abdomen bulge (Fig. 8.42). In addition, the thorax should not shift laterally relative to the pelvic girdle. The provocation of any pain is also noted at this time.

The pelvis is then compressed passively and the ASLR is repeated; any change in effort and/or pain is noted. The location of the compression can be varied to simulate the force that would be produced by optimal function of the deep muscles. Although still a hypothesis, clinically it appears that:

1. compression of the anterior pelvis at the level of the ASISs (Fig. 8.43A) simulates the force produced by contraction of lower horizontal fibers of transversus abdominis (TrA) and the internal oblique (IO) and the associated anterior abdominal fascia; whereas

2. compression of the posterior pelvis at the level of the PSISs (Fig. 8.43B) simulates that of the lumbosacral multifidus and the thoracolumbar fascia;

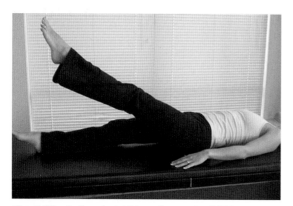

Fig. 8.39 • Active straight leg raise, optimal. This model is demonstrating an optimal strategy for an active straight leg raise. The only joint moving is the left hip joint. The thorax, lumbar spine, and pelvic girdle remain aligned and controlled throughout the task.

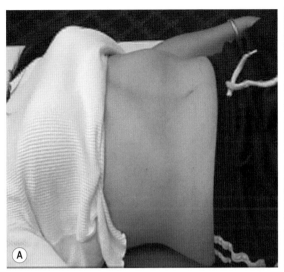
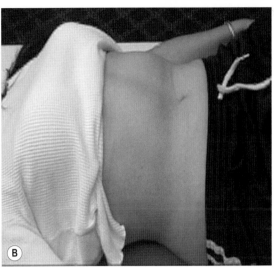
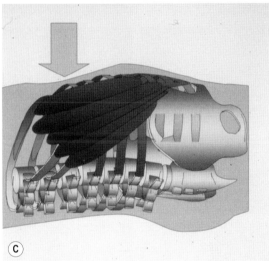

Fig 8.41 • Active straight leg raise, non-optimal. This model is demonstrating a non-optimal strategy for an active straight leg raise. (A) The abdomen at rest. (B) The abdomen during the ASLR. Note the narrowing of the infrasternal angle and the transverse abdominal crease that occurs as the thorax flexes relative to the pelvis. (C) Schematic drawing that reflects the consequences of overactivating the external obliques during this task. Note the depression of the upper abdomen, bulging of the lower abdomen, flexion of the thoracolumbar spine, and posterior pelvic tilt. Reproduced with permission from Dr. Paul Hodges.

3. compression of the anterior pelvis at the level of the pubic symphysis (Fig. 8.43C) simulates the action of the anterior pelvic floor and the endopelvic fascia in coordination with the lowest fibers of TrA and IO; whereas

4. compression of the posterior pelvis at the level of the ischial tuberosities simulates the action of the posterior pelvic wall and floor;

5. compression can also be applied obliquely through the pelvis (one side anteriorly and the

opposite side posteriorly). You are looking for the location where more, or less, compression reduces the effort necessary to lift the leg – the place where the patient comments 'that feels marvelous!'

When the patient presents with a diastasis rectus abdominis (RA), observe the difference in effort to lift the heavy leg when the lateral fascial edges of the RA are approximated (Fig. 8.43D). Although the response to patterns of pelvic compression do

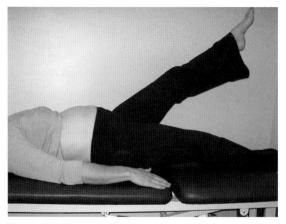

Fig. 8.42 • Active straight leg raise, non-optimal. This model is demonstrating a non-optimal strategy for an active straight leg raise. Note the excessive abdominal bulging. This strategy is often associated with breath-holding.

not always correlate exactly to impairments in the related muscles, the responses provide information about which net vectors of augmented or decreased compression across the pelvis are going to positively impact load transfer in the pelvis. For example, consider the following clinical scenario:

1. The patient reports that it is harder to lift the left leg and an impairment of the left deep fibers of multifidus (dMF) is noted. Your hypothesis could be that posterior compression of the pelvic girdle will decrease the effort required to perform this task.

2. Posterior compression of the pelvic girdle *increases* the effort required to lift the left leg and hypertonicity of the ipsilateral superficial fibers of multifidus (sMF) is noted. Your original

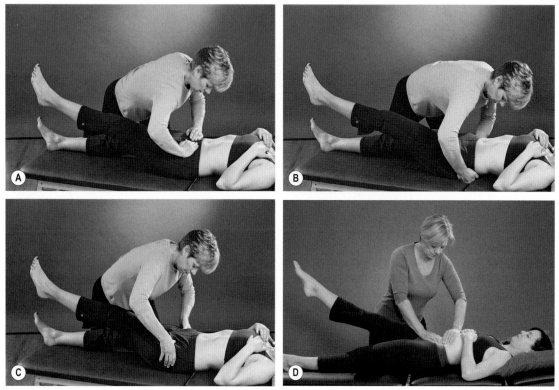

Fig. 8.43 • Active straight leg raise with specific pelvic compression. (A) Bilateral anterior compression of the pelvic girdle (approximating the anterior superior iliac spines (ASISs)) simulates the force provided by the horizontal fibers of transversus abdominis and the internal oblique and the associated anterior abdominal fascia. (B) Bilateral posterior compression of the pelvic girdle (approximating the posterior superior iliac spines (PSISs)) simulates the force provided by the lumbosacral multifidus and the thoracolumbar fascia. (C) Bilateral anterior compression that approximates the pubic symphysis simulates the force provided by the anterior pelvic floor and the endopelvic fascia, the lowest horizontal fibers of transversus abdominis and internal oblique. (D) Approximation of the left and right rectus abdominis towards the midline supports the linea alba and provides a firm anchor for the deep transverse abdominal muscles.

hypothesis is now negated and a new hypothesis could be that the sMF are excessively compressing the lumbopelvis (this is non-optimal) and further compression is not indicated *at this time*. Release of the sMF (Chapter 10) is indicated prior to training dMF (Chapter 11).

Clinical reasoning of the multiple test findings is always required to explain the findings from the ASLR test.

Note the key findings from ASLR task analysis in the outer ring of the Clinical Puzzle (strategies for function and performance).

Strategies for function and performance – summary

This concludes the section on task analysis for strategies for function and performance; however, it is important to remember that many other movements/postures can be assessed. The tasks or postures chosen for strategy analysis depend on the patient's story and what has meaning for them. In Chapter 12, complex task analysis will be further covered and ways to simulate meaningful tasks will be discussed.

The key for any task analysis is to apply the principles described in this section and then to record both the task and its findings (e.g. areas of loss of control, areas of loss of mobility, timing of loss of control between areas, impact of providing correction/facilitation of optimal biomechanics) in the outer

ring of the Clinical Puzzle. Once the areas of failed load transfer have been identified, along with other non-optimal features in postural orientation and/or postural equilibrium, further tests are required to determine which system(s) are responsible for the non-optimal strategy observed. Why is failed load transfer occurring? How does it relate to the pain experience? Is it poor motor control (impairment of the neural system), a stiff fibrotic joint (impairment of the articular system), excessive width of the linea alba (impairment of the myofascial system), or cognitive/emotional factors (fear or faulty beliefs of movement or fear of pain, i.e. features of the person in the middle of the puzzle)? The combination of information from the subjective history and the findings during the strategy analysis will direct the therapist to the systems to assess next. For example, if during a squat task, L4–5 was noted to give way into flexion (flexion hinge) before the hips flexed, and the hips had an altered movement axis in flexion (femoral head failed to center), the lumbar region is identified as needing further analysis as well as the hip, and this is listed in both the articular and neural pieces of the Clinical Puzzle (Fig. 8.44). The regional tests for the lumbar spine and hip will provide further information regarding the contribution of each puzzle piece/system (articular, neural, myofascial, or visceral) to the non-optimal strategy noted.

Chapter 9 will expand on how clinical reasoning is applied to multiple test findings in several case reports. First, the specific regional tests for the pelvic

Fig. 8.44 • The template of the Clinical Puzzle can be used to facilitate clinical reasoning 'on the fly,' and helps the clinician to prioritize subsequent regions and tests needed during the examination process.

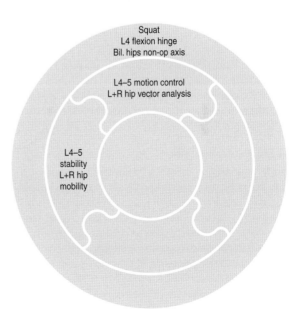

Squat
L4 flexion hinge
Bil. hips non-op axis

L4–5 motion control
L+R hip vector analysis

L4–5
stability
L+R hip
mobility

girdle, lumbar spine, and hip necessary for determining the contribution of the various pieces to the Clinical Puzzle require description. It is not necessary to perform all of the following tests, nor is it necessary to perform them in the order presented in this chapter. Once again, the specific findings from the task analysis and the patient's story will direct you to the region and the specific regional tests will identify the pieces within the region that are relevant. This requires continual hypothesis generation (Kerry et al 2008, Kerry 2009), as well as interpretation and reflection of the test results as the examination progresses. Jensen et al (2007), as well as Jones & Rivett (2004), argue that this is a key requirement to develop clinical expertise.

Regional tests – the pelvic girdle

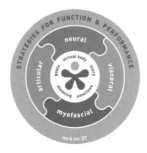

The pelvic girdle requires further analysis if, during any task, the strategy used causes asymmetrical movement of the left and right sides of the pelvis or loss of motion control at either the left or right SIJ or the pubic symphysis (non-optimal and inappropriate strategy). Clinical reasoning of the findings from multiple tests is necessary to understand the significance of the results of each individual test and this will be covered, in part, in this chapter and then in further detail through the case reports in Chapter 9.

The following tests examine the passive articular mobility as well as the integrity of the articular, myofascial, and neural systems to control translation of the joints of the pelvic girdle. Passive movement analysis requires an evaluation of two zones of motion, the neutral zone and the elastic zone (see Fig. 4.9), but first, positional analysis is required. When interpreting mobility findings, the position of the bone at the beginning of the test should be correlated with the subsequent mobility as alterations in joint mobility may merely be a reflection of an altered starting position. If the innominate is posteriorly rotated relative to the sacrum, then the amplitude of motion for this SIJ will be reduced compared to the other side and this should be interpreted as a normal finding as far as the joint is concerned.

Buyruk et al (1997) and Damen et al (2002b) have shown that asymmetrical stiffness (or laxity) of the SIJs correlates with, and is prognostic for, pelvic impairment and pain. As it is impossible to know exactly how *much* movement an individual should have, passive movement analysis relies on comparing one side to the other. If consideration is not given to the starting position of the joint, then the findings from the mobility tests are easily misinterpreted. The results from these tests are then considered with those from the active movement part of the one leg standing test (Fig. 8.17) to determine whether the joint is stiff, lax, fixated, or compressed.

Pelvic girdle: positional tests

When assessing the position of the innominate bones relative to each other, it appears to be more reliable to use the entire hand to gain information kinesthetically rather than visualizing one point of the bone (i.e. ASIS or posterior superior iliac spine (PSIS)). To the authors' knowledge, the reliability of kinesthetic positional testing has not been tested formally, yet throughout our courses we have consistently found that the students' findings are more reliable when the position of the pelvis is assessed this way.

With the patient lying supine, legs extended, palpate the anterior aspect of both innominates with the heels of the hands (Fig. 8.45). Let the rest of the hand mold to the innominate and, with eyes closed, gain an impression as to whether the pelvis feels twisted (intrapelvic torsion, IPT) or sheared in a craniocaudal or anteroposterior plane. Then, open your eyes and palpate the inferior aspect of the ASIS bilaterally and/or the superior aspect of the pubic tubercles (Fig. 8.46) to confirm or negate the initial impression. Make sure to keep your head and neck very still while making this judgment. Sideflexion of the craniovertebral joints changes perception and could alter the visual findings. See for yourself by trying this test. Hold your arms out in front of you and point your thumbs towards each other. Focus on a distant object between your thumbs, using your peripheral vision to sense the level of your left and right thumbs, and then hold them still as you sideflex your upper neck right and left and note what happens to the level of your

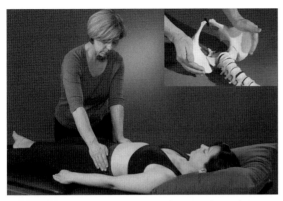

Fig. 8.45 • Pelvic girdle: positional tests – innominates (anterior). Use as much of your hands as possible and compare the kinesthetic findings with the visual when assessing the position of the innominates relative to each other.

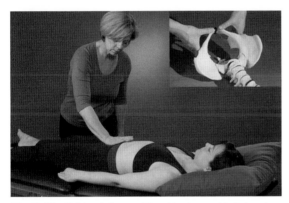

Fig. 8.46 • Pelvic girdle: positional tests – pubic tubercles. Use the heel of one hand and palpate the cranial aspect of the left and right superior pubic rami. Note any step, or shear, of the symphysis by sliding the heel of the hand to the left and right; appreciate this with your kinesthetic sense. Inset: confirm the kinesthetic impression by palpating the left and right superior pubic rami with either the thumbs or index fingers and compare the visual and kinesthetic findings.

thumbs. They go up and down! Imagine now that you are in a reliability trial and consistently kept changing the angle of your head. Unless everyone held their head sideflexed to the same side during all tests, it is likely that this variable could affect intertester reliability. Now there's an interesting study.

To assess the impact of hip position on pelvic position, have the patient flex their hips and knees and

note any change in the rotation between the innominates. Multiple force vectors arising from imbalanced hip muscles can significantly impact the position of the pelvis in the supine, prone, and neutral positions. This test helps to differentiate an intrinsic impairment from an extrinsic one (Figs 8.47A–D). Similarly, multiple force vectors arising from the thoracic and lumbar regions can impact the position of the pelvis and often manifest during forward bending of the trunk (Fig. 8.48A,B).

With the patient lying prone, palpate the posterior aspect of both innominates. Let your entire hand mold to the innominate and repeat the analysis from this position (Fig. 8.49). The findings should be similar to those in the supine position when the patient's hips and knees are extended. To assess the impact of knee position and/or the anterior lower extremity myofascial slings on pelvic position, have the patient flex their knees and note any change in position between the innominates (Fig. 8.50A,B).

The dorsal aspect of the inferior lateral angle (ILA) appears to be the most reliable place for assessing the position of the sacrum (direction of rotation between the innominates) (Fig. 8.51) as the sacral base depth can be influenced by the size and tone of multifidus. To determine the position of the sacrum, a comparison is made of the posteroanterior relationship of the ILA bilaterally. To find the ILA, begin by palpating the median sacral crest. Follow the crest inferiorly until you reach the sacral hiatus (unfused spinous processes of S4 and S5). From this point, palpate laterally until you feel the lateral edge of the sacrum; this is the ILA. A posterior left ILA is indicative of a left rotated sacrum.

At this point a determination regarding the physiological or non-physiological nature of the positional findings is made. A physiological right intrapelvic torsion (IPTR) will have the following findings:

(a) the left innominate will be anteriorly rotated relative to the right innominate; and

(b) the sacrum will be rotated to the right.

A physiological left intrapelvic torsion (IPTL) will have the following findings:

(a) the right innominate will be anteriorly rotated relative to the left innominate; and

(b) the sacrum will be rotated to the left.

All other positional relationships are non-physiological and *suggestive, but not confirmative,* of either an intra-articular shear lesion (articular system deficit) or a significant decrease in the resting

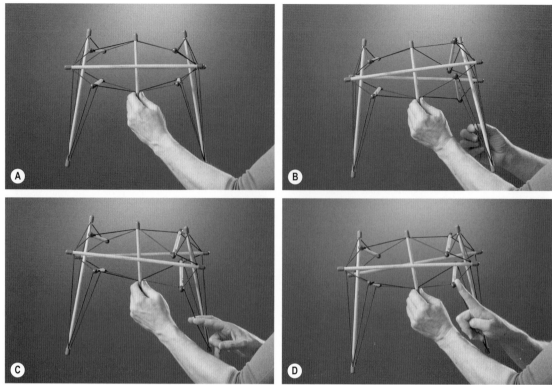

Fig. 8.47 • Pelvic girdle: positional tests – impact of muscle imbalance from the lower extremity. This tensegrity model (created by Tom Flemons of www.intensiondesigns.com) illustrates the effect that myofascial vector pulls (the elastics) can have on the bones (the wooden bars). (A) When the muscles connecting the pelvis to the lower extremity are in balance, the pelvis will be in a neutral position (no intrapelvic torsion (IPT)) and this position will not be impacted by flexing or extending the hips while supine or by bending the knees while in the prone position. (B) Hypertonicity of the superficial hip flexors can potentially rotate the ipsilateral innominate anteriorly and create an IPT. In this illustration, the model is oriented as if looking at the pelvis from behind, with tension increased in the right superficial hip flexors simulated by shortening the elastic. Significant hypertonicity of the superficial hip flexors can create an IPT, which is apparent even in the crook lying position (hips and knees flexed). Alternately, the torsion may not appear until the hips are extended while supine or the knees are bent while prone. (C) Hypertonicity of the superficial hip extensors can also create an IPT. These extrinsic force vectors tend to appear and disappear as the position of the lower extremity is varied. (D) Conversely, intrinsic intrapelvic muscle imbalances (simulating the force of the right deep posterior intrapelvic muscles) create torsions that are consistent and do not vary with altering the position of the lower extremity.

tone of the muscles that control motion of the SIJ (neural system deficit).

When one innominate appears to be sheared vertically relative to the other (also known as an upslip), the ischial tuberosities can be used to confirm the non-physiological position. To assess the position of the ischial tuberosities, palpate the inferior aspect of the ischial tuberosity bilaterally. Initially use the heels of both hands and then palpate the ischial

tuberosities with the thumbs (Fig. 8.52). Ensure that you are on the most *inferior* aspect of the tuberosity as a rotated innominate can change the apparent craniocaudal relationship between the left and right sides if you are palpating the dorsal aspect of the ischial tuberosity. Further tests (articular mobility) and considerations from the patient's story (history of trauma) are required to confirm the hypothesis of a shear lesion (upslip).

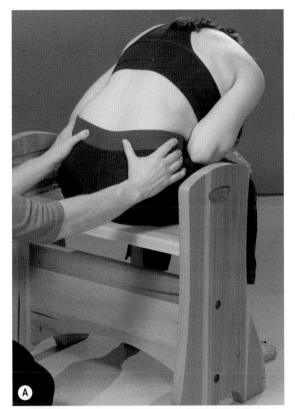

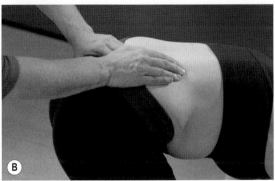

Fig. 8.48 • Pelvic girdle: positional tests – impact of neuromyofascial imbalance from the thoracolumbar spine. (A) Initially note the resting position of the pelvic girdle in a neutral sitting position; ensure that the hips are able to flex fully with a centered femoral head before performing this test. Have the patient bend forward and flex the entire thoracolumbar spine and note any change in the pelvic position. Unilateral hypertonicity of the paravertebral muscles can potentially rotate the ipsilateral innominate anteriorly and create an intrapelvic torsion, or create a lateral tilt of the pelvic girdle depending on the muscles involved. (B) This neuromyofascial imbalance will have been apparent during the forward bending test. Note the asymmetry in muscle tone in the model bends forward.

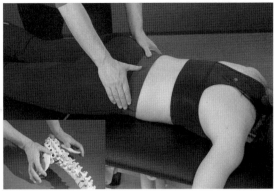

Fig. 8.49 • Pelvic girdle: positional tests – innominates (posterior). Use as much of your hands as possible when assessing the position of the innominates relative to each other.

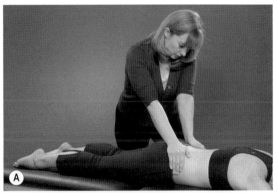

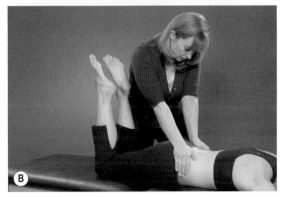

Fig. 8.50 • Pelvic girdle: positional tests – impact of neuromyofascial forces from the lower extremity. (A) In the prone position, note the presence/absence of any intrapelvic torsion (IPT). (B) Have the patient bend both knees and note any impact on the position of the pelvis relative to the lumbar spine; the pelvis may tilt anteriorly and thus extend the low back if the superficial hip flexors fail to lengthen adequately (tensor fascia latae, rectus femoris). In addition, note whether an IPT occurs during this task, and the range of knee flexion at which any changes occur.

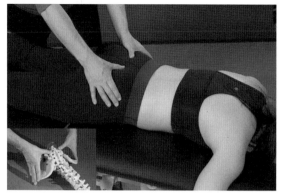

Fig. 8.51 • Pelvic girdle: positional tests – sacrum. Compare the dorsoventral relationship of the left and right ILA of the sacrum to determine the direction of sacral rotation. A dorsal left inferior lateral angle (ILA) suggests that the sacrum is rotated to the left. When physiological, the right innominate will be anteriorly rotated and the left innominate posteriorly rotated; this is an IPTL (intrapelvic torsion to the left).

Pelvic girdle: articular system mobility – sacroiliac joint

Once the resting position of the pelvic girdle is known, the passive mobility of the sacroiliac SIJ can be assessed and the findings compared to the starting position of the joint. If one innominate is rotated more posteriorly than the other, then the available range of motion at this SIJ should be less. Recall from Chapter 4 that posterior rotation increases tension in the ligaments of the SIJ and thus will reduce movement. If the innominates are not rotated relative to one another and the sacrum is in a neutral position, then the amplitude of motion between sides should be symmetrical.

The SIJ is capable of a small amount of translation that facilitates its angular motion (Chapter 4). When the SIJ is healthy, the innominate can be felt to glide passively a variable amount relative to the sacrum. There are no imaging studies or measurement tools that have yet been able to detect what the hand can feel. The direction of this glide is variable and depends on the individual's structure (Chapter 3). Consequently, the orientation of the plane of the joint must be found before any analysis of the zones of motion (neutral and elastic) is done. The results from the following tests must be compared with the positional test findings (see above) as well as the active mobility test findings (part of the OLS test

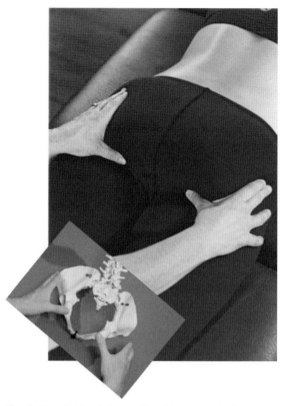

Fig. 8.52 • Pelvic girdle positional tests – ischial tuberosities. It is important to assess the position of the most inferior aspect of the ischial tuberosity (palpate the same place on both the right and left bones) as anterior rotation of the innominate causes the ischial tuberosity to move dorsocranially and can give the false impression of the innominate being sheared cranially (upslip).

described above (Fig. 8.17)) before any judgment can be made as to whether the joint is stiff, lax, fixated, or compressed.

With the patient in crook lying, support the knees over a bolster and place the arms by the patient's sides or across the abdomen. This is the best position to assess passive movement of the SIJs as the sacrum is counter-nutated in this position; it is the loose-packed position for the SIJ (Chapter 4) and thus the greatest amount of available motion will be felt. It is important to ensure that the patient is as relaxed as possible as it is known that even minimal activation of several muscles can change the stiffness of the SIJ (Chapter 4). The goal is to have the low back, pelvis, and hips in a neutral position; check to ensure that the PS is level with the ASISs (no posterior or anterior pelvic tilt) and then gently move the rib cage laterally from side to side to ensure the oblique abdominals and erector spinae muscles are not overactive. If it is not possible for the patient to relax the superficial muscles, this test may be deferred until these muscles are released as the findings will certainly be influenced by the altered muscle tension/tone.

SIJ: Neutral zone analysis in the anteroposterior plane. Once you are sure that the patient is relaxed and the pelvis is in a neutral position with respect to the thorax and the lower extremities, palpate the medial aspect of the posterior iliac crest (just above and medial to the PSIS) (Fig. 8.53) by sliding your cranial hand beneath the pelvis. Do not press too deeply into the multifidus muscle to avoid nutating the sacrum. With the heel of the other hand, palpate the ipsilateral ASIS and, with the rest of this hand, the iliac crest. The first step is to determine the plane

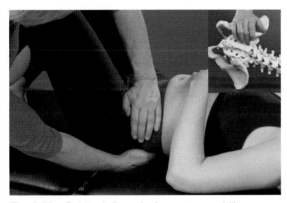

Fig. 8.53 • Pelvic girdle: articular system mobility – sacroiliac joint (SIJ): neutral zone analysis in the anteroposterior plane. The innominate should be capable of gliding parallel to the sacrum at all three aspects of the joint, superior, middle, and inferior. Take care to pay attention to the amount of force required to initiate motion of the innominate; this is the beginning feel. Once the resistance to motion increases (R1), the end of the neutral zone has been reached. Compare the quantity and quality of this motion at all three aspects of the SIJ to the opposite side and correlate the findings with the active mobility test (one leg standing, Fig. 8.18). A common mistake noted when teaching this very sensitive test is that therapists tend to be too 'heavy handed' and go through all the available joint motion before paying attention to what they are feeling. They then state that they cannot feel anything! The reason is that they are at R20 and have gone through both zones of motion and beyond, into rotating L5–S1 and above.

or orientation of the joint as there is a high degree of individual variance (Chapter 3). Apply a gentle oscillatory force in an anteroposterior direction varying the inclination from slightly medial to lateral. One of those planes will meet with the least amount of resistance and you will feel the innominate slide into your palpating fingers relative to the sacrum; this is the joint plane. Once the plane of the joint is found, apply a small anteroposterior translation force to the innominate paying particular attention to the beginning feel of the motion.

How hard do you have to push to initiate movement? How much movement is there? Does it feel the same when you focus the force to the top part of the joint (using more of the hypothenar eminence), the middle part of the joint (using more of the third metacarpal), and the inferior part of the joint (the thenar eminence)? In other words, is the glide parallel at all three parts or does there appear to be a part of the joint that is compressed preventing a parallel glide and inducing a rotation (either anterior or posterior)? Compare all of the kinesthetic sensations of the SIJ's passive motion behavior to the other side; this is a detailed analysis of the neutral zone (0–R1) of motion that involves much more than just assessing the amplitude of motion.

Hypertonicity of certain muscles can compress parts of the SIJ and prevent a parallel glide only at that part, and thus induce a rotation during the test. For example, the superior part of the SIJ can be compressed by increased tone of the superficial fibers of multifidus and this prevents a parallel glide at the superior aspect of the SIJ. In addition, instead of feeling a clear parallel glide, an anterior rotation of the innominate is induced during the test. If compression of the superior aspect of the SIJ is found, the next step is to palpate the superficial fibers of multifidus where they attach to the posteromedial aspect of the iliac crest to confirm/negate the hypothesis that hypertonicity of these fibers is contributing to the aberrant motion noted. With the patient lying prone, palpate the superficial fibers of multifidus where they attach to the medial aspect of the posterior iliac crest (see Fig. 3.48) and note any hypertonicity (Fig. 8.54A). Follow the hypertonic fascicle cranially to note its segmental origin (Fig. 8.54B). Fascicular hypertonicity is often associated with segmental or multisegmental atrophy of the deep laminar fibers of multifidus. Hypertonicity of the deep laminar fibers of multifidus may also be found. These fibers are palpated immediately lateral to the spinous process of the lumbar segment(s) or just lateral to the

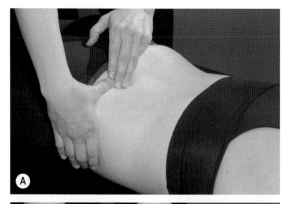

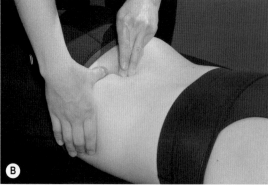

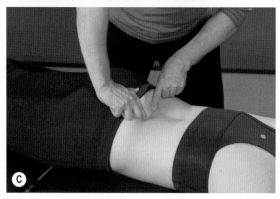

Fig. 8.54 • Pelvic girdle: palpation of the superficial fibers of multifidus. (A) Hypertonicity of the superficial fibers of multifidus that insert into the posteromedial aspect of the iliac crest can create a force vector, which compresses the superior aspect of the sacroiliac joint. Palpate the muscle perpendicular to the fibers and note the direction of the fascicle, as well as (B) the cranial segmental attachment. In parts (A) and (B) the specific hypertonic fascicle attaches from L4 to the iliac crest. (C) Segmental atrophy or inhibition of the deep laminar fibers of multifidus is often found at the level of the cranial attachment of the hypertonic superficial fibers of multifidus. Note the lack of tone/bulk on the right side of L4 in this subject.

median sacral crest from which the hypertonicity is arising (Fig. 8.54C). Press firmly, but gently into the tissue and compare the tone and bulk of these deep fibers to the opposite side, as well as to levels above and below.

The inferior part of the SIJ can be compressed by overactivation of ischiococcygeus that prevents a parallel glide at the inferior part of the SIJ and induces a posterior rotation of the innominate during this test. If compression of the inferior aspect of the SIJ is found, the next step is to palpate the ischiococcygeus (see Fig. 3.62B) from a point just lateral and inferior to the ILA (Fig. 8.55A) to its insertion into the ischial spine to confirm/negate that hypertonicity of this muscle is the cause of the aberrant motion noted. This can be done with the patient in either the prone (Fig. 8.55A) or supine (Fig. 8.55B) position.

Hypertonicity of the piriformis muscle (see Fig. 3.55A) tends to compress all three parts of the SIJ. All parts of the SIJ feel very resistant to motion and tender trigger points in piriformis confirm the cause. Piriformis is palpated just lateral to the sacrum and the sacrotuberous ligament (Fig. 8.56).

Clinical reasoning. If the SIJ is fibrotic and stiff (articular system impairment), both its active and passive range of motion will be reduced compared to the opposite side and the pelvis will not unlock on this side during loading tasks. If the SIJ is lax and loose (articular system impairment), the active motion is often reduced on this side, yet the passive range of motion is greater when sides are compared. The reduced active motion is likely due to a non-optimal bracing strategy that is trying to control the joint's motion. The strategy has rendered the joint rigid during tasks that require mobility, and is therefore non-optimal. Alternately the bracing strategy may persist in the supine position and the passive range of motion will also be reduced; the underlying laxity does not become apparent until tone in the muscles protecting the joint is released. If the SIJ is fixated (articular system impairment) no movement occurs either on active or passive mobility testing and the joint plane cannot be found, i.e. the joint almost feels fused. In addition, there is a history of significant trauma and the pelvic position is non-physiological and does not vary with movement. A compressed SIJ (neural system impairment) presents with the most inconsistent findings; in fact, the most consistent thing about a compressed SIJ is the inconsistency of the findings. Commonly, only one part of the SIJ is restricted, the axis of motion is altered, and subsequent tests that assess muscle tone

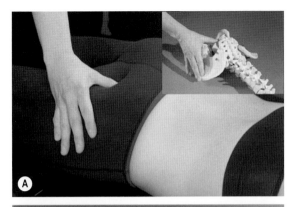

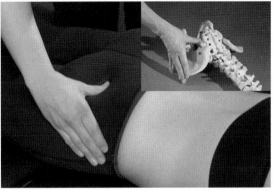

Fig. 8.56 • Pelvic girdle: palpation of piriformis. Palpate piriformis lateral to the sacrum between S2 and S4, superior to the inferior arcuate band of the sacrotuberous ligament. Explore the length of the muscle from the lateral aspect of the sacrum to its insertion into the greater trochanter, noting any areas of increased tone and/or tenderness.

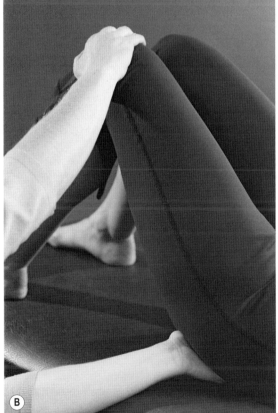

Fig. 8.55 • Pelvic girdle: palpation of ischiococcygeus. (A) Palpate ischiococcygeus immediately inferior to the inferior lateral angle of the sacrum and the inferior arcuate band of the sacrotuberous ligament and note the tone and presence of any tender trigger points within the muscle. (B) Ischiococcygeus can also be palpated with the patient in the supine position. Find the coccyx and then palpate for increased tone and tenderness in ischiococcygeus, which lies directly lateral to the coccyx and inferior to the inferior lateral angle.

(neural system tests) are necessary to confirm or negate the diagnosis of a compressed SIJ.

SIJ: Elastic zone analysis. Once the joint's behavior in the neutral zone is understood, continue to apply a posterior translation force to the innominate paying particular attention to the point where the resistance begins to rise and further force is required. You are moving towards the end of the joint's range and are in the elastic zone of the motion. How much resistance is there to motion in the elastic zone and is any pain provoked when gliding the innominate in this zone (R1–R2)? What is the end feel like? If pain is provoked during this test, other tests for pain provocation of the SIJ (see below) are indicated.

Clinical reasoning. The stiff SIJ imparts a very rapid rise in the resistance to motion and the end feel is quite firm, whereas the lax SIJ gives very little resistance in this zone and is often, though not always, painful. The compressed SIJ feels like you are 'pushing a boat up a river'; there is a springy sense to the resistance that varies with the application of force at different speeds. As myofascial compression occurs in the neutral zone (0–R1), the elastic zone cannot be accurately assessed in a compressed joint. It is also impossible to test the elastic zone of motion when the SIJ is fixated as all movement is totally blocked.

SIJ: Neutral zone analysis in the craniocaudal plane. There is a small amount of translation available in the craniocaudal plane at the SIJ in the non-weight bearing position (Fig. 8.57). The direction of this

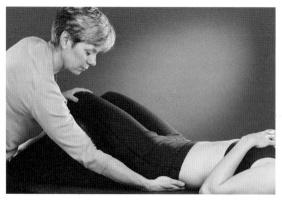

Fig. 8.57 • Pelvic girdle: articular system mobility – sacroiliac joint: neutral zone analysis in the craniocaudal plane. The innominate should glide parallel to the sacrum; the direction is variable.

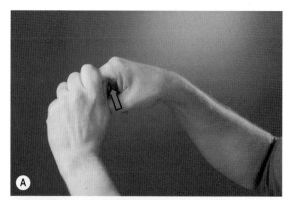

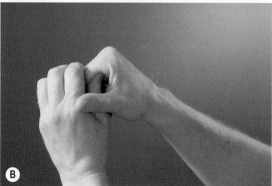

Fig. 8.58 • Integrity of the articular system restraints. All synovial joints have a variable amount of passive glide or translation between the articular surfaces; this glide facilitates physiological movement. (A) In the loose-packed position, the capsule and the ligaments are the least tense and therefore the amplitude of translation between the articular surfaces is the greatest. (B) In the close-packed position, the capsule and ligaments are taut and no passive translation should be possible. This confirms that the articular system restraints are intact.

glide is variable between sides and between subjects, and must be found before the neutral zone can be assessed. The amplitude and quality of the motion in the neutral zone should be symmetrical between sides.

Clinical reasoning. When the SIJ is stiff, the amplitude of neutral zone motion is reduced in both the anteroposterior and craniocaudal planes; the fixated joint prevents the joint plane from being palpable in both planes, whereas the compressed joint can present with variable findings (remember how inconsistent this impairment is). When the craniocaudal glide is present and clear, yet the anteroposterior glide feels somewhat 'stiff' at the superior, middle, or inferior (or all three) part(s), it is likely that the joint is compressed (neural system impairment) and not stiff (articular system impairment). When the SIJ is compressed it is not possible to test the integrity of the articular system restraints (i.e. ability of the passive restraints to resist translation or shear of the joint) as the hypertonic muscles prevent the joint from being close-packed.

Pelvic girdle: integrity of the articular system restraints – sacroiliac joint

All joints have a variable amount of translation to facilitate the physiological movement possible; the SIJ is no exception. Figure 8.58A illustrates the small amount of dorsal translation of the right second metacarpophalangeal joint when this joint is in the loose-packed position. When the joint is fully flexed and held in its close-packed position, no translation is possible as this position has tightened both the

capsule and the articular ligaments (Fig. 8.58B). The principles of this test can be applied to the SIJ to determine the integrity of the articular system restraints; this test determines whether there is a deficit in the joint's capsule and/or ligaments (i.e. the passive system).

The starting position for this test is the same as for testing neutral zone motion of the SIJ in the anteroposterior plane (see above). Find the plane of the SIJ, note the amplitude of movement available in the neutral zone, and then close-pack the joint. The SIJ is close-packed by nutating the sacrum and posteriorly rotating the innominate (Chapter 4). The sacrum is nutated by applying an anterior force with your dorsal hand while simultaneously rotating the innominate posteriorly (Fig. 8.59). Remember, the

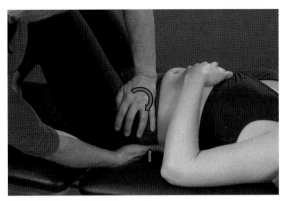

Fig. 8.59 • Pelvic girdle: integrity of the articular system restraints – sacroiliac joint (SIJ). When the sacrum is nutated and the ipsilateral innominate posteriorly rotated, the SIJ is close-packed and there should be no palpable anteroposterior translation. If movement can still be palpated, one cause may be the loss of integrity of the passive restraints. The arrows indicate the direction of force applied by the therapist's hands.

amplitude of motion is very small. Hold this position and repeat the anteroposterior glide; no movement should occur when the articular system restraints are intact. If movement is still present, consideration must be given to whether or not the history and other test findings support a diagnosis of a lax SIJ.

Clinical reasoning. If the patient is unable to control motion of the SIJ during loading tasks (unlocking noted in forward bend, squat, or one leg standing tasks), and the amplitude of passive motion of this joint is greater than that of the opposite side, and the joint's motion is not controlled by the articular system restraints (i.e. close-packing the joint does not reduce the amplitude of the neutral zone to zero), this suggests that there is an impairment of the passive restraints of the articular system. This patient may be able to compensate for this articular system impairment with training. If the neural and myofascial systems are functioning optimally, the following tests will help to predict whether a training program that follows the principles of The Integrated Systems Model approach will be beneficial.

Pelvic girdle: influence of the myofascial and neural systems on the sacroiliac joint

The influence of the myofascial and neural systems on the SIJ can only be tested if the deep muscle system is functioning optimally and the myofascial system is intact – in other words, if the patient is able

to coactivate the pelvic floor, the left and right transversus abdominis, and the left and right deep lumbosacral multifidus, and the fascia is able to transmit the force of this coactivation through the SIJ. If there are deficits in the activation of these muscles (absence or delay, etc.), training is required before this test can be done (Chapter 11). If there is loss of integrity of the myofascia (linea alba and/or endopelvic fascia) (Chapter 6), motion of the SIJ may still be present during this test even if the neural system is functioning well.

Palpate the available neutral zone motion of the SIJ on the impaired side (side of unlocking during loading tasks) and note the amplitude. Have the patient gently coactivate the deep muscles and, as they hold this gentle co-contraction, retest the neutral zone motion; there should be none. A gentle activation of the deep muscles should be sufficient to control all movement in the neutral zone.

Clinical reasoning. If the patient is unable to control motion of the SIJ during loading tasks (unlocking noted in forward bend, squat, or one leg standing tasks) and the myofascial and neural systems have no influence on the articular motion, it is the authors' experience that *at this time* physiotherapy treatment will not be successful for restoration of full function. Prolotherapy can help to restore the integrity of the passive system and is indicated at this time (Chapter 11). When the joint's mobility can once again be influenced by the myofascial and neural systems, the authors have found that treatment following the principles of The Integrated Systems Model approach is very effective. This highlights the need for multidisciplinary teams in clinical practice.

Pelvic girdle: integrity of the articular system restraints – pubic symphysis

The PS is a fibrous joint with minimal, if any, translation potential (<22mm (Chapter 4)). The articular system of the PS is assessed by attempting to specifically shear the joint in a craniocaudal direction. With the heel of one hand, palpate the superior aspect of the superior ramus of one pubic bone. With the heel of the other hand, palpate the inferior aspect of the superior ramus of the opposite pubic bone (Fig. 8.60). Fix one pubic bone and apply a slow, steady vertical translation force to the other. There should be almost no neutral zone motion, a very firm and rapid rise in resistance to motion, and no pain provoked with this test. Switch your hands and repeat the test.

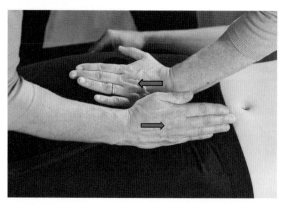

Fig. 8.60 • Pelvic girdle: integrity of the articular system restraints – pubic symphysis. Minimal, if any, craniocaudal translation (<2mm) should occur during this passive test. The end feel should be very firm and the test should not provoke pain. The arrows indicate the direction of force applied by the therapist's hands; the test should be repeated with the hands switched to test vertical translation of the other side.

Pelvic girdle: influence of the myofascial and neural systems on the pubic symphysis

If the patient's story suggests that further analysis of the PS is required, there are several functional tasks that could be included in the analysis of strategies for function and performance. Load transfer through the PS can be analyzed during any task; however, the following tasks provide more specific challenge to craniocaudal control of the PS. The PS is palpated at the superior pubic rami bilaterally as the patient either laterally tilts the pelvis (Fig. 8.61A) or lifts one leg slightly off the table (Fig. 8.61B). If the strategies for load transfer through the PS are optimal, no translation between the left and right superior pubic rami will occur during either of these tasks. Alternately, with the patient standing on a step or a stool, palpate the cranial aspect of the left and right superior pubic rami. Instruct the patient to hang one leg off the side without laterally tilting the pelvis (Fig. 8.61C). No craniocaudal translation should occur at the PS.

If there is FLT of the PS during any of these tests, the ability of the myofascial and neural systems to control motion at the PS should be evaluated. In supine position, while palpating the superior aspect of the right and left pubic rami, have the patient attempt a deep muscle system co-contraction and assess the impact of the resulting contraction.

If the myofascial and neural systems are impaired, translation or torsion of the PS may still occur. If an articular system impairment was previously identified, then the impact of the deep muscle system co-contraction on vertical translation of the PS is also assessed. Repeat the craniocaudal translation test (Fig. 8.60) and note the available motion. Have the patient gently coactivate the deep muscles and, as they hold this gentle co-contraction, retest the craniocaudal translation of the PS. If the myofascial and neural systems are functioning well, any positive translation found on passive testing should be controlled. This indicates that retraining of the deep system and integration into functional loading tasks has the potential to control the articular system deficit of the PS. If the myofascial and/or neural systems are impaired, motion will still be available at the PS. Further tests will reveal which components need to be treated (myofascial and/or neural), and once the relevant impairments are addressed (e.g. motor control of deep muscles, restoration of fascial integrity of the anterior abdominal wall, etc.), the ability of the myofascial and neural systems to control motion of the PS should be re-evaluated. In other words, once the patient is able to coactivate the pelvic floor, the left and right transversus abdominis (and the left and right deep lumbosacral multifidus), the impact of this contraction on the craniocaudal shear of the PS is re-assessed.

Pelvic girdle: pain provocation tests

Pain provocation tests have shown good intertester reliability (Laslett et al 2005, Laslett & Williams 1994, Robinson et al 2007) especially when combined test results are considered. They can also help to explain to patients why certain activities/exercises may provoke their condition. On occasion, it is necessary to treat the painful structure before function can be restored, particularly if the exercises being taught are aggravating a painful, inflamed structure.

Long dorsal ligament. This structure is often tender to palpation in patients with pelvic girdle pain. The patient is lying prone with the head neutral and arms by the sides. With one hand, palpate the iliac crest and follow it posteriorly to just inferior to the PSIS (see Fig. 3.27). This point is dorsal to the long dorsal ligament, which can be felt as a vertically oriented band. Note any tenderness to palpation. Continue to palpate the ligament with one hand and apply a counter-nutation force to the sacrum (Fig. 8.62). Note the increase in tension in

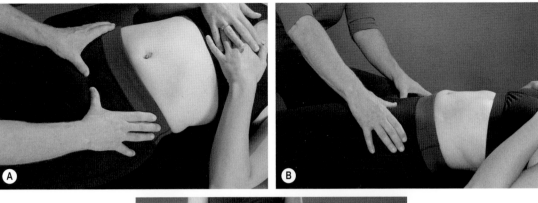

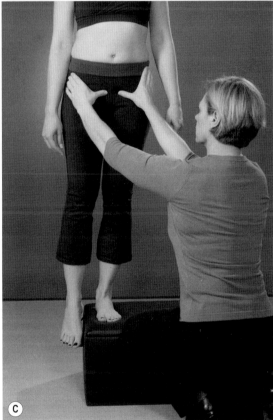

Fig. 8.61 • Pelvic girdle: specific tasks for analysis of load transfer through the pubic symphysis (PS). Control of the PS is assessed by noting the presence/absence of any craniocaudal translation during specific task analysis; the patient either (A) laterally tilts the pelvis or (B) slightly lifts one leg off the table. (C) Standing with one leg hanging is an alternate task useful for testing strategies for control of the PS. Note that if the patient has poor control, an intrapelvic torsion may occur during these tests and will create torsion at the PS, which will be felt; this is physiological and not the same as the craniocaudal translation that occurs with loss of the integrity of the articular system restraints. If failed load transfer of the PS occurs during any of these tasks, further analysis of the articular, myofascial, and neural systems is required.

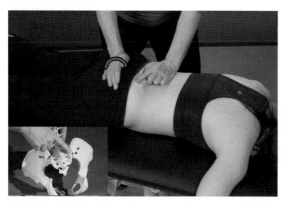

Fig. 8.62 • Pelvic girdle: pain provocation tests, long dorsal ligament. One hand palpates the long dorsal ligament (inset) while the other hand applies a counter-nutation force to the sacrum (arrow). If the ligament is a source of nociception, this test will provoke local pain.

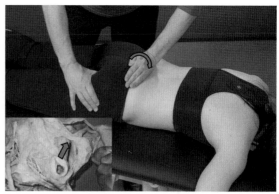

Fig. 8.63 • Pelvic girdle: pain provocation tests, sacrotuberous ligament. One hand palpates the inferior arcuate band of the sacrotuberous ligament (arrow on inset) while the other hand applies a nutation force to the sacrum (arrow). If the ligament is a source of nociception, this test will provoke local pain.

the long dorsal ligament and any increase in local pain. If this test is associated with increased pain, then this structure is a likely nociceptive source.

Sacrotuberous ligament. Although the sacrotuberous ligament can be injured during a fall on the buttock, this structure is less often a source of pelvic pain. The patient is lying prone with the head neutral and arms by the sides. Palpate the ischial tuberosity with one thumb. From this point, palpate medially and cranially until you reach the inferior arcuate band (medial band) of the sacrotuberous ligament (Figs 3.27, 8.63). It should feel like a taut guitar string when you pronate and supinate your forearm and roll your thumb over the ligament. Continue to palpate the ligament and apply a nutation force to the sacrum (Fig. 8.63). Note the increase in tension in the sacrotuberous ligament. If this test is associated with increased pain, then this structure is a likely nociceptive source.

Anterior distraction and posterior compression. This test is not intended to stress a particular structure, but rather tests for pain provocation when the pelvic girdle is compressed posteriorly and distracted anteriorly. With the patient lying supine, palpate the medial aspect of the ASIS bilaterally with the heels of the crossed hands (Fig. 8.64). Apply a slow, steady, posterolateral force through the ASISs, thus distracting the anterior aspect of the SIJ and PS and compressing the posterior structures. Maintain the force for 5 seconds and note the provocation and location of pain.

Posterior distraction and anterior compression. This test is not intended to stress a particular

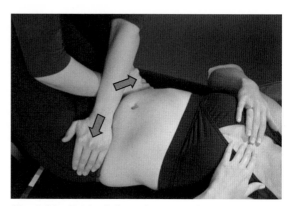

Fig. 8.64 • Pelvic girdle: pain provocation tests, anterior distraction and posterior compression.

structure, but rather tests for pain provocation when the pelvic girdle is compressed anteriorly and distracted posteriorly. If an intra-articular synovitis of the SIJ is present, this test also increases the patient's pain. With the patient sidelying, hips and knees comfortably flexed, palpate the anterolateral aspect of the uppermost iliac crest (Fig. 8.65). Apply a slow, steady, medial force through the pelvic girdle, thus distracting the posterior structures of the SIJ and compressing the anterior. Maintain the force for 5 seconds and note the provocation and location of pain.

Thigh thrust or P4 (posterior pelvic pain provocation) test. The P4 test (posterior pelvic pain provocation test) as described by Ostgaard et al (1994) begins with the patient supine and the hip and knee

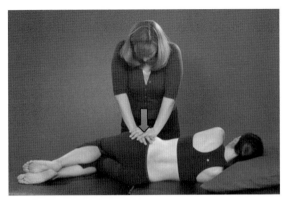

Fig. 8.65 • Pelvic girdle: pain provocation tests, posterior distraction and anterior compression.

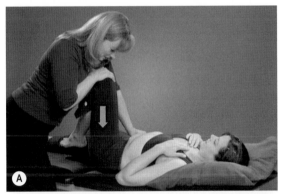

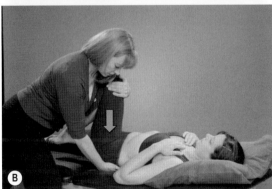

Fig. 8.66 • Pelvic girdle: pain provocation tests, thigh thrust or P4 (posterior pelvic pain provocation) test. (A) P4 test as suggested by Ostgaard et al (1994). (B) Modification of the P4 test: the sacrum is stabilized posteriorly before the anteroposterior shear is applied to the innominate through the flexed femur.

flexed. The pelvic girdle is stabilized through the contralateral innominate and a gentle posterior force is applied through the femur (Fig. 8.66A). When pain is provoked in the gluteal area on the ipsilateral side, the test is considered positive. A modification of this

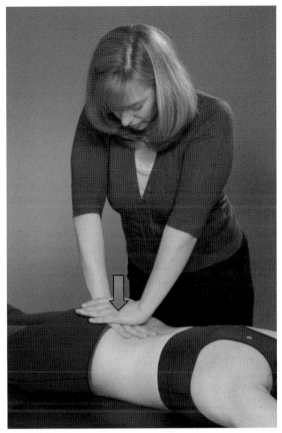

Fig. 8.67 • Pelvic girdle: pain provocation tests, sacral thrust.

test is to stabilize the sacrum posteriorly before applying the anteroposterior force to the SIJ through the femur and innominate (Fig. 8.66B). Maintain the force for 5 seconds and note the provocation and location of pain. The same information can be gained from the SIJ: elastic zone analysis test (see above).

Sacral thrust. With the patient prone, apply a pure posteroanterior force (not nutation) to the dorsal aspect of the sacrum (Fig. 8.67). Maintain the force for 5 seconds and note the provocation and location of pain.

Clinical reasoning. Laslett et al (2005) have found that when any two of the four non-specific provocation tests (distraction, compression, thigh thrust, sacral thrust) are positive, the SIJ is a source of pain. These patients often do not do well in a sacroiliac belt, nor do they respond at this stage of their recovery to exercises that further compress their pelvis. Medical management to relieve the synovitis is often required prior to commencing physiotherapy.

Regional tests – the lumbar spine

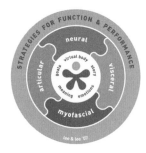

The lumbar spine requires further analysis if during any task the strategy used causes segmental or multi-segmental restriction of movement or loss of segmental motion control (flexion or extension hinge, loss of rotational control). Clinical reasoning of the findings from multiple tests is necessary to understand the significance of the results of each individual test and this will be covered, in part, in this chapter and then in further detail in Chapter 9.

Similar to the principles described in the previous section on the pelvic girdle, there are specific tests that examine the passive mobility as well as the integrity of the articular, myofascial, and neural systems for the joints of the lumbar spine. Passive movement analysis requires an evaluation of two zones of motion, the neutral zone and the elastic zone, and consideration must be given to the presence of any muscular tone that may prevent movement analysis of the joint at this time. Often neuromyofascial techniques (Chapter 10) are necessary to release the superficial muscle hypertonicity before an articular assessment of the lumbar spine can be performed.

When interpreting the mobility findings, the position of the bone at the beginning of the test should be correlated with the subsequent mobility as alterations in joint mobility may merely be a reflection of an altered starting position. If the L5 vertebra is rotated to the left relative to the sacrum, and the amplitude of motion for left rotation is reduced compared to the levels above, this should be interpreted as a normal finding as far as the joint is concerned. The following tests examine the position and mobility (including both neutral and elastic zone analysis) of the joints of the lumbar spine.

Lumbar spine: positional tests

To determine the position of L5 relative to the sacrum, the posteroanterior relationship between the L5 vertebra and the sacrum is noted. This can be done in neutral, full flexion, or full extension. For example, if there is a physiological left intrapelvic torsion (IPTL) in forward bending, L5 should be rotated to the left when its position is assessed in forward bend (Fig. 8.68). A passive mobility test of L5–S1 may be influenced by the IPT secondary to altered tension through the iliolumbar ligaments; this is not an articular restriction but rather a reduction of motion secondary to an altered resting position. Movement analysis of the lumbar spine is therefore best done after the pelvic girdle has been restored to a neutral position and any hypertonicity

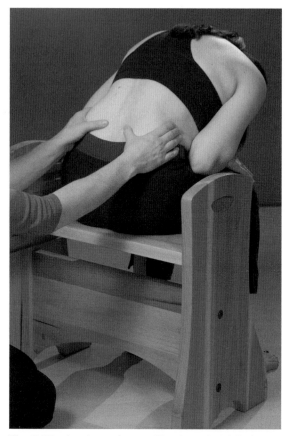

Fig. 8.68 • Lumbar spine: positional test in full flexion. Palpate L5 just lateral to the spinous process and note the direction of rotation compared to the inferior lateral angles of the sacrum. Note which bone is rotated the most to determine the resting position of the L5–S1 joint. If L5 is rotated further to the left than the sacrum, then L5–S1 is rotated to the left. If L5 is rotated to the left but less than the sacrum, then the L5–S1 joint is rotated to the right. The validity of this test is likely to be affected if there is any asymmetry in tone of multifidus, and thus findings from this test need to be confirmed/negated with other tests.

in the superficial muscles (erector spinae, superficial fibers of multifidus, internal oblique, quadratus lumborum) has been released.

Lumbar spine: articular system mobility – intervertebral lumbar joints

Flexion and extension of the lumbar spine should not be associated with any segmental or multisegmental sideflexion/rotation (Chapter 4) and a segmental mobility analysis is indicated if this is observed. Passive mobility of the lumbar spine is tested with the patient sidelying and the top hip and knee comfortably flexed. Localize the test to the specific segment by rotating the thorax down to the level above and flexing the lumbar spine up to the level below. Segmentally flex, extend, sideflex, and then combine sideflexion and rotation, paying attention to the beginning feel of each motion (Fig. 8.69). How hard

do you have to push to initiate movement in each direction? How much movement is there? What is the end feel of the motion like? Hypertonicity of the superficial, multisegmental, paraspinal muscles can compress the zygapophyseal joint(s) and prevent the superior glide that is required for flexion, sideflexion, and sideflexion/rotation.

Clinical reasoning. If the left zygapophyseal joint at L4–5 is fibrotic and stiff such that a superior glide is restricted, both active and passive segmental mobility will be impacted. Forward bending will reveal a left rotation at L4–5 and right lateral bending will reveal a kink in the multisegmental curve at L4–5. Passively, motion will be reduced into flexion and right sideflexion and the elastic zone of motion will be very resistant with a hard end feel. If the left zygapophyseal joint at L4–5 is fibrotic and stiff such that an inferior glide is restricted, backward bending will reveal a right rotation at L4–5 and left lateral bending will reveal a kink in the multisegmental curve at L4–5. Passively, motion will be reduced into extension and left sideflexion and, again, the elastic zone of motion will be very resistant and the end feel hard. A compressed zygapophyseal joint will often yield the same mobility findings but the quality of the beginning feel in the neutral zone as well as the quality of the end feel is characteristically different. Hypertonic muscles impart a springy quality to the movement with a less definitive stop to the motion. When this sensation is felt, immediately palpate the paraspinal muscles (Fig. 8.70) and note any trigger points or hypertonicity to confirm that the zygapophyseal joint is actually compressed and not

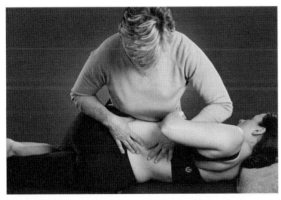

Fig. 8.69 • Lumbar spine: articular system mobility – intervertebral lumbar joints. Clinicians often ignore the multiple layers of muscle between the skin and the vertebral column when assessing mobility of the lumbar spine. The lumbar joints are often incriminated as being restricted when in fact it is impossible to assess them in the presence of hypertonic superficial muscles. In this situation, a generic distractive manipulation technique is often effective for restoring mobility due to the impact of a thrust technique on segmental muscle tone (Chapter 10). When performing passive mobility tests for the lumbar spine, pay attention to the amount of force required to initiate motion, be aware of the beginning feel and the specific direction of the resistance to motion (vector of force) as this is where you will feel the restriction produced by the hypertonic muscles. Explore segmental flexion/ extension, sideflexion, and sideflexion/rotation and correlate the findings with the active mobility tests, and the motor control patterns observed during task analysis.

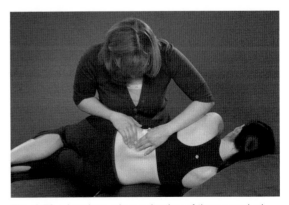

Fig. 8.70 • Lumbar spine: palpation of the paraspinal muscles. Palpate the multisegmental paraspinal muscles (lumbar longissimus, lumbar iliocostalis, quadratus lumborum) and note the presence of hypertonicity and/or tender trigger points.

stiff. If local pain is provoked while testing the elastic zone, specific tests for the integrity of the articular system restraints (see below) are indicated.

Lumbar spine: integrity of the articular system restraints

Segmental injuries are common in the lumbar spine and the structural changes that occur as a consequence of the trauma are often seen with imaging studies. However, MRI and CT cannot always provide information on how well motion is controlled at the injured segment by either the passive system (articular) or the active/control system (myofascial/neural systems). The following tests assess the integrity of the passive lumbar segmental restraints for rotation and translation.

Rotation: left rotation L4–5. With the patient right sidelying, left hip and knee slightly flexed, right hip and knee extended, palpate the left side of the spinous process of L4 with the cranial hand. With the long and ring fingers of the caudal hand, palpate the right side of the spinous process of L5 (Fig. 8.71). Left rotation, or left segmental torsion, is tested by fixing L4 and right rotating L5 about a pure vertical axis beneath the L4 vertebra (the L4–5 segment relatively left rotates). This is a

non-physiological rotation and results in osseous impaction of the right zygapophyseal joint and distraction of the left zygapophyseal joint within 2–3° of rotation. The end feel should be firm, the neutral zone small, and no pain should be provoked with this test.

Anteroposterior/posteroanterior translation: neutral and elastic zone analysis of L4–5. With the patient in sidelying, hips and knees flexed, cradle the lower extremities with your caudal/arm hand (Fig. 8.72). With your other hand, palpate the interspinous space of the segment being assessed. Flex the lumbar spine through the lower extremities until the L4–5 segment is in a neutral position (neither flexed nor extended). From this position, fix the spinous process of L4 and apply an anteroposterior translation force through the femurs and pelvis to translate L5 posteriorly beneath the fixed L4 (testing a relative anterior translation of L4 on L5). Note the amplitude of the neutral zone, the resistance of the beginning feel and the quality of the end feel (elastic zone), and compare these findings to the levels above and below. Note the presence/absence of any provoked pain throughout the test.

Subsequently, remove the fixation on the spinous process of L4 and, with the cranial hand, palpate the interspinous space between L4 and L5. With your caudal hand, palpate the spinous process of L5 and the median sacral crest of the sacrum; continue to

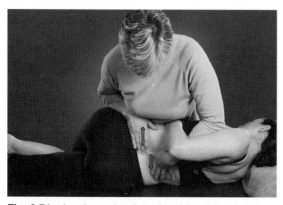

Fig. 8.71 • Lumbar spine: integrity of the articular system restraints, left rotation L4–5. It is common to see rotation injuries to the lumbar spine in clinical practice; this test assesses the integrity of the superior articular process. There is articular impaction of the contralateral (in this instance the right one) zygapophyseal joint as well as distraction of the capsule and ligaments of the ipsilateral zygapophyseal joint (in this instance the left one). When pain is provoked during this test, care must be taken to ensure motion control during any exercise/task/sport that requires rotation of the lumbar spine, and the thorax should be checked for rotational mobility.

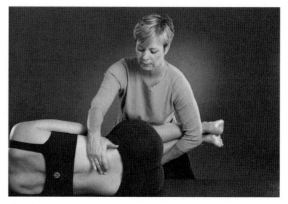

Fig. 8.72 • Lumbar spine: integrity of the articular system restraints, anteroposterior/posteroanterior translation: neutral and elastic zone analysis of L4–5. A small amount of horizontal translation should be present when the lumbar segment is tested in the neutral position. However, the passive restraints should control all translation when the segment is either flexed or extended. If motion persists, this suggests loss of integrity of the passive restraints of the articular system.

support the lower extremities with your abdomen/ thighs. Apply a posteroanterior translation force to L5 and the sacrum to translate L5 anteriorly beneath the L4, which is fixed by the weight of the trunk on the table. Take care to notice when L4 begins to move; this is the end of range for the L4–5 segment. Note the amplitude of the neutral zone, the resistance of the beginning feel, and the quality of the end feel (elastic zone) and compare these findings to the levels above and below. Note the presence/ absence of any provoked pain throughout the test.

When a joint is held in its close-packed position, no translation should be possible as this position tightens both the capsule and the articular ligaments (see Fig. 8.58B). The principles of this test can be applied to the joints of the lumbar spine to determine the integrity of the articular system restraints (the passive restraints).

Passively extend the specific lumbar segment being assessed, hold this close-packed position, and repeat the anteroposterior/posteroanterior translation tests described above. Repeat the tests with the segment fully flexed. No movement should occur in either the fully extended or flexed position when the articular system restraints are intact.

Clinical reasoning. If the patient is unable to control segmental motion of the lumbar spine during meaningful tasks (e.g. there is a segmental flexion hinge in forward bend (Fig. 4.13A) or segmental extension hinge in backward bend (Fig. 4.13B)), the amplitude of passive motion of this joint is greater than the levels above or below, and the motion is

not controlled by the articular system restraints when the joint is close-packed, this suggests that there is an impairment of the passive restraints of the articular system. This patient may be able to compensate for this articular impairment with training. If the neural and myofascial systems are functioning optimally, the following tests will help to predict whether a training program that follows the principles of The Integrated Systems Model approach will be beneficial.

Lumbar spine: influence of the myofascial and neural systems on the joints of the lumbar spine

The influence of the myofascial and neural systems on the joints of the lumbar spine can only be tested if the deep muscle system is functioning optimally and the myofascial system is intact. If there are deficits in the activation of the deep muscles, training is required before this test can be done (Chapter 11). If there is loss of integrity of the myofascia (linea alba and/or endopelvic fascia) (Chapter 6), motion of the lumbar segment may still be present during this test even if the neural system is functioning well.

Palpate the available anteroposterior/posteroanterior motion of the lumbar segment and note the amplitude. Have the patient gently coactivate the deep muscles and, as they hold this gentle co-contraction, retest the neutral zone motion; there should be none. A gentle activation of the deep muscles should be sufficient to control all movement in the neutral zone (Fig. 8.73A,B).

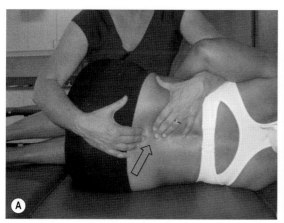 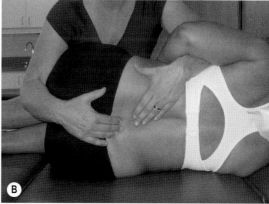

Fig. 8.73 • Lumbar spine: influence of the myofascial and neural systems on the joints of the lumbar spine. (A) Note the excessive posteroanterior translation available at L5–S1 (arrow). (B) When the myofascial and neural systems for the lumbar spine are functioning optimally, a gentle contraction of the deep system will be sufficient to control all segmental posteroanterior translation as is shown in this illustration.

Clinical reasoning. If the patient is unable to control motion of a lumbar segment during loading tasks (e.g. there is a segmental hinge or buckle noted in forward/backward bend, squat, or one leg standing tasks) and the myofascial and neural systems have no influence on the articular motion, it is the authors' experience that *at this time* physiotherapy treatment will not be successful for restoring function. Prolotherapy can help to restore the integrity of the passive system and is indicated at this time (Chapter 11). When the joint's mobility is once again influenced by the myofascial and neural systems, the authors have found that treatment following the principles of The Integrated Systems Model approach is highly effective. This highlights the need for multidisciplinary teams in clinical practice.

Regional tests – the hips

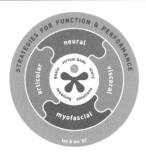

The hips require further analysis if during any task the strategy used causes restriction of movement or loss of motion control (altered axis of motion or non-optimal femoral head position). Clinical reasoning of the findings from multiple tests is necessary to understand the significance of the results of each individual test and this will be covered, in part, in this chapter and then in further detail in Chapter 9.

The following tests examine the position and passive mobility of the hip joint in the non-weight bearing position. As with the lumbar spine and pelvic girdle, motion analysis requires an evaluation of two zones of motion: the neutral zone and the elastic zone. However, before any interpretation of mobility can be made, the position of the femoral head with respect to the acetabulum must be determined. The hip joint is under the influence of several large muscles and an imbalance in myofascial tension or muscle tone can cause a displacement of the femoral head and thus restrict the joint's functional range of motion.

The hip: dynamic non-weight bearing positional tests

Dynamic non-weight bearing analysis of hip position begins with the patient in the crook lying position. Note the resting position of the pelvic girdle (presence or absence of an IPT) and then palpate (spring) the inguinal ligament bilaterally noting the symmetry of tension between the left and right sides. Palpate the left and right femoral head (2cm below the midway point between the ASIS and the PS) and note any prominence or tenderness. The femoral head should be barely palpable. Subsequently, palpate both the innominates and the femoral heads bilaterally (Fig. 8.74) and while maintaining gentle contact, instruct the patient to slowly extend their hips and knees. At the end of this task note any:

1. change in the femoral head position and whether the change is unilateral or bilateral;
2. change in the position of the pelvic girdle (appearance of an IPT); and
3. the position of the entire lower extremity (external or internal rotation).

As mentioned previously, the hip is often subjected to multiple force vectors from muscle imbalances and the net vector often results in displacement of

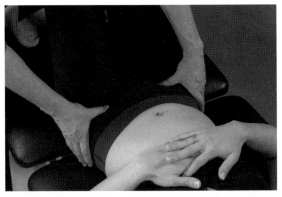

Fig. 8.74 • The hip: dynamic non-weight bearing positional tests. Non-optimal force vectors from hypertonic muscles can create malalignment of both the pelvic girdle and the femurs. The malalignment may or may not be evident in the crook lying starting position. Note any intrapelvic torsion or femoral head displacement and then instruct the patient to extend their legs and note any change in the alignment of the pelvic girdle and femoral heads. Further specific analysis (vector analysis) for relevant hypertonicity of the hip musculature is required to determine the cause of any noted malalignment.

the femoral head. This test is a quick screen for the presence of non-optimal force vectors that are further analyzed during the articular system mobility tests (see below).

The hip: articular system mobility – hip joint

As a reminder from Chapter 4, osteokinematically, flexion/extension occurs when the femur rotates about a coronal axis through the center of the femoral head and neck; the femoral head should remain centered within the acetabulum through the full excursion of motion. Although variable, approximately 100° of femoral flexion is possible, following which motion of the SIJ and lumbar spine occurs to allow the anterior thigh to approximate the chest. Approximately 20° of femoral extension is possible. When rotation of the femoral head occurs purely about this axis (i.e. without conjoined abduction/adduction or medial/lateral rotation), the motion is arthrokinematically described as a pure spin. No translation of the femoral head relative to the acetabulum should occur when the joint spins purely.

Like the pelvic girdle and the lumbar spine, movement analysis of the hip requires the evaluation of two zones of motion, the neutral zone and the elastic zone, and consideration must be given to the presence of any muscular tone that may prevent movement analysis of the joint at this time. Often neuromyofascial techniques (Chapter 10) are

necessary to release the superficial muscle hypertonicity before a complete articular assessment of the hip joint can be done. When analyzing the passive range of motion of the hip joint there are several things to note for each direction of motion tested including:

1. the range of free, non-resisted motion where the femoral head remains centered in the acetabulum (neutral zone of motion);
2. the presence of any vectors of force preventing free, non-resisted motion and the specific muscles that are causing these vectors. Compression of the hip joint is often associated with displacement of the femoral head well before the end of the joint's potential range. Functional range of motion is limited to that range where the femoral head remains centered;
3. the resistance of the elastic zone (only palpable if there are no hypertonic muscles creating vectors of force in the neutral zone of motion);
4. the quality of the end feel at the end of the elastic zone; and
5. the total range of motion of the hip joint at the end of the elastic zone.

With the patient lying supine, palpate the femoral head and the innominate (Fig. 8.75A). Support the lower extremity with the other hand/arm and passively flex the femur until posterior rotation of the ipsilateral innominate begins (Fig 8.75B,C); this is

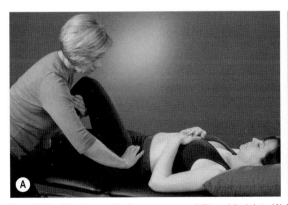
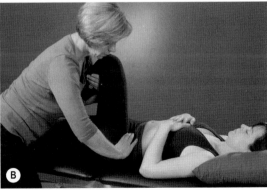

Fig. 8.75 • The hip: articular system mobility – hip joint. (A) Note the starting position of the femoral head. (B) Passively flex the femur and note the response of the femoral head. If it is anterior, does it center into the acetabulum or does it translate further anterior or does it remain the same? If it starts centered, does it displace anteriorly at a certain range? If it is centered, does it remain so throughout the range? Once the innominate begins to rotate posteriorly, the limit of functional hip flexion has been reached.

Continued

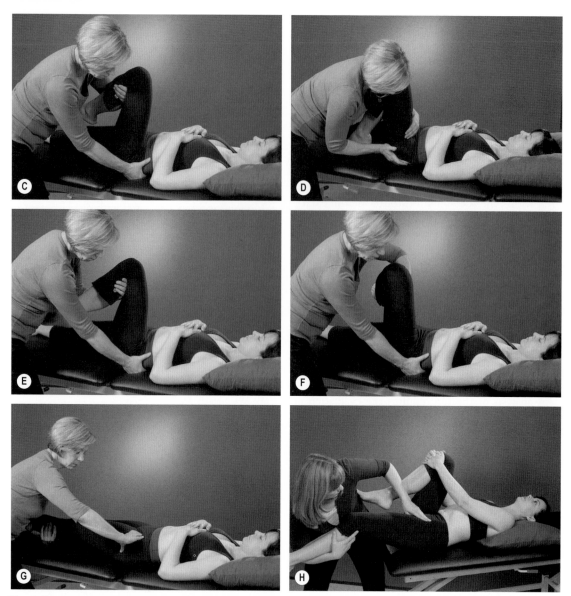

Fig. 8.75 – cont'd • (C) The motion of the innominate can be confirmed by palpating the posterior aspect of the bone. (D) Stop at the point when the femoral head is felt to displace anteriorly and palpate the muscles of the buttock and thigh. Note any increased activity/tone in any muscle that occurs at the point when the femoral head displaces. It is our experience that consistent increases in tone at certain points of range during a fully passive test are indicative of altered neural drive to the muscles and this is clinically relevant. This vector analysis test helps to determine which hypertonic or 'tight' muscles are relevant to the presenting problem(s). Multiple muscles may be creating the single net force vector and all will require release in order to restore optimal biomechanics of the hip. (E) Internal and (F) external rotation of the femur can be tested in varying degrees of flexion/extension. If the femoral head is anteriorly displaced, rotation will be affected. Consider the patient's story and meaningful tasks when choosing which hip movements to test. (G) Palpate the femoral head and the innominate and extend the femur. Note the response of the femoral head, the point at which anterior rotation of the innominate occurs (this is the limit of functional hip extension), and the presence of increased muscle activity/tone at the point of changed femoral head position or early end of range of motion. (H) Some meaningful tasks require analysis of full hip extension range of motion; this is accomplished by moving the patient to the side of the bed or to the end of the bed. This position allows easy testing of combined extension and adduction/abduction, internal/external rotation.

the limit of functional flexion of the hip joint. Next, note the position of the femoral head during this test. If the femoral head displaces anteriorly at any point during this test, note the range of motion at which this occurs; at that point in range, stop and palpate all of the muscles of the thigh and posterior buttock (rectus femoris, TFL, sartorius, adductors, quadratus femoris, gluts, piriformis, obturator externus, psoas, etc.), and note the presence of any increase in muscle activity or hypertonicity that correlates with the change in femoral head position (note that there is often more than one muscle creating the net non-optimal force vector) (Fig. 8.75D).

If free, non-resistant flexion is available, test internal and external rotation (Fig. 8.75E,F), feeling again for any increase in muscle tone/activity and non-optimal force vectors. Return to palpate the femoral head and innominate and passively extend the femur until anterior rotation of the ipsilateral innominate begins (Fig. 8.75G). Note the response of the femoral head during this test. If the femoral head displaces anteriorly at any point during this test, stop and palpate all of the muscles of the thigh and note the presence of any increase in muscle tone/activity (there is often more than one muscle creating the non-optimal force vectors). In order to test the full range of extension, the patient will need to be moved to the edge of the table or down the table (Fig. 8.75H), and the same analysis performed at the point where the femoral head axis changes.

Passive abduction/adduction can also be tested in varying degrees of flexion/extension. The functional range of motion is reached when the pelvic girdle bends laterally beneath the vertebral column. Test the hip in a variety of combined movements (flexion/adduction/internal rotation, extension/abduction/external rotation, etc.) to determine:

1. the combinations of movements that yield the greatest resistance; and
2. the most active and persistent force vectors and the muscles/myofascia creating them.

The hip: integrity of the articular system restraints

The following tests assess the integrity of the articular system restraints of the hip joint (i.e. the passive system). The intent is to stress all of the capsule and ligaments simultaneously. If the test is painless, then the subsequent tests, which help to differentiate the individual ligaments, are not required. Pay particular attention to the end feel of the combined movements

(should be firm) as well as to the provocation of any pain.

With the patient supine, lying close to the edge of the table, the ipsilateral femur is extended until anterior rotation of the innominate begins. The femur is then rotated medially to the limit of the physiological range of motion. The proximal thigh is palpated and a slow, steady, posterolateral force is applied along the line of the neck of the femur to stress the capsule and ligaments further (Fig. 8.76). No movement should occur when the articular system restraints are intact and no pain should be provoked.

Inferior band of the iliofemoral ligament. This ligament is taut when the femur is fully extended. If passive femoral extension elicits the greatest amount of pain, this ligament may be a nociceptive source.

Iliotrochanteric band of the iliofemoral ligament. With the patient supine, lying close to the edge of the table, the ipsilateral femur is slightly extended, *adducted*, and fully rotated laterally. The distal femur is fixed against the therapist's thigh and the proximal femur is palpated. A slow, steady distraction force is applied along the line of the neck of the femur and the provocation of local pain is noted.

Pubofemoral ligament. With the patient lying supine, the ipsilateral femur is slightly extended, *abducted*, and fully rotated laterally. The distal femur is fixed against the therapist's thigh and the proximal femur is palpated. A slow, steady distraction force is applied along the line of the neck of the femur and the provocation of local pain is noted.

Ischiofemoral ligament. This ligament primarily limits internal rotation as well as adduction of the

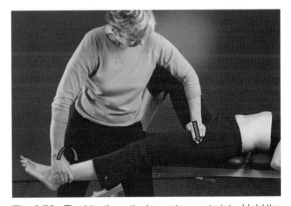

Fig. 8.76 • The hip: the articular system restraints. Hold the femur extended and medially rotated (left arrow) and apply a posterolateral distractive force to the proximal femur (right arrow). No movement should occur and no pain should be provoked.

flexed hip (Hewitt et al 2002). With the patient lying supine, the ipsilateral femur is flexed, adducted, and fully rotated *medially*. A slow, steady distraction force is applied along the line of the neck of the femur and the provocation of local pain is noted. This position can also create anterior impingement so noting the location of the pain is critical for differentiation.

The hip: impact of the myofascial and neural systems on the hip joint

If the muscles primarily responsible for controlling motion of the femoral head are functioning well, the femoral head should remain centered or seated during all loading tasks. This requires optimal functioning of the myofascial and neural systems for the hip. Assessing the patient's automatic strategy (task analysis) for controlling load through the hip at specific points in the range of motion can provide additional information for clinical reasoning and treatment. With the patient supine, position the femur passively such that the femoral head is centered in the acetabulum, fully supporting the weight of the leg. Continue to monitor the femoral head position and instruct the patient to hold the position of the leg as you remove your support. Note any displacement of the femoral head. This test can be done in a variety of positions and in all of them the femoral head should remain centered. If there is loss of femoral head centering, further tests are used to determine the underlying impairments (neural, myofascial, and/or articular systems).

If the underlying impairment(s) are in the neural or myofascial systems, the effectiveness of restoring these systems during the treatment process can be evaluated as follows. Position and support the hip in the range of motion where loss of control was identified. While palpating the femoral head, ask the patient to perform a contraction of the deep muscles of the LPH complex (determined by specific assessment, see below; training techniques are covered in Chapter 11). Remove support of the leg and note the impact of this pre-contraction on the control of the femoral head; if the myofascial and neural systems are being effectively restored the femoral head will now remain centered. Furthermore, if a passive system deficit has been identified (joint laxity), the effectiveness of the myofascial and neural systems to compensate for the passive impairment is evaluated by repeating the positive articular system restraints test *while* the patient holds their deep muscle system contraction. If the

myofascial and neural systems are functioning well, there will be no motion of the femur when the test is repeated with a contraction.

Clinical reflection time

At this point in the examination considerable information has been gained with respect to the articular system and all joints that potentially require mobilization and/or have impairments of their passive restraints should now be listed in the articular piece of the Clinical Puzzle. In addition, hypertonicity in specific muscles that are preventing full assessment of articular status, as well as impacting joint motion, will have been identified. These muscles are listed in the neural piece of the Clinical Puzzle along with the joint with which they are associated. What is not yet known is the status of the myofascial system (linea alba and endopelvic fascia) and the neural system (motor control of the deep and superficial muscles of the abdominal canister specifically pertaining to the sequencing and timing of activation), and the contribution of these systems to the non-optimal strategy noted during meaningful task analysis.

The abdominal canister

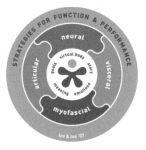

Function can be significantly compromised when a joint's motion is not controlled through its full range. In the joint's neutral zone, the passive system cannot contribute to motion control and it is the responsibility of the control system to provide strategies that prevent buckling of the 85 joints in the abdominal canister (see Fig. 4.34) while allowing the required movements during a multitude of tasks of varying loads, mobility, predictability, and perceived risk (Chapter 4) (see Figs 4.35, 8.1). This next section will cover the assessment tests and clinical reasoning for the myofascial and neural systems of the Clinical Puzzle. These tests are required if, during any task, the strategy used results in loss of motion control and failed load transfer at any of the joints of the abdominal canister and if either:

1. the articular system tests (previously covered under regional tests) are negative; or
2. the articular system tests are positive and suggestive of a lax joint and consideration is being given to the effect of training to restore control.

Clinical reasoning of the findings from multiple tests is necessary to understand the significance of the results of each individual test as it pertains to the hypothesis generated and this will be covered, in part, in this chapter and then in further detail through the case reports in Chapter 9.

In health, the deep muscles should co-contract in response to a command that begins with intention. This system is preparatory (Chapter 4) and should respond prior to the activation of the superficial muscles, especially in conditions where the task is predictable. Therefore, imagining or thinking about (preparing), but not actually doing, a movement appears to be a more effective way of accessing the appropriate neural pathways to the deep muscles. To our knowledge, there are no studies that have investigated the use of imagery such as 'imagine a guy wire connecting the ASISs' versus 'doing commands' such as 'hollow your abdomen or draw your navel to your spine' for their efficacy in isolating responses from the deep muscles of the abdominal canister. Clinical expertise suggests that the cues given by the clinician can significantly impact the response of the deep and superficial muscles and that the imagery cues suggested below are more effective in isolating a deep response than 'doing' commands.

Abdominal wall – palpation

In order to clinically analyze the response of transversus abdominis (TrA) to a verbal cue or command, it must be palpated or observed via ultrasound imaging. A common mistake seen when teaching clinicians to assess this muscle is the failure to reach the appropriate depth in the abdomen before beginning the assessment. If the clinician is palpating the abdomen at the depth of the internal oblique (IO), the underlying response of TrA is often missed. If the external oblique (EO) is hypertonic, the tension of its fascia (which overlays TrA) will often prevent the clinician from being able to reach the layer of TrA and this very common substitution strategy can be misinterpreted as a contraction of TrA. Therefore, assessment

of the abdominal wall begins with palpation and observation of each layer (layer palpation).

With the patient in supine or crook lying (knees supported over a bolster), palpate the superficial fascial layer of the lower abdomen below the level of the umbilicus to the PS. The skin should move freely in all directions; note the presence of any surgical scars and the mobility of the skin and the superficial fascia. With both thumbs, palpate the abdomen approximately 7cm (2.5in) medial to and slightly inferior to the ASIS, and slowly press through the superficial fatty layer to reach the fascia of the EO (Fig. 8.77). Gently press into this layer and note the presence and symmetry of any tension (gently spring the fascia of the EO and compare the left and right sides for symmetry). Next, observe if it is easy to pass through the EO fascia to reach the layer of the IO (Fig. 8.78). The IO is quite muscular here and feels like a moist sponge cake. Explore the tone of the IO layer, as well

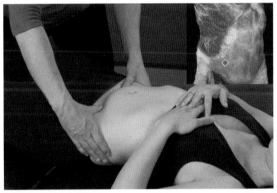

Fig. 8.77 • Abdominal palpation: external oblique (EO). Note the depth of the therapist's thumbs in this illustration as well as the fascia of the EO in the anatomical inset. At this depth, no activation of transversus abdominis (TrA) can be felt and this is a common mistake when assessing the response of TrA to verbal cuing. When the EO contracts, a superficial tension of its fascia will be felt and it is important not to mistake this for a contraction of TrA. If you do not have access to ultrasound imaging, this substitution strategy can be determined as follows. When the patient is relaxed, perform a 'ribcage wiggle' by gently translating the lower ribcage to the left and right. Give the patient the cue to contract and, if you feel tension in response to your cue that you believe is TrA, repeat the ribcage wiggle while the contraction is held. If the EO has contracted, the ribcage will be restricted, but if TrA did indeed contract, the ribcage will remain free to move. Anatomical picture reproduced with permission from Acland and the publisher Lippincott Williams & Wilkins, 2004.

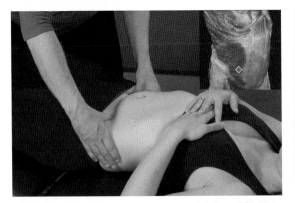

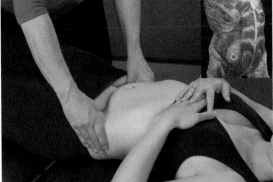

Fig. 8.78 • Abdominal palpation: internal oblique (IO). Note the increased depth of palpation of the therapist's thumbs compared to the depth for palpation of the external oblique. At this depth, activation of the IO is easily felt; however, any prior recruitment of the transversus abdominis (TrA) may be missed. Because the IO is muscular here (see inset), its activation will cause a broadening of the muscle that will be felt as a bulge or pressure that pushes the thumbs out of the abdomen. It is very common for an IO contraction to be mistaken for a proper TrA contraction, because it is easy to feel, especially when patients think they have to 'really feel the contraction' with their fingers. An isolated TrA contraction is much more subtle and generally patients are less able to feel it; therefore we use other 'self-tests' for patients to check if they are doing the correct or incorrect training (see Chapter 10). Anatomical picture reproduced with permission from Acland and the publisher Lippincott Williams & Wilkins, 2004.

Fig. 8.79 • Abdominal palpation: transversus abdominis (TrA). Note the increased depth of palpation required to assess transversus abdominis compared to the internal oblique and external oblique. Once the appropriate depth is reached, the thumbs are gently drawn apart (adducted) until a line of tension is felt (take up the slack in the fascial system). When the TrA contracts it will be immediately felt in the tensed fascia, and the fingers will be taken along the 'fascial ride,' which is felt as a drawing of the thumbs laterally and into the abdominal wall (see inset). Anatomical picture reproduced with permission from Acland and the publisher Lippincott Williams & Wilkins, 2004.

as the ability to pass through this layer to reach the fascia that separates it from TrA. Compare the left and right sides. A hypertonic IO will feel firm and more resistant to your thumb (stale sponge cake or full balloon) and will not allow you to pass easily through the muscle to the layer of the TrA. At this level of the abdomen, the most posterior part of the IO layer is the fascia of TrA (Fig. 8.79). Once you reach this layer (take care not to go any deeper into the peritoneum), apply gentle tension to the TrA fascia by adducting your thumbs (draw the TrA fascia laterally). You should be able to feel a linear tension force between your thumbs that makes a shallow 'v' parallel to the line of the inguinal ligaments. All of the slack has now been taken up in the fascia of TrA and the linea alba and you are ready to assess the response of this deep muscle to a verbal cue/command.

In a healthy system, TrA is known to co-contract with the pelvic floor (Chapter 4) and evaluation of

this co-contraction begins with a cue that involves the pelvic floor. One of the following three cues should evoke a symmetrical, equally timed response of TrA:

1. 'Slowly and gently squeeze the muscles around your urethra as if to stop your urine flow.'
2. 'Slowly and gently draw your vagina (or testicles) up into your body.'
3. 'Imagine there is a wire connecting your anus to the back of your pubic bone. Slowly and gently connect along this line and think about drawing your anus up and forward.'

When TrA co-contracts with the pelvic floor in response to any of these cues, a deep, light tension will be felt in the TrA fascia and the abdomen will hollow drawing the thumbs inward and lateral. No movement of the thorax, lumbar spine, or pelvic girdle should occur. In our experience, asking the patient to hollow the abdomen is less effective than the previous cues for eliciting an isolated deep muscle co-contraction response. If there is no response of TrA to any of these three cues try the following abdominal cues:

1. 'Imagine there is a wire connecting your hip bones anteriorly [ASISs] from the left to right side.

Think about generating a force which would draw these two bones together.'

2. Alternately, cue the patient to 'imagine there is a wire connecting your hip bones anteriorly [ASISs] from the left to right side and think about drawing the two bones *apart*.'

3. 'Feel my fingers in your abdomen and the tension they create in your tissue. Connect to my fingers and try to create the same tension that draws your stomach in and out.'

Abnormal responses include an:

1. absent response of TrA to any cue given; or
2. asymmetrical response of the left and right TrA.

Common non-optimal responses include:

1. activation of EO, which is felt as tensioning of the superficial fascia of the abdominal wall (Fig. 8.80A). Ultrasound imaging can be used to confirm that the tension felt is not coming from TrA (Fig. 8.80B);

2. activation of IO without an earlier contraction of TrA. This will feel like a muscular broadening or bulge, which pushes your thumbs out of the abdomen and is a normal response IF TrA activated first (deep tension with lateral draw felt first) (Fig. 8.80C). If you are not at the right depth to feel TrA or if the contraction happens too quickly you may miss the earlier activation; this is where ultrasound imaging is helpful (see below);

3. coactivation of both TrA and IO together. This is often missed as once the IO contracts it is not possible to feel what TrA is doing. Once again, this is where ultrasound imaging is helpful.

Abdominal wall – ultrasound imaging

Ultrasound imaging is a safe, invaluable method for observing and measuring the deep muscles of the trunk that are not otherwise easily assessed. When a clinical reasoning process is used to analyze the findings from the ASLR test, abdominal wall palpation tests, and the ultrasound imaging tests, decisions regarding both the myofascial and neural systems of the Clinical Puzzle are enhanced. Almost all of the ultrasound images and video clips presented in this edition are oriented according to imaging convention. In other words, the images are such that the patient's right side is on the left side of the image (mirror image). This is a change from the third edition and is consistent with conventional imaging protocols. The new images and video clips in this current edition were collected using the MyLab25 (Biosound Esaote) (Fig. 8.81A).

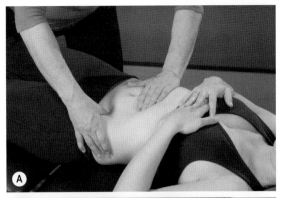

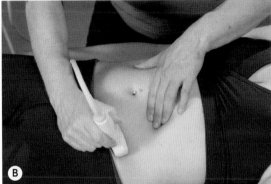

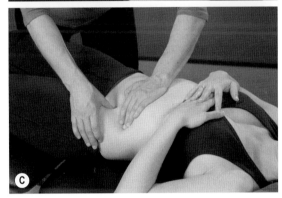

Fig. 8.80 • Abdominal palpation: non-optimal responses for the transversus abdominis (TrA). (A) When the external oblique (EO) activates instead of TrA, a superficial tensioning of the EO fascia can be felt and narrowing of the infrasternal angle can be seen. The contraction can also be felt along the costal margins of the rib cage. In addition, activation of EO will render the rib cage rigid and resistant to mediolateral motion (decreased ribcage wiggle). (B) If fascial tension is felt in both the anterolateral aspect of the lower and upper abdominal wall, ultrasound can help to differentiate whether the activation is coming from TrA or EO. This figure illustrates the probe placement and palpation for this test. (C) If a distinct muscular bulge is felt during palpation for TrA activation, confirm that this is the internal oblique (IO) by ultrasound imaging or by palpating the vertical fibers of the IO as illustrated here.

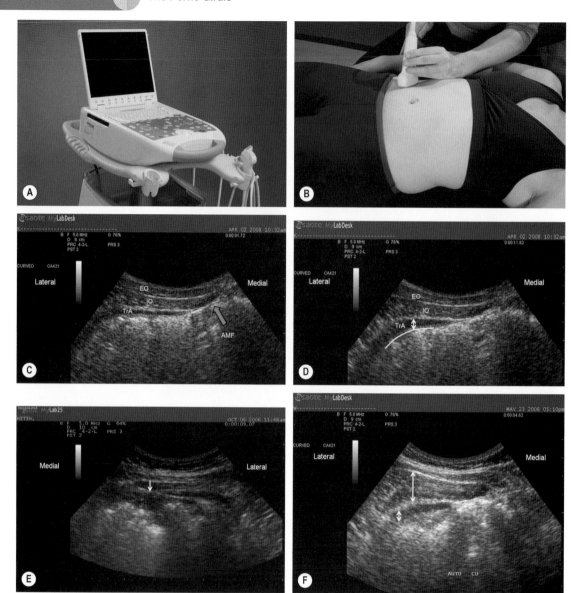

Fig. 8.81 • Ultrasound imaging: anterolateral abdominal wall. (A) The MyLab25 ultrasound imaging unit used to collect the new ultrasound images and video clips in this text (Biosound Esaote). (B) Probe placement for imaging transversus abdominis. The exact location of the probe needs to be manipulated according to what is seen on the ultrasound screen. For conventional imaging, the marker on the probe is oriented to the patient's right and the image captured is a mirror image of the abdomen such that the right transversus abdominis (TrA) is on the left side of the ultrasound screen. (C) Ultrasound image of the right anterolateral abdominal wall at rest. AMF, anterior midline fascia. (D) Ultrasound image showing an optimal isolated contraction of the right TrA. Note the broadening as well as the lateral slide of TrA beneath the internal oblique (IO) as well as the corseting of the muscle (curved line). Note the tapering of the medial aspect of both the IO and the TrA. The optimal response can be seen on Video 8.2 🖱. (E) When the IO contracts before TrA (with or without an associated TrA contraction) it appears to broaden into the relatively slack TrA fascia creating a bulbous medial aspect. Alternately, IO can slide laterally over the TrA. This can be seen on Video 8.3a,b 🖱. (F) Ultrasound image of the right abdominal muscles during a curl-up task. Note the coactivation of both TrA and IO in this image. This optimal response can be seen on Video 8.4a 🖱. A non-optimal response can be seen on Video 8.4b 🖱. Watch how the deep system 'shuts off' and appears to slide medially beneath the IO during this curl-up task. Now watch Video 8.4c 🖱. In this clip, the TrA never contracts and IO slides laterally over the top of it during this curl-up task.

Continued

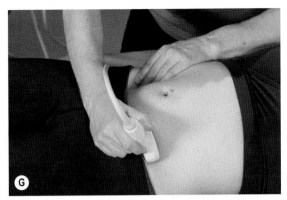

Fig. 8.81 – cont'd • (G) Ultrasound imaging and palpation can be used in combination to watch one side of the abdominal wall and the feel the other. This test provides information on the symmetry of activation of the left and right sides.

With the patient in crook lying, knees supported over a bolster, expose the abdomen from the xyphoid to the PS. Using a 5MHz curvilinear probe, place the well-gelled ultrasound transducer transversely on the anterolateral aspect of the abdomen with the transducer marker oriented to the patient's right side (Fig. 8.81B). Vary the angle and location of the transducer until there is a clear transverse image of the TrA, IO, and EO, and in particular be sure to include the most medial aspect of TrA where it blends with the anterior midline fascia (Fig. 8.81C). The depth control and gain can be adjusted so that the muscle layers are more easily observed; be sure to adjust the focus to the layers of interest.

Prior to assessing the response of the abdominals to verbal cuing, note any movement of the muscles during quiet breathing. Activity of the TrA should be minimal during quiet breathing (Hodges & Gandevia 2000a); however, when there is an increase in the chemical drive (increased carbon dioxide levels) or mechanical drive (articular or myofascial restrictions in the thorax), TrA is the first abdominal muscle recruited to assist expiration. Hypertonicity of TrA can also be observed at this time (the muscle will appear to be contracted).

Subsequently, observe the response of the abdominal muscles to the following cues:

1. 'Slowly and gently squeeze the muscles around your urethra as if to stop your urine flow.'
2. 'Slowly and gently draw your vagina (or testicles) up into your body.'
3. 'Imagine there is a wire connecting your anus to the back of your pubic bone. Slowly and gently connect along this line and think about drawing your anus up and forward.'
4. 'Imagine there is a wire connecting your hip bones anteriorly [ASISs] from the left to right side. Think about generating a force which would draw these two bones together.'
5. 'Imagine there is a wire connecting your hip bones anteriorly [ASISs] from the left to right side and think about drawing the two bones apart.'

Optimally, the TrA will slide laterally beneath the IO, broadening and corseting around the trunk (Fig. 8.81D, Video 8.2 🖱) before any broading of the IO is seen. Ideally one hand is used to palpate the same side that you are imaging; note whether or not you feel an IO bulge before you see TrA contract on the ultrasound image. In some patients, palpation will identify IO contraction sooner than it is seen on the ultrasound as there is a minimum threshold of EMG activity in the abdominal muscles for architectural change on ultrasound to occur. As the patient increases the level of contraction (more effort), the IO should contract and will be seen to broaden. The shape of the medial aspect of both the TrA and IO is interesting to note. When TrA contracts first, it appears to tense the anterior midline fascia such that when the IO contracts both muscles appear to taper medially. When the IO contracts first (with (Fig. 8.81E, Video 8.3a 🖱) or without an associated TrA contraction), it appears to broaden into the relatively slack TrA fascia creating a bulbous medial aspect. It can also appear to slide laterally over the top of the TrA, instead of TrA sliding underneath the IO (Video 8.3b 🖱).

Subsequently, note the response of the abdominal wall during a head and neck curl-up. This task will require all of the muscles of the abdominal wall to coactivate, and therefore activation of TrA during this task is difficult to assess via direct palpation. It is easily observed via ultrasound imaging (Fig. 8.81F, Video 8.4a,b,c 🖱).

Ultrasound imaging provides information on the response of the deep muscles to a verbal cue; however, it cannot discern whether the activation is symmetrical as only one muscle is being observed. Palpation of one TrA while imaging the other can add further information to the bilateral palpation tests described above (Fig. 8.81G).

Clinical reasoning

Training the anterior abdominal wall (restoring an optimal activation response) is indicated if the ASLR test improves with anterior compression or an oblique compression of the pelvic girdle *and* if on palpation and ultrasound imaging deficits in the response of the abdominal wall (including TrA, IO, and EO) are noted. When no response of TrA is palpable and yet on ultrasound imaging an optimal response is noted, an assessment of the midline anterior abdominal fascia (myofascial system) is indicated before it is possible to predict if training is able to restore function.

Midline anterior abdominal fascia – palpation

According to Rath et al (1996), the inter-recti distance halfway between the PS and umbilicus should measure no more than 0.9cm, 2.7cm just above the umbilicus and 1.0cm halfway between the umbilicus and the xyphoid (in the under 45 years age group). The inter-recti distance can be reliably measured using dial calipers (Boxer & Jones 1997) or ultrasound imaging (Coldron et al 2008), and in a recent pilot study it was noted that several healthy nulliparous women, as well as men, had inter-recti distances larger than these measures (Lee D, unpublished). Clinically, it appears that the inter-recti distance is less relevant to a patient's recovery than the ability of the deep muscles to generate tension through the midline abdominal fascia (Chapter 6 and see case reports Christy & Melissa, Chapter 9 🖱). The following tests examine the integrity of the linea alba and its ability to transfer

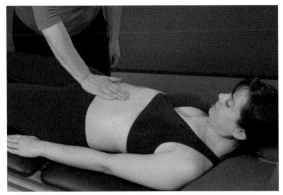

Fig. 8.82 • Abdominal palpation: midline anterior abdominal fascia. The linea alba should transfer forces between the left and right rectus abdominis (RA) during a head and neck curl-up task. Consequently, increased tension of the linea alba should be felt with minimal, if any, separation of the left and right RA.

the forces produced by the abdominal wall and thus force close the joints of the lumbar spine and pelvic girdle.

With the patient in crook lying, palpate the linea alba in the midline from the xyphoid to the pubic symphysis. Note the presence or absence of fascial tension in this rest position. Instruct the patient to do a slow head and neck curl-up and palpate the response of the linea alba (Fig. 8.82). Does it widen, narrow, or remain the same? Does the tension change in the linea alba during the curl-up (decrease or increase)? Is there any invagination or protrusion of the abdomen in the midline during this task (Fig. 8.83A,B). Explore the entire length of the linea alba and note the changes throughout its length during the curl-up task.

Midline anterior abdominal fascia – ultrasound imaging

With the patient in crook lying, knees supported over a bolster, expose the abdomen from the xyphoid to the PS. Using a 10–12MHz linear probe, place the well-gelled transducer over the midline anterior abdominal fascia (Fig. 8.84A). The level of the abdomen imaged depends on the palpation findings; choose the level where the least tension is felt during the curl-up task. Manipulate the angle until there is a clear image of the medial edge of the left and right RA and the intervening linea alba (Fig. 8.84B). Note the echogenicity of the linea alba at rest, the

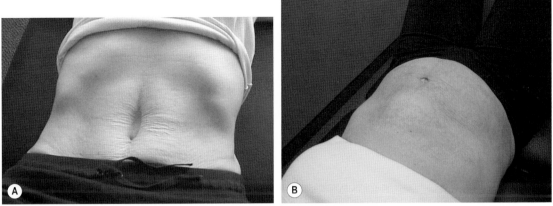

Fig. 8.83 • Abdominal palpation: midline anterior abdominal fascia, linea alba. (A) This patient has a diastasis rectus abdominis and during a head and neck curl-up the linea alba invaginates into the abdominal cavity. It is a reflection of the strategy she is using to perform this task. Note the widening of the lower rib cage. (B) This patient also has a diastasis rectus abdominis and during a head and neck curl-up the linea alba protrudes out of the abdominal cavity. Note the doming of the midline abdomen. Again, this reflects the strategy she is using to perform the curl-up task.

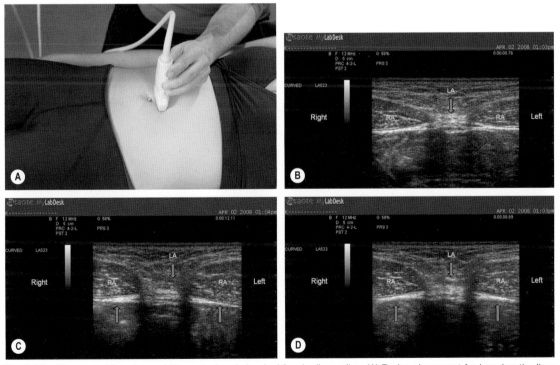

Fig. 8.84 • Ultrasound imaging: midline anterior abdominal fascia, linea alba. (A) Probe placement for imaging the linea alba just above the umbilicus. (B) Ultrasound image of the linea alba (LA) and medial aspect of the left and right rectus abdominis (RA) at rest. (C) Ultrasound image of the linea alba during a curl-up task (no pre-cuing yet an automatic recruitment of TrA occurred). Note the echogenicity of the posterior rectus sheaths (upward arrows) and the continuity of this force through the linea alba. (D) Ultrasound image of the linea alba during a curl-up task with a cue to pre-contract the deep muscles. Note the change in angle of the fascia under RA. On Video 8.5a,b 🖱 the first curl-up is automatic; the subject then precontracts the deep muscles (note the lateral pull through the left and right RA) prior to performing the second curl-up.

inter-recti distance, and the breadth or width of the left and right RA. The inter-recti distance and the width of the recti can be measured using the internal measurement system of the ultrasound unit during all of these tasks.

Note the changes in the linea alba during the following tasks:

1. Head and neck curl-up task with no cue to pre-contract the deep muscles. The inter-recti distance may increase or decrease; this appears to depend on the abdominal level, the strategy used for this task, and the laxity/integrity of the linea alba. A key change to note is the echogenicity of the linea alba, which should increase (i.e. the white line should get brighter or maintain the same brightness); notice also any change in shape of both the RA and the linea alba (Fig. 8.84C, first part of Video 8.5a,b 🖱).

2. Cue a contraction of the deep muscles and have the patient maintain this co-contraction while performing the head and neck curl-up task. The posterior fascia of the rectus sheaths as well as the linea alba can be seen to 'brighten' and there is an observable lateral force from the left and right sides during the pre-contraction phase of this task (Fig. 8.84D, second part of Video 8.5a,b 🖱). The tension of the healthy linea alba appears to increase as this lateral force occurs. Note any difference in the echogenicity of the linea alba, the inter-recti distance, and the shape of the linea alba between these two tasks. Video 8.5b is of the linea alba of a postpartum woman during a head and neck curl-up task. She does not automatically pre-contract the deep system during this task and when cued to do so the difference in the shape and width of the linea alba is easily seen. Without a pre-contraction of the deep system, the linea alba appears to sag between the left and right RA (first part of the clip). When she pre-contracts the deep system, the sagging is no longer evident (second part of the clip). There is a clear difference in what appears to be the ability to generate tension in the linea alba between the two strategies. She also notes a significant difference in the effort to perform the task; more effort is required without the pre-contraction of the deep system.

Move the probe to either the left or right RA and repeat both tasks 1 and 2 above (Fig. 8.85A–D, Video 8.6 🖱). When the deep muscles are functioning

optimally, minimal difference will be noted in the width of RA, as in a healthy system a pre-contraction of the deep muscles will occur automatically without cuing. When there is a delay or absence of activation of TrA, the width or broadening of RA appears to increase significantly during this task; an asymmetrical recruitment of TrA causes asymmetry in the width of the two recti. With a symmetrical pre-contraction of TrA, the broadening of the recti is symmetrically reduced. The hypothesis is that TrA tenses the posterior fascia of the rectus sheaths as well as the intermediate zone of transverse fibrils of the linea alba (Fig. 3.45) and limits the broadening of the RA. Theoretically, this would allow for more force to be transferred through the fascial system when RA contracts in a pretensed container. Examples of ultrasound images seen in patients with diastasis rectus abdominis can be seen in Chapter 6 (see Video 6.2 🖱) and Chapter 9 (see case reports Christy & Melissa, Chapter 9 🖱).

The last thing to observe with ultrasound imaging is the ability of the left and right TrA to increase tension in the midline structures. Begin by applying ample ultrasound gel to the patient's abdomen from left to right side at the level to be imaged. Start on the right side and image TrA. Cue the patient to activate the deep system with whatever cue you have found is most effective for them (i.e. connect), and observe the response. If the response is optimal, move the location of the transducer to the right RA and repeat the cue to connect and observe the response in the right RA and the related fascia. Move the transducer to the linea alba and repeat the cue to connect, then image the left RA and related fascia, and then finally move the transducer to the left TrA. Optimally, a contraction of the left and right TrA can be seen to increase tension along the entire length of the fascia to and across the midline even when there is a separation of the recti (Video 8.7 🖱). We consider this to be a 'functional diastasis rectus abdominis.'

Clinical reasoning

If the midline abdominal fascia is able to generate sufficient tension to control the joints of the low thorax, lumbar spine, and pelvic girdle through the contraction of the deep muscles, then training will likely be effective for restoring function. If, however, the fascia is not able to generate sufficient tension, training will not be effective and surgery to restore the anatomical integrity of the midline anterior

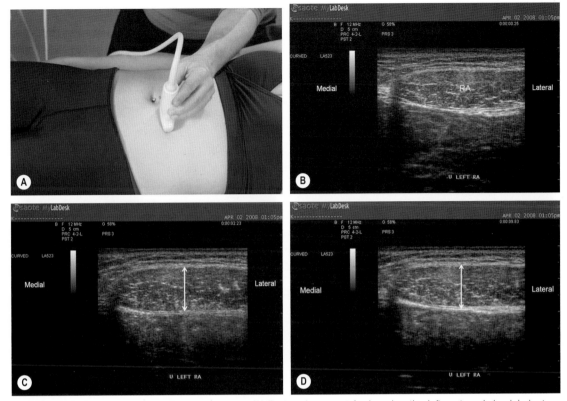

Fig. 8.85 • Ultrasound imaging: rectus abdominis. (A) Probe placement for imaging the left rectus abdominis just above the umbilicus. (B) Ultrasound image of the left rectus abdominis at rest. (C) Ultrasound image of the left rectus abdominis during a curl-up task (no pre-cuing). Note the broadening of rectus abdominis. (D) Ultrasound image of the left rectus abdominis during a curl-up task with a cue to pre-contract the deep muscles. Note that there is very little difference in the shape of rectus abdominis in either (C) or (D) or any difference in the amplitude of the broadening as the deep system is functioning optimally and is automatically recruited during the curl-up task with or without cuing. Watch Video 8.6 to see this in action. In a functional abdominal wall a co-contraction of the left and right transversus abdominis will tense the fascial envelope of the left and right rectus abdominis as well as the linea alba even when there is a diastasis of the recti, and this can be seen via ultrasound imaging (Video 8.7).

abdominal fascia is indicated (see case reports Christy & Melissa, Chapter 9 and Video 6.2).

The pelvic floor – ultrasound imaging

A specific examination of the pelvic floor is indicated if the patient presents with urinary incontinence (Chapter 6), prolapse, pelvic floor/perineal pain, or a sensation of pressure on the pelvic floor, or if no response is elicited in TrA when a cue is given to contract the pelvic floor. The pelvic floor is a critical part of the abdominal canister (Chapter 4), and should not be ignored by orthopedic clinicians. Similarly, it is only one part of the abdominal canister and pelvic floor therapists need to consider the other components when working with patients with either incontinence or lumbopelvic pain (Lee 2004, Lee & Lee 2004b, Lee et al 2008a). The pelvic floor is assessed either internally or by ultrasound imaging, but preferably both. As neither author (DL or LJL) is a certified pelvic floor therapist, the specifics of assessing the pelvic floor internally will not be covered here. Both authors regularly use ultrasound imaging to view the function of the pelvic floor and refer to a certified pelvic floor therapist when indicated. Once again, this highlights the need for multidisciplinary and interdisciplinary teams.

The endopelvic fascia and the muscles of the pelvic floor can be assessed with 2D ultrasound imaging from either an abdominal or perineal approach. Different information is gained from each view of the pelvic floor. To image the bladder, it must be moderately, but not completely, full. Instruct the patient to void and then drink 500mL of fluid 1 hour before the examination. This will standardize the amount of fluid in the bladder for subsequent examinations.

The pelvic floor – ultrasound imaging: transverse abdominal approach. This approach is valuable for assessing symmetry of activation of the left and right sides of the pelvic floor as the response of both sides can be seen simultaneously. The disadvantage of this view is that there is not a bony landmark to measure motion against and therefore the absolute direction of motion is indeterminate.

With the patient in crook lying, knees supported over a bolster, expose the abdomen from the xyphoid to the PS. Using a 3.5MHz curvilinear well-gelled probe, orient the ultrasound transducer (marker to the patient's right) transversely across the midline just superior to the PS and vary the angle until there is a clear image of the urinary bladder (Fig. 8.86A,B). Adjust the depth control so that a complete image of the bladder is on the screen and adjust the focus to the level of the endopelvic fascia. Note the shape/profile of the resting bladder and then observe the response of the endopelvic fascia as well as the bladder to the following cues:

1. 'Slowly and gently squeeze the muscles around your urethra as if to stop your urine flow.'
2. 'Slowly and gently draw your vagina (or testicles) up into your body.'
3. 'Imagine there is a wire connecting your anus to the back of your pubic bone. Slowly and gently connect along this line and think about drawing your anus up and forward.'

Optimally, the endopelvic fascia will tense as the pelvic floor muscles contract and the result is a net vector that results in a midline lift of the bladder (Fig. 8.86C, Video 8.8 🖱). Note:

1. the change in the shape/profile of the bladder (the presence or absence of any lift and its location (midline, left, or right), or any deformation of the bladder); and
2. any apparent descent of the bladder. A true determination of bladder descent cannot be made from this approach as many factors can make the bladder appear to descend on the ultrasound screen. Bladder descent is best imaged with the perineal approach;
3. note the sustainability of the contraction (watch for fatigue and a slow letting go of the lift; this is suggestive of an endurance deficit of the pelvic floor).

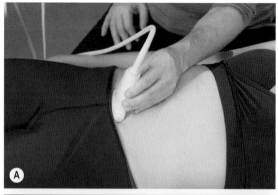

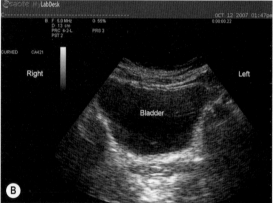

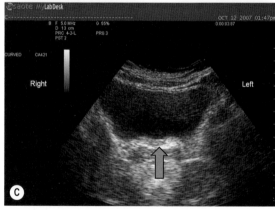

Fig. 8.86 • The pelvic floor – ultrasound imaging: transverse abdominal approach. (A) Probe placement for imaging the bladder and pelvic floor in the transverse abdominal view. (B) Ultrasound image of the bladder prior to a cue to contract the pelvic floor. (C) Ultrasound image of the same bladder during a cue to contract the pelvic floor. Note the indenting of the bladder at the inferior aspect of this image (arrow). This is an optimal response and can be seen on Video 8.8 🖱.

The pelvic floor – ultrasound imaging: parasagittal abdominal approach. The benefit of this approach is that the left and right sides of the pelvic floor can be imaged separately to confirm/negate the impressions from the transverse view. There is still the disadvantage of not having a bony landmark to measure motion against, thus the need for the perineal view.

With the patient in crook lying, knees supported over a bolster, expose the abdomen from the xyphoid to the PS. Using a 3.5MHz curvilinear well-gelled probe, orient the ultrasound transducer (marker to the patient's head) in the midline sagittal plane just superior to the PS and then to the left and right of midline (orient the probe from superolateral to inferomedial when not in the midline (parasagittal)) (Fig. 8.87A). Vary the angle until there is a clear image of the urinary bladder and the urethrovesical neck (Fig. 8.87B). Adjust the depth control so that a complete image of the bladder is on the screen and adjust the focus to the level of the endopelvic fascia. Note the shape/profile of the resting bladder and then observe the response of the endopelvic fascia as well as the bladder to the following cues:

1. 'Slowly and gently squeeze the muscles around your urethra as if to stop your urine flow.'
2. 'Slowly and gently draw your vagina (or testicles) up into your body.'
3. 'Imagine there is a wire connecting your anus to the back of your pubic bone. Slowly and gently connect along this line and think about drawing your anus up and forward.'

Optimally, the endopelvic fascia will tense as the pelvic floor muscles contract and the result is a net vector that results in a lift of the bladder (Fig. 8.87C, Video 8.9). Note:

1. the change in the shape/profile of the bladder (the presence or absence of any lift and its location relative to the bladder and neck of the urethra, any deformation of the bladder); and
2. any apparent descent of the bladder. A true determination of bladder descent cannot be made from this approach as many factors can make the bladder appear to descend on the ultrasound screen. Bladder descent is best imaged with the perineal approach;
3. the sustainability of the contraction (watch for fatigue and a slow letting go of the lift; this is suggestive of an endurance deficit of the pelvic floor).

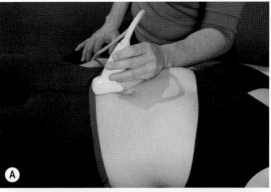

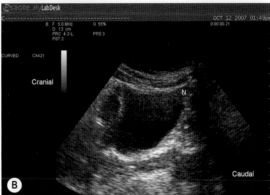

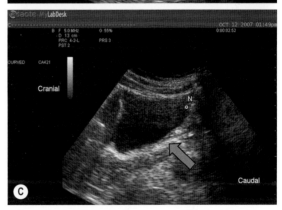

Fig. 8.87 • The pelvic floor – ultrasound imaging: parasagittal abdominal approach. (A) Probe placement for imaging the bladder and pelvic floor in the parasagittal abdominal view. (B) Ultrasound image of the bladder in the parasagittal view prior to a cue to contract the pelvic floor. N, neck of the bladder. (C) Ultrasound image of the same bladder during a cue to contract the pelvic floor. Note the lift of the bladder (arrow) that occurs during this contraction. This is an optimal response and can be seen on Video 8.9 .

The pelvic floor – ultrasound imaging: perineal approach. This approach to imaging the pelvic floor and the organs of the pelvis yields the greatest amount of information and is always indicated when treating women with pelvic organ prolapse with or without urinary incontinence. The responses of the bladder, the neck of the urethra, and the anorectal angle are easily seen during multiple tasks in both the supine and standing positions. The authors wish to acknowledge the research (Peng et al 2006, 2007), clinical expertise, and personal clinical instruction of Ruth Jones (Lovegrove) (PT, PhD, Stanford University) who not only taught us how to image the pelvic floor properly with this approach but also provided ongoing mentorship as we learned to interpret the clinical findings.

With the patient in crook lying, hips and knees flexed, the perineum is exposed and the patient draped for comfort. To facilitate interpretation, invert the image on the ultrasound screen. A 3.5MHz curvilinear probe is prepared for imaging by applying gel to the surface of the probe and then covering the probe with a powder-free glove (Fig. 8.88). All of the air should be removed from the glove, which is firmly held around the probe ensuring that an adequate layer of gel remains between the probe and the glove. Apply another layer of gel over the top of the glove and check the ultrasound screen for any artifacts (black streaks). Continue to manipulate the gel until all of the artifacts are gone. With a gloved hand, apply the probe to

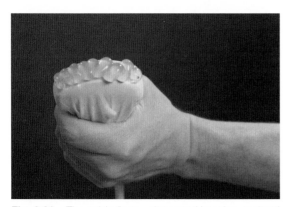

Fig. 8.88 • The pelvic floor – ultrasound imaging: perineal approach. The transducer probe is prepared by applying a thick layer of ultrasound gel to the surface, then covering this with a powder-free latex glove, ensuring there is no air between the gel and the glove, and then applying a second layer of gel over top of the glove.

the midline of the perineum with the marker oriented towards the anus. Vary the angle of the probe until there is a clear image of the PS, urinary bladder and neck of the urethra, and the anorectal angle (Fig. 8.89A).

Note the shape/profile of the resting bladder relative to the position of the PS and then observe the response of all of the structures to the following cues:

1. 'Slowly and gently squeeze the muscles around your urethra as if to stop your urine flow.'
2. 'Slowly and gently draw your vagina (or testicles) up into your body.'
3. 'Imagine there is a wire connecting your anus to the back of your pubic bone. Slowly and gently connect along this line and think about drawing your anus up and forward.'

An optimal contraction of the pelvic floor will tense the endopelvic fascia and result in a lift (net vector) that is cranioventral. The anorectal angle will move up and forwards towards the neck of the urethra (Fig. 8.89B, Video 8.10). Subsequently, note the response when the patient is instructed to bear down or perform a closed-glottis Valsalva (Fig. 8.89C, Video 8.11) and then a cough (Fig. 8.89D, Video 8.12). The bladder should remain supported by the pelvic floor during both of these tasks; minimal descent of the pelvic organs, perineal body, or rectum should be seen.

Non-optimal responses include:

1. No visible movement of the anorectal angle occurs during a cue to contract the pelvic floor.
2. A vector of lift that is not directed towards the neck of the urethra (Video 8.13) during a cue to contract the pelvic floor. This patient presented with stress urinary incontinence. The vector of lift that occurs with her pelvic floor contraction is almost directly cranial and therefore does not force close the urethra.
3. Descent of the bladder below the level of the PS during a closed glottis Valsalva (Video 8.14). This is the same patient during a closed glottis Valsalva. Note the descent of the bladder below the level of the PS, a likely sign of a myofascial deficit and/or non-optimal activation of her pelvic floor during this task.
4. Descent of the bladder below the level of the PS during a cough (Video 8.15). This is a different patient who 2 years prior had a

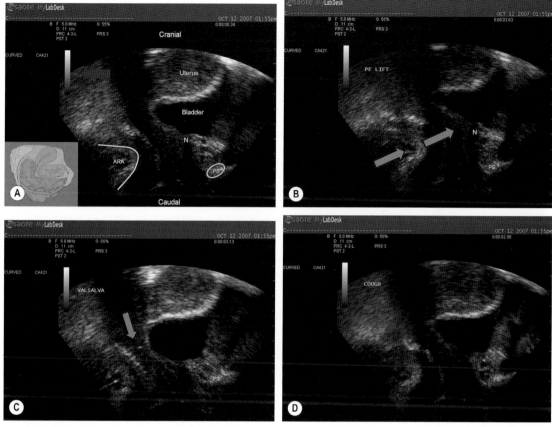

Fig. 8.89 • The pelvic floor – ultrasound imaging: perineal approach. (A) Ultrasound image of the pelvic organs as seen with the perineal approach prior to a contraction of the pelvic floor. PS, pubic symphysis; ARA, anorectal angle; N, neck of the bladder. (B) Ultrasound image of the pelvic organs as seen with the perineal approach during a contraction of the pelvic floor. The vector of lift (arrow) is anterior and superior. This is an optimal response and can be seen on Video 8.10. (C) Ultrasound image of the pelvic organs during a closed glottis Valsalva. Optimally, the bladder will not descend below the level of the PS. A functional response to a closed glottis Valsalva can be seen on Video 8.11 . (D) Ultrasound image of the pelvic organs during a cough; the optimal response can be seen on Video 8.12 .

hysterectomy and was now presenting with stress urinary incontinence. She had transvaginal tape (TVT) surgery 6 weeks prior to this ultrasound assessment. She was still incontinent when she coughed and this clip shows that, while the urethra is clearly suspended, the posterior structures are not supported during a cough.

Deep fibers of multifidus – palpation

While the deep fibers of multifidus (dMF) are not anatomically contained within the abdominal canister, they play a significant role in segmental motion control of the lumbar spine and control of the pelvis (Chapter 4), and thus are part of the functional abdominal canister. Although ultrasound imaging has been used extensively in research to measure changes in the size of the dMF following injury (Chapter 5), clinically it appears that palpation is more sensitive especially when minimal activation occurs. Both methods of assessment will be covered in this section.

With the patient in prone lying, palpate the dMF immediately lateral to the spinous process of the lumbar segment(s) or just lateral to the median sacral crest (see Fig. 8.54C). Press firmly, but gently, into the tissue and compare the tone of these deep fibers to the opposite side as well as to levels above and below. Note if there is any hypertonicity of the erector spinae increasing tension in the thoracolumbar fascia and limiting access to the deepest fibers

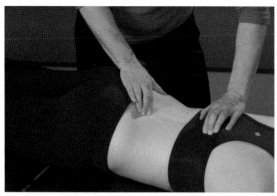

Fig. 8.90 • Deep fibers of multifidus – palpation. This subject has a hypertonic fascicle of the thoracic longissimus arising from the eighth thoracic segment (cranial hand), which is significantly increasing the tension in the thoracolumbar fascia limiting the therapist's ability to assess the deep fibers of multifidus at L4 (caudal hand). This fascicle will need to be released/relaxed before further assessment of the segmental tone at L4 is possible.

(Fig. 8.90). This muscle may need to be released before further assessment of the function of multifidus is possible.

If all of the deep muscles of the abdominal canister are working synergistically, co-contraction appears to occur with a cue to connect to any part of the system. One of the following three cues should evoke a symmetrical, equally timed response of the dMF:

1. 'Slowly and gently squeeze the muscles around your urethra as if to stop your urine flow.'
2. 'Slowly and gently draw your vagina (or testicles) up into your body.'
3. 'Imagine there is a wire connecting your anus to the back of your pubic bone. Slowly and gently connect along this line and think about drawing your anus up and forward.'

When the dMF co-contracts with the pelvic floor in response to any of these cues, a deep swelling or pressure into the palpating finger(s) will be felt. No movement of the thorax, lumbar spine, or pelvic girdle should occur. In our experience, asking the patient to 'make this muscle swell' is less effective than the imagery cues for eliciting an isolated deep muscle co-contraction response. If there is no response to any of these three cues try the following cues:

1. 'Imagine there is a wire connecting your hip bones posteriorly [PSISs] from the left to right side. Think about generating a force which would draw these two bones together.'

2. 'Imagine there is a wire from the back of your pubic bone running through your pelvis to your low back where I am pressing. Connect along this wire or line and then gently suspend this vertebra up towards your head.' 'Imagine this vertebra is like the lid of a teapot and gently lift the lid.' 'Imagine suspending this vertebra 1mm above the one below it to create space between the vertebrae.'

Abnormal responses include:

1. absent response of the dMF to any cue given; and/or
2. asymmetrical response of the left and right dMF.

Common substitution strategies include:

1. activation of superficial fibers of multifidus; and/or
2. the erector spinae, which is felt as tightening of the superficial fascia of the lumbopelvis.

Deep fibers of multifidus – ultrasound imaging

With the patient in sidelying, position the lumbar spine in neutral; support the waist with a towel if necessary. Using a 10–12MHz linear probe, place the well-gelled ultrasound transducer longitudinally over the articular pillar with the marker oriented to the patient's head or transversely over the articular pillar with the marker oriented to the patient's right. In the longitudinal view, vary the angle of the transducer until there is a clear image of the lumbar multifidus, sacrum, and articular processes of L5–S1, L4–L5, and L3–L4. In the transverse view, vary the angle of the transducer until there is a clear image of the spinous process, lamina, and the deep and superficial fibers of multifidus. The depth control can be adjusted so that the muscle layers are more easily observed; be sure to adjust the focus to the layers of interest (Fig. 8.91A–D).

Either view can be used to subsequently observe the response of the dMF to the following cues:

1. 'Slowly and gently squeeze the muscles around your urethra as if to stop your urine flow.'
2. 'Slowly and gently draw your vagina (or testicles) up into your body.'
3. 'Imagine there is a wire connecting your anus to the back of your pubic bone. Slowly and gently connect along this line and think about drawing your anus up and forward.'
4. 'Imagine there is a wire connecting your hip bones posteriorly [PSISs] from the left to right side.

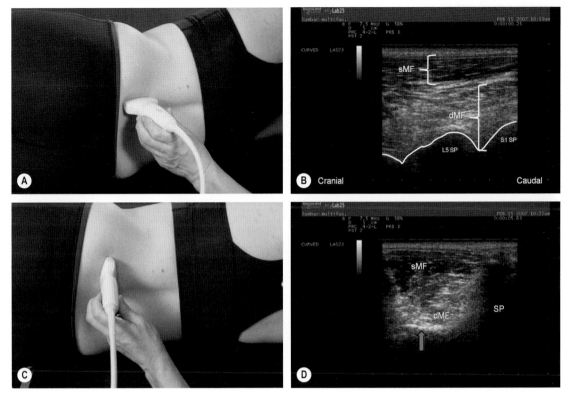

Fig. 8.91 • Deep fibers of multifidus – ultrasound imaging. (A) Probe placement for imaging multifidus longitudinally in the sagittal plane. Orient the probe with the marker towards the patient's head. (B) Ultrasound image (longitudinal view) of the deep and superficial muscles at the lumbosacral junction. See Video 8.16 🖱 to view an optimal isolated contraction of the deep fibers of multifidus (dMF) in the longitudinal orientation. (C) Probe placement for imaging multifidus transversely. Orient the probe with the marker to the patient's right. (D) Ultrasound image (transverse view) of the deep and superficial muscles at L4–5. SP, spinous process; arrow, lamina. See Video 8.17 🖱 to view an optimal isolated contraction of the deep fibers of multifidus in the transverse view. When the erector spinae or superficial fibers of multifidus contract with or without the dMF a concurrent broadening of all muscles will be seen (longitudinal view Video 8.18, transverse view Video 8.19 🖱) and often extension of the lumbar spine will occur.

Think about generating a force which would draw these two bones together.'

5. 'Imagine there is a wire from the back of your pubic bone running through your pelvis to your low back where I am pressing. Connect along this wire or line and then gently suspend this vertebra up towards your head (lift the teapot lid).'
'Imagine suspending this vertebra 1mm above the one below it to create space between the vertebrae.'

When the dMF co-contracts with the pelvic floor in response to any of these cues, a broadening of the muscle will be seen with no activation of the superficial fibers (Video 8.16 longitudinal view, Video 8.17 transverse view 🖱). An absent response will result in no activation or change in breadth of the muscle

on ultrasound imaging. When the erector spinae or superficial fibers of multifidus contract with or without the dMF a concurrent broadening of all muscles will be seen (Video 8.18 longitudinal view, Video 8.19 transverse view 🖱) and often extension of the lumbar spine and/or thoracic spine will occur.

Transversus abdominis and deep fibers of multifidus – palpation

Coactivation of TrA and the dMF in response to a cue to contract the pelvic floor can be assessed in either the prone (Fig. 8.92A) or supine (Fig. 8.92B) position. With one hand, palpate TrA at the appropriate depth, and with the other hand palpate dMF. Cue the patient to contract the pelvic floor with whatever cue is known to result in an optimal contraction (see

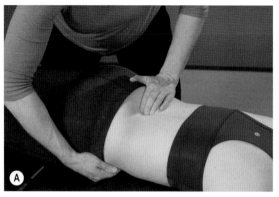
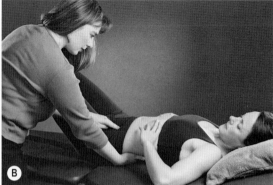

Fig. 8.92 • Transversus abdominis (TrA) and deep fibers of multifidus (dMF) – palpation. Coactivation of TrA and dMF can be assessed in (A) the prone or (B) the supine position. Ensure that the appropriate depth is located before cuing a co-contraction. Feel for absence and/or timing delays in activation. This test can be modified to assess TrA bilaterally, dMF bilaterally, right TrA and right dMF, or left TrA and left dMF.

The pelvic floor – ultrasound imaging) and note the response of TrA and dMF. This is certainly a test where four hands would be useful. The left and right TrA should coactivate with the left and right dMF; move your hands accordingly to assess the synergy of activation.

Clinical reasoning

The findings from the ASLR test (including the response to specific compression of the pelvic girdle) are often (but not always) correlated to the responses of the deep muscles of the abdominal canister. It is common to find the following combination of test findings. Positive ASLR:

1. with effort decreased with bilateral anterior compression and either a unilateral or bilateral deficit of TrA;

2. with effort decreased with bilateral posterior compression and either a unilateral or bilateral deficit of dMF;

3. with effort decreased with bilateral anterior compression at the level of the PS and either a unilateral or bilateral deficit of the pelvic floor and/or unilateral or bilateral deficit of TrA;

4. with effort decreased with an oblique compression (left anterior and right posterior) and a deficit of the left TrA and right dMF; or

5. with effort decreased with an oblique compression (right anterior and left posterior) and a deficit of the right TrA and left dMF.

When a negative ASLR test is found (no change in effort when compression is applied to the pelvic girdle) there are often either no deficits in the deep muscles of the abdominal canister, or there is an excessive superficial muscle recruitment strategy (IO, EO, RA, ES, sMF) with underlying deep muscle deficits such that there is too much compression from the superficial activity and more compression across the pelvic girdle is not beneficial. Alternately, the primary cause for the noted deficit in the ASLR is not intrinsic to the pelvis. This is commonly seen in the thorax or hip-driven pelvic impairment (see case report Julie G, Chapter 9 Video JG22).

The diaphragm

The diaphragm forms the roof of the abdominal canister (see Fig. 4.34) and its function is intimately related to the lumbopelvic complex as well as to the thorax. Hypertonicity of the EO, IO, RA, and ES commonly restricts mobility of the lower thorax and prevents optimal diaphragmatic breathing. At this point in the objective examination, a determination should already have been reached regarding the presence or absence of hypertonicity of EO, IO, RA, and/or ES. To assess the impact of an overactive superficial muscle on the ability of the diaphragm to expand the lower thorax, palpate the rib cage in varying positions (standing, sitting, lying supine, prone, or child's prayer pose) (Fig. 8.93A–D) and note the symmetry of both the amplitude and timing of expansion of the rib cage, and correlate these findings with the presence of any hypertonicity in the muscles overlying the rib cage. When the EO, IO, RA, and ES are co-contracted, minimal expansion

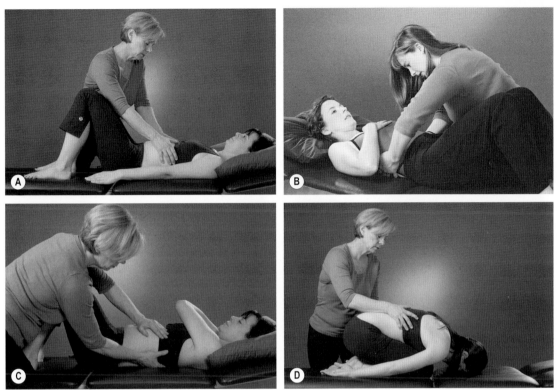

Fig. 8.93 • The diaphragm. Palpation of the rib cage for lateral costal expansion and release during respiration. (A) This subject is a back-gripper and when she breathes in the erector spinae limits the opening of the posterior rib cage and the thorax tilts posteriorly on inspiration. As there is no overactivity of the superficial abdominals, the anterior aspect of the rib cage expands symmetrically. Limitation of posterolateral expansion is determined by palpation, shown in (B). (C) This handhold is useful when assessing unilateral expansion during inspiration. The subject's arm is across her chest for photographic purposes only and should be by her side to avoid increasing tension through the scapular muscles and impacting the breathing findings. (D) The child's prayer pose (yoga) is very useful not only for assessing the ability of the posterior rib cage to move with inspiration but also for treatment. Overactivity of the erector spinae significantly restricts the posterior thorax during inspiration.

of the rib cage occurs during inspiration and most movement occurs in the upper anterior part of the chest (apical breathing).

Psoas – palpation

Psoas is a deep muscle of the abdominal canister (see Fig. 4.34) and hypotheses abound regarding its role in stabilizing both the spine and the hip. Clinical expertise suggests that it is an important muscle for both segmental control of the lumbar spine as well as the hip joint, in addition to its role as a hip flexor. Timing delays in recruitment during hip flexion tasks are commonly seen in patients presenting with 'clicking hips,' and are associated with hypertonicity of the superficial hip flexors. The following test is used to assess the recruitment timing of psoas during a hip flexion task.

With the patient in crook lying, palpate the psoas by gently sliding your cranial hand along the iliacus (begin at the ASIS) ensuring that you are deep to the viscera and not pushing directly through the organs (Fig. 8.94). Slide this hand medially, and approach the lateral aspect of the psoas muscle. To confirm that this is indeed the muscle, gently resist hip flexion with the other hand; an immediate broadening of psoas is easily felt if your hand is in the right place. With the other hand, palpate the hypertonic hip flexor (or adductor) previously found during the regional tests for the hip. Instruct the patient to slowly begin to lift the ipsilateral foot off the table and note which muscle activates first, the hypertonic hip flexor/adductor or the psoas. An optimal recruitment pattern is for psoas to activate prior to the superficial hip flexor or adductor.

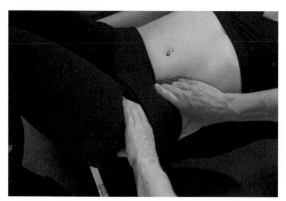

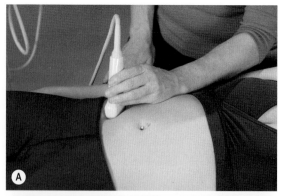

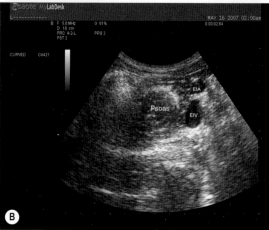

Fig. 8.94 • Psoas – palpation. Clinical expertise suggests that during hip flexion tasks psoas should activate prior to the superficial hip flexors and/or adductors. The therapist's cranial hand is palpating psoas and the caudal hand the rectus femoris. As the patient initiates a lift of the foot off the table, the therapist notes which muscle activates first; it should be psoas.

Psoas – ultrasound imaging

With the patient in crook lying, knees supported over a bolster, expose the abdomen from the xyphoid to the PS. Using a 3.5–5MHz curvilinear probe (the frequency used will depend on the patient's girth, i.e. how deep the muscle is), place the well-gelled ultrasound transducer transversely on the anterolateral aspect of the abdomen adjacent to the medial aspect of the ilium with the transducer marker oriented to the patient's right side (Fig. 8.95A). Vary the angle and location of the transducer until there is a clear transverse image of the psoas (Fig. 8.95B). The depth control can be adjusted so that the muscle layers are more easily observed – be sure to adjust the focus to the layers of interest.

Observe the response of psoas to the following tasks/cues:

1. 'Slowly lift your foot off the table.'
2. 'Imagine there is a guy wire that connects your hip (palpate the greater trochanter) through the head of the femur deep into the hip socket (acetabulum). Think about generating a force that would draw the hip deeper into the socket.'

Optimally, the psoas will contract and this will be seen as a broadening of the muscle (Video 8.20 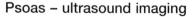). Correlate the ultrasound findings with the palpation findings.

Fig. 8.95 • Psoas – ultrasound imaging. (A) Probe placement for imaging the right psoas muscle. Look for the pulsation of the external iliac artery to landmark psoas. (B) Ultrasound image of psoas. EIA, external iliac artery; EIV, external iliac vein. The optimal response can be seen on Video 8.20 .

Interconnected myofascial muscle slings

The superficial muscles of the abdomen and lower extremity are essentially part of an interconnected myofascial sling system, comprising several muscles and their related fascia, which produce forces along the sling(s). A muscle may participate in more than one sling and the slings may overlap and interconnect depending on the task being performed. The hypothesis is that the slings have no beginning or end, but rather connect to assist in the transference of forces. It is possible that the slings are all part of one interconnected myofascial system and the particular sling that is identified during any motion is merely due to the activation of selective parts of the whole sling.

The identification and treatment of a specific muscle dysfunction (weakness, inappropriate recruitment, shortening) is important when restoring optimal strategies for load transfer. It is important to test for muscle strength and length and it is assumed that all readers will have a basic understanding of how to test this. A key point to remember when testing a muscle's strength is this: just because a muscle *seems* weak to specific testing does not mean that the muscle tissue itself is impaired and responsible for the reduced force production on muscle testing; it merely implies that the sling is not able to resist the force you are applying. Manual muscle testing (Kendall et al 1993), although quite specific, still tests the function of several muscles working together. A positive 'strength' test could be due to impairments in the neural system (lack of innervation, altered timing of the muscle synergists required, lack of recruitment of one or any muscle along a sling, non-optimal control of the bones to which the muscle(s) attach), impairments in the myofascial system (muscle tears, fascial tears, scarring), and/or an underlying loss of the articular system restraints where the muscles attach.

In addition, it is assumed that the reader has a basic understanding of how to assess and treat a true contractile muscle lesion or sprain. Grade 1 and Grade 2 muscle sprains are painfully strong when resisted isometrically, as opposed to Grade 3 sprains (i.e. complete ruptures), which are relatively painfree and weak when resisted isometrically. Of course, there exists an entire spectrum of dysfunction between the two extremes. It must be remembered that contractions of muscles induce compression forces across joints and also increase tension in the various ligaments to which they attach. Therefore, a pain response may not be indicative of a muscle strain at all, but rather the pain may be coming from a joint that reacts to compression or from a ligament that is painful to stretch.

Neurological conduction and mobility tests

These tests examine the conductivity of the motor and sensory nerves relative to the lumbosacral plexus as well as the mobility of the dura through the intervertebral foramina. The reader is referred to Butler (2000) and Shacklock (2005) for a more in-depth review of neural and dural mobility.

Motor conduction tests

The L2 to S2 motor nerve roots are evaluated clinically via the peripheral muscles they innervate. Although there are no true peripheral myotomes in the lower quadrant (one muscle solely innervated by one nerve root), specific muscles known as *key muscles* are primarily innervated by one motor nerve and their function is a reflection of the neurological innervation. Initially, a maximal contraction is elicited from the key muscle and the quantity and quality of strength are compared to the opposite side. If the muscle tests are strong, six submaximal contractions are elicited to detect accelerated fatigability – a common finding of neurological impedance.

The motor nerves and the key muscles that are evaluated include:

L2 psoas major, adductors;

L3 adductors, quadriceps;

L4 quadriceps, tibialis anterior;

L5 extensor hallucis, extensor digitorum, peronei;

S1 hamstrings, gastrocnemius;

S2 hamstrings, gluteus maximus.

Sensory conduction tests

The L1–S2 sensory nerve roots are evaluated clinically via the dermatomes they innervate. Dermatome maps can be confusing and conflicting as many are inaccurate and based on flawed studies. Lee et al (2008b) conducted a thorough systematic review of all dermatome maps, chose the studies with high methodological standards, and then overlaid the maps accepting the regions that agreed and deleting those that did not. The resultant map 'represents the most consistent tactile dermatomal areas for each spinal dorsal nerve root found in most individuals, based on the best available evidence' (Lee et al 2008b) (Fig. 8.96). The large blank areas on this new map reflect areas where overlap and variability were found.

Detailed examination of the distal extent of the dermatome is useful in detecting early neurological interference. One of the first signs of sensory dysfunction is hyperesthesia within a specific dermatome. This sign tends to occur long before sensation becomes reduced or obliterated completely, and its existence is often a surprise to the patient.

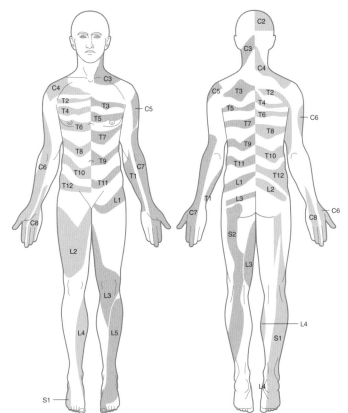

Fig. 8.96 • The evidence-based dermatome map representing the most consistent tactile dermatomal areas for each spinal dorsal nerve root found in most individuals, based on the best available evidence. The dermatomal areas shown are NOT autonomous zones of cutaneous sensory innervation as, except in the midline where overlap is minimal, adjacent dermatomes overlap to a large and variable extent. Blank regions indicate areas of major variability and overlap. S3, S4, and S5 supply the perineum but are not shown for reasons of clarity. Redrawn from Lee et al, 2008b.

Reflex tests

The spinal reflexes are evaluated via the myotactic response to stretch of the key muscle innervated by the root in question. They include the following:

L3, L4 quadriceps (i.e. knee jerk);

L5, S1, S2 gastrocnemius (i.e. ankle jerk).

The integrity of the spinal cord is evaluated by the plantar response test.

Vascular tests

These tests screen the circulatory status of the lower extremity. Careful observation of the skin color, texture, response to dependency and elevation, and the length of time for superficial wounds to heal should be noted. The femoral, popliteal, and dorsalis pedis arteries are palpated and auscultated in the femoral triangle, popliteal fossa, and dorsum of the foot, respectively. If a deep vein thrombophlebitis is suspected, the response to passive dorsiflexion of the ankle should be noted (Homan's sign)

and the region carefully palpated for heat and/or tenderness.

Adjunctive tests

X-rays make good policemen but poor counselors, in that while the straight radiography may exclude serious bone disease and significant mechanical defect, it does not often provide much guidance about how to treat the patient.

Grieve 1981.

The primary reason for obtaining the results of adjunctive tests is to rule out serious pathology and to discover the presence of anatomical anomalies prior to treatment.

Some adjunctive tests include the following:

1. radiography (X-rays);
2. discography;
3. myelography;
4. radiculography;

5. epidurography;
6. tomography;
7. transverse axial tomography;
8. computed transverse axial tomography;
9. radiographic stereoplotting;
10. interosseous spinal venography;
11. cineradiography and fluoroscopy;
12. thermography;
13. nerve root infiltration;
14. electrodiagnosis;
15. intervertebral disc manometry;
16. cystometry;
17. radioactive isotope studies;
18. ultrasonography;
19. nuclear magnetic resonance.

With respect to the SIJ, Lawson et al (1982) reported on the benefits of computed axial tomography (CT scanning techniques) as opposed to conventional radiography in the detection of mild erosions and narrowing of the joint. Because of the

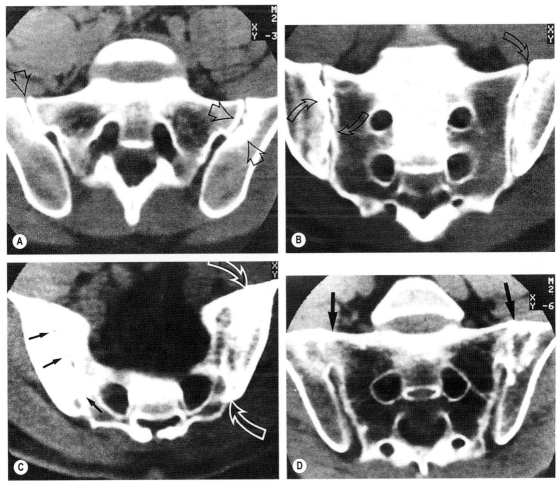

Fig. 8.97 • (A) A computed tomography scan (transverse plane) of a patient with Reiter's disease. This image clearly reveals the focal sclerosis (arrows), narrowing, and erosion of the sacroiliac joint associated with this disease. The depth of the joint is clearly visualized. (B) A computed tomography scan (vertical plane) of a patient with Reiter's disease illustrating narrowing, erosion, and focal sclerosis (arrows) of the articular surfaces of the sacroiliac joints. (C) A computed tomography scan of a patient with ankylosing spondylitis. Note the total ankylosis of the right sacroiliac joint (open arrows). (D) A computed tomography scan of a patient with ankylosing spondylitis. Note the bilateral bony ankylosis of the sacroiliac joints. Reproduced with permission from Lawson et al and the publisher Raven Press, 1982.

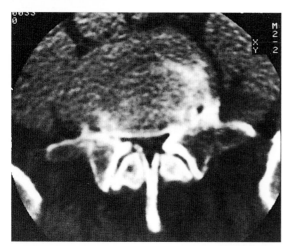

Fig. 8.98 • A computed tomography scan of the L5–S1 segment illustrating central stenosis secondary to enlargement of the zygapophyseal joints bilaterally. Reproduced with permission from Kirkaldy-Willis and the publisher Churchill Livingstone, 1983.

1. asymmetry of the posterior zygapophyseal joints;
2. congenital absence of a pedicle;
3. accessory laminae;
4. osseous bridging of the transverse processes;
5. dysplasia or absence of the spinous process of the L5 or S1 vertebrae (spina bifida);
6. dysplasia of the pars interarticularis;
7. spina magna of the L5 vertebra;
8. trapezoidal L5 vertebra, lumbarized S1 vertebra – partial or complete;
9. sacralized L5 vertebra – partial or complete;
10. anomalous adventitious joint between the transverse process of the L5 vertebra and the ala of the sacrum;
11. asymmetrical height of the ala of the sacrum with one side higher than the other, creating a sacral tilt;
12. calcified iliolumbar ligament (Grieve 1981).

The findings noted on adjunctive testing of the LPH complex must be correlated with the findings noted on clinical examination if their significance is to be understood. Rarely can treatment be directed by the results of these tests alone.

three-dimensional spatial orientation of the SIJ, CT scanning was superior in obtaining visualization of the joint space. Thus, the diagnosis of inflammatory sacroiliitis, which is based on the identification of joint narrowing, sclerosis, ankylosis, or erosion, was facilitated. Figure 8.97A–D illustrates the visualization of both the synovial and the ligamentous portions of the SIJ that is possible with this adjunctive test. Several MRI images of the LPH complex are illustrated in Chapter 3.

CT scanning techniques can reveal congenital and/or acquired anatomical changes in the lumbar spine (Fig. 8.98). The dimensions of the central spinal canal as well as the lateral recess are clearly visualized and often confirm or deny the clinical findings of physical trespass.

The lumbosacral junction is often the site of congenital anomalies, which may or may not be significant to the clinical picture. Their presence, however, should be ascertained. The anomalies seen at this level include:

Summary

There is an infinite number of tests that could be assessed for every patient met in the clinic; however, those included in this chapter form the foundation of a thorough examination of the LPH complex. Other patient-specific tests will be introduced in subsequent chapters as selected cases are presented and clinically reasoned. Clinical expertise evolves from disciplined, reflective practice and includes both skill acquisition (getting better at doing the various tests and techniques) and clinical reasoning (getting better at doing the right thing at the right time). This chapter has focused on 'how to do things'; let's move on to consider 'the right thing at the right time' and meet some patients who have given us permission to share their stories with you.

Clinical reasoning, treatment planning, and case reports

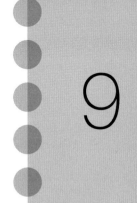

9

Diane Lee   Linda Joy-Lee

CHAPTER CONTENTS

Introduction 255

Lumbopelvic–hip pain and impairments –
figuring out the Clinical Puzzle 258

Treatment principles for an integrated
evidence-based program 260

Components of the treatment program . . . 260

Case reports 270

Summary 282

Introduction

Every day in clinical practice, health care practitioners meet patients seeking help for their loss of function (disability) and pain. While we watch for research evidence to guide our practice, treatment must go on. Clinicians are keenly aware of the need to be effective in clinical practice and many feel that this requires being evidence-based. In Chapter 7, evidence-based clinical practice (EBP) was discussed and by now the reader will understand that we adhere to Sackett's definition that includes clinical expertise as a significant component of EBP (see Fig. 7.4). It is unlikely that there will ever be enough research evidence for every situation met in clinical practice. Sackett et al (2000) note that:

> External clinical evidence can inform, but can never replace individual clinical expertise, and it is this expertise that decides whether the external evidence applies to the patient at all, and if so, how it should be integrated into a clinical decision.

Most clinicians resonate with Sackett et al's definition of EBP and agree that clinical expertise is necessary to bridge the gap between what science

suggests (propositional knowledge) and what we need to know practically (non-propositional knowledge) to treat patients with disability and pain. Which brings us to the next question – what is clinical expertise? According to Cleland et al (2008):

> Clinical expertise refers to the clinician's proficiency and acuity when making judgments and applying clinical skills in the care of individual patients.

According to Ericsson & Smith (1991), 'expertise has been defined as having the ability to do the right thing at the right time.'

Clinical expertise, therefore, has two components, skill acquisition (do the right thing) and clinical reasoning (at the right time) (Fig. 9.1). In Chapter 8, the fundamental tests for assessing the lumbopelvic–hip complex (skill acquisition), and a small amount of clinical reasoning, were presented. This chapter will outline the treatment principles for the management of lumbopelvic–hip disability and pain, and go further into narrative, hypothesis-oriented (hypothetic-deductive), and interpretive reasoning (Jensen et al 2007, Jones & Rivett 2004, Kerry 2009) for the various subjective and objective findings through a series of case reports. Jones & Rivett (2004) credit Higgs & Jones (2000) as defining clinical reasoning as a process

> in which the therapist, interacting with the patient and significant others . . . structures meaning, goals and health management strategies based on clinical data, client choices and professional judgment and knowledge. It is this thinking and decision making associated with clinical practice that enable therapists to take the best-judged action for individual patients. In this sense, clinical reasoning is the means to 'wise' action.

A variety of reasoning processes are used simultaneously throughout the therapeutic relationship

DOI: 10.1016/B978-0-443-06963-5.00009-2

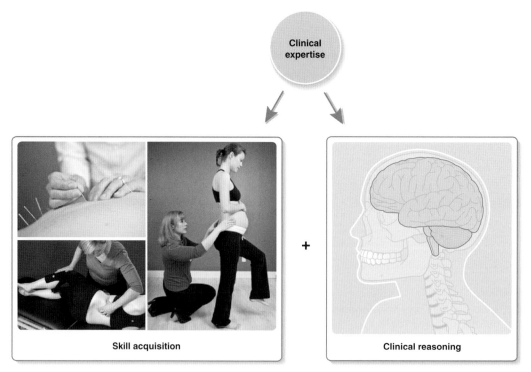

Clinical expertise

Skill acquisition

+

Clinical reasoning

Fig. 9.1 • Clinical expertise is comprised of two components, skill acquisition (the ability to do the right thing) and clinical reasoning (at the right time).

with the intent of making the wisest decisions. Understanding the patient as a person requires knowing their perspective and experience of the problem, including how it is affecting their life (sensorial, cognitive, and emotional dimensions (Chapter 7)). This is derived through narrative reasoning that gathers information from the patient as well as from referring professionals and, if necessary, the patient's family. As the story unfolds, guided by directed enquiries, the therapist begins to understand the patient's beliefs, expectations, motivations, and attitudes or, as Mezirow (1990) states, their 'meaning perspective.' This perspective evolves from an accumulation of personal, social, and cultural experiences. The meaning perspective may facilitate or retard recovery; thus, it is important to understand.

As experience is gained, expert clinicians often use pattern recognition for decision-making when faced with cases that are not complex and with which they feel very familiar. For example, 30 years ago it was common to hear expert clinicians, who were leaders and teachers, make broad statements, such as 'I have seen thousands of patients with pelvic girdle pain and impairment and I always find that the innominate is rotated anteriorly. All you need to do is rotate the

innominate posteriorly and the problem will be fixed and the pain will go away.' For obvious reasons, this mode of reasoning has a high potential for error. The logical basis for pattern recognition is known as induction and the form of reasoning is called inductive reasoning. It is based solely on a practitioner's experience and observations in clinical practice and the logic is at risk for being in error.

> Consideration of the problems of induction is nothing new. The argument against inductivism was highlighted in the work of a 20th century philosopher called Karl Popper. His claim was that adherence to an inductivist approach is erroneous and limited and that in order for a more accurate approximation to what is correct to be made, a deductive approach should be taken.
>
> Popper 1980, from Kerry 2009.

Hypothesis-oriented reasoning (Jones & Rivett 2004), also known as hypothetic-deductive reasoning (Jensen et al 2007, Kerry 2009, Kerry et al 2008), attempts to refute or support an original hypothesis by considering all of the data from the subjective and objective examination. The logical basis for hypothesis-oriented reasoning is deduction or deductive logic. This form of reasoning reaches conclusions from premises believed to be true (possibly facts). The strength of the conclusion is based on the level of truth of the premises. For example, if the hypothesis is that loss of integrity of the passive structures of the right sacroiliac joint (SIJ) is responsible for the failed load transfer noted on the right side of the pelvis during right single leg loading, then at least two tests pertaining to the right SIJ should support this hypothesis. If the amplitude of motion of the right SIJ is greater than the left and the end feel of the elastic zone is 'softer' on the right (premise 1), and when the SIJ is close-packed there is still movement in the neutral zone (premise 2), deductive logic would support the initial hypothesis. Although there remains room for error in this mode of reasoning, it is more likely that the answer is closer to the truth. It is thought to be a more robust form of enquiry (Kerry 2009). The strength of the conclusion (validity) depends on the strength of the premises – at least in hypothetic-deductive reasoning the premises can be tested! Only the strongest hypotheses will survive and make it to the next stage of assessment as nothing is ever 100% certain or valid in clinical practice.

Abductive reasoning or logic considers multiple observations (some of which may be true and some for which there may be multiple explanations and therefore are not necessarily true) and generates hypotheses that are most likely and probable to explain them. In clinical practice, an objective examination comprises several observations, and there are multiple possible hypotheses and explanations for most conditions. Often the clinician uses a combination of hypothetic-deductive and abductive logic simultaneously to decide on the best explanation and, consequently, the best plan for treatment. For example, consider the scenario outlined above. If in addition to the first two premises:

1. the amplitude of neutral zone (NZ) motion of the right SIJ is greater than the left SIJ and the end feel of the elastic zone (EZ) is soft; and

2. close-packing the right SIJ did not result in zero motion in the NZ;
a third and fourth tests found;

3. decreased resting tone and marked atrophy of the right lumbosacral multifidus; and

4. the patient had generalized connective tissue laxity (hypermobility) and very loose joints;

then abductive logic would support another possibility for the failed load transfer of the right side of the pelvis noted in single leg loading. Instead of incriminating the articular system as the primary impairment (e.g. articular laxity), a case could be made for

incriminating the neural system (e.g. altered motor control leading to non-optimal strategies for function and performance). The management of an articular versus a neural system impairment is very different; the first may require prolotherapy for restoration of function and performance whereas the latter would likely resolve with a motor learning program.

The more findings there are to support a hypothesis, the more likely the hypothesis is right. As all hypotheses are tested, the clinician reflects and interprets the results of all findings using interpretive reasoning to decide on the treatment plan (Fig. 9.2). Interpretive reasoning considers the results from the assessment as well as any relevant research evidence. In order to successfully perform all types of reasoning in the clinical context, therapists need to have well-organized knowledge including propositional (knowledge ratified by research trials), non-propositional (professional craft or 'knowing how' knowledge) and personal (knowledge gained from personal experiences (Chapter 7) (Jones & Rivett 2004)).

Critical reflection requires one to examine assumptions and reflect on the validity of decisions made (Edwards & Jones 2007). Reflective practice is the way clinicians learn, transform, or evolve from their experiences. Reflecting on 'what went right' and 'what went wrong' involves thinking about your thinking, and requires a clinician to be open to challenges to their own paradigms, ideas, and perspectives. Metacognitive reflection is the term used for reflective thinking at this higher level (Jones & Rivett 2004). This highlights the need for clinicians to be *adaptive* and willing to change, modify, or reject their paradigms as new information, from both clinical experience and science, becomes available.

It is interesting to note that, as clinical expertise develops, the clinician may feel that they are making decisions based on 'gut instinct,' and yet evidence suggests that this 'blink' decision is actually based on multiple and repeated experiences of reflective practice and pattern recognition over time (Gladwell 2005). How long does it take to develop clinical expertise? Some may argue that years of practice are necessary. However, if there is little or no reflection in those many years, it is unlikely that clinical expertise will develop. Alternately, with awareness, conscious and methodical critique and reflection, we feel that expertise can be gained in relatively short periods of time. As noted by Butler (2000),

> . . . there are clinicians who have had 20 years experience in 20 years of clinical practice; there are others who have 20 years of experience in one year of clinical practice.

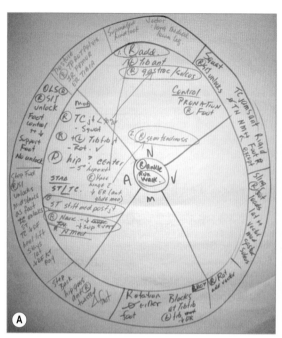

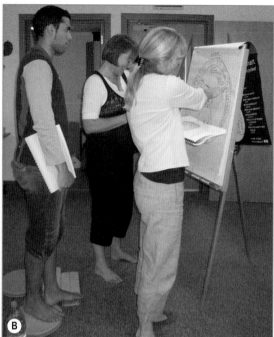

Fig. 9.2 • During our courses, the Clinical Puzzle is used to chart the key findings from both the subjective and objective examination. Students then reflect and use interpretive reasoning to develop hypotheses pertaining to all the findings. Clinical expertise is rapidly developed with this collaborative discussion and reasoning of multiple puzzles (cases).

The latter has reasoned, learned, experimented with management techniques, remained open, been aware of the outcomes movement, and has read widely.

Butler 2000.

Clinical reasoning is an ongoing learning process . . . and is integral to life-long learning, reflective practice and continual professional development

Kerry 2009.

The case reports in this chapter will illustrate a variety of reasoning used throughout the assessment process and our hope is that they will facilitate further development of your clinical expertise. The specific treatment techniques (skill acquisition) required for implementing the treatment plans in these case reports are detailed in Chapters 10, 11, and 12.

Lumbopelvic–hip pain and impairments – figuring out the Clinical Puzzle

What does the story of a patient with lumbopelvic–hip (LPH) pain and/or disability sound like? Are there pain patterns and behaviors that link to specific underlying impairments? In Chapter 5, some common clinical presentations pertaining to specific structural changes in the LPH complex were discussed; however, these presentations failed to consider the cognitive and emotional dimension of each patient's experience. Two patients with similar structural and mechanical impairments, yet different thoughts and beliefs about what is going on (cognitive dimension), and different emotional states tagged to that concern (emotional or affective dimension – optimism, trust, confidence, hope, fear, anxiety, depression, anger, and/or loss of hope), would have very different presentations. It is imperative to consider the contribution of all three dimensions of the patient's experience when planning treatment if the best outcome is to be achieved.

All patients with failed load transfer through the LPH complex demonstrate non-optimal strategies during meaningful tasks (forward bending, backward bending, squat, step forward, prone hip extension, sitting, running, rowing, dancing, etc.). The reasons for the non-optimal strategy are variable and clinical reasoning (hypothesis-oriented, interpretive, and reflective) is essential for differentiating the causes. Impairments in any of the systems of the Clinical

Puzzle (see Fig. 7.11) can either singularly, or in combination, cause failed load transfer of the lumbar spine, pelvic girdle, and/or hip.

When assessing the strategies used for the performance of various tasks, questions and hypotheses will arise pertaining to one or more of these systems. The Clinical Puzzle is used to record, or chart, these questions. For example, if during the one leg standing test the mobility of L5–S1 is in question, it is listed in the articular piece of the puzzle, and if during the same task motion control of the left SIJ is in question, it is listed in both the articular and neural pieces of the puzzle. This ensures that key tests are not missed during the objective examination and that the hypotheses are derived from abductive logic. During the process of the examination, the Clinical Puzzle is used to reflect on the findings (interpretive reasoning) to determine how they relate to the patient's clinical presentation. What is the most likely explanation for the patient's presenting pain and disability that incorporates the findings of the tests, given the information already gained in the subjective examination (mechanism of injury/onset of problems, aggravating positions/activities, relieving positions/activities, imaging studies, cognitive and emotional features, etc.)? Clinical reasoning 'on the fly' involves ongoing formation of hypotheses and the evaluation of these hypotheses in order to retain or reject them *while the objective examination continues*. Certain features of the patient's story may lead to the generation of two or three hypotheses that could possibly explain the patient's presentation. With the information gained from each clinical test, the therapist is determining whether the findings are supporting or negating the initial hypotheses; think of this as a mental score sheet for each hypothesis. If the initial hypotheses are not being supported by the findings, the therapist may need to generate new hypotheses that then lead the clinician to perform other clinical tests in order to confirm or negate the new hypotheses. This process is often occurring subconsciously, and is happening alongside the assessment of the patient's cognitive and emotional responses to the assessment and treatment process, which are also integrated into the hypothesis formation and testing.

Although there may be observable impairments in several systems, the goal of the assessment and clinical reasoning process is to determine which pieces of the puzzle (and which specific impairments in those systems) are the most relevant to the clinical picture. Overall, during the process of the assessment, a multifaceted picture of the patient will unfold. By the end of the examination the therapist should have a solid hypothesis that links findings from all pieces of the puzzle (physical (articular, neural, myofascial, visceral), cognitive, and emotional). This means that the clinician can describe a rationale for which structures and mechanisms are creating the pain experience, why certain structures and activities have become painful, and how the pain experience relates to loss of function and inability to participate in meaningful activities. The results of the clinical reasoning process can be summarized in the puzzle. The clinical puzzles with each of the case reports in this chapter illustrate the initial phases of the clinical reasoning process. Note that not all findings from subsequent system tests are included in the puzzle; as a learning tool, we suggest you refer to the text and video clips and complete the puzzle as appropriate for each case. Take a moment to generate your own hypotheses as the case unfolds.

When treatment is directed to the most relevant impairments (physical, cognitive, and emotional), successful resolution of the pain and disability, along with attainment of functional goals, usually follows. This highlights the importance of re-assessment in management, as the response to treatment serves to validate or negate the therapist's original hypothesis about the sources of the presenting problem.

If one considers all of the possible combinations of impairments and the associated findings that can lead to pain and/or loss of function, the LPH complex can seem complicated. In reality, when sound reflective, critical thinking, and logic are coupled with a thorough examination, the primary impairment and initial treatment plan emerges. As treatment evolves over several sessions, the focus often changes as the patient's journey towards function occurs. Reflective practice helps to direct treatment as clinical puzzles are dynamic and change over time. What may begin as a primary articular impairment (e.g. joint fixation) may become a primary neural impairment (e.g. non-optimal motor programs for specific tasks) once the joint's mobility is restored. The case reports presented in this chapter illustrate multiple different presentations of LPH pain and disability. They demonstrate how the various aspects of clinical reasoning are used throughout the therapeutic process to determine the primary and secondary impairments and direct the initial treatment plan.

Treatment principles for an integrated evidence-based program

The ultimate goal of the evidence-based approach, The Integrated Systems Model, is to change strategies for function and performance; that is, to change the way patients live, move, and experience their bodies. From a pain perspective, training optimal strategies can change the pain experience via several possible mechanisms. In most cases, there are likely multiple mechanisms that interact and change inputs into the body-self neuromatrix (see Fig. 7.9) and result in decreased pain. Biomechanically, training optimal strategies facilitates the unloading of painful structures by equally distributing load through the kinetic chain to balance compression, shear, and tensile forces during both static and dynamic tasks. For patients whose pain is primarily tissue-related (peripherally mediated (Chapter 7)), that is, related to overload, exhausted adaptive potential, and irritation of nociceptive structures, changing postural and movement strategies will decrease pain by addressing the source of inappropriate loading on the pain-generating structures. From a CNS processing perspective, letting go of old strategies and behaviors, and replacing them with new ones, requires a multidimensional process that impacts emotional, social, environmental, and cognitive dimensions as well as physical dimensions. Key elements include:

1. education;
2. increasing the understanding of the barriers (physical, emotional, and cognitive) to recovery that are patient-specific;
3. giving positive feedback;
4. restoring hope; and
5. desensitizing painful movements and contexts with graded exposure and activity;

all of which contribute to removing threat and creating a new brain map – in essence, 'deleting' neural networks that are part of the patient's unique pain experience, thus opening the door for new neural networks to be created.

From a functional perspective, training optimal strategies creates maximum efficiency and synergy within and between systems in the body (see Fig. 8.1), so that the patient experiences ease of movement, confidence in their body, and a sense of grace and power when they move. Optimal strategies create beautiful, fluid movement. Athletes will often describe the feeling of 'being in the zone' or 'in the flow' that comes when a state of relaxed, but intense, focus is attained during periods of high performance. Giving patients this new experience in their body, and making them aware of *how they feel in their body* (interoception) with the new strategy as compared to the old strategy, provides positive feedback and further motivation to continue to engage and commit to the rehabilitation process.

So how do we facilitate change? This question has challenged philosophers, theologians, and scientists for centuries. How much change is possible? What is the influence of underlying pathoanatomical changes such as joint degeneration and brain injury? Exciting advances in the field of neuroscience and experiences of clinicians and scientists alike give us increasing understanding and optimism in answering these questions, in that the nervous system is shown to be continually 'learning to learn' (Doidge 2007), and that it has an immense capacity to change and evolve across the human lifespan. It is evident that there are many 'ways in' to the human mind and body that enable and facilitate the changing of behavior. The therapist can use a diverse range of manual techniques and application of biomedical knowledge (propositional), but also needs to have skills in listening, counseling, and teaching patients (non-propositional), as well as the ability to internally reflect and critique their own biases and perspectives that may be facilitating or hindering the recovery process for the patient (personal knowledge). Overall, the primary role of the therapist is one of a *facilitator* or *coach*; the ultimate responsibility for the patient's recovery lies with the patient, as only the patient can make the changes necessary for attaining optimal function. Given all this, creating an effective treatment program may seem a complex and difficult task; however, when a broad perspective is taken, the process can be broken down into two basic components.

Components of the treatment program

Treatment according to The Integrated Systems Model has two main components (Fig. 9.3):

1. remove the non-optimal strategy by addressing barriers and creating new options for movement to set the stage for learning new strategies; and
2. train a new strategy that is based on meaningful tasks.

Fig. 9.3 • The two primary components of the treatment program according to The Integrated Systems Model.

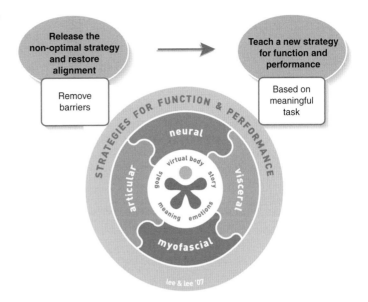

Remove the non-optimal strategy by addressing barriers

In our many interactions with therapists around the world, a common experience is that therapists find it difficult to teach some patients new movement tasks/exercises and strategies. For example, we are often asked, 'What is the best cue for teaching someone how to isolate transversus abdominis?' In our experience, there is not one 'best cue' for all patients; the challenge is to find the best cue for each patient. Furthermore, the most common oversight in cases where patients are having difficulty learning new strategies is that the therapist has neglected to address all of the barriers that are perpetuating the use of the non-optimal strategies. This can be compared to trying to save a new file on a full hard drive; without deleting the old files there is no room for the new files. A further analogy would be trying to upgrade software without deleting components of the old version, leaving competing elements in the system that make the new versions unable to run. Our experience is that once the old strategy and the barriers to change are removed, training new patterns of recruitment of muscles and total body movement strategies occurs with relative ease. One or two verbal cues combined with manual facilitation helps the patient 'find' the new pattern.

The challenge for clinicians is that barriers can be multiple and varied even across patients with similar pain presentations and similar biomechanical impairments. They can exist across several domains (physical, cognitive, behavioral, psychosocial, emotional, cultural, and contextual), especially in complex clinical cases. In the example above, a physical barrier would be a dominant internal oblique, such that when the patient tries to recruit transversus abdominis, the internal oblique is recruited first and with a large amount of activity (compared to what is required for the task) (Video 8.3a,b 🖱). In this case, trying to teach the patient to recruit transversus abdominis without downtraining or releasing the internal oblique (see Figs 10.33–10.37) is asking the patient to perform an exceedingly difficult task, and will likely result in failure and disillusionment with the process. Cognitively, if the patient does not understand the relevance of the exercise to their goals and values, it will not be successful because the patient is not committed to the process. This second scenario may in fact be a therapist-induced barrier if the therapist has neglected to explain the meaning and relevance of the isolation practice to the patient. This may be due to a lack of appreciation of the importance of educating patients (therapist belief), lack of time (environmental pressures), or an inability to create links and a story to explain how the isolation practice does indeed relate to the patient's goal of running a marathon (poor communication skills), for example. The non-reflective practitioner, however, will simply label the patient as 'non-compliant,' as they will lack the introspective skills to see their contribution to the patient's cognitive barrier.

To successfully address barriers and create the environment for patients to explore new strategies for function, the clinician 'requires a rich blend of biomedical, psychosocial, professional craft and personal knowledge, together with diagnostic, teaching, negotiating, listening and counseling skills' (Jones & Rivett 2004). In some cases, referral to more experienced clinicians or complementary therapies in a multidisciplinary team may be required. However, there are many ways to address barriers, and experienced clinicians may subconsciously choose from a variety of approaches based on trial and error over many years of clinical practice. What follows is an overview and discussion of specific ways to address common cognitive, emotional, environmental, and physical barriers that are encountered when treating patients with LPH pain and dysfunction. This is by no means an exhaustive list; references are given for further discovery in specific areas.

Addressing barriers: characteristics of the therapist

Although many therapists may be keenly aware of knowledge and skill performance areas on which they need to improve, it is less common for therapists to reflect upon the role that their own beliefs and attitudes play in facilitating or hindering change in their patients. Do you believe that your patients can change? Do you believe that you have the skills to help them change? For some therapists, teaching patients to change their postural and movement strategies seems like a daunting task. 'My patient has walked like this/run like this/sat like this for the last 10/20/30 years...how can you expect them to change? It is really hard to change long standing habits.' But is it truly hard to change? Your answer to this question will have a significant impact on your ability to help your patients change. If you as a therapist believe that change will be difficult or impossible for your patient, then this is more likely than not to be your experience (which will in turn reinforce your belief system). Studies have shown that 'perceived prognosis influences real outcomes' (Miller & Rollnick 2002).

> If you treat an individual as he is, he will stay as he is, but if you treat him as if he were what he ought to be and could be, he will become what he ought to be and could be.
>
> Johann Wolfgang von Goethe, from Miller & Rollnick 2002.

One of the features necessary for change to occur is that patients have faith and hope in the process (Miller & Rollnick 2002); if *you* have no hope for them, how can you expect that they will?

Of course, having the skills and knowledge to help patients is also essential. But with the ever-expanding scientific and clinical evidence base in all areas relevant to assessing and treating pain and dysfunction in human beings, it is unrealistic to think that any one therapist will know everything there is to know about how to best manage every clinical situation that may present. The awareness of this fact often leads many well-trained and highly skilled therapists to doubt their abilities. This lack of confidence can then be a barrier for a patient's recovery; they will sense the insecurity, which will then undermine the patient's confidence in the process. Although it is important to recognize your limitations and to refer onwards to more experienced or specialized practitioners if needed, it is important to know and work within your strengths with confidence. Being perceived as an expert can have a significant impact on patient outcomes (Jensen et al 2007).

There is a multitude of other characteristics of the therapist that can be barriers to the patient's recovery process; we do not intend to provide a comprehensive review of the subject, but rather we hope to stimulate thought and introspection so that individual therapists can be more aware of their unique perspectives, biases, and experiences. These can influence not only treatment outcomes but also the therapist's own levels of satisfaction and enjoyment in their work.

Addressing barriers: characteristics of the person in the center of the Clinical Puzzle

Systemic factors. This category includes anything that affects the general health of the patient and the quality and function of connective tissue. Systemic diseases such as Ehlers–Danlos syndrome, ankylosing spondylitis, and rheumatoid arthritis will have particular relevance to neuromusculoskeletal dysfunction, but general lifestyle habits such as smoking, nutrition, and hydration will also affect the ability of tissues to heal and respond to incremental loading and training. Stress is known to have wide-ranging effects, including impairment of nutrient absorption, fatigue, immune suppression, and neural degeneration (David 2005, Gifford 1998, Jones & Rivett 2004, Melzack 2001, 2005). Thus, approaches such as meditation and breathing exercises can influence the pain experience by facilitating better coping strategies and reducing stress. Cardiorespiratory conditions such as asthma, emphysema, and chronic respiratory infections are particularly relevant as respiratory function, spinal control, and continence are closely linked (Chapters 4, 5, 6). Change related to different life stages, such as puberty and menopause, or hormonal imbalance due to environmental and lifestyle factors (e.g. long-term use of the birth control pill, fertility medications), can have a significant impact on LPH pain and the contribution of the visceral system to the presenting problem(s). Depending on the health care setting, the physiotherapist may be the first health professional from which the patient seeks help. Therefore, it is always important that the therapist obtain information to determine if any red flags for serious pathology warrant referral to the appropriate medical professional (see Boissonault 1995).

In general, addressing barriers that relate to systemic factors requires that the therapist be aware that there may be significant global contributors to the patient's presenting problem. The therapist's role is to give appropriate advice (within their scope and expertise), encourage and support the patient as they seek information and explore solutions, and refer to other health practitioners for further investigation and/or treatment. This requires that the therapist be widely read in many areas related to health, and that they build a network of health professionals to refer to and collaborate with.

Meaning perspective. There are many ways to address barriers that are related to the patient's meaning perspective. Some patients may require referral to the appropriate health professional to help them deal with effects related to trauma (e.g. post-traumatic stress) or physical abuse that are related to their pain and disability. Alternately, even though most physiotherapists do not have formal training in areas such as cognitive psychology, many aspects related to a patient's meaning perspective and emotional state can be positively influenced if the therapist can establish a suitable therapeutic relationship and create an appropriate environment for exploring and learning. A safe and supportive environment is key for patients to be able to express and explore their thoughts, ideas, and feelings. Expressing empathy 'through skillful reflective listening . . . to understand the client's feelings and perspectives without judging, criticizing, or blaming' can help create the desired environment (Miller & Rollnick 2002). The key catalyst for change is often awareness; as the patient becomes cognizant of the barrier that their thoughts, beliefs, and/or emotions are creating, they are able to discover new perspectives and potential solutions.

Methods of communication such as 'motivational interviewing' (Miller & Rollnick 2002) provide useful guidelines to create these environments.

> A general goal of motivational interviewing is to enhance the client's confidence in his or her capability to cope with obstacles and to succeed in change.
>
> Miller & Rollnick 2002.

Miller and Rollnick identify three key features that underlie the spirit of motivational interviewing: collaboration, evocation, and autonomy. On collaboration they note:

> The method of motivational interviewing involves exploration more than exhortation, and support rather than persuasion or argument. The interviewer seeks to create a positive interpersonal atmosphere that is conducive but not coercive to change.

On evocation:

> . . . the interviewer's tone is not one of imparting things (such as wisdom, insight, reality) but rather of eliciting, of finding these things within and drawing them out from the person . . . a drawing out of motivation from the person.

On autonomy:

> The overall goal is to increase intrinsic motivation, so that change arises from within rather than being imposed from without and so that change serves the person's own goals and values.
>
> Miller & Rollnick 2002.

The reader is referred to the book *Motivational interviewing: preparing people for change* (Miller & Rollnick 2002) for further exploration of these topics.

Becoming a skilled teacher is also an essential component for addressing a patient's understanding of their condition and pain experience, and the changes in behavior needed for recovery. Thus, increased understanding about education and learning theory are other areas for therapists to explore in order to increase their effectiveness in facilitating change (Higgs 2004). With respect to low back pain, Moseley (2002) has shown that a combination of physiotherapy and education regarding the neurophysiology of pain is effective in producing both symptomatic and functional change in the moderately disabled chronic group. It is interesting that health professionals often believe that patients will not understand the neurophysiology of chronic pain and therefore hold back this valuable information (Moseley 2003b). This is an example of a barrier to change created by the therapist's beliefs. The books *Explain pain* (Butler & Moseley 2003) and *Understand pain, live well again* (Pearson 2007) provide tools for therapists to help patients understand their pain experience and are recommended resources. They are available at www.noigroup.com and www.lifeisnow.ca.

Overall, it is essential that during the assessment and treatment process, the therapist can clearly identify the most significant features of the patient's meaning perspective that are creating a barrier to change and recovery. For some patients it may be their understanding of pain; for others it may be a loss of hope and lack of confidence in the ability of any health professional to help. These different barriers will require different information to facilitate a new meaning perspective. The potential diversity and combinations of restricting beliefs, expectations, motivations, and attitudes make it impossible to have a blanket approach to dealing with this category of barriers. Also note that life events, such as the death of a family member, can change the patient's emotional state and levels of stress at any point in the treatment process. These new events need to be factored into the effect on the patient's ability to participate in the rehabilitation process and the management strategy may have to be adapted given the new circumstances.

Addressing barriers: physical impairments – the rest of the Clinical Puzzle

Physical impairments relevant to the physiotherapy examination are classified according to the rest of the Clinical Puzzle (see Table 7.4a–d). Through the clinical reasoning process and careful analysis of the evolving puzzle, the primary system(s) driving the patient's non-optimal strategies for function and performance will become evident. Understanding the underlying impairment then allows the clinician to choose the most appropriate treatment techniques to release the old strategy. For example, if the primary impairment is altered motor control (neural system impairment), which is resulting in increased muscle tone and excessive compression of the inferior pole of the SIJ, but poor control of the same SIJ during vertical loading, the preferred treatment technique will be one that decreases excessive tone in the muscles that compress the inferior pole of the SIJ, and then to retrain the muscles that are better designed to control loading through the SIJ. Alternately, if the primary impairment is joint fibrosis that

is creating excessive compression of the SIJ joint (articular system impairment), the preferred treatment technique will be a grade IV sustained mobilization of the SIJ to address the restrictive articular structures. This does not, however, mean that the patient with the stiff, fibrotic SIJ will not have impairments in the neural system. Given the role that receptors in the ligaments, capsule, and fascia play in providing accurate proprioceptive information to the central nervous system, this patient will likely need to train a better strategy for function. The key is to time the implementation of the exercise program and other needed techniques appropriately, based on the information gained from the clinical reasoning process. This highlights the problems with designing research studies based only on pain presentation that then compare one modality or treatment technique with another. Patients often need a combination of techniques that address the relevant impairments in the appropriate order. In general, it is extremely rare not to have a neural system component to a patient's presentation, as impairments in the other pieces, if present for even short periods of time, create altered motor control. But the neural system impairment may or may not be the primary reason for altered strategies for function. Prescribing exercises to change motor control (addressing the neural system impairment) when there is an underlying articular restriction (fibrosis or fixation) will often result in failure at the exercises and an inability to change strategies, as well as increased pain and disability, in the worst-case scenario.

Alternately, if there is poor motion control due to the loss of integrity of the joint's ligaments and capsule (articular system impairment), the patient will alter motor control (neural system impairment) to compensate. Again, this is a case of altered motor control secondary to the articular impairment; that is, addressing the motor control impairment will not address the primary reason for the patient's problem and thus will not lead to resolution of the problem. However, removing the compensatory strategy is still an important step in the management program, as the non-optimal motor control usually creates malalignment and non-optimal force vectors of compression and tension that can perpetuate pain and poor function. Often the presence of a compensatory strategy makes it difficult to fully assess the function of the articular system (Chapter 8), and it is only when increased tone in the muscles involved in the substitution pattern is released that the articular structures can be confidently assessed. Releasing the compensatory strategy also allows for the teaching of a new strategy, which may need to be combined with prolotherapy in order to improve the integrity of the passive structures.

What follows is an outline of techniques that can be used to address the different impairments and remove the physical barriers to teaching a new strategy. These techniques will be further described in terms of 'how to' perform them in Chapter 10 (skill acquisition).

Impairments in the articular system (see Table 7.4a). For the fibrotic stiff joint, passive articular mobilization techniques are the most effective. The technique is graded according to the irritability of the articular tissues. Long-standing fibrosis requires a sustained grade 4+ passive mobilization. For the joint that is fixated (see Chapter 10 for a discussion on current thoughts regarding the possibility of joint fixation in the lumbopelvis), a passive articular manipulation technique is necessary to restore the joint's mobility.

When the driver behind the non-optimal strategy for function and performance is a loss of integrity of the articular restraints, and the deep muscles cannot compensate and control motion in the neutral zone, the articular impairment presents a barrier to restoring function. Prolotherapy (Cusi et al 2010, Dorman 1994, 1997) is indicated in these situations. Prolotherapy involves the injection of an irritant solution into the joint's ligaments that creates an inflammatory reaction. The subsequent migration of fibroblasts into the inflamed tissue promotes the production of collagen, which increases the stiffness of the ligament. Typically, the capsule/ligaments are injected every 2–6 weeks and the treatment is repeated for three to six sessions. The role of the therapist during this process is to ensure that motion of the joint is controlled with an external support (SIJ belt or tape) to prevent excessive shearing of the joint and to ensure that optimal alignment is maintained (balance the force vectors to maintain optimal joint alignment, see Chapter 10). As prolotherapy is often painful, the therapist also provides essential cognitive and emotional support during this process. Once activation of the deep muscles begins to affect motion in the neutral zone of motion (i.e. the joint glide can be reduced by a co-contraction of the deep muscles), anatomical recovery has begun. Training new and more optimal strategies for functional tasks can now begin.

Impairments in the myofascial system (see Table 7.4b). Many forms of myofascial release techniques can be used to increase mobility in the myofascial slings and in the fascial interfaces between muscles if there is restriction in this system. Scarring, adhesions, or increased laying down and bonding of connective tissue due to repetitive loading patterns can alter the force vectors (i.e. mechanical lines of tension and compression) that muscles create when they are activated (either with increased resting tone or dynamically). These non-optimal vectors can create resistance and difficulty when training new patterns of posture and movement and, thus, need to be addressed if present.

In some cases, loss of integrity in the myofascia (e.g. muscle strains, fascial tears, etc.) is present and driving non-optimal strategies for function and performance. If there is sufficient loss of integrity such that loads cannot be transferred through the myofascial structures (e.g. in some cases of diastasis rectus abdominis, or tears of the endopelvic fascia), or if there are adhesions that are extensive or entrapping painful structures (e.g. ilioinguinal nerve entrapment in some cases of hockey groin syndrome), surgery is indicated to restore integrity to the tissue or to release the adhesions.

Impairments in the neural system (see Table 7.4c). To downtrain, inhibit, or release hypertonic muscles, there are many techniques that decrease tone via neurophysiological mechanisms. Altering the drive to the alpha-motoneuron may occur at the spinal cord level or from higher centers. The choice of release technique will depend on a variety of factors and will be discussed in Chapter 10. Suitable techniques include:

1. release with awareness (Chapter 10);
2. self-release with awareness, stretch with awareness, active mobilization or muscle energy techniques (Chapter 10), functional or craniosacral techniques (not covered in this text);
3. grade I–III oscillatory joint mobilization (not covered in this text);
4. high acceleration, low amplitude muscle recoil technique (Chapter 10);
5. joint mobilization and high acceleration, low amplitude thrust (manipulation) (Chapter 10);
6. dry needling/intramuscular stimulation (IMS) (Chapter 10);
7. techniques to restore optimal breathing (Chapter 10);
8. movement approaches that incorporate breathing, relaxation, and movement with awareness (Chapters 10, 11, 12); and
9. finding the optimal lumbopelvic pyramid and training neutral spine strategies (Chapter 11).

Impairments in the visceral system (see Table 7.4d). Addressing underlying visceral disease may require medical intervention and thus it is essential that the clinician be aware of non-mechanical patterns of pain and indicators of visceral disease. For mobility and fascial/ligamentous restrictions in the visceral system, the reader is referred to methods such as those developed by Jean-Pierre Barral, known as visceral manipulation (www.barralinstitute.com).

Train a new strategy based on meaningful tasks

The key components of teaching new strategies for function and performance are:

1. waking up and coordinating the deep and superficial muscle systems (Chapter 11);
2. training a new strategy for posture (Chapter 12); and
3. training a new strategy for movement (Chapter 12).

The specific background and the techniques will be covered in later chapters; here we will discuss some key principles to consider when developing the treatment program.

General principles

Optimize neuroplasticity. Training a new strategy for motor components, as well as for cognitive, behavioral, and emotional components, relies on the ability of the patient to *learn* the new strategy. The underlying mechanism for any learning (motor skills, perceptual, cognitive) is brain plasticity (Merzenich et al 1996).

> Brain plasticity refers to the lifelong capacity for physical and functional change; it is this capacity that explains how experience induces learning throughout life.
>
> Mahncke et al 2006.

Previously, it was thought that the brain was only plastic in infancy and childhood; it is now well established that neural maps in the brain change throughout life.

> … the brain is plastic; that is, the brain is capable of reorganization, including developing new short-range interconnections, at any age throughout adult life.
>
> Mahncke et al 2006.

Research in neuroscience and experimental psychology, as well as clinical approaches in neuro-rehabilitation, provide us with insight into the key components necessary for the laying down of new neural networks and driving brain change (Doidge 2007, Mahncke et al 2006, Merzenich et al 1996, Morris et al 2006, Moucha & Kilgard 2006). As Merzenich et al (1996) notes,

> Cognitive neuroscience studies also reveal the most effective strategies for driving brain change. The subject must be attentive and motivated. The training must be progressive and adapted to each training subject. The training schedule must be repetitious and intense.
>
> Merzenich et al 1996.

The underlying neurophysiological mechanisms that 'drive brain change' are beyond the scope of this text; however, the essential clinical components emerge in the literature. The most effective strategies include consistent features, and are:

1. highly focused attention and awareness. Studies have shown that 'paying close attention is essential to long-term plastic change' (Doidge 2007). If tasks are performed without awareness and focus, brain maps change, but the changes do not last. Therefore, if you want to make lasting strategy changes, exercises have to be performed with a fully engaged brain, focused in the moment (not while watching the evening news, for example);
2. massed practice that is task-oriented. The exercise can be component movements of the goal task if the patient cannot perform at the level of task complexity required for the functional movement. Morris et al (1996) refer to this as 'shaping,' whereby a motor objective is approached in small steps by successive approximations. Although high numbers of repetitions are the goal, the pattern and timing of the firing of the neurons is also key. 'Neurons that fire together, wire together; neurons out of sync fail to link' (Doidge 2007, Hebb 1949, Merzenich et al 1996). This speaks to the need for practicing quality of movement in as much quantity as possible; 'practice makes permanent, not perfect.' It is essential to show patients ways to determine when they have lost the quality of movement and then to stop practice for that session;
3. using tasks that have meaning and providing positive feedback. Tasks that have meaning will capture patients' attention, and factors such as attention, reward, and novelty are known to enhance plasticity by increasing the release of

specific neurotransmitters such as dopamine and acetylcholine (Mahncke et al 2006). Positive feedback could be considered a form of 'reward' that enhances neuromodulatory function;

4. providing specific patterns of sensory stimulation related to the task. It is known that 'sensory input determines the form of cortical reorganization' and that 'perceptual learning and cortical plasticity are specific to attended sensory features' (Moucha & Kilgard 2006). These findings from physiological studies provide a possible explanation for our clinical observation that the location, timing, and modulation of sensory (tactile) cuing can make significant changes in the strategy used for task performance. Together with verbal cues and encouragement, they provide a powerful stimulus to facilitate change;

5. plateaus in progress are normal and are actually only 'apparent' plateaus. These are 'part of a plasticity-based learning cycle – in which stages of learning are followed by periods of consolidation. Though there [is] no apparent progress in the consolidation stage, biological changes [are] happening internally, as new skills [become] more automatic and refined' (Doidge 2007).

It is important to educate patients that this is normal and to be expected, so that they do not get discouraged by the apparent slowing of progress.

Finally, consider that science continues to provide more and more evidence that our manual therapy techniques have effects via neurophysiological mechanisms (Chapter 10). The changes from various forms of 'manual magic' can last for varying duration, but generally are not sustained, which is consistent with neuroplasticity principles. That is, the changes in muscle tone, available range of motion, and pain that we can effect with manual techniques provide us with a window to then lay down new brain maps. This has implications for how clinicians allocate their treatment session time, and indeed how long appointment times should be. The most effective time to perform massed, focused practice is immediately following the manual release techniques, with the specific guidance, feedback, and encouragement of the clinician in a one-on-one setting. Sending patients home after a quick demonstration with a photocopied 'exercise sheet,' with little practice done in the clinic, is much less likely to create lasting change.

Reinforce 'letting go' of the old strategy. In order to facilitate the formation of new brain maps, it is essential to stop patients from using the old maps. During the process of removing the non-optimal strategies, the clinician will have learned which tactile and verbal cues and images are most effective in helping the patient 'let go' of holding key muscles, postural patterns, and movement patterns. It is essential that the clinician continue to use these verbal and tactile cues at the same time as the new strategies are taught. For example, if a patient tends to be a back-gripper, and overuses the erector spinae during tasks, the cuing sequence for learning a new strategy would involve first cuing to 'let the muscles in your back relax and melt,' followed immediately by the cue for using a different muscle such as transversus abdominis, 'Now think of a line connecting the two bones in the front of your pelvis and drawing them together.' It is also important that you help the patient understand that, in order to live and move differently in their body, knowing how to 'let go' of the old strategy is just as important as learning 'how to do' a new strategy.

Educate the patient. There are many different ways that patients perceive and understand the word 'training' or 'exercise.' It is essential that patients understand that training a new strategy is not related to approaches they may have been exposed to in community gym settings that are about strength, power, or endurance of muscles. Basically, the clinician needs to portray that this is a new approach to 'exercise,' which is about changing the way the brain is programmed, and about how the brain accesses different programs for posture and movement. Thus, *quality* of movement is key, and is not to be lost at the expense of *quantity*. It is helpful to remind patients that the program is not really about exercise, but rather about 'changing the way you live in your body.' Discussing the known changes that occur in the motor control system with pain and injury (see Chapters 4 and 5) is also useful to highlight that the patient's main deficit is not one of muscle strength but one of recruiting the right muscles at the right time and in the right coordination with other muscles. If, indeed, there are strength losses due to deconditioning and disuse, it is still first desirable to train the correct patterning and synergy of the muscle system, and then to work on strength and endurance parameters in functional movements, which can also occur in conjunction with a progressive program for increasing cardiovascular fitness relevant to patient goals. In Chapter 11 we discuss how to use load, perceived effort, and resisted tests to illustrate the impact of proper recruitment synergies and the effect that the deep muscles can have on strength output so that patients can experience and understand the role of optimal motor control (interoceptive facilitation).

Be specific and choose tasks with meaning. Ensure that any 'exercise' you prescribe has relevance to the patient's needs and goals. This affects all dimensions of their experience (sensorial, cognitive, and emotional), and is not just related to biomechanical factors. Breaking down functional tasks into component movement blocks is a way of building towards functional patterns; be sure to discuss and demonstrate to the patient how the training task you are prescribing relates to either their aggravating activities or their goals. Furthermore, in order to ensure that the treatment program addresses the key impairments that are driving the non-optimal strategy, the clinician must design the program around:

1. the segment(s) of poor control;
2. the direction(s) of poor control;
3. the levels or regions of restricted mobility;
4. the overactive/dominant superficial muscles;
5. the inactive/inappropriately recruited muscles;
6. specific muscle length/strength imbalances; and
7. characteristics of the goal tasks such as cardiovascular requirements, load requirements, mobility requirements, level of predictability, etc.

Any training task given to the patient should always be assessed in light of the impact it has on the hypothesized pain-generating structures and mechanisms, as well as whether or not it is addressing key deficits identified in the assessment.

Wake up and coordinate the deep and superficial muscle systems

Increasing evidence supports the need for, and effectiveness of, isolation training for the deep muscles of the lumbopelvic canister (Chapter 11). Which muscles to train depends on the findings from the assessment. For some patients, starting with training a co-contraction of transversus abdominis and deep multifidus may be indicated. We still consider this 'isolation' training as it is focusing on the deep muscle system in isolation from the superficial muscle system. Chapter 11 covers how to train the deep system along with ways that

patients can self-monitor and self-progress their training routine as they learn to build better patterns for coordinating the deep and superficial muscle systems.

Postural training and movement training

Training new strategies for aggravating or goal-related postures and movement tasks (i.e. meaningful tasks) begins as early as possible in the treatment program. As soon as there is any letting go of the non-optimal strategies, components of new postural and movement strategies can be taught. For example, as unilateral butt-gripping is released, the patient can be taught how to sit symmetrically and equally on the ischial tuberosities, and to seat the femoral head in the sitting position. This will facilitate optimal intrapelvic alignment and a centered hip joint, and often relieves groin and/or posterior pelvic girdle pain in sitting. It is not necessary to correct all components of the posture or movement task right away; starting with two or three key alignment points or control points is enough to begin to train a new strategy. Chapter 12 will provide further specifics on how to train new strategies for posture and movement tasks.

Role of supports: sacroiliac belts and taping

Sacroiliac belts. A sacroiliac belt can be a useful adjunct for external support of the LPH complex at this time in the therapeutic process. Although the mechanisms of how belts and tape work remain unclear, it is known that the stiffness of the SIJ is enhanced when a generic belt is worn just below the anterior superior iliac spines (ASISs) (Damen et al 2002b). There are many sacroiliac belts on the market and most will be effective in providing some degree of compression/support to the pelvic girdle (Vleeming et al 1992a). However, patients often require more or less compression than a general belt can supply and it is often difficult to specify the location of the compression (bilateral anterior, bilateral posterior, unilateral anterior, and/or unilateral posterior) with a general belt. This led to the development of The Com-Pressor, a patented belt that allows compression to be applied specifically to different aspects of the pelvic girdle (Lee 2002) (Fig. 9.4A).

The Com-Pressor SI belt is used in conjunction with 'waking up the deep system' and 'training a

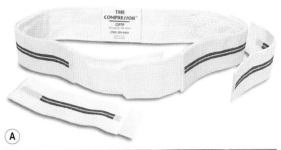

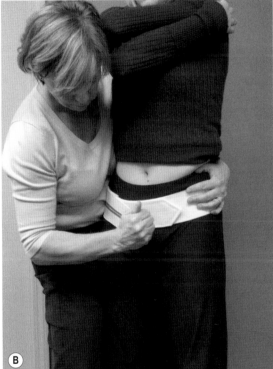

(A)

(B)

Fig. 9.4 • (A) The Com-Pressor is a patented sacroiliac belt designed to provide specific support to the pelvic girdle. The application of the tensile straps is determined by the findings of the active straight leg raise test. (B) The straps are applied with the patient standing, firmly anchoring the strap at the lateral aspect of the pelvis first and then stretching the strap and applying the other end to the midline either anteriorly or posteriorly.

new strategy for posture and for movement,' and is thought to provide both mechanical support and proprioceptive input to remind the brain which muscle(s) need facilitation. It is also likely that by providing the 'missing vectors' of support, the patient is less likely to return to non-optimal substitution strategies. How does the belt do this? The Com-Pressor supports the pelvis through the tension of

four very strong elastic straps. The straps are attached to an underlying body belt (Fig. 9.4B) that is applied around the pelvis just below the ASISs if the need is to compress the SIJs (Damen et al 2002a,b), and just above the greater trochanters if the need is to compress the pubic symphysis (Vleeming et al 1992). The location(s) of the compression strap(s) is variable and depends on the specific needs of the patient determined by the active straight leg raise (ASLR) test (Chapter 8). Further details on how this belt is integrated into the treatment program and specifically applied can be found throughout the case reports and will be discussed further in Chapter 11.

Tape. 'Missing vectors' can also be provided with tape applied directly to the skin over the pelvis. It is essential to apply the tape in standing, after release of the non-optimal strategy, and based on the clinical reasoning process used with the ASLR to decide where to apply compression. Tape is often better to use during activities or sports where the belt may move around, or where uniforms or other clothing will not accommodate the belt. Therapists who have taken our courses have also reported using tape over the Com-Pressor belt to augment specific vectors and maintain its position during vigorous sports activity. Cover-Roll is used as a base layer, and then Leukotape is applied while the therapist provides compression to the pelvis in the needed direction (Fig. 9.5; see case report Christy, Chapter 9, and Video 12.13 🖲).

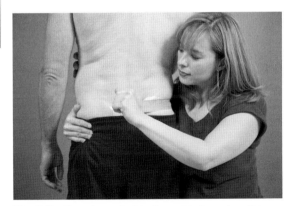

Fig. 9.5 • Tape is applied to the pelvis based on the findings from the active straight leg raise test. A base piece of Cover-Roll tape is applied in the direction of the appropriate vector. This therapist is applying compression across the pelvis using her right shoulder and a counter-pressure with the right hand to create posterior compression across the right side of the pelvis; Leukotape is applied while the compression is maintained.

Case reports

In the book, *The brain that changes itself,* Doidge (2007) notes the importance that well-known neuroscientist V. S. Ramachandran places on individual patient cases. Ramachandran believes that individual cases have everything to contribute to science and is quoted as saying,

> Imagine I were to present a pig to a skeptical scientist, insisting it could speak English, then waved my hand, and the pig spoke English. Would it really make sense for the skeptic to argue, 'But that is just one pig, Ramachandran. Show me another, and I might believe you!'

In addition to adding to science, case reports assist in constructing links between propositional, non-propositional or craft, and personal knowledge (Jones & Rivett 2004). What follows are the case reports of several patients all of whom presented with LPH pain in a variety of locations, some derived through trauma (sport and pregnancy) and some through maladaptive habits after macro- or microtrauma. All of them complained of increased pain with vertical loading tasks (standing, sitting, walking, and/or running) and all had been dealing with their pain and disability for at least 6 months.

The intention is to illustrate through these case reports how The Integrated Systems Model and clinical reasoning are used to understand the various findings (i.e. form hypotheses) and how the Clinical Puzzle facilitates both this reasoning process and subsequent management. The Integrated Systems Model provides a framework and helps to subgroup patients with LPH pain and impairment so that treatment is more likely to be effective. We would like to take a moment to acknowledge and thank the real people in these stories who gave us permission to share their journeys with you. Be sure to watch the online videos that accompany the case reports as you read the stories for more clinical reasoning 'on the fly.'

Only one case report is published in the hard copy of this text, the rest will be found in the ebook online (🖱). There are over 200 video clips online associated with this text and they illustrate many, if not all, of the tests found in Chapter 8 as well as the release techniques found in Chapter 10 and the training practice found in Chapters 11 and 12.

Laura – postpartum pelvic control impairment with associated stress urinary incontinence (neural system impairment)

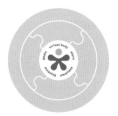

Laura's story

Laura was a 40-year-old mother of two children (ages nine and four) who presented with increasing concerns regarding her persistent pelvic girdle pain and incontinence. The pelvic girdle pain began during the fifth month of her second pregnancy. Both of her children were delivered vaginally; she had a small episiotomy with the first and no apparent pelvic floor trauma with the second. Laura reported having intermittent stress urinary incontinence (SUI) as a young gymnast during sudden vertical loading tasks (e.g. landing a vault). The SUI became more frequent after the birth of her children. Her current primary complaints included:

1. pain over the region of the right SIJ aggravated by sitting and combined plane loading tasks (walking, running, and forward bending); and

2. stress urinary incontinence that limited her ability to run (2 minutes maximum). She also experienced urinary leakage when sneezing and felt that this was worse when her bladder was full.

On specific questioning of her respiratory function, she also noticed intermittent holding of her breath and excessive yawning throughout the day. She felt that her primary problem was a weak pelvic floor and felt guilty that she was not doing enough strengthening or 'Kegel' exercises. Of note, her mother had urinary incontinence and two surgeries had not resolved her problem. Laura expressed concern that she would follow her mother's journey.

Laura was not currently engaged in any regular physical activity, finding that her duties as a physiotherapist and a mother kept her very busy. Her goal was to feel less tired during the day and to be able to run without incontinence. Based on her story,

Fig. 9.6 • Laura's complete Clinical Puzzle. Return to this figure as you read and consider the findings from Laura's story. L = left, R = right, IPTL = intrapelvic torsion left, TPRL = transverse plane rotation left, FB = forward bending, ✓ = optimal findings, BB = backward bending, SIJ = sacroiliac joint, RPF = right pelvic floor, OLS = one leg standing, RHL = right harder than left to lift, 1° c/o = primary complaints, Aggr = aggravating tasks, mob = mobility, R<L = right less than left, ↓RR = decreased right rotation, Imp = improves, LEO = left external oblique, RRF = right rectus femoris, Radd = right adductors, RsMF = right superficial multifidus, RThEs = right thoracic erector spinae.

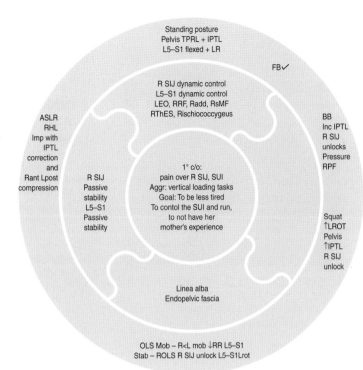

Standing posture
Pelvis TPRL + IPTL
L5–S1 flexed + LR

FB✓

R SIJ dynamic control
L5–S1 dynamic control
LEO, RRF, Radd, RsMF
RThES, Rischiococcygeus

ASLR
RHL
Imp with
IPTL
correction
and
Rant Lpost
compression

R SIJ
Passive
stability
L5–S1
Passive
stability

1° c/o:
pain over R SIJ, SUI
Aggr: vertical loading tasks
Goal: To be less tired
To contol the SUI and run,
to not have her
mother's experience

BB
Inc IPTL
R SIJ
unlocks
Pressure
RPF

Squat
↑LROT
Pelvis
↑IPTL
R SIJ
unlock

Linea alba
Endopelvic fascia

OLS Mob – R<L mob ↓RR L5–S1
Stab – ROLS R SIJ unlock L5–S1Lrot

the meaningful tasks chosen for strategy analysis were standing posture, forward bending, squat (stand to sit), and one leg standing. Her Clinical Puzzle began by entering her primary complaints and goals in the center (Fig. 9.6).

Narrative reasoning at this point

Sensorial dimension: Pelvic girdle pain and stress urinary incontinence are common complaints for a significant number of postpartum women and the location and behavior of Laura's pelvic girdle pain was consistent with an inability to transfer load effectively through the musculoskeletal and visceral components of the pelvic girdle. Her pain appeared to be predominantly peripherally mediated.

Cognitive dimension: Laura believed that her main problem was a weak pelvic floor caused by the vaginal delivery of her children. This belief would need some collaborative discussion during the treatment sessions once a reason for her incontinence was understood. This symptom had more meaning for her than her pelvic girdle pain.

Emotional dimension: She harbored some guilt that she was not doing her exercises and worried that, as her mother was incontinent in spite of two surgeries, she would be too.

Strategies for function and performance

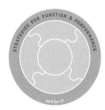

Standing posture

In standing, Laura's pelvis was rotated to the left in the transverse plane secondary to a unilateral anterior pelvic sway on the right (Fig. 9.7, Video LC1 🖰). This rotation was associated with an intrapelvic torsion to the left (IPTL) and a flexed, left rotated L5–S1. There was slightly more tension in the right inguinal ligament compared to the left; however, the right femoral head did not appear to be anteriorly displaced relative to the acetabulum. When her pelvis was manually brought to a neutral centered position, a vector of force resisting this motion was felt from the short adductors of the right hip (Video LC2 🖰). As you watch this video,

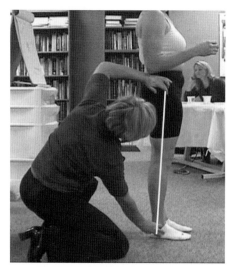

Fig. 9.7 • Laura's standing posture. Note the anterior displacement of the right greater trochanter relative to the right lateral malleolus. The pelvis is swayed anteriorly with respect to the pedal base.

note the position of her thorax as her pelvis is centered (thorax rotates to the right). The cause of this will become clear later.

Forward bending

Laura was able to forward bend with no increase in pelvic girdle pain. Her femoral heads remained centered in the acetabulum, the left intrapelvic torsion of her pelvis reduced to neutral, and the SIJs remained controlled throughout the task (Video LC3). At this time, this task was performed with an optimal strategy.

Backward bending

During backward bending, the left transverse plane rotation of the pelvis, as well as the IPTL, increased secondary to the appearance of two other vectors of force, one from the right rectus femoris (RF failed to eccentrically lengthen during this task) (Fig. 9.8A, Video LC4). and the other from the left external oblique. The right side of the pelvis unlocked quite early in this task (Fig. 9.8B). Laura reported feeling increased pressure in the right side of her pelvic floor when she bent backward. It is interesting to note that she did not complain of any pain during tasks that required backward bending of the trunk although she did report difficulty with

her continence during running, a task that requires unilateral hip extension.

Reflection and hypothesis development at this point

Several force vectors were acting on Laura's pelvis during both static standing and backward bending. The resultant net force vector was creating a rotation of her pelvis to the left (thorax to the right), an IPTL, and unlocking of the right side of the pelvis. The muscles identified so far that were potentially contributing to this malalignment and non-optimal movement strategy were the short adductors of the right hip, the left external oblique, and the right rectus femoris. Were these non-optimal force vectors impacting other loading tasks? More tests of loading were necessary to answer this question and to develop a hypothesis for the findings noted; meanwhile the findings from these tasks were recorded in Laura's Clinical Puzzle in the outer circle (Fig. 9.6).

One leg standing

Laura's ability to stand on one leg and flex the contralateral hip was evaluated next. She found it more difficult to stand on the right leg. With respect to intrapelvic mobility during this task (ability of the innominate to posteriorly rotate relative to the sacrum), asymmetry of motion was noted in that the right innominate appeared to posteriorly rotate less than the left (Video LC5). In addition, right rotation of L5–S1, which should occur as the right innominate posteriorly rotates, did not occur.

During left single leg loading the left side of the pelvis and hip remained controlled, whereas during right single leg loading the right side of the pelvis unlocked and L5–S1 rotated to the left (Video LC6). The loss of control at L5–S1 occurred *after* the right side of the pelvis unlocked. The right rectus femoris and tensor fascia latae appeared hyperactive during right single leg standing; however, the femoral head remained centered during this task.

Squat

During a squat, the left transverse plane rotation of the pelvis increased, as did the IPTL, and once again the right side of the pelvis unlocked.

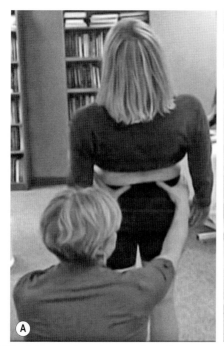
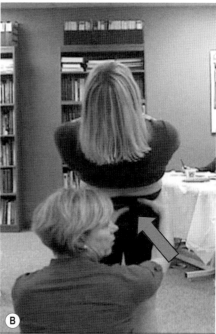

Fig. 9.8 • (A) The left transverse plane rotation of Laura's pelvis as well as the intrapelvic torsion to the left increases during backward bending. (B) The right side of the pelvis unlocks very early during this backward bending task.

Reflection and hypothesis development at this point

Multiple tasks (right one leg standing (ROLS), squat, backward bending (BB)) revealed poor control of L5–S1 and the right SIJ. Two hypotheses that could explain these findings are:

1. loss of integrity of the passive system restraints of both L5–S1 and the right SIJ (articular system impairment); and/or
2. loss of dynamic control of both L5–S1 and the right SIJ (neural system impairment).

Further tests were required for the articular system of both of these joints (passive restraints) as well as the neural system (dynamic control) to determine which hypothesis is more likely; these joints were recorded in Laura's Clinical Puzzle in both the articular system and the neural system piece of her Clinical Puzzle for further analysis (Fig. 9.6).

Active straight leg raise

In the supine position, Laura's pelvis continued to rest in an IPTL, which indicated that the vectors of force that were creating the malalignment in standing persisted in supine (i.e. there is maintained activity in muscles despite a change in task). During the ASLR task, she found it more difficult to lift the right leg off of the table, and when compression was applied to her pelvis without first correcting the intrapelvic torsion (Video LC7) there was minimal change in the effort required to lift the right leg. When the pelvic position was manually corrected (right innominate posteriorly rotated and the left innominate anteriorly rotated), and then an oblique compression force applied to the anterior aspect of the right innominate and the posterior aspect of the left innominate, the effort required to lift the right leg was markedly reduced.

Interpretive reasoning at this point

The findings from the active straight leg raise test suggested that her program should begin with releasing the vectors of force that were creating the malalignment of her pelvis before any training of the muscles of the lumbopelvic–hip complex (release the old strategy before training a new one).

The myofascial system

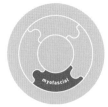

The fascia of the anterior abdominal wall plays a key role for the transfer of forces across the anterior midline. All postpartum women who present with pelvic girdle pain and/or urinary incontinence require an evaluation of the integrity of the linea alba as this structure is considerably stretched during pregnancy. Laura's linea alba had tolerated this stretch quite well; the inter-recti distance was within average limits both at rest and during a curl-up task (Video LC8) throughout its entire length. In addition, the linea alba had a firm posterior fascial barrier; the midline anterior abdominal fascia was intact, and therefore should be responsive to a contraction of the left and right transversus abdominis (TrA) (the fascia should be able to transmit forces generated by the muscle's contraction).

The neural system

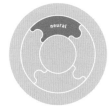

A clinical evaluation of the response of the deep and superficial muscle systems to a verbal cue was assessed. While palpating the lower abdominal wall, increased tension was felt superficially on the left, although a deeper level of palpation (to the level of TrA) was still possible. Subsequently, the response of the left and right TrA to a verbal cue to contract the pelvic floor was assessed; no response from TrA, IO, or EO was felt with this cue. However, when an abdominal cue was given (e.g. imagine a guy wire connecting your two hip bones (ASISs) and gently connect along this line), the left TrA responded in isolation from the left IO and EO whereas the right did not (Video LC9). An ultrasound imaging unit was not available at this time to confirm the palpation findings. Given the tension noted in

the left superficial abdominal wall, attention was then directed to the left external oblique (Video LC10). Rotation of her thorax was notably restricted both to the left and to the right; however, left rotation was more restricted and the vector of resistance was felt to be coming from the left anterior abdominal wall. Subsequent palpation for hypertonicity in the left anterior abdominal wall revealed increased resting tone in a specific fascicle of the left EO and the diaphragm at the left seventh and eighth ribs (Video LC10).

With respect to the deep fibers of multifidus, there was no response to any verbal cue in the right deep fibers of multifidus at L5–S1 and hypertonicity was noted on palpation of the right superficial fibers of multifidus from L3 to the iliac crest as well as the right thoracic erector spinae.

With respect to her pelvic floor, it was not possible to know if the verbal cue was actually affecting a response from the levator ani as neither an internal nor ultrasound imaging evaluation was possible at this time; Laura was a participant of one of our courses and, as mentioned previously, an ultrasound unit was not available. She was advised to see DL in the clinic in 3 weeks' time for follow-up and to assess the function of her pelvic floor (perineal UI).

Reflection and hypothesis development at this point

Collectively the vectors produced by hypertonicity of the superficial muscles (the left external oblique, right thoracic erector spine, right rectus femoris, and right adductor) were inducing right rotation of the thorax/left rotation of the pelvis and consequently the IPTL. With respect to the deep muscles, neither the right TrA nor the right dMF at the lumbosacral junction was responsive to either a pelvic floor or abdominal cue. An analysis of the pelvic floor would add more clarity to the clinical picture – a much needed piece at this time.

The strategies that Laura used during multiple loading tasks failed to control the right SIJ and L5–S1 (loss of rotational control). Why? So far, we know that Laura's abdominal myofascial system was intact and that she had a significant impairment in the neural system of the LPH complex that was likely contributing to these non-optimal strategies. Was there also an underlying impairment in the articular system (right SIJ, L5–S1)? To answer this question the passive restraints at L5–S1 and the right SIJ required analysis, as did their dynamic control.

The articular system

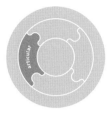

Sacroiliac joints

The right sacroiliac joint was compressed superiorly by hypertonicity of the right superficial fibers of multifidus (noted above to run from L3 to the iliac crest) and inferiorly by hypertonicity of the right ischio-coccygeus (confirmed by palpation) (Video LC11). Release of these force vectors was required before an assessment of the integrity of the passive restraints of the right SIJ could be done and were entered into the neural system piece of Laura's Clinical Puzzle (Fig. 9.6).

Lumbar joints

A 'softer' end feel (resistance) to posterior translation in flexion at L5–S1 was noted. The end feel of posterior translation in extension at L5–S1 was firm and consistent with levels above (Video LC12). This suggests that the passive restraints that control full segmental flexion at L5–S1 were compromised. However, clinical experience suggests that, when there is decreased resting tone and/or atrophy of the deep fibers of multifidus, this test is often falsely positive. When the test is repeated after restoring function to the deep fibers of multifidus, it is often negative, thus ruling out a passive restraint, or articular system, impairment. Dynamically, L5–S1 was poorly controlled when a flexion force was applied to the trunk with the joint in its neutral position.

Clinical impression derived from hypothesis development, reflection, interpretive reasoning, and abductive logic

From this initial assessment, the hypothesis was that Laura had a pain disorder that was peripherally mediated due to poor control of the right SIJ and L5–S1, and according to The Integrated Systems Model her primary impairment was in the neural system. What remained to be assessed was the function of her pelvic floor (neural system function and integrity of the endopelvic fascia (myofascial system)). In addition, the integrity of the ligaments of the right SIJ was still uncertain (articular system). If this hypothesis was correct, restoring the function of the neural system (specifically the activation of the deep fibers of multifidus) should change the findings of the articular system restraints test for L5–S1; this should be retested at a later session to provide further confirmation of the initial hypothesis. The findings were explained to Laura and the hypothesis proposed as to how they could collectively be causing both her pelvic girdle pain and incontinence. Following the principles of The Integrated Systems Model approach, the following initial treatment plan was implemented, keeping in mind that the primary symptom with meaning for her was stress urinary incontinence.

Initial treatment

Remove the non-optimal strategy by addressing barriers

The following muscles were released with a combination of techniques including positional release, release with awareness, and manual therapy (high acceleration, low amplitude thrust (HALAT) specific to L3–4) (Chapter 10):

1. right short adductors and rectus femoris;
2. right ischiococcygeus (positional release, release with awareness);
3. right superficial fibers of multifidus from L3 to the iliac crest (positional release, release with awareness, HALAT to L3–4); and
4. right thoracic erector spinae (high acceleration muscle spring technique) and external oblique/ diaphragm (positional release and stretch) (Video LC13).

Subsequently, the position of Laura's pelvis in standing was restored to neutral (but not the thorax), the active mobility of the right SIJ was restored and the strategy used for both single leg loading (OLS test) and squatting was initially optimal (no unlocking of the right side of the pelvis) (Video LC14); however, when the task was repeated, the right side of the pelvis tended to unlock. A clear parallel glide was now present at all three parts of the right SIJ, which could then be taken into a close-packed position to test the integrity of the passive restraints (articular system); they were found to be intact.

Her pelvis could now rest in a neutral position in supine lying.

Subsequent repeat analysis of the response of the deep muscle system to a verbal cue revealed a persistent delay of the right TrA and minimal activation of the right deep lumbosacral multifidus.

Train a new strategy based on meaningful tasks

Wake up the deep system. Subsequent to releasing these vectors of force, Laura was taught to co-contract the deep muscle system using imagery to facilitate the motor programming (Video LC15 🖱). An anterior pelvic floor cue (squeeze the muscles around your urethra) still did not elicit a response from either the left or right TrA, but a cue to lift the vagina and a cue to connect the anus to the back of the pubic bone did. However, the best cue for co-contraction of the left and right TrA was an abdominal cue (e.g. connect the ASISs).

None of these cues resulted in activation of the right dMF at the lumbosacral junction. However, a suspension cue for L5–S1 resulted in an isolated response of the right dMF. The resultant 'chord' cue (best cue for co-contraction synergy of all the deep muscles) was to first gently suspend L5 off of S1 and then follow this with an image to connect the ASISs anteriorly. The best cue for adding in/on the pelvic floor would be determined following the ultrasound examination 3 weeks later. Ideally, it would have been done at this point (first treatment).

When practicing this isolation co-contraction at home, Laura was advised to watch for any return of the IPTL and instructed on how to release the likely cause (right short adductors), if present (Video LC16 🖱) before her training practice. Ensuring that her pelvis was in neutral alignment, she was instructed to isolate the co-contraction and then to breathe normally for 10 seconds and to repeat this isolation task 10 times for three sets (the evidence for this protocol is presented in Chapter 11 (Tsao & Hodges 2007, 2008)). It is important to 'rewire the neural network' with a strategy that incorporates breathing into the task.

Integrate this motor program into functional tasks and reassess strategies for function and performance. Laura was then taught how to integrate the co-contraction of the deep muscles into loading tasks (Videos LC17, LC18 🖱) with an optimal strategy that ensured she was able to transfer loads through the LPH complex efficiently and safely in spite of predictable and unpredictable internal and external perturbations (Chapters 11, 12). Once again, the hypothesis of how altered motor control could be causing her pelvic girdle pain and incontinence was discussed with ample opportunity for any questions or concerns she had. Her compliance and commitment to this movement practice was essential for rewiring the neural network and her long-term success.

Follow-up 3 weeks later

After this first treatment, Laura reported feeling much better for 2–3 days and that the location of her pain had changed from the region of the right SIJ to the right superolateral buttock and groin. As neither a pain score nor a functional abilities score (PSFS) was obtained during the initial evaluation, this can only be considered a subjective report and may be biased or invalid. She also noted that for 2 weeks she did not yawn at work, and that this had only recurred over the previous few days.

A key missing neural and myofascial piece of the Clinical Puzzle from the first assessment was an analysis of her pelvic floor function (ability to activate in response to a verbal cue and the integrity of the endopelvic fascia). In addition, all postpartum women require a screen of the linea alba and its response to a curl-up task. This is best assessed via ultrasound imaging (Chapter 8) and was done first to complete her Clinical Puzzle.

The pelvic floor

Perineal ultrasound imaging was used to assess the function of Laura's pelvic floor during various tasks. When given three different cues to contract the pelvic floor:

1. squeeze the muscles around the urethra;
2. lift the vagina;
3. imagine a line connecting the anus to the back of the pubic bone and connect along this line;

the vector of the resultant lift was noted to be non-optimal (towards the middle of the bladder as opposed to the neck of the urethra) (Fig. 9.9A,B, Video LC19 🖱). A posteroinferior displacement of the bladder occurred during a Valsalva when it was performed without a precontraction of the pelvic floor. The displacement could be controlled when the pelvic floor was activated before the Valsalva maneuver. The same displacement of

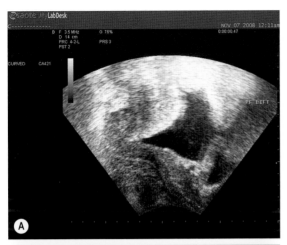

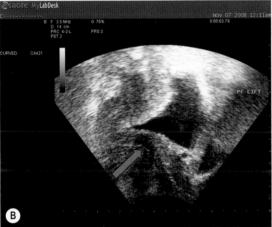

Fig. 9.9 • Perineal ultrasound image of the pelvic organs. (A) Resting image of Laura's pelvic organs from a perineal view. (B) The vector of lift from a contraction of Laura's pelvic floor. Note how the arrow is directed towards the middle/back of the bladder as opposed to the neck of the urethra; this is a non-optimal vector of lift.

the bladder was seen during a cough, and a precontraction of the pelvic floor did not control this displacement.

The abdominal wall

Subsequently, a clinical and an ultrasound imaging evaluation of the abdominal wall and deep lumbosacral multifidus revealed the following. It was now easy to reach the layer of TrA through the abdominal wall; the tension of the left side noted in the first examination was no longer present. Laura was now able to recruit the deep muscles synergistically

Reflection and hypothesis development at this point

During the first assessment, no verbal cue to contract the pelvic floor resulted in a response from the transversus abdominis (TrA). The hypothesis at that time was that Laura was possibly not activating her pelvic floor. The findings from this test negate that hypothesis as Laura was able to contract her pelvic floor with all three verbal cues; however, the vector of lift was non-optimal. This may be due to adhesions between/within the pelvic floor muscles and/or endopelvic fascia or a non-optimal recruitment strategy of the various muscles comprising the pelvic floor. An internal examination would be required to differentiate these causes. Of concern was the posterior displacement of the bladder during both the Valsalva and cough maneuvers. A precontraction of the pelvic floor prior to the Valsalva (the Knack) did control the bladder descent, whereas it did not when she coughed. This examination suggests that there was laxity of the endopelvic fascia (poor bladder support) and further tests via internal examination were necessary to confirm/negate this hypothesis. An appointment with a certified pelvic floor therapist was scheduled. The fact that this pelvic floor contraction did not result in a response of the TrA suggests that the reflex connection between the two muscles was disordered and that a pelvic floor cue would not be the best cue to initiate a synergistic response of the deep muscles.

(left and right TrA and left and right dMF) in isolation from the superficial abdominals and the erector spinae (Video LC20). However, during a curl-up task (Fig. 9.10A), both TrAs appeared to be inactive and the internal oblique actually slid lateral over the top of the TrA (Fig. 9.10B, Video LC20). In other words, although she could activate the deep muscles, the strategy she chose for the curl-up task did not activate the left or right TrA.

What was the impact of this strategy on the linea alba? Just above the level of the umbilicus, the interrecti distance was 0.96cm, well within suggested normal limits (Fig. 9.11A) (Chapter 6). During a curl-up task, minimal tension appeared to develop in the linea alba (Fig. 9.11B, Video LC21); the linea alba appeared to 'droop' between the left and right rectus abdominis. When she precontracted the TrA and then did a curl-up, tension was evident in the linea alba (Fig. 9.12, Video LC22) and a screen of her ability to isolate a deep muscle system contraction revealed that she still had a tendency to co-contract the left IO with the left TrA.

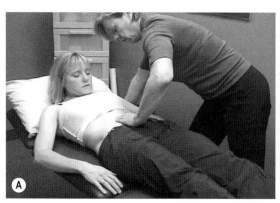
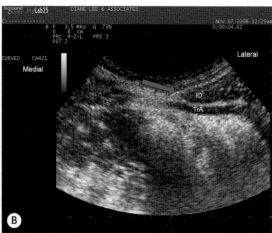

Fig. 9.10 • Abdominal wall – curl-up task. (A) Palpation of the linea alba during a curl-up task. (B) Ultrasound image of the left abdominal wall during a curl-up task (no cue to precontract the transversus abdominis (TrA)). Note how the internal oblique has slid laterally over the top of the TrA.

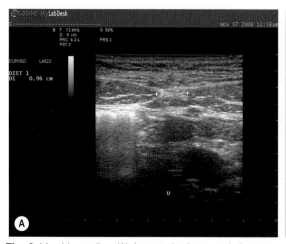
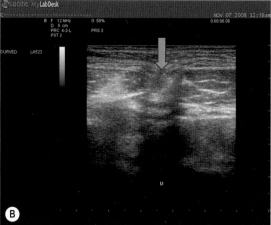

Fig. 9.11 • Linea alba. (A) At rest, the inter-recti distance was 0.96cm just above the umbilicus, a width that is within normal limits. (B) During a head and neck curl-up task the linea alba appears to droop between the left and right rectus abdominis as opposed to increasing in tension.

Standing posture

Her pelvis was no longer rotated to the left in the transverse plane, although she tended to sway her pelvis anteriorly bilaterally. Her thorax, in general, was translated to the left and specifically the eighth thoracic ring was translated to the left (rotated to the right) and the fifth thoracic ring was translated to the right (rotated to the left).

Load transfer tasks

There was symmetry of motion between the left and right sides of the pelvis during one leg standing with contralateral hip flexion and no unlocking of either side of the pelvis; however, poor control of the thorax was noted during this task (Video LC23). Backward bending no longer increased the left transverse plane rotation of her pelvis and the right side of the pelvis did not unlock. Laura no longer felt any increase in pressure in the right side of her pelvic floor during this task. Forward bending was now provocative for pain at the lumbosacral junction and, although her pelvis moved well, a non-optimal strategy was noted at the eighth thoracic ring (T7–8 and left and right eighth ribs). This ring translated further

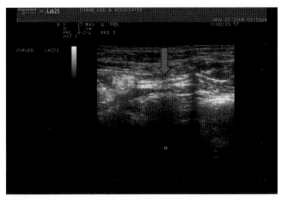

Fig. 9.12 • Linea alba response to a precontraction of transversus abdominis prior to the curl-up task. Note the increase in tension of the linea alba (arrow).

to the left and rotated to the right and the onset of this loss of control occurred simultaneously with the onset of her lumbosacral pain (Video LC24). This finding was relevant to the management of her low back and groin pain as function of the abdominal canister is significantly impacted by the behavior of the oblique abdominal muscles, which arise from the fifth to twelfth thoracic rings. Of note, correcting and supporting the eighth thoracic ring *did not* change the pain behavior or her ability to forward bend, suggesting that this is *not* the primary impairment (and suggests that the eighth thoracic ring is compensatory; note the position of the upper thorax into left rotation when the eighth thoracic ring is corrected during forward bend).

During a squat the right side of the pelvis still unlocked quite late in the task (Video LC25). When the task was performed while standing on rotation discs (taking away the ground reaction forces), the left transverse plane rotation of the pelvis recurred, the right side of the pelvis unlocked, and the eighth thoracic ring translated to the left and rotated to the right (Video LC25). As with the forward bending task, correcting the eighth thoracic ring translation did not change the findings of this task.

In addition to the left eighth thoracic ring translation, a translation of the fifth thoracic ring (T4–5 and left and right fifth ribs) to the right (with associated left rotation) was found. Correcting the position and biomechanics of the fifth thoracic ring improved not only the range of motion for right thoracopelvic rotation, but also restored her ability to fully flex and extend either leg in sitting (full slump) with

no lumbosacral pain (Video LC26). When the myofascial force vectors restricting the fifth thoracic ring were released, Laura was able to fully rotate and flex her thoracolumbar spine without ring support and without pain. Although she could squat on the rotation discs with no rotation of her pelvis, she still needed to work on her thoracic control (Video LC26). Assessment and treatment of the 'thoracic ring' (an approach developed by Linda-Joy Lee) is beyond the scope of this text, even though it is essential to include here for a full understanding of how this case managed. For more information on how we assess and treat the thorax please see www.discoverphysio.ca.

Reflective reasoning for subsequent treatment and homework practice

The findings from the perineal ultrasound imaging examination were reviewed with Laura and she was advised that, although the endopelvic fascia appeared to be stretched, she could control the position and movement of her uterus and bladder with a properly timed pelvic floor contraction during slow tasks, which increased her intra-abdominal pressure. She was given advice on how to protect the health and support of these organs by using 'the Knack' prior to a cough or sneeze and was also advised to continue the co-contraction deep muscle system training previously prescribed. After collaboration with her, a follow-up consultation with a pelvic floor therapist was booked to evaluate the presence/absence of any adhesions or tears of the endopelvic fascia and specifically to evaluate the ability of each part of the levator ani (pubococcygeus, puborectalis, puboviceralis, iliococcygeus) to contract. The goal was to see if the vector of the pelvic floor lift could be improved, thus giving more support to the neck of the bladder and the urethra.

Optimal strategies for standing, forward bending, squatting, and rotation were reviewed with a focus on imagining the thorax floating or being suspended above the pelvis (in particular the fifth and eighth thoracic rings) (Lee & Lee 2008b). She was advised to play with these images and feel the impact of various images and positions on her lumbosacral pain and her incontinence. It was essential to learn (in both her body and brain) why it was important not to transfer loads with her pelvis posteriorly tilted if long-term continence was to be assured.

Two weeks later, Laura emailed to say that she had started running again (she had been advised not to do that yet) and that she ran for 4 consecutive days for 15–25 minutes. She reported that her 'rib cage felt good; the best news is that I didn't leak, however my SI pain returned with a vengeance.' It was apparent that she was still using non-optimal strategies for running but better strategies for her continence.

Follow-up 1 month later

Laura lives 2.5 hours from the clinic and, in addition to being a full time mother, is a very busy physiotherapist, thus frequent visits were not an option. She reported that her pain had persisted in the area of the right gluteals although the intensity and frequency was less. She found that using an elliptical trainer gave her relief of this pain (4–5 minutes of use was sufficient) and that certain yoga poses (especially those involving single leg standing on the right leg) were still aggravating within a short period of time. She continued to note less yawning and more energy in general, and felt her continence was fairly good with only intermittent leakage accompanying a sneeze or cough.

Pelvic floor examination

For this visit, she was scheduled to see Johanne Sabourin (a physiotherapist certified in pelvic floor diagnostics and treatment and an associate at Diane Lee & Associates), as well as Diane Lee for a follow-up ultrasound and biomechanical evaluation. From the internal pelvic consultation Johanne noted the following:

1. decreased sensation of the right vaginal wall;
2. decreased anal and bulbocavernosus reflexes;
3. fascial adhesions/restrictions affecting the mobility of the pelvic and coccygeal nerve plexi and the right obturator nerve;
4. a 'low' bladder and a slight rectocele; and
5. that a contraction of the pelvic floor muscles did not result in a cranioventral lift.

Johanne released the fascial restrictions of the nerves and their plexi manually with internal techniques not covered in this text and noted an immediate improvement in the vector of the pelvic floor lift, as well as an improvement in the mobility of the nerve plexi.

Subsequently, a perineal ultrasound evaluation (Video LC27 – compare to Video LC19) confirmed that the vector of lift during a cue to contract the pelvic floor was now directed more

towards the neck of the bladder. During the Valsalva task, there was much less descent of the bladder and, notably when she coughed without a precontraction of the pelvic floor, a slight descent of the perineal body could be seen, whereas when she employed the Knack (precontraction of the pelvic floor and the transversus abdominis), complete support of the bladder and perineal body was seen.

Load transfer tests

As previously noted during the last follow-up visit, her pelvis was in a neutral posture and she was able to recognize when she would lose this optimal, centered position and stand in an anterior pelvic sway. During the one leg standing test, symmetry of active SIJ motion was present, neither side of the pelvis unlocked during single leg loading, and rotation of L5–S1 was controlled (Video LC28). Backward bending also revealed an optimal strategy (no pelvic asymmetry, no unlocking of either side of the pelvis). Similarly during a squat task, there was no intrapelvic torsion and no unlocking of either side of the pelvis. Forward bending was no longer provocative for pain in the lumbosacral region, and there was no lateral translation/shift or rotation of either the eighth or fifth thoracic rings. In supine position, there was no difference in effort to lift either leg unless compression was applied to the pelvic girdle. Compression of the pelvis resulted in increased effort to lift the right leg and this suggests that further compression was not necessary.

In sitting, rotation of the thorax was more symmetrical; the eighth and fifth thoracic rings rotated congruently with those above and below and thus did not impede motion. In addition, the slump test was now negative.

Articular and neural systems

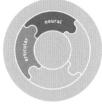

The right SIJ remained uncompressed; a clear parallel glide of the innominate relative to the ipsilateral sacrum was present (Video LC29). In addition, the deep muscle system responded synergistically in response to a verbal cue to connect the ASISs together. This was evident both via palpation and ultrasound imaging, although imaging revealed that there was a tendency for the left IO to co-contract with the TrA. During analysis of a curl-up task, the motor control strategy was still non-optimal in that the deep system was still not being recruited automatically on either the left or right sides. When the task was performed with a precontraction of the deep system (connect and then curl-up), Laura noticed a reduction in the effort required.

Articular, neural, and myofascial systems

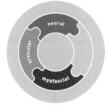

When a contraction of the deep muscle system occurred, the effect of this contraction was evident (via ultrasound) in the linea alba, as well as the left and right rectus abdominis muscles (Video LC30). During the curl-up task (no precontraction of the deep system), the linea alba still appeared to 'droop,' and once again when she precontracted the deep system prior to the curl-up this strategy appeared to generate tension in the linea alba. Activation of the deep muscle system also restricted all movement in the neutral zone of the left and right SIJ as well as L5–S1.

Reflective reasoning for subsequent treatment and homework practice

Collectively, these findings suggest that the deep system was capable of controlling motion of the joints of the pelvis; however, the strategy chosen by the central nervous system was not yet optimal for some tasks. To build a new motor pattern, focused attention and massed practice is required (Chapters 11, 12). Laura was reminded of this and encouraged to continue to use the deep muscle system cognitively, especially during single leg loading tasks. Her home practice was reviewed (integrating deep system activation into squats, lunges, step forward/back, elliptical training, etc.), and she was advised to be cognizant of her strategies in her yoga classes during poses that required single leg loading on the right. Once she is able to automatically recruit the deep system synergistically and in coordination with the superficial system, less attention will be required and it is anticipated that she will achieve full function without pain or loss of continence. Her pain was lessening, her continence was

improving (sensorial dimension of her experience), she understood why and how her pain and incontinence occurred (cognitive dimension of her experience), and she now realized that her journey need not be the same as her mother's (cognitive and

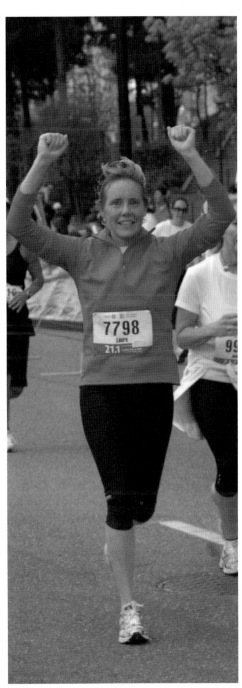

Fig. 9.13 • Laura successfully completes the half marathon in Vancouver.

emotional dimensions of her experience). She was empowered by the necessary knowledge and movement training and was aware of how to load her lumbopelvis such that she moved better, felt better, and was better. An email from Laura 3 months later:

> Just wanted to give my success story update. I ran 10 miles last week without SI pain! No leaking either though I still must be careful if I sneeze with bladder full. I started running mid February and have gradually progressed. I will be running the Vancouver half marathon on May 3rd! Thank you for all your help.

Laura completed the half marathon with no leakage and no pelvic girdle pain (Fig. 9.13).

Summary

The nervous system is 'plastic,' not 'elastic,' and change is always possible. Where 'elastic' bounces back, 'plastic' has the ability to be reshaped and reformed, much like the nervous system. We highly recommend the book *The brain that changes itself* by Norman Doidge (2007) for further information on neuroplasticity of the nervous system and how imagery and other techniques can be used to facilitate the development of different neural firing patterns. Doidge often states that 'neurons that fire together, wire together.' In all of the cases presented in this chapter, rewiring of neural firing patterns is an element of the treatment program. There are several more case reports associated with this chapter; these can be found online. Be sure to read/watch them all to see their diversity and to understand the clinical reasoning process necessary for prescriptive treatment planning.

The following chapters will present specific techniques (skill acquisition) for releasing joints, muscles, fascia, etc. (Chapter 10) followed by training for the deep and superficial muscle systems (Chapter 11) and then a final chapter to integrate it all into function (Chapter 12).

Techniques and tools for addressing barriers in the lumbopelvic–hip complex

Diane Lee   Linda-Joy Lee

10

CHAPTER CONTENTS

Introduction 283

Addressing barriers: characteristics of the person in the center of the Clinical Puzzle . . . 285

Addressing barriers: physical impairments . . . 285

Techniques for releasing the neural and myofascial systems 290

Techniques for mobilizing the articular system 312

Techniques for releasing the viscera 320

Active technique for correcting pelvic alignment 321

Summary 321

Introduction

Treatment for most patients' pain and disability (i.e. non-optimal strategies for function and performance) begins with addressing the barriers (physical, cognitive, and/or emotional) that are preventing better strategies(see Fig. 9.3). The intent of this chapter is to describe and illustrate the specific treatment techniques, tools, and home practice that are helpful for achieving this goal (skill acquisition). The clinical reasoning with respect to when, and for whom, these techniques are useful has been covered in detail in Chapter 9. Chapter 11 will focus on the first part of the second component of the program – how to train new strategies based on meaningful tasks.

Education is a key component throughout this collaborative approach. Motivating people to make changes in their life, whether it is changing their sitting posture or changing their beliefs, begins with explaining why these changes are necessary. At the end of your assessment, the most 'likely and lovely' hypothesis supported by key findings should have been developed. From this hypothesis, a treatment plan is developed that includes addressing any barriers to recovery (physical, cognitive, emotional), and treating specific impairments to facilitate retraining and restoration of meaningful tasks. Before you begin treatment, take the time to explain your hypothesis as well as your expectation of the steps and timeline necessary to achieve the patient's goals. Answer any questions and refer to your website(s) (Interest Box 1) or other resources for more information if necessary.

Be sure to enlist the patient's commitment to the treatment plan you are proposing; collaborative programs are more likely to succeed. Ask them to tell you what they now understand about their problem; this is a great way to hear how they have interpreted your hypotheses and the proposed treatment program. If the patient does not understand why they need to make changes, they will not likely 'buy in' or commit to the process necessary for long-term recovery. In other words, without an understanding and willingness to focus their attention and accumulate massed practice, they will not likely rewire the neural networks and change their non-optimal strategies. Think of yourself primarily as the patient's coach, or educator, and use your tools (manual therapy, dry needling, electrotherapy) only when necessary to facilitate change (in joint mobility, muscle tone, muscle length, posture, movement, etc.). Create a learning environment in your treatment room and try to foster an approach that empowers the patient to take control of what is happening (or not happening) in their bodies. Once they start

DOI: 10.1016/B978-0-443-06963-5.00010-9

Interest Box 1

Websites with useful information supporting *The Integrated Systems Model*
  www.discoverphysio.ca, www.dianelee.ca
  www.synergyphysio.ca

to feel the difference in how their body responds to load and movement by merely *thinking* differently, you have successfully removed a major barrier to their recovery. They now have the choice to live differently in their bodies; keep reminding them of this.

If during a subsequent visit they say, 'I felt better for a few days after our last session but my pain has all come back so I guess your treatment is not working,' it is clear that they have not embraced a fundamental principle of this program. Recovery is their responsibility; it is up to them, not you. Our response to this comment would be something along the lines of 'Hang on, you were better for a few days and that means I did my job, I helped to create the opportunity for you to feel better; however, whatever you did in those few 'better' days caused the pain to recur. Let's have a chat about some things you were doing in that time to see if I can help *you* identify what *you* didn't pay attention to that facilitated the return of your symptoms.' Get it?

The motto of Diane's physiotherapy clinic (http://www.dianelee.ca) is to 'Empower through Knowledge, Movement and Awareness' and the motto of LJ's clinic (http://www.synergyphysio.ca) is to 'Move Better, Feel Better, Be Better' (Fig. 10.1). We feel strongly that patients need to embrace their own recoveries, and we see ourselves as guides through the process. Sometimes, an entire treatment session may be spent 'just talking' and that is acceptable if the conversation helps to address current barriers to recovery (see case report Julie K, Chapter 9 🖰). Too often, clinicians feel that they need more treatment techniques and/or exercises to help patients feel better; in our experience less is often more.

So, as you read the rest of this chapter and review the video clips online, remember that being an effective clinician is not about having hundreds of treatment techniques in your tool box, although you do need to have some; it is about knowing when to use the right one at the right time, and having the skill to perform/teach them well (clinical expertise). The right treatment will often facilitate an immediate awareness of something being different/better and opens the opportunity for teaching/learning new movement and/or postural strategies (move better) that allow your patient to feel better and be better, and that can be tremendously empowering.

Before discussing how to address barriers, the words 'exercise', 'training', 'practice' and 'manual therapy' require consideration. The word 'exercise' is a bit like 'stability' (Ch. 4) with several different meanings. To many patients, it is a noun whose definition is,

> an activity requiring physical effort, carried out especially to sustain or improve health and fitness: exercise improves your heart and lung powerloosening-up exercises (New Oxford American Dictionary).

This definition suggests that all exercises require effort and that time is set aside for 'doing exercises' and does not suggest that it is important to carry anything forward from the 'exercise' into functional tasks. An alternate definition (also from the New Oxford American Dictionary) is,

> a process or activity carried out for a specific purpose, especially one concerned with a specified area or skill: an **exercise in** public relations.

This definition is more in line with what is necessary to rewire neural networks and build new, and more optimal, movement strategies. Because of the potential for misinterpretation, we have chosen, for the most part, to use the words 'training' and 'practice' in this text instead of the word 'exercise'. Training means to

> Verb: teach a particular skill or type of behavior through practice and instruction over a period of time
>
> Adjective: (**trained**) cause (a mental or physical faculty) to be sharp, discerning, or developed as a result of instruction or practice.

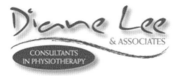

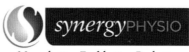

Fig. 10.1 • The mottos for Diane Lee's and Linda-Joy Lee's physiotherapy clinics are integrated into the education aspects of all treatment programs.

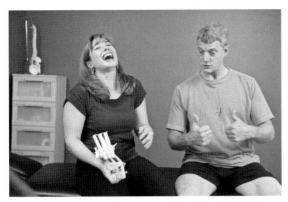

Fig. 10.2 • Education is a powerful tool in rehabilitation; there is much to learn from your patients – do not miss the opportunity to see the experience through their filters.

As a reminder from chapter 7, rewiring neural networks requires focused attention and massed practice and we feel that the word 'training' and 'practice' more accurately reflect this. As for 'manual therapy', this term refers to any technique that is done with the hands regardless of depth, amplitude or velocity.

Addressing barriers: characteristics of the person in the center of the Clinical Puzzle

Systemic factors

On occasion, systemic, or non-mechanical, factors appear to be the primary driver of the pain mechanism. In this case, the inclusion of, and sometimes referral to, an appropriate medical practitioner is essential for recovery.

Meaning perspective (cognitions and emotions)

If there are dominant psychosocial factors driving the pain mechanism, referral to a professional skilled in cognitive behavioral training may be indicated. However, for most patients, the psychosocial factors associated with their pain and disability can be addressed and influenced if the right therapeutic environment and relationship is created (Chapter 9).

A safe, non-threatening environment is essential if patients are to express and explore their thoughts, ideas, and feelings (Fig. 10.2). Often, the key catalyst that creates a change in the patient's beliefs and attitudes is simply becoming aware of the barrier that their thoughts, beliefs, and/or emotions are creating (thought viruses (Butler & Moseley 2003)). Becoming aware empowers one to make a choice and a change (develop a new neural network). As a reminder from Chapter 9, the books *Explain pain* (Butler & Moseley 2003) (www.noigroup.com) and *Understand pain, live well again* (Pearson 2007) (www.lifeisnow.ca) provide tools for therapists to help patients understand their pain experience and are recommended resources. Often a good hypothesis, developed from a thorough physical assessment, can explain non-resolving symptoms and quickly shatter cognitive barriers, especially when validated by a treatment program that reduces pain and improves function within predicted timelines.

Addressing barriers: physical impairments

There are many techniques that decrease muscle tone and restore joint motion, including: articular mobilization (Grades 1, 2, 3), manipulation (high acceleration, low amplitude thrust or Grade 5), soft tissue release (myofascial release, counter-strain, positional release, functional techniques, muscle energy, trigger point release), and dry needling/intramuscular stimulation (IMS). The exact mechanisms underlying the efficacy of these techniques are unclear. It is thought that they all work by altering neural drive to the alpha moto neuron at the level of the spinal cord (Fig. 10.3) or by altering the drive from the brain (higher centers).

Soft tissue techniques for the release of hypertonic muscles are not new. Osteopathic physicians and physical therapists have long used strain–counter-strain, muscle energy, functional (positional release), and trigger point techniques for reducing muscle tone. In our experience, doing these techniques *to* a patient appears to have a short-term benefit, whereas using imagery to engage the patient's awareness during any, or all, of these techniques creates a more lasting effect. There appears to be a learning component when the patient's awareness is integrated into the release technique, perhaps due to rewiring neural networks. This approach/

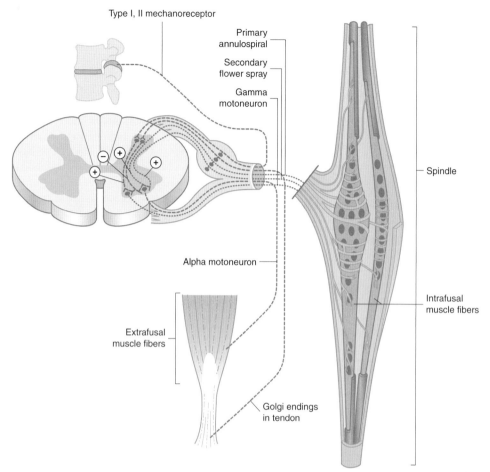

Type I, II mechanoreceptor

Primary
annulospiral

Secondary
flower spray

Gamma
motoneuron

Spindle

Alpha motoneuron

Intrafusal
muscle fibers

Extrafusal
muscle fibers

Golgi endings
in tendon

Fig. 10.3 • The resting tone of a muscle is influenced and controlled by many neural feedback loops involving the brain, spinal cord, and peripheral receptor systems. Afferent input can be altered by changing the position of the joint and its associated muscles, tendons, and fascia. The result can be a decrease in the efferent output to the extrafusal muscle fiber(s), and consequently a decrease in muscle tone. This is called a positional release. Imagery and awareness can activate the higher centers that have a descending inhibitory influence on the efferent output to the extrafusal muscle fiber(s) and can further reduce the resting tone of a muscle. We call this 'release with awareness' (Lee & Lee 2004a) and find that combining the two techniques is a very effective way to reduce muscle tone.

technique is called *release with awareness* (Lee & Lee 2004a) and requires focused attention. It ultimately gives the patient control over the hypertonic state of the muscle(s). When the most effective image or cue for release is found, it provides the patient with a new skill that they can then integrate into:

1. specific stretching practice (*stretch with awareness*); as well as
2. specific muscle recruitment training (Chapter 11); and
3. specific movement practice that is relevant to their meaningful task (Chapter 12).

It is incredibly empowering for patients to feel the change in their pain and the immediate improvement in mobility that *release (or stretch) with awareness* can create. The technique is clinically applicable whenever, and wherever, hypertonicity from altered motor control or increased neural drive is present. The hypothesis is that focused attention and awareness facilitates learning of how to dampen neural drive from higher centers. When aiming to restore joint mobility, we find that releasing neuromuscular barriers first is an effective way to truly assess what is happening in the underlying articular system. Once the superficial and potentially compressive muscles are released/relaxed, specific joint mobilization techniques (Grade 4) effectively restore the mobility of the articular structures, namely the joints, peri-articular ligaments, and fascia. This chapter will describe how to perform the following techniques (skill acquisition):

1. *release with awareness*;
2. dry needling;
3. specific joint mobilization;
4. specific high acceleration, low amplitude thrust; and
5. *stretch with awareness*.

Some of these techniques can be learned from a book (1, 3, 5), whereas others require course work and certification for the safety of the patient (2, 4). A few principles require review before the techniques are described.

Principles of *release with awareness* techniques

Release with awareness is based on some of the same principles as functional, counter-strain, positional, and trigger point release techniques. The awareness part of the technique is what differentiates it from the others, and we believe that this component involves multiple networks in the brain, including the centers for learning and memory. If neural networks are to be rewired, learning has to be part of the technique. Alternately, releasing the non-optimal muscle activity patterns can be thought of as 'deleting' or 'erasing' current neural networks. The principles of the *release with awareness* technique are to:

1. Position the joint/muscle so as to shorten the hypertonic fascicle, and then:
   (a) monitor the area of increased muscle tone (can be fascicle specific) with gentle pressure; as you
   (b) move the joint so as to shorten the origin and insertion of the hypertonic muscle. When multiple agonist/antagonist muscles are hypertonic, monitor two or three muscles simultaneously and find a position of the joint that reduces the tone in all of the monitored muscles;
   (c) to facilitate further shortening of the hypertonic fascicle, approximate it intramuscularly with the palpating hand if possible. This can be done before or after step (b).
2. It is then imperative to wait for a reduction in tone to occur as the spinal cord responds to the reduced

input from the primary annulospiral endings of the muscle spindles in the hypertonic fascicle(s) and altered input from the relevant mechanoreceptors in the joints, muscles, and fascia. This usually occurs within 15–20 seconds. This is the positional component of the release technique.

3. Once a reduction in tone is felt in the monitored muscle/fascicle, cue the patient to further release or soften the muscle with both verbal and manual cues that suggest 'letting go.' The cues aim to evoke activation of the higher centers in the brain that can influence and reduce the tone of the muscle. The verbal cues are almost always associated with images that soften, melt, give way, and let go. When the patient is successful, another level of release will be felt within the muscle and through the joint that is being compressed. This is the awareness component of the release technique and can be clearly sensed by both the therapist and, usually, the patient. In all cases, give the patient positive feedback, such as, 'That's it, yes, keep letting go just like that' so that they can learn what images and sensations they need to create in their body to cause the release in their muscles. This facilitates increased awareness of what they need to think/do to facilitate more relaxation and is essential for learning the skill so that it can be applied during other activities. Appropriate positive feedback is also likely to enhance neuroplasticity (see Chapter 9).

4. Once the maximum release is obtained, the muscle is then taken passively through its full range either by stretching or lengthening the fascicle directly (intramuscular technique) or by moving the joint so as to stretch/lengthen the fascicle. As you lengthen the muscle, 'listen' to its response to avoid any recurrence of the hypertonicity. The second part of this technique addresses any intramuscular myofascial barriers or restrictions.

5. Teach the patient a home practice that reinforces what they have learned with you about how they can self-release their hypertonic muscles. This practice often helps to control pain and maintain mobility, and should generally be done before any retraining of the deep muscles or movement training.

Principles of dry needling techniques

Dry needling of painful points with acupuncture needles has been used historically by many practitioners and has recently (1990s) been introduced to physiotherapists in Canada by Dr. Chan Gunn

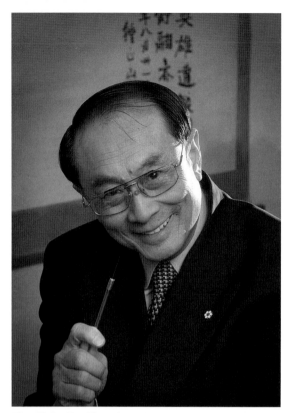

Fig. 10.4 • Dr. Chan Gunn, innovator and founder of Intramuscular Stimulation and the Institute for the Study and Treatment of Pain (www.istop.org).

(Fig. 10.4) (Gunn 1996). An early pioneer of dry needling, Dr. Gunn developed his radiculopathy model based on his clinical experience while treating injured workers with multiple musculoskeletal complaints. He called this technique IMS (intramuscular stimulation) to differentiate the radiculopathy model from the myofascial trigger point model (Simons et al 1999).

The underlying premise of Dr. Gunn's model is that myofascial pain is always the result of either peripheral neuropathy or radiculopathy. The hypotheses for this approach were developed from Cannon and Rosenblueth's Law of Denervation (1949), which states that

> othe function and integrity of innervated structures is dependent upon the free flow of nerve impulses. When the flow of nerve impulses is restricted, all innervated structures, including skeletal muscle, smooth muscle, spinal neurons, sympathetic ganglia, adrenal glands, sweat cells, and brain cells become atrophic, highly irritable, and supersensitive.

When using dry needling in the method of GunnIMS, treatment always includes dry needling of the peripheral muscle at either its sensitized motor point or its musculotendinous junction, as well as the paraspinal muscles (including to the depth of the multifidi) of the associated spinal segment.

Practitioners who use dry needling according to the myofascial trigger point model specifically target active trigger points in myofascial tissues. Simons et al (1999) note that trigger points in myofascial tissues may be active (trigger local or referred pain without being stimulated) or latent (require stimulation to trigger local or referred pain); however, they may alter muscle activation patterns and limit range of motion. The exact mechanisms underlying myofascial trigger point development and elimination with dry needling remains unclear. Shah et al (2005) note that there is an increased concentration of substances that modulate nociception (e.g. bradykinin, substance P, interleukin-1, etc.) at active trigger point sites, and that a marked reduction of these chemicals occurs almost immediately after a local twitch response is evoked using dry needling. Theories abound and the reader is referred to two excellent articles by Simons & Dommerholt (2006) and Dommerholt et al (2006) for an in-depth review on the research into this technique.

We have found dry needling/IMS to be an extremely useful tool when used in conjunction with manual release techniques (especially *release with awareness*) and followed with home practice that includes *self-release with awareness* and *stretch with awareness*. We use both the GunnIMS model and the myofascial trigger point model. If hypertonicity is found in both a peripheral muscle and an associated, segmental, paraspinal muscle (e.g. adductor longus and L2–3 superficial multifidus), it is recommended that both sites be released with a *release with awareness* technique followed by dry needling if necessary. If a latent or active trigger point in a peripheral muscle is not associated with segmental, paraspinal muscle hypertonicity, then only the peripheral muscle is released and needled. If you are interested in using dry needling technique in your clinical practice, certification is required. The Institute for the Study and Treatment of Pain (www.istop.org) is the organization that certifies qualified practitioners for GunnIMS.

Principles of specific joint mobilization techniques

Once the muscles have been released, the true mobility of the underlying joint can be assessed. The neutral zone of motion should now be clear (devoid of any myofascial influences/compression) and the elastic zone will reveal the direction and quality of the specific vector of restriction (end feel). When a joint is sprained and a synovitis occurs, the capsule may become restricted and, although specific patterns of restriction have been reported for every joint (Cyriax 1954), it is common to find a wide variety of patterns for each joint.

Joints that present with restrictions in the capsule and the associated ligaments often have multiple vectors of force limiting motion, and mobilization in several directions is often required. Joints that have not been subjected to an intra-articular synovitis or capsulitis can also become restricted, especially when the joint has been compressed by overactivation of muscles for prolonged periods. In both situations, it is important to assess the specific vector, or direction, of resistance and focus the specific mobilization technique to this vector. Distraction of the joint's capsule combined with a vector-specific Grade 4 or 4+ mobilization (sustained hold at the barrier) is our preferred technique for releasing restrictions in the peri-articular tissues. Range of motion practice combined with *self-release with awareness* and *stretch with awareness* practice is then given to maintain the mobility gained with the manual technique.

Principles of high acceleration, low amplitude thrust (HALAT) techniques

It has been established that manipulating the lumbar spine can reduce pain (Assendelft et al 2003, Koes et al 2001). Flynn et al (2002), with a clinical prediction rule (CPR) in its early development, recommended five key factors that could predict who would benefit from manipulation of the low back; they are:

1. duration of current episode of low back pain <16 days;
2. extent of distal symptoms: not having symptoms distal to the knee;
3. Fear-Avoidance Beliefs Questionnaire Work subscale score <19 points;
4. segmental mobility testing: at least one hypomobile segment in the lumbar spine;
5. hip internal rotation range of motion: at least one hip with >35° of internal rotation range of motion.

Fritz et al (2005) considered the association between two of the above five factors, duration and extent of symptoms (1 and 2), and noted that these two factors alone were associated with a good prognosis for use of

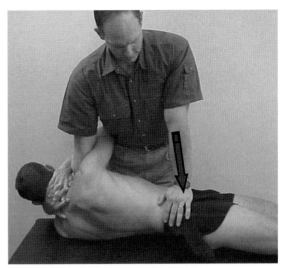

Fig. 10.5 • This picture is from Fritz et al (2005) and illustrates the technique used to develop a clinical prediction rule for deciding when manipulation should be employed for patients with low back pain. It is readily apparent that this is a non-specific technique and that multiple joints may 'pop' with its use. Reproduced with permission from Fritz et al and the publisher BMC, 2005.

a manipulative technique. What kind of manipulative technique? Does specificity matter? Figure 10.5 is reproduced from Fritz et al (2005) and illustrates the general nature of their investigated manipulative technique. This has resulted in heated debate between this group (Flynn, Childs, Fritz) and experienced clinicians, who believe that manipulation of the spine should be specific to be safe and effective (McLaughlin 2008, Pettman 2006). All that can be said from the evidence is the following: if your patient has had their pain for less than 16 days and the pain does not radiate below the knee they will benefit from a manipulation of their lumbar spine regardless of its specificity. If your patient has had their pain longer than 16 days and the pain radiates further, then they may not. There is not much need for debate with this clinical prediction rule as most patients presenting to private physiotherapy practices have been living with their pain experience for more than 2 weeks, and something more than a non-specific manipulation technique is likely going to be required to restore their function and reduce their pain.

High acceleration, low amplitude, thrust techniques have their place in a multimodal program and over the last 10–15 years there has been a significant paradigm shift with respect to the understanding of how these techniques work to relieve pain and restore mobility. The biomechanical theories of the past are giving way to new theories supported by evidence once again in the field of neuroscience (Indahl et al 1995, 1997, 1999, Kang et al 2002, Pickar 2002, Sung et al 2005). According to Pettman, an internationally renowned clinician highly experienced in the use and teaching of these techniques:

> Despite advances in visual diagnostic techniques, purely mechanical causes of spinal articular restrictions have never been demonstrated. This casts serious doubt that the therapeutic basis of manipulation is mechanical . . . the 'joint cavitation' theory seems invalid and we also know that a 'pop' is not necessary for a successful result . . . The bulk of evidence suggests that there is a fundamental neurophysiologic response to manipulation.
>
> Pettman 2006.

Further evidence to support the hypothesis that articular techniques can evoke muscular responses comes from studies done on Swedish pigs and cats. When the ventral aspect of the SIJ of a Swedish pig was stimulated, a response in the gluteus maximus and quadratus lumborum occurred; whereas, when the dorsal aspect of the SIJ was stimulated, a response in the lumbosacral multifidus occurred (Indahl et al 1999). Stimulating the articular capsule of the lumbar zygapophyseal joint in a Swedish pig evokes a response in the deep fibers of multifidus unilaterally, whereas stimulating the intervertebral disc evokes a response in multifidus bilaterally (Indahl et al 1995) and this response did not occur when the zygapophyseal joint was injected with an anesthetic (lidocaine). Sung et al (2005) investigated the factor of speed on the afferent discharge from Golgi tendon organs and muscle spindles in the paraspinal muscles of cats and noted that when the speed of the technique approached that of a HALAT technique, there was a simultaneous increase in the discharge from these receptors. Clearly, the articular and muscular systems are linked through the neural system and one can impact the function of the other.

Is it essential for the technique to be specific or not? The current scientific evidence says no; clinical expertise says, sometimes, yes. Our experience has been that specific HALAT techniques require less force and are, therefore, safer. HALAT techniques are associated with some risk and, when used inappropriately and/or unskillfully can do harm. Therefore, we support the clinicians who advocate specificity, not because we support the biomechanical model, but because the technique is more controlled and safer. The techniques presented in this chapter are highly specific and are used in combination with other manual techniques, neuromuscular training, and movement training for best outcomes.

All practitioners who wish to learn HALAT techniques (manipulation) must be trained and certified to do so. In Canada, postgraduate certification in manual and manipulative therapy is available for physiotherapists through the Canadian Academy of Manipulative Therapists, a division of the Canadian Physiotherapy Association (www.manipulativetherapy.org). For a complete dissertation and update on the history, principles, and practice of HALAT techniques in physiotherapy practice, the reader is referred to Pettman (2006, 2007) and Paris (2000).

Principles of *stretch with awareness* techniques

Once the neural drive to a muscle has been dampened (addressing neural barriers) and the muscle's ability to lengthen restored (addressing neural and myofascial barriers), the patient is taught to maintain the new resting tone and length through appropriate home practice. Traditional exercises for stretching specific muscles can be modified into 'sling stretches' that lengthen a continuous myofascial line comprising several muscles and the fascial connections between them. The imagery cues that facilitated relaxation of the muscle(s) during the *release with awareness* technique are integrated such that the neural tone is reduced as the myofascia is lengthened (*stretch with awareness*). Small release balls can replace the therapist's hands to provide afferent information to the CNS about what and where to release. Yoga straps, or the wall, can be used to support the lower extremity such that attention may be focused on releasing/lengthening the relevant sling of muscles. Later, the release cues are integrated into specific deep muscle training (Chapter 11) and meaningful task training (Chapter 12); therefore, spending some time on sharpening the skill of selective sling lengthening and 'letting go' independent of task performance is worthwhile in the early stages of rehabilitation.

Techniques for releasing the neural and myofascial systems

Combined release techniques for the muscles compressing the hip joint

It is not uncommon to find two or three muscles of the hip that are hypertonic and collectively creating a net vector of force that decentralizes the femoral

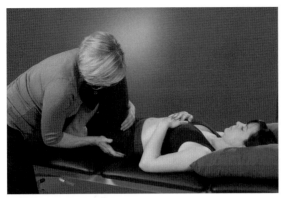

Fig. 10.6 • Combined release technique for the left tensor fascia latae and gluteus medius. Both muscles are monitored as the hip is positioned such that the femoral head centers. This position usually results in a dampening of the resting tone of any/all hypertonic muscles of the hip. See the text for further details on the use of this combined release technique.

head. Each muscle can be released individually or multiple muscles, and their net vector, can be released with a combined technique. Dry needling can also be used to release specific hypertonic fascicles that persist after the *release with awareness* technique. Hypertonicity in the superficial hip muscles is released first to facilitate access to the deeper muscles (obturator externus and obturator internus, quadratus femoris, gemelli, etc.). See Chapter 9, Videos MQ12, MQ14 and 10.1, 10.2 🖱 for demonstrations of these techniques.

Starting position – positional release. With the weight of the leg fully supported, palpate the hypertonic muscles in the anterior, posterior, medial, or lateral aspect of the hip joint/groin assessed as being responsible for the non-optimal femoral head position (Figs 10.6, 10.7). The muscles could include rectus femoris, tensor fascia latae, sartorius, gluteus medius, gluteus minimus, long or short adductors (pectineus, adductor brevis, adductor longus, gracilis, adductor magnus), psoas, iliacus, piriformis, quadratus femoris, and/or the superior/inferior gemelli. Gently monitor the response of one, two, or three of these muscles (specifically the ones found to be hypertonic on assessment) as you move the femur into more flexion/extension, abduction/adduction, medial/lateral rotation. Find the spot where there is the least amount of tone in all monitored muscles. Maintain this articular position and then gently shorten the specific hypertonic fascicle by approximating the origin and insertion with your fingers (intramuscular shortening)

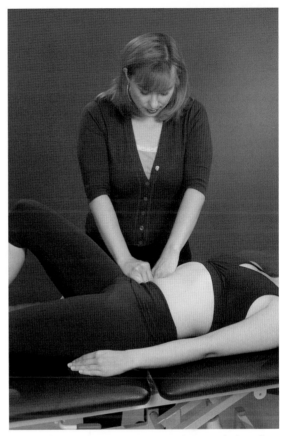

Fig. 10.7 • Specific intramuscular release technique for psoas. Palpate psoas from the anterior aspect of L2 to L4 and look for a tender hypertonic point. Be sure to approach the muscle from beneath the ascending or descending colon; come in from the lateral aspect of the abdomen as opposed to directly in the midline. Approximate the muscle using an intramuscular technique and wait for the resultant dampening of tone. Use verbal cues such as 'let my fingers sink into your belly, let your back relax and lengthen, imagine your leg falling away from your body, etc.' to facilitate the release. Once maximum release has been obtained, specifically lengthen the fascicle and have the patient extend the leg on that side.

(Fig. 10.8). Hold both the articular and intramuscular positions and wait for the resultant dampening of tone to occur (positional release). This will feel like a subtle softening of the muscles.

Adding awareness – cues to patient. Manual cue – apply light downward pressure on the femur in the direction that would center the femoral head. Use words to facilitate the relaxation or letting go of the hypertonic muscles and posterior seating of the femoral head. Some effective images/cues

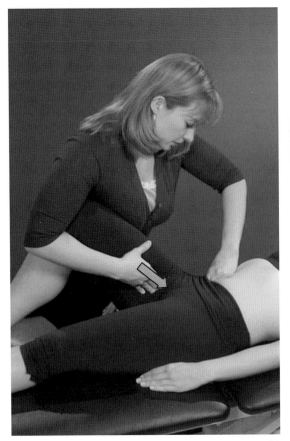

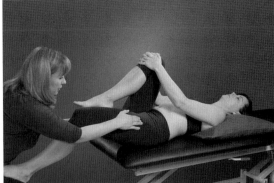

Fig. 10.9 • Combined intramuscular release, *release with awareness* and *stretch with awareness* technique for vastus lateralis (VL) and adductor magnus (AM). The technique begins by positioning the hip joint where the muscles are relaxed; support the foot on your thigh. Monitor the tone in VL and AM and shorten the hypertonic fascicles with an intramuscular technique (approximate either end of the hypertonic fascicle), wait for the dampening response, and then cue a release. Once the maximum release is obtained, specifically lengthen the fascicles of both muscles with either hand and extend the hip simultaneously using verbal cues to encourage them to keep the VL and AM soft and relaxed.

Fig. 10.8 • Combined intramuscular release, *release with awareness* and *stretch with awareness* technique for the right psoas and the short adductors. This is an example of how two muscles can be released simultaneously. The right hip is positioned such that both the psoas and the short adductors slightly relax (hip flexion and slight adduction). One hand focuses on the psoas and the other on the short adductors. Shorten the adductors using an intramuscular technique (arrow on the adductors), cue a release of the psoas ('let my fingers sink into the muscle') and wait for a dampening response from both. Once maximum release is obtained, specifically lengthen the fascicles of both muscles with either hand and ask the patient to lengthen the leg, encouraging them to keep the psoas and the short adductors soft and relaxed.

include: 'Let my fingers sink gently into these muscles, let your leg go heavy, relax your hip and see if you can let your thigh bone slide back towards the table like a telephone pole sinking in a mud bank; soften the muscles around your groin/pubic bone, let the pubic bone open like the wishbone of a turkey, etc.' Any words and images that cue relaxation can be tried. As the patient discovers how to release these

muscles you will feel the hip joint decompress, the femoral head center, and the muscles soften. Encourage them with words like, 'That's it, you've got it' to reinforce learning.

Restoring length – after release. Once the neural component has been released, lengthen the fascicle manually (myofascial component) and then take the hip joint through a full range of motion that lengthens the hypertonic muscle (Fig. 10.9). Continue to use words to encourage relaxation/release and continue to monitor the relevant muscles for any recurrence of hypertonicity.

Recheck femoral head position. If the technique has been successful, the femoral head will now be centered and remain so throughout the full passive range of motion of the hip joint (unless there are deeper vectors still present; see next section). Test the new functional range of hip motion and repeat the *release with awareness* technique for any muscles that are still impacting any part of the range of motion of the hip joint.

Dry needling – residual hypertonic fascicles. Persistent hypertonicity can be addressed using dry needling or IMS. Figure 10.10A–F illustrates the possible insertion points for using this technique to further release/relax the superficial muscles of the hip.

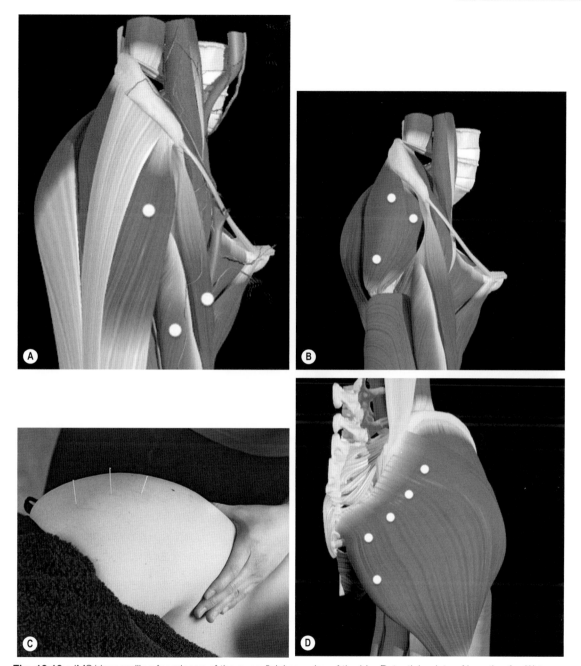

Fig. 10.10 • IMS/dry needling for release of the superficial muscles of the hip. Potential points of insertion for (A) tensor fascia latae, rectus femoris, sartorius, (B) gluteus medius and minimus, and (C) the gluteal group. (D) It is common to find multiple tender hypertonic points along the superior fascial insertion and the inferomedial border of gluteus maximus.

Continued

Home practice. To maintain the release gained, the patient is instructed to continue to practice at home. It is important that they understand that this practice is crucial for developing new strategies for function, and that the more time they can dedicate to the release of these muscles the faster the rewiring of the neural network will occur (massed practice). If they ask you how many times a day they need to 'do these exercises', they have not understood the concepts of this program. Remind them that this is like learning a new language

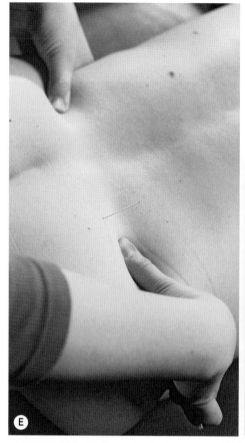

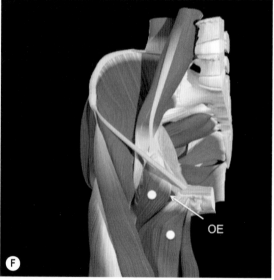

Fig. 10.10—cont'd • (E) Needle in situ for one point of gluteus maximus. (f) The short adductors are commonly hypertonic in patients presenting with posterior or anterior (groin) pelvic girdle pain. This illustration shows the common insertion points for IMS/dry needling of the adductor group. OE = obturator externus. Note the opening between pectineus and adductor longus through which obturator externus can be palpated. The anatomical pictures in this group of figures are from Primal Pictures Ltd. (www.primalpictures.com).

and that this practice is actually getting them ready to exercise (strengthen and condition).

Small balls and support straps (yoga straps) are useful home tools for this work. The patient can use a small ball (or their hand) to apply gentle pressure to any hypertonic muscle in the buttock or thigh while simultaneously thinking of the effective image or cue that facilitated relaxation of the muscle in the clinic (Fig. 10.11). When releasing the muscles in the buttock, the leg is often supported on a chair.

For releasing and lengthening the superficial muscles of the posterior, medial, or lateral thigh at home, the patient is supine with the leg supported either by a yoga strap or on a wall (Fig. 10.12A,B, Videos 10.2, 10.3). Both the supine (10.13A) and prone (Fig. 10.13B) position can be used for releasing and lengthening the superficial muscles of the anterior thigh and psoas. The practice involves the use of images/cues to relax/

lengthen the relevant muscles as the hip/femur/tibia is taken through increasing ranges of motion (*stretch with awareness*). Some patients can be taught to monitor either the femoral head or the innominate to feel for non-optimal displacement of either bone during this home practice (Fig. 10.13C). Consider the principles and goals of the practice and modify the specifics according to the patient's needs.

Specific release techniques for the deeper muscles compressing the hip joint

Obturator externus is very deep and can only be palpated once the short adductors (pectineus, adductor brevis, and longus) have been released. There is a palpable opening between pectineus and adductor

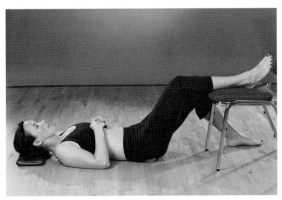

Fig. 10.11 • Home practice for release of the posterior buttock. A small release ball is a useful home tool for relaxation and dampening of tone in the muscles of the posterior buttock. In this illustration, the patient has placed the ball over the upper, lateral gluteal muscles. The leg is supported and the patient thinks about the cues that facilitated relaxation of these muscles in the clinic such as 'let the muscles under the ball soften, relax, melt, and think about allowing the weight of the femur to sink into the back of your buttock much like a telephone pole sinking in a mudbank.' The ball can also be placed more medially to assist the release of piriformis and medioinferiorly for ischiococcygeus.

longus just lateral to the pubic tubercle through which obturator externus can be palpated (Fig. 10.10F, see case report Christy, Chapter 9, Video CD9).

Starting position – positional release. Position the hip into 90° of flexion and support the femur against your body. Gently palpate the obturator externus between the pectineus and adductor longus muscles. When hypertonic, the obturator externus muscle can be exquisitely tender. Apply gentle pressure to the muscle and slowly externally rotate/abduct/flex/extend the hip until you find the position of the hip where the muscle feels a bit softer. Maintain this articular position and wait for the resultant dampening of tone to occur (positional release). This will feel like a subtle softening of the muscle.

Adding awareness – cues to patient. Manual cue – apply light pressure into the muscle and cue the patient to release/relax, to allow your fingers to sink into their groin, to let the hip come away from the pelvis. As they discover how to release/relax you will feel the hip joint decompress and the obturator externus soften. Encourage them with words like 'that's it, you've got it' to reinforce the learning.

Restoring length – after release. Once the neural component has been released, lengthen the muscle by internally rotating the hip joint through its full range of motion. Continue to use words to encourage

relaxation/release and monitor the obturator externus for any recurrence of hypertonicity.

Recheck femoral head position. If the technique has been successful, the femoral head will now be centered and remain so throughout the full passive range of motion of the hip joint.

Home practice. Teach the patient where to palpate the obturator externus while lying in a crook lying position (the flexed hip and knee can initially be supported to facilitate relaxation of the superficial muscles of the hip). While applying gentle pressure to the muscle, have them remember the image/cue that released/relaxed the muscle and teach them to be aware of the difference in the sense of compression of the hip joint when the muscle is relaxed versus hypertonic. Teach them to feel for the femoral head position in the supine, crook lying position and to check this position after their home practice. Empower them with the skills to release themselves and to understand how to identify when a release technique is necessary.

Obturator internus (OI) is also very deep and only the most inferior part can be palpated externally. Hypertonicity of this muscle is common in women with stress urinary incontinence and is often associated with hypertonicity of the levator ani muscle group. We feel that OI should be considered as part of the three-dimensional pelvic floor that connects the left and right greater trochanter through the fascial connections to the levator ani (see Fig. 3.55C) (Lee & Lee 2007).

Starting position – positional release. With the patient in crook lying, support the hips and knees over a bolster. With one hand, palpate the inferior aspect of the OI muscle on the medial aspect of the inferior ramus of the pubis and/or the ischial ramus. With your other hand, palpate the ipsilateral knee. Apply gentle pressure to the muscle to monitor its tone and then slowly externally rotate the ipsilateral hip joint through the knee. Apply a gentle downward force along the length of the femur so as to center the femoral head. Maintain this articular position and wait for the resultant dampening of tone to occur (positional release). This will feel like a subtle softening of the muscle.

Adding awareness – cues to patient. Manual cue – apply light pressure into the muscle and cue the patient to release/relax, let the 'sitz bones' go wide, and let the hip come away from the pelvis. As they discover how to release/relax you will feel the hip joint decompress and the OI soften.

Restoring length – after release. Once the neural component has been released, lengthen the muscle by internally rotating the hip joint through its full range of motion. Continue to use words to encourage

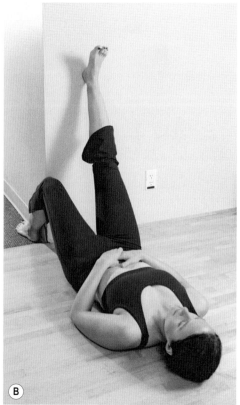

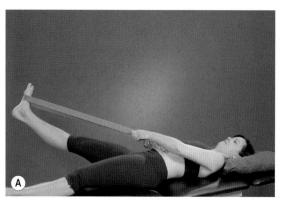

Fig. 10.12 • Home practice for release of the superficial muscles of the hip. (A) In this home practice, the patient is using a yoga strap to support her right leg as she abducts the lengthened lower extremity to a position where a comfortable stretch is felt in the targeted muscle group. She is also monitoring her abdominal wall to integrate a practice that coordinates the deep and superficial abdominal muscles during this task (Chapter 11). This ensures that movement of the abdominal canister is controlled as the leg is moved independently from the trunk. For the release part of this practice, instruct the patient to remember the cues that resulted in relaxation of the target muscle and to think about 'reaching the heel long' without losing the connection of the femoral head in the acetabulum. This 'reaching' cue often results in further dampening of the superficial muscles and greater range of motion. (B) For some, the leg is too heavy for the strength of their arms and they are unable to use the yoga strap. In this case, the wall can be substituted for the strap. This works well for the long muscles of the posterior thigh (hamstrings) and less well for the adductors as the weight of the leg has to be controlled when abducted (Video 10.3 🖱).

relaxation/release and monitor the OI for any recurrence of hypertonicity.

Recheck femoral head position. If the technique has been successful, the femoral head will now be centered and remain so throughout the full passive range of motion of the hip joint.

Home practice. Small balls work well to facilitate relaxation or release of the OI muscle. While lying supine with the leg supported on a chair, the small ball is placed just medial to the ischial tuberosity. The patient thinks about the cues that facilitated relaxation of the OI in the clinic and checks the efficacy of their practice by noting the response of the femoral head position and the freedom and amplitude of the post-practice range of internal rotation of the hip.

Once all of the muscles of the hip have been released and the femoral head remains centered through the full range of passive flexion/adduction/abduction and rotation, the pelvic rock exercise (with or without a gym ball) becomes very useful for home practice (Fig. 10.14A,B with a gym ball, see Video 12.18 🖱).

Specific release techniques for muscles compressing the sacroiliac joint

There are four key muscles that when hypertonic can compress and limit both passive and active mobility of the SIJ. Each muscle (together with the forces

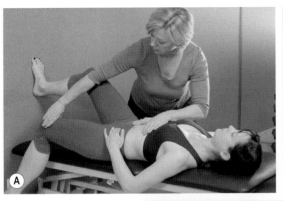

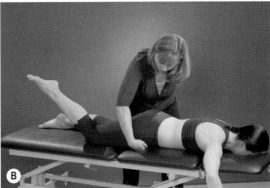

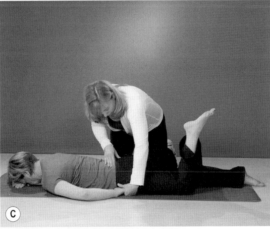

Fig. 10.13 • Home practice for releasing the superficial muscles of the hip. (A) In this illustration, the supine patient is palpating the left femoral head (left hand) to ensure it remains centered, as well as their pelvic girdle (right hand) to ensure it remains neutral, as they slowly extend the left hip and release the anterior superficial muscles of the left hip. (B) In this illustration, the therapist is monitoring both the pelvis and the femoral head for either an IPT or femoral head displacement (anterior translation or rotation) as the patient lengthens the anterior superficial muscles of the hip by bending the knee. In both (A) and (B), verbal and manual cues are used to assist the release. (C) The patient can be taught to monitor their pelvis (for a tilt or torsion) and/or their femoral head(s) to ensure an optimal strategy is used during this home practice. In this illustration, the therapist is monitoring the left SIJ (for unlocking) with her right hand and instructing the patient to monitor the femoral head with her left.

produced by fascia) appears to compress a specific part of the SIJ:

1. ischiococcygeus can compress the inferior part of the joint, prevents a parallel glide between the innominate and sacrum, and creates an axis that results in posterior rotation of the innominate when gentle anteroposterior (AP) pressure is applied to the innominate;

2. piriformis can compress all three parts of the SIJ, preventing a parallel glide at all parts of the joint (superior, middle, and inferior); and the

3. superficial fibers of multifidus and

4. erector spinae can compress the superior part of the joint, preventing a parallel glide between the

innominate and sacrum and creating an axis that results in an anterior rotation of the innominate when gentle AP pressure is applied to the innominate.

Ischiococcygeus

Starting position – positional release. With the patient in crook lying, support the hips and knees, preferably over a bolster. With the index and middle fingers of your caudal hand, palpate the ischiococcygeus just lateral to the coccyx and inferior to the inferior arcuate band of the sacrotuberous ligament (see Fig. 3.62B); alternately, explore the ischiococcygeus just inferior and medial to the inferior lateral angle

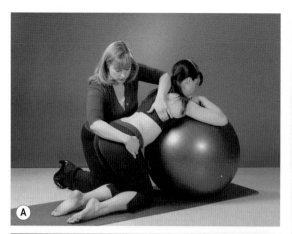

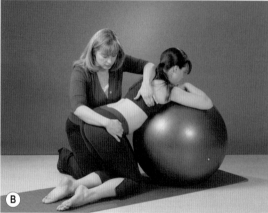

Fig. 10.14 • Home practice for maintaining mobility of the hip in the partial weight bearing position. (A) Instruct the patient to start with the femurs directly beneath the pelvis (femoral heads centered) and the thoracolumbar spine in neutral. The thorax can be supported over a gym ball to make the task easier. From this position, instruct the patient to gently rock backwards by folding, or hinging, at the hips symmetrically (optimal hip flexion with no loss of femoral head centering). In this illustration, the therapist is monitoring flexion of the right hip and ensuring that the thoracopelvic position remains neutral. (B) A progression for this task is to then have the patient move their hips to one side (abduct one hip and adduct the other) (to the left in this illustration) and then to the other. They can explore the entire circumductive range of motion, and when any resistance is encountered use imagery and cues to facilitate a release of whatever muscle is limiting the smooth excursion of motion.

(ILA) of the sacrum. Look for a tender point in the muscle. With the heel of this hand palpate the lateral aspect of the ischial tuberosity, and with your cranial hand palpate the ilium (Fig. 10.15). Apply gentle pressure to the muscle to monitor its tone and then slowly

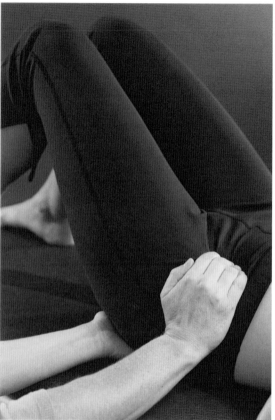

Fig. 10.15 • Specific *release with awareness*, combined with *stretch with awareness*, technique for ischiococcygeus. In this illustration, the therapist is monitoring the left ischiococcygeus with the fingers of the left hand while the heel of this hand approximates the ischium towards the coccyx (shortens the fibers). The therapist's right hand facilitates the movement of the innominate through the ilium.

approximate the ischium towards the coccyx with the heel of your hand (shorten the origin and insertion of the muscle). You can also add slight anterior rotation of the innominate (with your opposite hand) to facilitate maximal positional release of this muscle. Maintain this articular position and wait for the resultant dampening of tone to occur (positional release). This will feel like a subtle softening of the muscle.

Adding awareness – cues to patient. Manual cue – maintain light pressure into the muscle and cue the patient to release/relax. Images of letting the 'sitz bones' go wide or of letting the tailbone float are often effective. As they discover how to release/relax you will feel the pelvis decompress and the ischiococcygeus soften.

Restoring length – after release. Once the neural component has been released, lengthen the muscle by abducting the innominate (pull the ischium laterally and push the ilium medially). Continue to use words to encourage relaxation/release and monitor the ischiococcygeus for any recurrence of hypertonicity.

Recheck passive range of motion of the SIJ. If the technique has been successful, the innominate will now be able to glide freely relative to the sacrum in a parallel manner; the inferior part of the joint will no longer be compressed. Further release of piriformis and/or the superficial fibers of multifidus may be required for restoring the full range of SIJ motion.

Dry needling – residual hypertonicity. Persistent hypertonicity can be addressed using dry needling or IMS. Figure 10.16A,B and Chapter 9, Video CD9 🖱 illustrate the point used for IMS/dry needling to further release/relax ischiococcygeus.

Home practice. Small balls work well to facilitate relaxation or release of the ischiococcygeus muscle. While lying supine with the leg supported on a chair, the small ball is placed just lateral to the coccyx over the tender, hypertonic point. The patient thinks about the cues that facilitated relaxation of the muscle in the clinic.

Piriformis

Starting position – positional release. With the patient in crook lying, support the hip against your body. With one hand, palpate the piriformis just lateral to the sacrum and cranial to the inferior arcuate band of the sacrotuberous ligament (see Figs 3.55A,

3.62A). Look for a tender point in the muscle. Apply gentle pressure to the muscle to monitor its tone and then slowly rotate/abduct the femur to facilitate maximal positional release of this muscle (Fig. 10.17). Although this muscle has been noted to change its direction of rotation above 60° of hip flexion (Kapandji 1970), when it is hypertonic it appears to remain an external rotator regardless of the range of hip flexion. Shortening the muscle, therefore, almost always requires external rotation of the femur and a variable amount of hip flexion and abduction. Maintain the articular position that yields the greatest amount of relaxation and wait for the resultant dampening of tone to occur (positional release). This will feel like a subtle softening of the muscle.

Adding awareness – cues to patient. Manual cue – maintain light pressure into the muscle and cue the patient to release/relax. Images of letting the hip decompress (come laterally) are often effective. As they discover how to release/relax, you will feel the pelvis and hip joints decompress and the piriformis soften.

Restoring length – after release. Once the neural component has been released, lengthen the muscle by internally rotating and flexing/adducting the femur. Continue to use words to encourage relaxation/release and monitor the piriformis for any recurrence of hypertonicity.

Recheck passive range of motion of the SIJ. If the technique has been successful, the innominate will now be able to glide freely relative to the sacrum in a parallel manner; all parts of the joint will no longer be compressed.

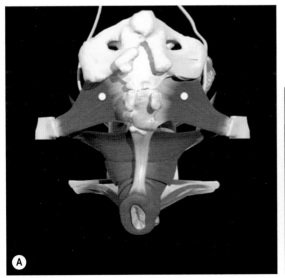
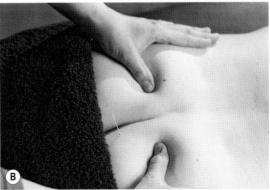

Fig. 10.16 • IMS/dry needling for release of the muscles compressing the SIJ. (A) Point of insertion for ischiococcygeus. From Primal Pictures Ltd. (www.primalpictures.com). (B) Needle in situ for ischiococcygeus.

299

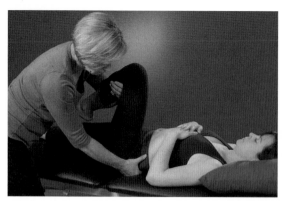

Fig. 10.17 • Specific *release with awareness*, combined with *stretch with awareness*, technique for piriformis. The piriformis muscle is monitored with one hand while the other seeks the position of the hip that facilitates its relaxation. Cue the patient with images of softening, melting, let the hip relax in the socket, and when you feel the hip and SIJ decompress, slowly take the hip joint into flexion/adduction and internal rotation. Watch for any anterior impingement of the hip, with or without groin pain, that likely signals a recurrence of the hypertonicity.

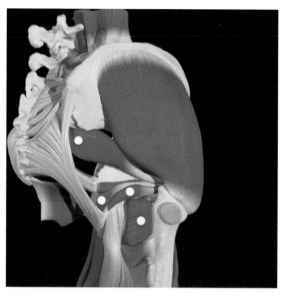

Fig. 10.18 • IMS/dry needling potential points for release of the deep posterior hip muscles: piriformis, obturator internus, inferior gemelli, and quadratus femoris. From Primal Pictures Ltd. (www.primalpictures.com).

Dry needling – residual hypertonicity. Persistent hypertonicity can be addressed using dry needling or IMS. Figure 10.18 and case report Christy, Chapter 9, Video CD9 🖱 illustrate the point used for dry needling to further release/relax piriformis.

Home practice. Small balls work well to facilitate relaxation or release of the piriformis muscle. While lying supine with the foot supported on a wall or chair, the small ball is placed over the tender point in piriformis. The patient thinks about the cues that facilitated relaxation of the muscle in the clinic and checks the efficacy of the release by noting the improved ability to move their hip into internal rotation and adduction while in the flexed position.

Superficial fibers of multifidus

Hypertonicity of the superficial fibers of multifidus (sMF) can compress multiple segments of the lumbar spine as well as the superior part of the sacroiliac joint (see Fig. 3.49). It is often associated with an underlying deficit of the deep fibers of multifidus that may be segmental or multisegmental. Palpate the hypertonic fascicle in sMF and follow it to the highest (most cranial) lumbar segment. You will now have identified the cranial and caudal extent of the hypertonic fascicle. See Chapter 9, Videos MQ13, 10.4 🖱 for a demonstration of the following technique.

Starting position – positional release. With the patient sidelying with the muscle to be released on

the uppermost side, localize the technique to the appropriate lumbar segments (e.g. L2 → SIJ) by rotating the thorax down to the first level above the hypertonic fascicle (e.g. L1-2). Support, and control, the thorax by winding your cranial arm through the patient's upper arm. Flex the patient's upper hip and knee, and place this foot behind the bottom knee. Palpate the hypertonic fascicle within the superficial fibers of multifidus and locate the tender point. Shorten the fascicle by sideflexing the lumbar spine through the thorax and pelvis and approximating either end of the hypertonic fascicle (intramuscular shortening). Hold both the articular and intramuscular positions and wait for the resultant dampening of tone to occur (positional release) (Fig. 10.19). This will feel like a subtle softening of the muscle.

Adding awareness – cues to patient. Some effective images/cues for releasing the superficial fibers of multifidus include: 'Let my fingers sink into your back, try to let the bones of your back relax into the table, or hang like a hammock, think about opening up space between your pelvis and your ribcage.' As they discover how to relax this muscle you will feel it soften further. Remember to encourage them as they learn to connect and release; this helps to reinforce that they are actually doing something essential and useful.

Restoring length – after release. Once the neural component has been released, lengthen the fascicle

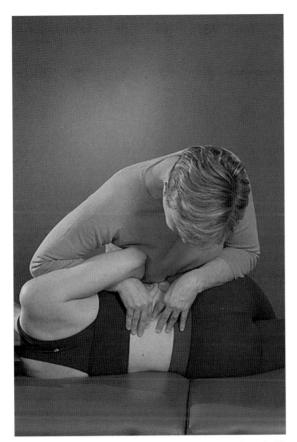

Fig. 10.19 • Specific *release with awareness*, combined with *stretch with awareness*, for the superficial fibers of multifidus. Shorten the fascicle specifically by approximating the iliac crest towards the appropriate spinous process. Monitor the hypertonic point and cue the patient verbally and manually to soften, release, relax. Once the maximum release has been obtained, specifically lengthen the fascicle with either an intramuscular technique (use your hands) or positional technique (sideflex to the contralateral side using your body).

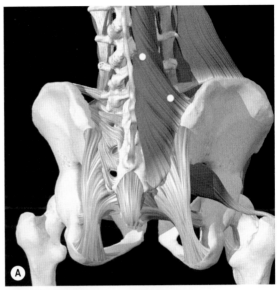

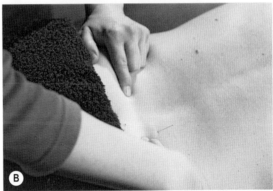

Fig. 10.20 • IMS/dry needling for release of the superficial fibers of multifidus (sMF). (A) Potential points of insertion for IMS/dry needling of the sMF. From Primal Pictures Ltd. (www.primalpictures.com). (B) Needle in situ at an inferior point.

manually (myofascial component – intramuscular stretch) as you take the lumbar spine through a full range of motion that lengthens the hypertonic muscle (contralateral sideflexion). Continue to use words to encourage relaxation/release and continuously monitor the fascicle for any recurrence of hypertonicity.

Recheck range of motion of the SIJ and the lumbar spine. If the technique has been successful, the innominate will now be able to glide freely relative to the sacrum in a parallel manner; the superior part of the joint will no longer be compressed on passive mobility testing. The specific mobility tests of the lumbar spine that had previously been restricted should now have full motion restored, unless there

is an underlying articular impairment (which will now be easily identified). In addition, now that all parts of the SIJ have been decompressed, the innominate should be able to posteriorly rotate relative to the sacrum on the non-weight bearing side, and the L5 should rotate to the non-weight bearing side during the one leg standing with contralateral hip flexion test.

Dry needling – residual hypertonic fascicles. Persistent hypertonicity can be addressed using dry needling or IMS. Figure 10.20A,B illustrates the points used for dry needling to further release/relax the superficial fibers of multifidus.

Home practice. In a four-point kneeling position, or prone over a ball, movements through full range

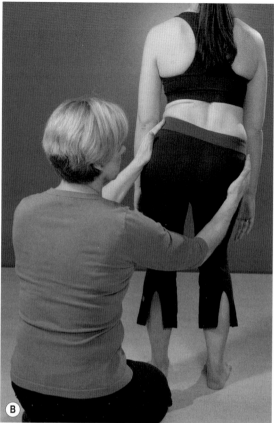

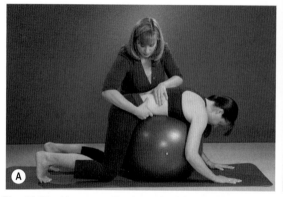

Fig. 10.21 • Home practice for maintaining the release of the superficial fibers of multifidus. (A) With the patient supported prone over a ball, provide verbal and tactile cues to facilitate relaxation of the sMF and lengthening of the lumbar spine (e.g. 'Let the weight of your pelvis hang off the ball'). This can also be an effective position for self-release of the erector spinae muscles. (B) The 'Pelvic Salsa' is a useful home practice for 'freeing' the pelvis and teaching dissociated movement of the pelvis, hips, and lumbar spine. It requires the patient to be able to lengthen/relax the adductors/abductors of the hip and lateral flexors of the lumbar spine. Have the patient semi-squat and ensure that the femur heads are centered and the lumbar spine is neutral. Have the patient follow your hands as your encourage lateral tilting, with no rotation or anterior/posterior tilting, of the pelvis. This practice helps to break rigid patterns of posture and movement.

of motion for lumbar flexion and sideflexion can be taught to maintain the length of the superficial fibers of multifidus (Fig. 10.21A). This can also be done in standing to facilitate dissociation of the pelvis/hip and lumbar spine (Fig. 10.21B).

Release techniques for multisegmental muscles compressing the lumbar spine

In addition to the superficial fibers of multifidus, hypertonicity of the longissimus thoracis pars lumborum, iliocostalis lumborum pars lumborum, and/or the quadratus lumborum can compress the lumbar

spine (and superior pole of the SIJ) and prevent segmental motion. The principles for release are the same as those described for releasing the superficial fibers of multifidus; the response of the hypertonic point in the relevant muscle is monitored as the lumbar spine is positioned such that the hypertonic fascicle/muscle is shortened. Cues to release/relax are given, the response noted, and the muscle is subsequently taken into a full stretch. It is common for multiple joints of the lumbar spine to 'pop' or 'cavitate' during the stretch part of this technique. Passive segmental flexion and sideflexion of the lumbar spine should be improved and the release of these muscles now allows further assessment of the articular system of the lumbar spine (mobility of the zygapophyseal joints (Chapter 8)).

Release techniques for superficial muscles compressing the thorax and abdomen

Erector spinae

The thoracic components of the erector spinae (longissimus thoracis pars thoracis and iliocostalis lumborum pars thoracis) are powerful compressors of the posterior joints of the thorax and lumbar spine, and through the attachment to the thoracolumbar fascia can also compress the SIJs (see Fig. 3.48A). A common, non-optimal, postural strategy seen in dancers is 'back-gripping' secondary to overactivation of the erector spinae. The thorax is posteriorly tilted (extended), the pelvis is anteriorly tilted, and the lumbar spine is

compressed between the two (Fig. 10.22A,B). Unilateral hypertonicity of these muscles can create a long multisegmental curve in the thorax and lumbar spine and an intrapelvic torsion (Fig. 10.22C). When combined with poor intrapelvic control, unlocking of the pelvis can occur (thorax-driven pelvic impairment, see Case report Julie G 🖱). The specific release and retraining of segmental control of the rings of the thorax is beyond the scope of this text (Lee 2003, Lee & Lee 2008b); however, it is important to know how to release the superficial back muscles to restore optimal function of the lumbopelvic–hip complex.

High acceleration, low amplitude recoil technique. Starting position – positional release. With the patient prone, place a small compressible ball (e.g. overball (Fig. 10.23A)), or a pillow, under the chest. Palpate

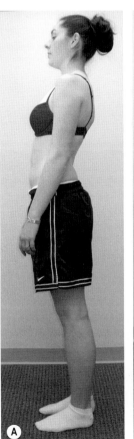
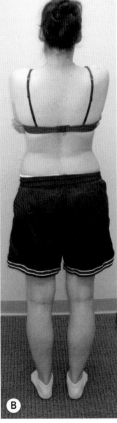
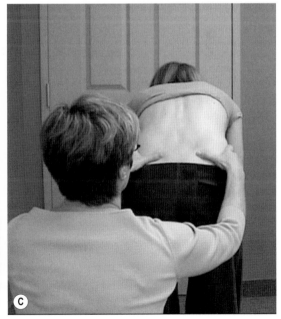

Fig. 10.22 • (A) The lateral profile of a back-gripper. This young woman habitually overactivates her erector spinae to position her thorax relative to her pelvis. Her abdominal wall is lengthened, her lumbar spine is shortened, and her thorax is posteriorly tilted. (B) From behind, note the excessive extension and resultant buckle at L3–4. (C) This young woman (see Case report Julie K, Chapter 9 🖱) has hypertonicity of the right erector spinae that fails to relax to allow eccentric lengthening in forward bending. The resultant force vector has produced a rotoscoliosis in her thorax and lumbar spine and an intrapelvic torsion.

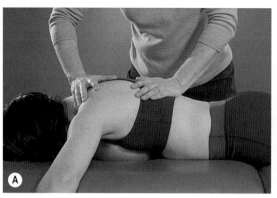 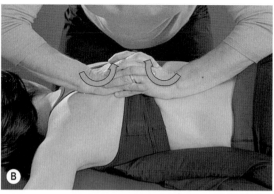

Fig. 10.23 • High acceleration, low amplitude recoil technique for release of the thoracic portion of the erector spinae (ES). (A) A soft overball can be placed under the chest to position the thorax in slight extension relative to the pelvis (slightly shorten the origin and insertion of the ES), and to create flexion of the thorax to provide the feeling of 'opening' of the posterior ribcage. (B) Alternately, use a pillow to flex the thorax and position it in slight posterior tilt relative to the lumbar spine. Capture the cranial and caudal end of the hypertonic fascicle(s) with the heels of your hands and interlock your fingers. Apply enough posteroanterior pressure to reach the layer of the ribs (do not compress the rib cage anteriorly) and shorten the ES as you sideflex the thorax. Ensure that your elbows are aligned and do not press any further anteriorly into the chest for the rest of the technique. Rapidly approximate the heels of your hands (adduct your shoulders) and simultaneously come off the chest (arrows) (see second part of Video 10.5 🖰). Immediately follow this technique with a specific intramuscular stretch of the relevant fascicles of ES.

the cranial and caudal extent of the hypertonic fascicle within the erector spinae and apply the heels of your left and right hand to either end of this fascicle. Interlace your fingers, extend your wrists, and align your elbows (Fig. 10.23B). Gently press into the muscle until you reach the 'layer of the ribs.' Capture both the muscle and the ribs and gently approximate both hands (sideflex the thorax and shorten the origin and insertion of the hypertonic fascicle).

Adding awareness – cues to the patient. Instruct the patient to let their chest soften into the ball/pillow and slowly let the air leave their chest.

Recoil. Once maximum shortening/release is obtained, quickly adduct your shoulders, approximate your wrists, and come off the chest (see case report Laura, Chapter 9, Video LC13 and Video 10.5 🖰). Take care not to go *into* the thorax with more posteroanterior pressure. If hypertonicity is found bilaterally, repeat this technique on the other side.

Hold/relax, or muscle energy, technique – starting position. With the patient sitting with their arms lightly crossed, palpate the cranial end of the hypertonic fascicle. Lengthen the fascicle by sideflexing and rotating the thorax (Fig. 10.24) to the motion barrier. Take care not to create more hypertonicity by moving quickly, or too far. Once the barrier is reached, instruct the patient to gently rotate either towards or away from you. Have them hold this gentle contraction for 3–5 seconds and after they relax

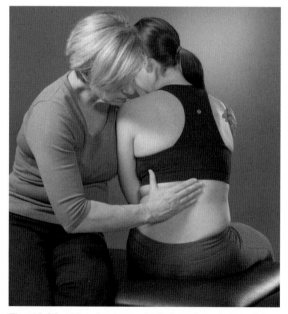

Fig. 10.24 • Muscle energy technique for release of the thoracic portion of the erector spinae. This is a direct technique followed by hold, or contract, and relax. Position the thorax such that the hypertonic muscle is somewhat lengthened. Monitor the fascicle and apply a resistance to rotation through the patient's shoulder (either towards or away from you). Hold the contraction for 3 seconds, relax, take up the extra length allowed by the hold–relax, and repeat three to four times.

completely take the thorax further into sideflexion/rotation to further lengthen the hypertonic fascicle. Repeat the technique three to four times.

Restoring length – after release. Once the neural component has been released, lengthen the specific fascicle and/or the entire erector spinae manually (myofascial component) with a moderately strong stretch (Fig. 10.25A,B).

Recheck range of motion of the thorax and lumbar spine and hypertonicity. If the technique has been successful, the thorax and lumbar spine will flex further and lateral bending to the opposite side will be improved. Importantly, the chest will be freer for respiration and rotation tasks.

Dry needling – residual hypertonic fascicles. Persistent hypertonicity can be addressed using dry needling, or IMS. Figure 10.26A,B illustrates the points

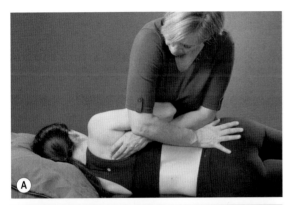

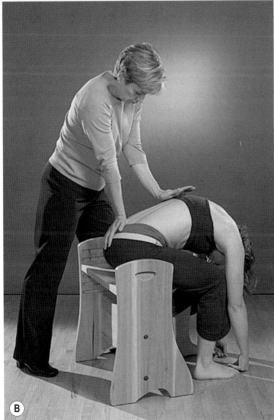

Fig. 10.25 • Specific stretch for the erector spinae. After the fascicles have been released stretch the myofascia in either (A) sidelying or (B) sitting.

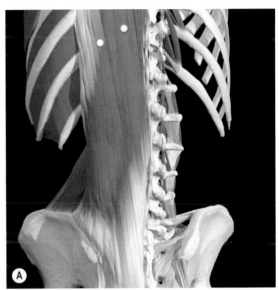

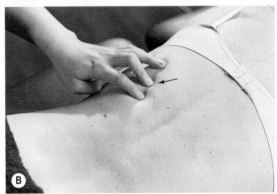

Fig. 10.26 • IMS/dry needling potential points for release of the thoracic portion of the erector spinae. (A) From Primal Pictures Ltd. (www.primalpictures.com). (B) When needling iliocostalis lumborum pars thoracis (insertion of erector spinae into the ribs), particular care needs to be taken to ensure the needle does not penetrate the thoracic cavity. With one hand, palpate the intercostal spaces above and below the rib of interest and be sure to direct the needle towards the rib. For longissimus thoracis pars thoracis, insert the needle directly over the transverse process of the thoracic vertebra.

used for dry needling to further release/relax persistent fascicles of the erector spinae. Unless you are very confident of your surface anatomy, all needling in the thorax should be contained to between the transverse and spinous processes. See case report Julie K, Chapter 9, Video JK8 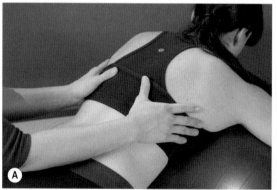 for a demonstration of this technique.

Home practice. Breath work can be used in the child's prayer pose position, or prone over a gym ball (Fig. 10.27A–C) to maintain the myofascial length gained from this technique. Instruct the patient to 'send their breath' to the areas of their thorax/back that require release. More home practice and cues for restoring optimal diaphragmatic breathing and releasing the chest are described in Chapter 11.

External oblique

The external oblique (EO) is a powerful compressor of the chest and, as a reminder from Chapter 3 (see Fig. 3.41), it is the largest abdominal with eight digitations arising from the external surfaces and inferior borders of the lower eight ribs (ribs 5–12) interdigitating with fibers of serratus anterior and latissimus dorsi. It is common to find this muscle hypertonic when it is used as part of a non-optimal strategy for transferring loads between the thorax and pelvis (e.g. a chest-gripping strategy). It is often hypertonic in women with stress urinary incontinence (Chapter 6), although hypertonicity of this muscle is not exclusive to this group. It is also common to find specific fascicles of the EO hypertonic and limiting motion of just one or two thoracic rings. This has significant implications for tasks requiring rotation of the thorax, as well as for function of the diaphragm and respiration.

Starting position – positional release. With the patient supine, hips and knees flexed, palpate the specific hypertonic fascicle of the EO (Fig. 10.28, case report Laura, Chapter 9, Video LC13 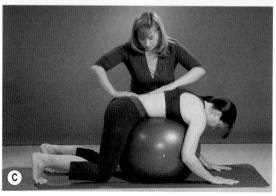).

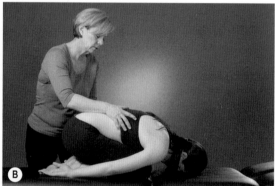

Fig. 10.27 • Home practice for release of the erector spinae. (A) With the patient prone over a gym ball, use your hands to manually cue where they are to send their breath for home practice. (B) The child's prayer pose from yoga is also a useful position for opening or lengthening the back if the patient has sufficient hip and knee flexion. (C) Lying prone over a curved structure, such as a gym ball, can also assist relaxation and lengthening of a hypertonic/tight erector spinae. Remind the patient to use any cues previously found helpful to optimize self-release.

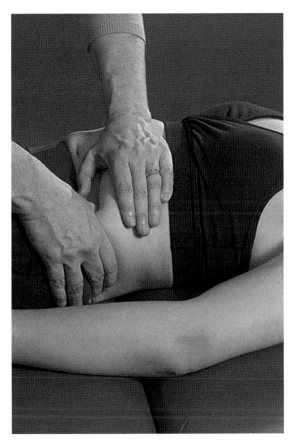

Fig. 10.28 • Specific *release with awareness* technique for the external oblique – supine. Monitor the tender point in the external oblique and shorten the hypertonic fascicle by approximating the specific rib(s) towards the linea alba. Cue a release ('let your abdomen soften and my thumb sink through the muscle') and then specifically lengthen/stretch the fascicle by taking the rib(s) away from the linea alba.

Shorten the fascicle by approximating the associated rib obliquely towards the linea alba and contralateral side of the pelvis. The fascicle can also be shortened directly with an intramuscular technique. Hold the fascicle in this shortened position and wait for the resultant dampening of tone to occur (positional release). This will feel like a subtle softening of the muscle.

Adding awareness – cues to patient. Cue the patient by saying 'let my fingers sink into your abdomen, let your rib cage relax and widen.'

Restoring length – after release. Once the neural component has been released, lengthen the fascicle manually (myofascial component – intramuscular stretch) between the associated rib and the linea alba.

Continue to use words to encourage relaxation/release and monitor the fascicle for any recurrence of hypertonicity. The lengthening of this anterior oblique sling can be taken further to include the contralateral adductor (Fig. 10.29A – cue a release first) and lower leg (Fig. 10.29B,C – take into a full myofascial stretch of the sling).

Recheck range of motion of the thorax and lumbar spine and hypertonicity. If the technique has been successful, the trunk (thorax and lumbar spine) will rotate further and the infrasternal angle will have widened. Importantly, the chest will be freer for respiration and rotation tasks.

Home practice. For releasing the chest bilaterally, have the patient either supine (Fig. 10.30A) or sitting. For releasing the chest unilaterally, have the patient in sidelying with the side to be released uppermost (Fig. 10.30B). Instruct the patient to 'send their breath' to the areas of their thorax/chest that require release and integrate the imagery cues that were previously found to be effective. Remind them to check their ability to rotate/translate their chest relative to the pelvis frequently during the day and to use their breath to release any acquired increase in resting tone.

Alternate technique for release. This technique can also be done in sitting (Fig. 10.31). Monitor the hypertonic fascicle either in the upper abdomen or along the line of the rib, shorten the fascicle, wait for the initial dampening response, cue a release ('let this rib soften into my hand, let my fingers soften into your belly,' etc.), and conclude the technique with a specific fascicular stretch using thoracic rotation.

Home practice for sling stretch with awareness. A strap, or the wall, is used to support the lower extremity. It is often useful to combine the specific cues for individual muscle release into an integrated cue for lengthening of the sling. For example, to lengthen the left anterior oblique sling from the foot to the rib cage, have the patient support the right lower extremity in a strap with the left hand (Fig. 10.32), or on the wall. They can palpate either the right short adductors or the left EO with their other hand. First, have them think about the cues that resulted in softening/relaxation of the adductors and the EO. Then, while maintaining this relaxed state, have them gently reach the heel long without losing control of either the pelvis or the thorax. A cue to imagine that the bones of their lower extremity are like a bobby pin inside a macaroni tube (their muscles), and to think of sliding the bobby pin down the

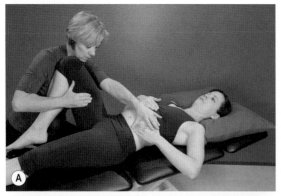

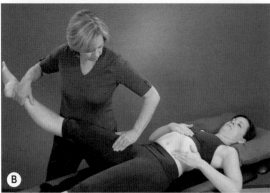

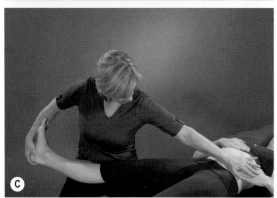

Fig. 10.29 • Combined release for the anterior oblique sling (external oblique (EO) and the contralateral adductors). (A) After the EO and the contralateral adductors have been specifically released, a combined technique can be done. Monitor the tone in both the EO and contralateral adductor, cue a release, and then (B) slowly lengthen the sling by abducting the flexed hip. In this illustration, the patient is monitoring the tone of the left EO as the therapist monitors the tone in the contralateral adductors during this task. (C) A full myofascial stretch of this sling includes dorsiflexion of the ankle, extension of the knee, abduction of the hip, and opening of the contralateral thorax.

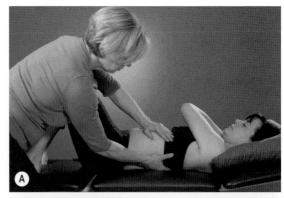

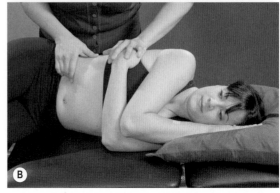

Fig. 10.30 • Home practice for using the breath to release/relax the external oblique. With the patient either (A) supine or (B) sidelying, use your hands to manually cue where they are to send their breath for home practice. In order for the chest to expand laterally, the brain must somehow release/relax the external oblique.

tube, is often effective in further relaxation and lengthening of this myofascial sling. Have them take the lower extremity further into the stretch, breathe into any tensed/tight spots, and repeat three to four times.

Internal oblique

Hypertonicity of the internal oblique (IO) is common in the upper and middle fibers that run superomedially, as well as the lower fibers that run inferomedially (see Fig. 3.40). The low horizontal fibers are released with an intramuscular technique, whereas the upper and middle fibers are released with a positional technique. *Release with awareness* is integrated with all of the techniques.

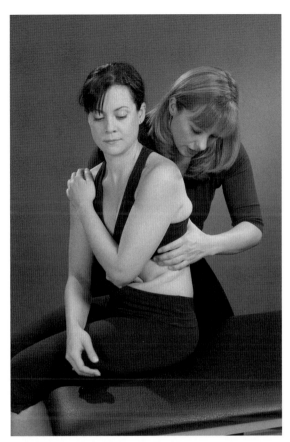

Fig. 10.31 • Specific release technique for the left external oblique (EO) – sitting. This is an illustration of the myofascial stretch portion of this release technique. The therapist is anchoring a fascicle of the left EO in the abdomen and then rotating the specific thoracic ring (segment) to the left to lengthen it.

Internal oblique, lower fibers – intramuscular release. With the patient supine, hips and knees supported over a bolster, palpate the medial and lateral extent of the hypertonic fascicle of the IO. Approximate the medial end towards the iliac crest (towards its origin) and hold the fascicle in this shortened position.

Adding awareness – cues to patient. Wait for the resultant dampening of tone to occur and then add awareness by cuing the patient to 'allow the belly to soften, to let my fingers sink into your abdominal wall.'

Restoring length – after release. Once the neural component has been released, lengthen the fascicle manually (myofascial component).

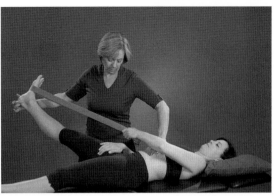

Fig. 10.32 • Home practice for release of the anterior oblique sling. In this home practice, the patient is using a yoga strap to support her right leg as she abducts the lengthened lower extremity to a position where a comfortable stretch is felt in the monitored muscle group, the adductors. This is an extension of the 'restoring length after release' technique (Fig. 10.29A–C), and is modified as necessary for home practice.

Recheck the response to verbal cue to isolate a contraction of transversus abdominis. If the technique has been successful, the optimal isolated response of transversus abdominis to a verbal cue is often, but not always, restored.

Home practice. Prior to training the deep system (Chapter 11), the patient should release the low horizontal fibers of the internal oblique (if hypertonic) by repeating this technique. Teach them how to find the hypertonic fascicle and how to feel for its release/relaxation through touch, fascicular shortening, and imagery. The IO layer should feel like a moist sponge cake and not a stale brownie (Chapter 8)!

Internal oblique, middle and upper fibers – positional release. The middle and upper fibers of the internal oblique are often hypertonic and when they are dominant during an automatic task, such as a curl-up, the rib cage and the infrasternal angle tends to widen. It is common to find a tender point in the upper and/or middle fibers of the IO halfway between the iliac crest and the ninth or tenth rib in the mid-axillary line (Fig. 10.33A,B, Video 10.6 🖱). These fibers tend to hold the lower ribs in posterior rotation and restrict expiration and contralateral rotation of the lower thorax. They can also create an intrapelvic torsion.

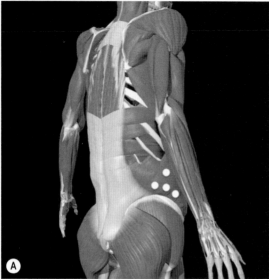

Starting position – positional release. With the patient in sidelying with the muscle to be released on the uppermost side, support and control the thorax by winding your cranial arm through the patient's upper arm. Flex the patient's upper hip and knee and place this foot behind the bottom knee. Palpate the hypertonic fascicle and shorten it by rotating/sideflexing the thorax (Fig. 10.34). Hold this position and wait for the resultant dampening of tone to occur (positional release). This will feel like a subtle softening of the muscle.

Adding awareness – cues to patient. Cue the patient to 'let the muscle in your waist soften, let your pelvis roll backwards, let my fingers sink into your waist, let your ribs relax into my hand.' Remember to encourage them as they learn to connect and

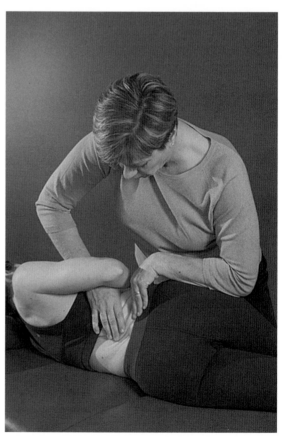

Fig. 10.33 • Locating a tender, hypertonic point in the internal oblique. (A) Location of common tender, hypertonic points in the upper and middle fibers of the internal oblique. From Primal Pictures Ltd. (www.primalpictures.com). (B) Palpation of tender points in the upper and middle fibers of the internal oblique.

Fig. 10.34 • Specific *release with awareness*, combined with *stretch with awareness*, technique for the upper and middle fibers of the internal oblique. Monitor the hypertonic point, shorten the origin and insertion of the hypertonic fascicle with ipsilateral sideflexion/rotation, wait for the dampening response, cue a release, and then take into a full myofascial stretch (contralateral sideflexion/rotation).

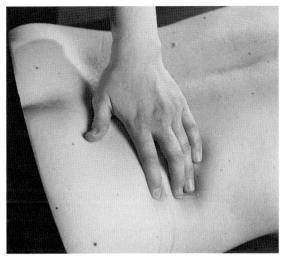

Fig. 10.35 • IMS/dry needling for release of the middle fibers of the internal oblique.

release; this helps to reinforce that they are actually doing something very essential and useful.

Restoring length – after release. Once the neural component has been released, lengthen the fascicle by taking the thorax into contralateral rotation/side-flexion in a direction that lengthens the hypertonic muscle. Continue to use words to encourage relaxation/release and monitor the fascicle for any recurrence of hypertonicity.

Recheck range of motion of the thorax. If the technique has been successful, rotation of the lower thorax to the opposite side will be improved, as will expiration of the lower rib cage.

Dry needling – residual hypertonic fascicles. Persistent hypertonicity of the IO can be addressed using dry needling, or IMS. Figure 10.35 illustrates the points used for dry needling to further release/relax persistent fascicles of the middle fibers of the IO.

Home practice. In a crook lying position with the hips and knees flexed, have the patient palpate the hypertonic fascicle in the waist and remember the image/cue that facilitated relaxation of the fascicle. Instruct them to slowly rotate their knees and pelvis towards the hypertonic side maintaining full contact of both sides of their thorax with the table (Fig. 10.36). Teach them to note when any increase in activation of the IO occurs; the muscle should remain relaxed during this motion. Small balls can also be used to facilitate relaxation of the EO and/or IO (Fig. 10.37A,B). Have the patient place a small, soft ball in the abdomen over the tender, hypertonic point and then lay prone. Cue the patient to use the image that was found effective during the release

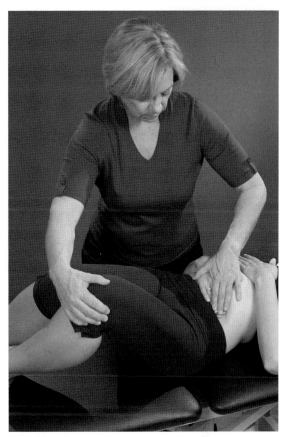

Fig. 10.36 • Home practice for release of the middle fibers of the internal oblique. Have the patient rotate their pelvis relative to the thorax so as to lengthen the monitored internal oblique. Remind them to use the cues/images that were effective for relaxing/releasing this muscle as they rotate.

with awareness technique to practice dampening the tone of the superficial abdominals. Note that this is also a useful self-release for psoas hypertonicity once the abdominals have been released.

Rectus abdominis

Rectus abdominis is often hypertonic in individuals who do repetitive curl-ups or abdominal 'crunches' as part of their exercise program, and can be asymmetrically hypertonic in individuals with pubic symphysis dysfunction and/or pain. It is best released with an intramuscular technique followed by a *stretch with awareness* practice.

Starting position – intramuscular release. With the patient supine, hips and knees supported over a bolster, palpate the cranial and caudal extent of the

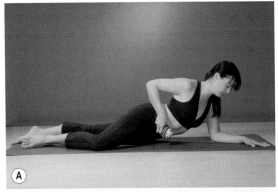

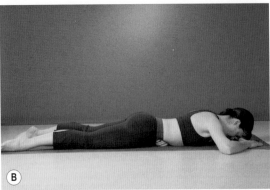

Fig. 10.37 • Home practice for release of the superficial abdominals – external and internal oblique. A small release ball is a useful home tool for relaxation and dampening of tone in the superficial abdominal muscles. Here, the patient (A) is placing a small ball over the anterolateral abdomen (over the hypertonic fascicles) and then (B) relaxing the abdomen so that the ball gently sinks in. Cues/images and breathing are used to facilitate this relaxation/release. There should be no pain, and no resultant bracing of the abdominal wall, during this practice.

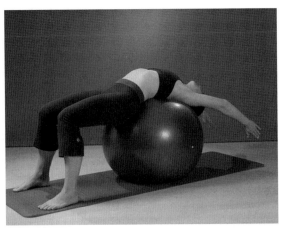

Fig. 10.38 • Home practice for lengthening the abdominal wall. This is a useful practice for chest-grippers. If balance is an issue, have them place the ball between a wall and a chair to secure the ball. They can use their arms to support their head and neck as they lengthen the front of the abdomen/chest or alternately, as in this illustration, they can lengthen the continuous myofascial slings into the arms by elevating them overhead. Integrate cues for release and breath work to get the most from this practice.

hypertonic fascicle. Approximate the two ends and hold the fascicle in this shortened position.

Adding awareness – cues to patient. Wait for the resultant dampening of tone to occur and then add awareness by cuing the patient to 'allow the belly to soften, let my fingers sink into your abdominal wall, open the space between your pelvis and your ribcage.'

Restoring length – after release. Once the neural component has been released, lengthen the fascicle manually (myofascial component).

Home practice. If the rectus abdominis is hypertonic and short it can be released and lengthened by laying supine over the curvature of a gym ball (Fig. 10.38), or in prone with a 'sloppy' push-up (the chest is pressed up with the arms while leaving the pelvis on the floor). Instruct the patient to palpate the hypertonic band(s) in this position, to use imagery to facilitate a release/relaxation, and to use their breath to relax/lengthen the midline of the abdominal wall and chest.

Techniques for mobilizing the articular system

Mobilization techniques for the stiff, fibrotic hip joint

Hypertonicity of the deep and superficial muscles of the hip can hide a true, stiff joint. The characteristic 'hard end feel' of a stiff, fibrotic joint can be felt once the muscles of the hip have been released. Techniques that distract the capsule are an effective way to mobilize fibrotic joints and are even more effective when they are vector specific. See case report Mike, Chapter 9, Video MQ15 for a demonstration of this technique.

Lateral distraction of the hip – starting position. With the patient supine, hip and knee flexed, place a mobilization strap around the proximal thigh and secure it around your pelvis (Fig. 10.39). A towel

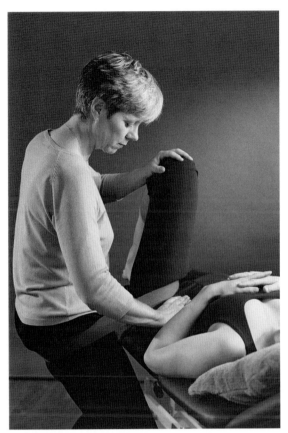

Fig. 10.39 • Passive mobilization technique for the stiff, fibrotic hip joint. The mobilization strap helps to apply the technique along the specific vector of resistance. A sustained Grade 4 mobilization technique is used to mobilize the adhered connective tissue within the fibrotic capsule.

or extension/abduction/internal rotation); the key is to release all of the vectors creating compression of the joint. Find the greatest vector of resistance and explore all directions and limits of the functional range of motion. Ensure that the femoral head remains centered throughout the technique (palpate it anteriorly), and release any hypertonic muscles that arise at any time.

Mobilization with movement (also known as a Mulligan mobilization or active release technique). After the passive technique has released the connective tissue, active mobilization with movement is useful. Maintain the lateral distraction of the hip along the line of the greatest vector of resistance and have the patient actively move further into, and out of, a variety of combined hip movements.

Recheck the functional range of motion of the hip joint. If the technique has been successful, the femoral head will now be centered and remain so through an increased range of motion of the hip joint. Test the new functional range of hip motion (range where the femoral head remains centered) and repeat the mobilization technique, if necessary.

Home practice. Integrate the new functional range of motion into a home practice that has meaning for them (i.e. squat, lunge, etc.) (Video 10.7 🖱 see Chapter 12). The 'Pelvic Salsa' is a lovely way to maintain the range gained in a treatment session (see Fig. 10.21C). Pelvic rock in four-point kneeling, or supported on a gym ball (see Fig. 10.14A,B), is also a useful movement task for maintaining the mobility gained and coordinating hip and pelvic girdle motion. Home practice for integrating hip mobility into tasks requiring extension will be covered later.

between the belt and the patient's thigh can be used for comfort. With one hand, palpate the femoral head and support the lower extremity with the other.

Vector mobilization. Take the hip joint to the motion barrier of flexion, adduction, and internal rotation (no pain should be provoked and the femoral head should remain centered in the acetabulum). Hold this femoral position and find the vector that provides the greatest resistance to lateral distraction by leaning back slightly into the mobilization strap. Explore a variety of angles and feel for the stiffest, most resistant vector. Once found, stop oscillating and sustain a strong, but painfree, lateral distraction force (Grade 4) in the line of this vector until you feel the connective tissue release. The hip joint can also be mobilized into other combinations of restriction (i.e. flexion/abduction/external rotation

Mobilization techniques for the stiff, fibrotic sacroiliac joint

This section describes the specific therapy indicated for restoring mobility of the sacroiliac joint following a traumatic sprain of the joint, as it is this injury that often leads to a stiffness and fibrosis if not properly managed. If the injury results in an intra-articular synovitis, several pain provocation tests will be positive (Chapter 8) and the goal of treatment at this time is to reduce the load through the joint such that healing can occur. The SIJ is a difficult joint to rest as most postures/positions compress the joint. Clinically, it appears that the best resting position for the painful SIJ is sidelying with the painful side uppermost and the hip and knee supported on a

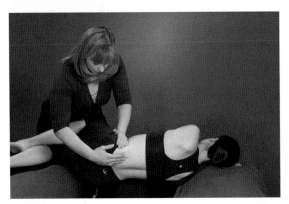

Fig. 10.40 • Passive mobilization technique to maintain mobility of the SIJ. In this illustration the therapist is supporting the patient's left femur on her abdomen and the left innominate in both of her hands. The SIJ can be taken through its full range of motion (4–6°) using a circumductive motion of both hands (rotate the innominate posteriorly and anteriorly).

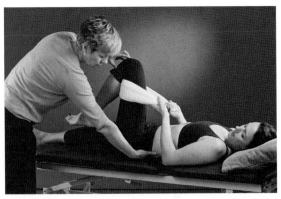

Fig. 10.41 • Home practice for maintaining range of motion in an inflamed SIJ. At home, instruct the patient to use either their hands or a towel to support the thigh and to then bring the knee towards the chest only until they feel a resistance to this motion (the first barrier). They can then apply a gentle hold/relax technique to have the hamstrings facilitate posterior rotation of the innominate. All home practice should be painfree.

pillow. Weight bearing activities, such as walking, standing, and sitting, should be minimized during the first few days. A cane can help to reduce loading through the pelvis when walking. Sacroiliac belts increase compression of the joint and often increase pain during this stage of healing.

As the pain and inflammation settle, passive (Fig. 10.40) and active range of motion of the SIJ should be encouraged. For home practice, have the patient pull their knee towards their chest to posteriorly rotate the innominate relative to the sacrum (Fig. 10.41). If the patient presents several weeks or months after the initial injury, it is possible that the SIJ has become stiff and fibrotic. The innominate is often positioned in anterior rotation relative to the sacrum, and the joint does not unlock during vertical loading tasks. Active posterior rotation is reduced compared to the opposite side, as is the passive joint mobility. The neutral zone is reduced compared to the other side, and the end feel in the elastic zone of motion is firm. It is common for this patient to report a change in location of their pain, with the regions above and below the restricted SIJ now painful (low back, groin, contralateral pelvis) instead of the SIJ. Once again, distraction of the joint according to specific vector analysis of the direction of greatest resistance is the mobilization technique of choice.

Distraction of the SIJ – starting position. With the patient supine, hip and knee flexed, palpate the medial aspect of the ilium and posterior superior iliac

spine (PSIS). With the other arm/hand support the femur, flex the hip, and posteriorly rotate the innominate relative to the sacrum until the motion barrier is perceived both with your posterior hand and with the flexing femur (Fig. 10.42). Adduct and wiht internally rotate the femur to the motion barrier of the hip. If this motion provokes pain in the groin and/or displaces the femoral head anteriorly, release the hypertonic muscles of the hip that are displacing the femoral head prior to mobilizing the SIJ. If the hip can be taken into flexion/adduction/internal rotation with no impingement in the groin, the technique can proceed.

Vector mobilization. Maintain the barrier of posterior rotation of the SIJ and flexion/adduction/internal rotation (IR) of the hip and distract the SIJ by applying a dorsolateral force along the length of the femur. Vary the direction of this force to find the specific vector of greatest resistance. Once found, sustain this force, do not oscillate, and wait for the connective tissue to release; the SIJ will distract posteriorly. Ensure that the muscles that can potentially compress the SIJ (superficial fibers of multifidus, piriformis, and ischiococcygeus) remain relaxed by using verbal cues (e.g. 'let your sitz bones go wide as I press down on your leg, let your buttock soften and your back relax').

Recheck the passive and active range of motion of the SIJ. The sacroiliac joint is capable of only a small amount of motion, and therefore it should be possible to restore all of its mobility in one treatment. If the technique has been successful, the passive

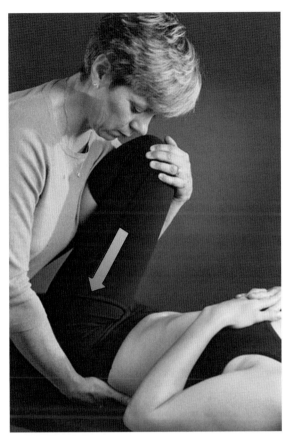

Fig. 10.42 • Passive mobilization technique for the stiff, fibrotic SIJ. After the SIJ is taken to the barrier for posterior rotation, the femur is slightly adducted and internally rotated. From here, the specific vector of resistance that is restricting motion of the SIJ is determined by applying a dorsolateral force (arrow) in a variety of directions; look for the vector of greatest resistance. Once this vector is found, a sustained Grade 4 mobilization technique is used to release the fibrotic connective tissue.

anteroposterior glide between the innominate and sacrum should be restored, parallel, and symmetrical. There is rarely any need for a home practice to maintain the range of motion gained.

Manipulation (high acceleration, low amplitude thrust) technique for the SIJ

There are many ways to manipulate the sacroiliac joint, and most techniques are chosen according to a biomechanical paradigm. If the innominate is felt to be fixated in a superior direction (also known as an

innominate upslip or sacral downslip), the suggested technique is to pull the innominate down. If the innominate is felt to be fixated in anterior rotation, the suggested technique is to posteriorly rotate it, and if fixated in posterior rotation, anteriorly rotate it. Previous editions of this text supported this approach; however, paradigms shift as scientific evidence and clinical expertise evolves and it appears that a skillfully applied, distractive manipulation technique can correct all of these 'positional faults.' As mentioned previously, there is an ongoing debate between clinicians, as well as between clinicians and researchers, as to the ability of the SIJ to sublux or become fixated. So, how should the story and objective findings of the individual whose mobility and function are restored with a specific manipulation, or HALAT technique, be interpreted (e.g. see case report Julie G, Chapter 9 🖱)? Julie presented with a history of multiple direct traumas to her pelvic girdle (a fall on her buttock, a car accident, a sudden vertical force up her leg), a non-physiological position of the three bones of the pelvic girdle (a right anteriorly rotated innominate relative to the left and a right rotated sacrum), and an extremely compressed (no palpable motion) left SIJ. Her ASLR test was negative in that, although she found it harder to lift her left leg, no compression of the pelvic girdle made the task easier. One specific manipulation of the left sacroiliac joint changed all of these findings (Video JG5 🖱). Was the joint truly 'out,' 'subluxed,' or 'fixated,' or merely excessively compressed?

In these individuals, when the integrity of the articular system restraints is tested post-manipulation, the ligaments/capsule appear to be somewhat compromised in that mobility is still possible when the joint is close-packed. This suggests that there is an underlying articular system impairment, and perhaps the strategy used to stabilize the joint prior to the manipulation involved co-contraction of multiple muscles, which effectively rendered the joint rigid in a non-physiological position. Although we are not sure of the exact mechanism underlying this particular condition, we do appreciate that there is a place for knowing how to apply a high acceleration, low amplitude thrust technique to the SIJ as the technique effectively restores the joint's mobility, for whatever reason.

Posterior distraction of the left SIJ – high acceleration, low amplitude thrust – starting position. With the patient in right sidelying and the lower leg extended and the upper hip and knee flexed, rotate the thorax and lumbar spine until L5–S1 is felt to be

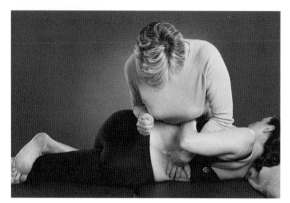

Fig. 10.43 • Specific manipulation technique for the SIJ (HALAT) (see Video JG5 🖱️).

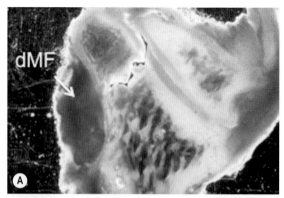

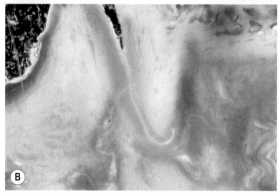

Fig. 10.44 • Unsuspected fractures involving the lumbar zygapophyseal joint following motor vehicle accidents (MVAs) (Twomey et al 1989). (A) Dr. Twomey gave Diane this beautiful dissection after both were keynote speakers in Hong Kong in 1992. The dissection comes from research published by Drs Twomey and Taylor in the 1980s while investigating fractures of the lumbar spine that were not visible on X-ray after severe MVAs. In this individual, an avulsion fracture of the mammillary process is evident and extends into the joint. Note the attachment of the deep fibers of multifidus (dMF). Contraction of these fibers would distract the fracture and this is possibly why the brain inhibits its activation in the early stages of this injury. (B) This dissection illustration is another gift from Dr. Twomey and beautifully shows an intra-articular fracture through the superior articular process of a lumbar zygapophyseal joint.

fully rotated to the left. With the cranial hand, firmly stabilize L5 and the sacrum. With the forearm, internally rotate the left innominate *about a pure vertical axis through the pelvic girdle* to gap or distract the posterior aspect of the SIJ (Fig. 10.43). The technique can be focused to the S1, S2, or S3 segment; find the stiffest vector of resistance.

Vector manipulation. From this position, a high acceleration, low amplitude thrust is applied through the left innominate to distract the posterior aspect of the left SIJ. The joint may not cavitate (pop or make a noise); this is not essential for the technique to be successful.

Recheck active and passive mobility of the SIJ. If the technique has been successful, the SIJ mobility will be restored. Further analysis is now required to assess the integrity of the articular, myofascial, and neural systems. The ASLR test will determine whether an external support is required and exactly where the compression straps should be applied (Chapter 11).

Home practice. This will depend on the findings from the subsequent assessment of the articular, myofascial, and neural systems.

Mobilization techniques for stiff, fibrotic joints in the lumbar spine

This section describes the specific therapy indicated for restoring segmental lumbar mobility (including the zygapophyseal joints and the intervertebral disc) following a traumatic sprain, as it is this injury that often leads to a stiff, fibrotic segment if not properly managed. Rest is rarely indicated for the acutely sprained back. Patients are encouraged to remain as active/mobile as possible. However, if there is a

suspected fracture of the zygapophyseal joint (Fig. 10.44A,B), there will be associated inhibition of the deep fibers of multifidus and healing of the bone must precede training of this muscle. The resting position for the painful low back is supine with the hips and knees semi-flexed and supported over a wedge. Once healing has progressed to the stage where load is tolerated, gentle movements through range should be encouraged (pelvic tilting in either the supine (Fig. 10.45) or four-point kneeling position).

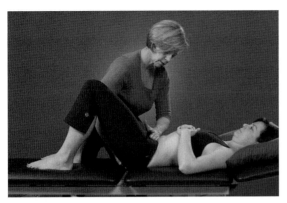

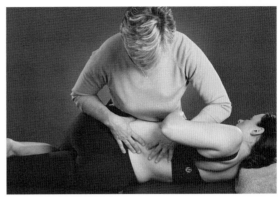

Fig. 10.45 • Home practice for maintaining range of motion after an acute sprain of the low back. Instruct the patient to tilt the pelvis posteriorly so as to flex the joints of the low back and then to tilt the pelvis anteriorly to extend them. Remind them to keep the amplitude of this practice within the painfree range.

Fig. 10.46 • Passive mobilization technique for the stiff, fibrotic lumbar joint. The treatment of choice is specific distraction of the lumbar three-joint complex along the most resistant vector. Once this vector is found, sustain the Grade 4 force until you feel the connective tissue release. Integrate with verbal and manual cues as necessary.

When pain is persistent and an individual's strategy for transferring loads has been non-optimal for some time (co-contraction of multiple trunk muscles that renders the low back stiff and rigid), the joints can also become stiff and rigid. This is not apparent until the multisegmental muscles of the back are released with techniques described above. It is common to find one segment hypermobile into either flexion or extension (flexion or extension hinge) (see Fig. 4.13A,B) and the segments above or below hypomobile. In treatment, the goal is to distribute the load throughout the lumbar spine, to mobilize the stiff segments, and to teach the patient to control motion at the hypermobile segment. The following techniques are useful for mobilizing the stiff, fibrotic joints of the lumbar spine.

Specific distraction of joints of the lumbar spine – starting position. With the patient sidelying with their hips and knees slightly flexed, localize the technique by rotating the thorax and lumbar spine to the level above the segment to be mobilized. Flex the uppermost hip, knee, and lumbar spine to the segment below the one to be mobilized and instruct the patient to simultaneously reach the lower leg towards the end of the table. The foot of the upper leg then rests against the popliteal fossa of the lower leg. The segment of interest should still be in a neutral position. Stabilize the thorax with your upper (cranial) arm and the pelvis/low lumbar spine with your lateral thorax and lower (caudal) arm. Your hands should be free to monitor/palpate the segment to be mobilized.

Vector mobilization. The specific vector of resistance is sought by segmentally sideflexing/rotating/flexing/

extending the joint (Fig. 10.46). Find the vector of greatest resistance, sustain the force, and wait for the connective tissue to release. The zygapophyseal and intervertebral joints will distract when the vector releases. Repeat the vector analysis and the mobilization if necessary. Ensure that all muscles that can potentially compress the joint (superficial fibers of multifidus, longissimus thoracis pars lumborum, iliocostalis lumborum pars lumborum, and/or quadratus lumborum) remain relaxed by using verbal and manual cues. A gentle hold/relax cue can also be integrated into this technique should a myofascial vector arrive.

Recheck the passive range of motion of the lumbar spine. The amplitude of motion for the lumbar joints is small and one mobilization technique should suffice to restore full range. The active range of motion may still appear limited if the strategy chosen still renders the spine rigid. As long as the passive mobility has been restored, the potential exists for retraining a better strategy for movement and control (Chapters 11, 12).

Home practice. The range of motion of the lumbar spine can be maintained by:

1. posterior, anterior, and lateral tilting of the pelvis in the supine position (Fig. 10.45); or
2. by using the 'Pelvic Salsa' practice in the standing position (see Fig. 10.21B);
3. using task-related movements that require the relevant lumbar spine range of motion (Chapter 12).

While teaching in Germany, Diane was introduced to the Salsero-chair, an invention of Edwin Jaeger

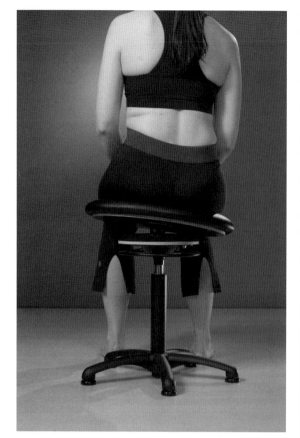

Fig. 10.47 • Edwin Jaeger invented this unique Salsero-chair for his own rehabilitation after a dance injury led to a prolapse of an intervertebral disc in his low back. It is challenging to find your center while seated on this multidirectionally unstable stool. It is different from sitting on a gym ball and specific motions of the pelvis beneath the lumbar spine and thorax are needed to rotate the stool clockwise and counter-clockwise. Although this can easily aggravate an early injured and painful lumbar spine, it is a great tool for restoring mobility and proprioceptive sense of lumbopelvic position once rehabilitation has moved to later stages of healing and retraining.

(Fig. 10.47), and has found it useful for retraining both mobility and positional sense for the lumbopelvis.

Manipulation (high acceleration, low amplitude thrust) techniques for the lumbar joints

An intra-articular meniscoid of a moderately degenerated zygapophyseal joint (Fig. 10.48A–C) can become stuck during flexion and rotation of the trunk if segmental motion is poorly controlled (the acute, locked back). A high acceleration, low amplitude thrust, or manipulation, technique is useful for this condition and it is thought that the technique relocates the meniscoid.

Specific distraction HALAT to relocate a lumbar zygapophyseal joint meniscoid – starting position. With the patient sidelying with their hips and knees slightly flexed, localize the technique by rotating the thorax and lumbar spine to the level above the segment to be manipulated. Flex the uppermost hip, knee, and lumbar spine to the segment below the one to be manipulated and instruct the patient to simultaneously reach the lower leg towards the end of the table. The foot of the upper leg then rests against the popliteal fossa of the lower leg. Stabilize the thorax with your upper (cranial) arm and the pelvis/low lumbar spine with your lateral thorax

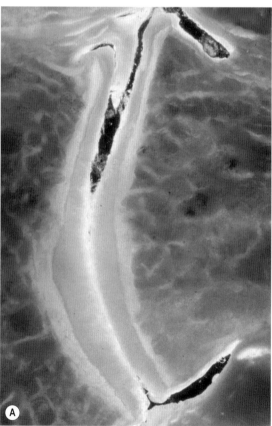

Ⓐ

Fig. 10.48 • (A) This is a coronal section through a healthy lumbar zygapophyseal joint; note the meniscoid inclusion. This dissection is another gift from Dr. Twomey.

Continued

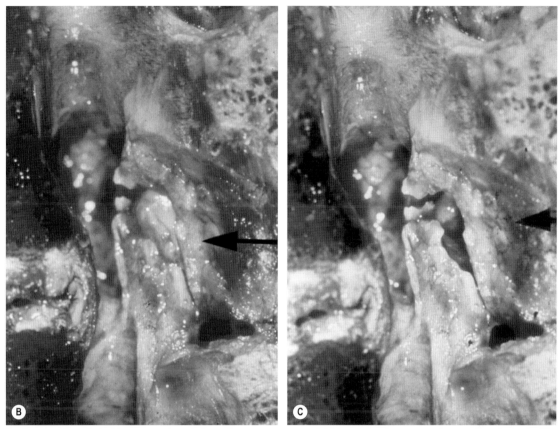

Fig. 10.48 – cont'd • (B) With degeneration, these inclusions can become thick and fibrotic and occasionally 'stuck' outside of the joint. The patient then presents with a flexed and laterally deviated posture. This is a sagittal section of a lumbar spine from Kirkaldy-Willis et al (1978) and is reproduced with permission. Note the thickening of the meniscoid inclusion. (C) This is the same dissection as (B) with the meniscoid inclusion removed; note the degeneration of the joint surfaces.

and lower (caudal) arm. Your hands should be free to monitor/palpate the segment to be manipulated.

Vector manipulation. Rotate the impaired segment in the pure transverse plane so as to distract the sagittal part of the zygapophyseal joint (Fig. 10.49); a firm barrier will be met almost immediately. From this position, distract the joint further with a very fast (high acceleration), small (low amplitude) thrust applied directly into axial rotation of the segment. In our experience, this manipulation technique must be specific to be effective for this condition.

Recheck the passive range of motion of the lumbar spine. If the technique has been successful, there will be an immediate restoration of passive segmental flexion and sideflexion/rotation. There will also be significant inhibition of the deep fibers of multifidus that

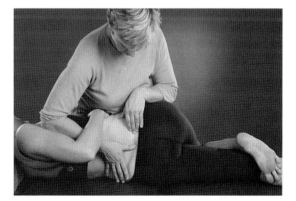

Fig. 10.49 • A very specific articular manipulation (HALAT) is essential for reducing a 'stuck' meniscoid in the lumbar zygaphophyseal joint.

will require retraining ('waking up' – Chapter 11) if recurrence is to be prevented. Further analysis is now required to assess the articular, myofascial, and neural systems.

Home practice. This will depend on the findings from the subsequent assessment of the articular, myofascial, and neural systems.

Specific distraction HALAT of the zygapophyseal joint for neuromyofascial release – starting position. With the patient sidelying with their hips and knees slightly flexed, focus the technique by rotating the thorax and lumbar spine to the level above the segment to be manipulated. Flex the uppermost hip, knee, and lumbar spine to the segment below the one to be manipulated and instruct the patient to simultaneously reach the lower leg towards the end of the table. The foot of the upper leg then rests against the popliteal fossa of the lower leg. Stabilize the thorax with your upper (cranial) arm and the pelvis/low lumbar spine with your lateral thorax and lower (caudal) arm. Your hands should be free to monitor/palpate the segment to be manipulated.

Vector manipulation. From this position, find the direction of the most resistant vector *for that segment* (flex/extend, sideflex/rotation). Cue the patient to release/relax and, at the moment you begin to feel the joint release, apply a very fast (high acceleration), small (low amplitude) thrust directly along the line of the resistant vector (Fig. 10.50, see case report Mike, Chapter 9, Video MQ13). This technique may produce a general response (multiple segments may release/have increased mobility), yet is very

specific in its application and only one joint should cavitate (pop).

Recheck the passive range of motion of the lumbar spine. If the technique has been successful, there will be an immediate restoration of both passive and active motion of the lumbar segment. This technique often, but not always, 'normalizes' the resting tone of both the deep and superficial fibers of multifidus; in other words, it can help to inhibit the sMF and 'wake up' the dMF. Manipulation of the spine also been reported to 'improve the contraction' of transversus abdominis (Gill et al 2007).

Home practice. The range of motion of the lumbar spine can be maintained by:

1. posterior, anterior, and lateral tilting of the pelvis in the supine position (Fig. 10.45);
2. using the 'Pelvic Salsa' practice in the standing position (Fig. 10.21b); or
3. using the Salsero-chair (Fig. 10.47); or
4. using task-related movements that require the relevant lumbar spine range of motion (Chapter 12).

Techniques for releasing the viscera

Addressing underlying visceral disease may require medical intervention, and thus it is essential that the clinician is aware of non-mechanical patterns of pain and indicators of visceral disease. Pain arising from the viscera appears to reflexly inhibit the deep muscles of the abdomen; therefore the restoration of optimal strategies for posture and movement will require that this system be addressed. The treatment of visceral disease is outside the scope of physiotherapy practice and when suspected should be referred to the patient's physician. However, it is not uncommon to find lack of mobility between the organs themselves and between the organs and the musculoskeleton as a consequence of inflammation, surgery, and/or trauma. These restrictions can also alter strategies for posture and movement, and treatment for this is definitely within the scope of physiotherapy practice (see case report Jennifer, Chapter 9), yet is not commonly taught. Jean-Pierre Barral has developed a comprehensive curriculum for the assessment and treatment of visceral impairments and the reader is referred to the Barral Institute for further information on this subject (www.barralinstitute.com).

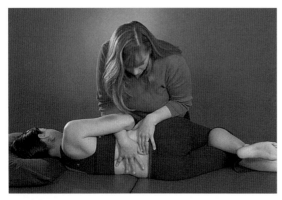

Fig. 10.50 • Specific articular manipulation (HALAT) technique for release of a lumbar zygapophyseal joint. Compare the localization of this technique to that in Fig. 10.5.

Active technique for correcting pelvic alignment

This is a useful technique to correct any residual intrapelvic torsion before beginning training of the deep muscle system (Chapter 11). In the supine lying position, if the pelvis rests in an IPTR, the following technique/home practice is chosen. Simply reverse the side of the technique for an IPTL.

Correction technique. The patient is supine, with their hips and knees flexed. With the long and ring finger of one hand, palpate the left sacral sulcus, just medial to the PSIS. The limit of posterior rotation of the left innominate is reached by passively flexing the left femur until the motion barrier for posterior rotation of the left innominate is perceived. From this position, the patient is instructed to resist further hip flexion, which is gently increased by the therapist. The isometric contraction is held for up to 5 seconds, followed by a period of complete relaxation. The innominate is then passively taken to the new barrier of posterior rotation. The hold–relax is repeated three times followed by re-evaluation of the intrapelvic alignment.

Home practice. The patient can be taught to do this technique at home using a towel (see Fig. 10.41). The patient engages the motion barrier of posterior rotation of the innominate by flexing the left femur and then gently contracts the hip extensors against the resistance of the towel. The contraction is held for up to 5 seconds, followed by a period of complete relaxation. The femur is then flexed further, thus taking the innominate to the new motion barrier of posterior rotation. The pelvis should be in neutral alignment before beginning the home practice for isolation training of the deep muscle system.

Summary

This chapter has described and illustrated several techniques for releasing many muscles and joints of the LPH complex. Be specific with the articular techniques and imaginative and creative with the cues for neuromyofascial release as they appear to be culturally and geographically sensitive. Once the patient learns how to perform these release techniques for themselves (*self-release with awareness*), the rewiring of the neural networks has begun. Sometimes, function can be restored (optimal strategies chosen for all tasks and pain reduced) using only the techniques described in this chapter. More often, there is still some work to be done to build new neural networks (train a new strategy), and to strengthen and condition the body in ways relevant to the patient's meaningful task. In the next chapter, we will discuss how to 'wake up' the deep muscle system of the LPH complex. These techniques are needed if, after all of these releases, the deep system remains inhibited or impaired. The final chapter will then integrate all of this into more advanced techniques, restoration of total body strategies for function and performance, and home practice.

Tools and techniques for 'waking up' and coordinating the deep and superficial muscle systems

11

Linda-Joy Lee   Diane Lee

CHAPTER CONTENTS

Introduction 323

Principles for training new strategies for
function and performance 323

Role of supports: sacroiliac belts and
taping 328

Finding the best position to start training
the deep muscle system of the abdominal
canister 329

'Waking up' and building the neural
network for the deep muscle system
of the abdominal canister 333

Finding the 'chord' cue – coactivation
of the deep muscle system of the
abdominal canister 353

Coordinating the deep and superficial
muscle systems 355

'Waking up' and building the neural network
for coordinating the deep and superficial
muscle systems of the hip joint 363

When to refer for prolotherapy 365

Summary – where are we at and
what's left? 366

Introduction

Once the physical, cognitive, and/or emotional barriers that are contributing to non-optimal strategies for function and performance begin to release and let go (Chapter 10), it is time to work on building optimal strategies (see Fig. 9.3). The key components for building new strategies are to:

1. 'wake up' and coordinate the deep and superficial muscle systems;

2. train new strategies for posture and movement based on the patient's meaningful tasks, needs, and goals.

This chapter will cover the first key component, how to 'wake up' and coordinate the deep and superficial muscle systems of the lumbopelvic–hip (LPH) complex, and Chapter 12 will then integrate this work into more advanced movement tasks combining cues for release and alignment (Chapter 10) with cues for function and performance during multiple complex tasks. First, let us revisit the principles of this part of the treatment program (Chapter 9) (Box 11.1) and then we will get into the specifics.

Principles for training new strategies for function and performance

Optimize neuroplasticity

Training a new strategy for function and performance relies heavily on principles from neuroscience and the neuroplastic capabilities of the brain. A reminder from Chapter 9: 'neurons that fire together, wire together.' If new motor programs are to be built, the following key conditions must be met:

1. focused attention and awareness during every single practice session; as well as

2. massed practice. In the initial stages of building a new neural network, it is critical to use the new network frequently; as well as have

© 2011, Elsevier Ltd.
DOI: 10.1016/B978-0-443-06963-5.00011-0

Principles for retraining new strategies for function and performance

1. Optimize neuroplasticity.
2. Reinforce 'letting go' of the old strategy.
3. Educate the patient.
4. Be specific.
5. Wake up the deep muscle system.
6. Integrate into posture and movement training in meaningful tasks.

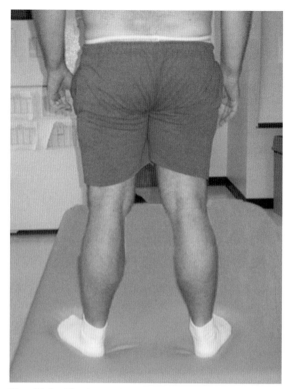

Fig. 11.1 • The butt-gripper is easily identified by the posteroinferior bunching of fabric (of shorts or tights) caused by the drawing in of the deep external rotators of the hip and posterior pelvic floor. Note the habitual external rotation of the lower extremities, a common lower extremity posture associated with butt-gripping.

3. specific patterns of sensory input, facilitation, and cuing related to the task. The location, timing, and modulation of tactile cuing can make significant changes in the strategy used, and contribute to aligning the 'virtual body' with the real body, along with creating a new 'flow of awareness.' Finally;

4. the tasks must have meaning and be reinforced with positive feedback.

If these key conditions are met during every treatment and home practice session, the environment for neuroplasticity will be optimized and new neural networks will be developed quickly.

Reinforce 'letting go' of the old strategy

In order to facilitate the formation of new brain maps, it is essential to stop using the old maps. During the process of removing the non-optimal strategies (Chapter 10), the clinician will have learned which tactile and verbal cues/images are most effective in helping the patient 'let go' of holding key muscles, postural patterns, and movement patterns. It is essential that the clinician continue to use these verbal and tactile cues at the same time as the new strategies are taught.

For example, if the patient tends to be a butt-gripper (Fig. 11.1), and sitting is a meaningful task (i.e. pain increases when they sit for prolonged periods and they require sitting for work), then how they move from standing to sitting (squat) is a key functional movement (meaningful task) to assess. If during a squat this patient cannot release/relax piriformis and ischiococcygeus unilaterally, they will sit with an intrapelvic torsion and this is a non-optimal position strategy for sitting (Fig. 11.2A). To correct this strategy for

sitting, the cuing sequence would begin with a 'release and align cue' – 'Let your sitz bones go wide and let your femurs sink into the sockets.' This would be followed immediately by a 'connect cue' for using the deep system such as, 'Imagine a guy wire from your anus to the back of your pubic bone (pelvic floor) and connect along this line and then think of a line connecting the two bones in the front of your pelvis and draw them together (transversus abdominis).' It is important to coactivate this deep system and not build patterns that activate each muscle separately, as the evidence suggests that they should work together (Chapter 4). We consider each muscle of the deep system to be like a note in a musical scale, and encourage the development of what we call 'chord cues.' Once they have thought about what they need to release/relax and then thought about when they need to engage, or connect, they can then be allowed to squat or move (release, align, connect, and then move = RACM) (Fig. 11.2B,C). Further verbal and

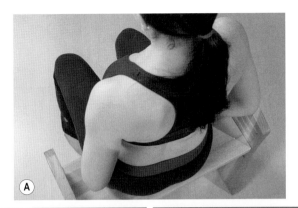

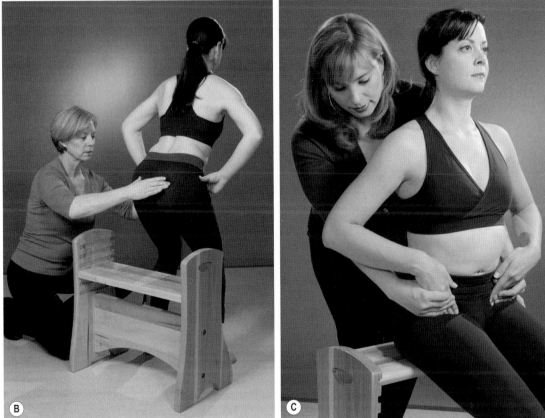

Fig. 11.2 • (A) Note the asymmetrical sitting posture. The pelvis is rotated in the transverse plane and is also in an intrapelvic torsion. This sitting posture is non-optimal and began with a non-optimal strategy for a squat (stand to sit). (B) Stand to sit training – cues for release of the piriformis and ischiococcygeus allow the left femoral head to seat and the pelvis to anteriorly tilt symmetrically over the femoral heads. It is more likely that the pelvis will 'arrive on the stool' in a neutral position with this strategy. (C) The therapist shows the patient how to ensure that the femoral heads are centered symmetrically in the seated position.

tactile cues are given as they squat to guide the movement ensuring optimal alignment and technique (Chapter 12). There are multiple video demonstrations of the progression of this instruction in the case reports in Chapter 9 and these can be found online.

Educate the patient

As mentioned in Chapters 9 and 10, education is a key component throughout this collaborative program. There are many different ways that patients perceive and understand the word 'training' or 'exercises,' which is why in Chapter 10 we used the word 'practice.' It is essential that patients understand that training a new strategy is not related to approaches they may have been exposed to in community gym settings that are about strength, power, or endurance of muscles. Basically, the clinician must portray that we need to first change the programs the brain uses for posture and movement and then 'exercise' the new program for strength, power, endurance, etc. Therefore, *how* a movement is performed is critical, and the *quality* is not to be lost at the expense of *quantity*. It is helpful to remind patients that the program is not really about exercise, but rather about 'changing the way you live in your body.' It is also useful to discuss the known changes that occur in the motor control system with pain and injury (Chapters 4 and 5), and to highlight that the main deficit is not one of muscle strength but one of recruiting the right muscles at the right time and in the right coordination with other muscles. If there is loss of strength due to de-conditioning and disuse, it is still first desirable to train the correct recruitment pattern and synergy of the muscle systems, and then work on strength and endurance in functional movements. This can occur in conjunction with a progressive program for increasing cardiovascular fitness relevant to the patient's goals.

In this chapter we will describe how to use load, perceived effort, and resisted tests to illustrate the impact that proper recruitment synergies can have on strength so that patients can experience and understand the role of optimal motor control. This is called 'load effort task analysis.' The more attention they pay to their experience when using different strategies, the faster the new neural networks will build (if they choose to do so).

Be specific

Ensure that any home practice you prescribe has relevance to the patient's needs and goals. Breaking down functional tasks into component movement blocks is a way of building towards functional patterns; be sure to discuss and demonstrate to the patient how the training task you are prescribing relates to either their aggravating activities or their goals. Furthermore, in order to ensure that the treatment program addresses the key impairments that are driving the non-optimal strategy, design the program around:

1. the segment(s) or joint(s) of poor control;
2. the direction(s) of poor control;
3. the levels or regions of restricted mobility;
4. the overactive/dominant superficial muscles;
5. the inactive/inappropriately recruited muscles;
6. specific muscle length/strength imbalances; and
7. characteristics of the goal tasks such as cardiovascular requirements, load requirements, mobility requirements, and level of predictability.

Any training task should be considered in light of the impact it has on the hypothesized pain-generating structures, as well as whether or not it is addressing key deficits identified in the assessment.

'Wake up' the deep muscle system

Chapters 4 and 5 reviewed the current evidence with respect to activation (timing and amplitude of muscle activity) of the muscles of the deep and superficial systems of the abdominal canister during both predictable and unpredictable perturbations of the trunk. In health, it appears that both the deep (TrA, PF, and the diaphragm) and superficial (EO, IO, RA, ES) muscles anticipate the pending load and increase their activation prior to the perturbation. What appears to differentiate the deep from the superficial muscles is that the deep muscles increase their activation prior to the load regardless of the direction of the perturbation (non-direction specificity). The behavior of both the deep and superficial muscle systems is altered in patients with LPH disability and pain (Chapter 5), and it is thought that restoring optimal recruitment of the deep and superficial muscle systems is important for restoring function and performance. Clinicians often ask during our courses:

1. What is the best way to restore optimal recruitment of the deep and superficial muscle systems?
2. When the optimal pattern is attained in the clinic, how many repetitions does one have to do per day, and for how long, to maintain it?
3. Does this new pattern become automatically integrated into the patient's functional tasks? What is the best way to make it automatic, that is, 'make it stick?'

Tsao & Hodges (2007) have addressed a couple of these questions and have shown that the type of exercise prescribed does matter if the non-directional specificity response of the deep muscle system to perturbations of the trunk is to be restored. Subjects with non-specific, persistent low back pain (LBP) and consistent delays in the onset of TrA in response to trunk perturbations via rapid arm movements were investigated. One group was given a single session of isolation training for TrA and a second group was given sit-up training. The isolation training consisted of performing a submaximal contraction (5% RMS_{max}) of TrA separate from the superficial abdominals, but not from the pelvic floor, with feedback provided by ultrasound imaging. They were instructed to keep breathing throughout the isolation task. Three sets of 10 contractions (holding each contraction for 10 seconds) were performed and a 2-minute rest allowed between each set.

The sit-up training was done in crook lying and the sit-up was only performed until activation of TrA was 5% RMS_{max}. Both groups performed the same number of repetitions and sets. Immediately after this training session, the timing of TrA onset was re-measured during rapid arm movements of flexion and extension (Fig. 11.3). The isolation training group showed an earlier activation of TrA for all directions of perturbation to the trunk, whereas

the sit-up group showed an earlier recruitment of all the abdominal muscles during arm flexion and a further delay in the onset of TrA during arm extension. Therefore, non-directional specificity for recruitment of TrA was *not* restored in the sit-up training group, whereas it was improved in the isolation training group. So, the type of training does appear to be important for restoring optimal recruitment for *multiple* directions of loading. Note that both the isolation training and the sit-up training caused changes in the way the central nervous system (CNS) controls the trunk muscles; however, the changes resulting from the isolation task are the desired outcome because they resemble the way the CNS controls the muscles in painfree populations.

So, if it only takes 30 repetitions to rewire the neural network the next question is, 'How long will the new program last?' In a second study, Tsao & Hodges (2008) had nine subjects with non-specific LBP attend for four sessions of assessment and/or training (initial, 2 weeks, 4 weeks, and 6 months). Isolation training for TrA was provided at the initial and 2-week sessions and they were advised to continue with this

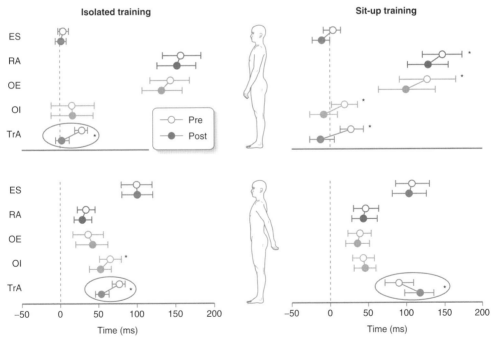

Fig. 11.3 • Group data are shown following isolated transversus abdominis training (left panel) and sit-up training (right panel), for trials of arm flexion (upper panel) and extension (lower panel). Dotted line indicates onset of deltoid electromyography (EMG) and negative values denote earlier EMG activation relative to the deltoid. Onset of EMG and 95% confidence intervals are shown for trials before (open circle) and after (closed circle) training. Note the earlier activation of the TrA after training in both directions of arm movements with isolated training, but only for flexion with sit-up training.
Reproduced with permission from Tsao & Hodges (2007) and *Experimental Brain Research*.

practice twice daily for 4 weeks (their compliance was measured). They did not continue with the training after 4 weeks. The authors noted 81% compliance with the training protocol and improvements in the patient-specific functional scores and self-reported pain scores at both 4 weeks and 6 months and concluded:

> Specifically, four weeks of this type of training [isolation training] of the TrA in people with recurrent LBP is associated with long-term improvements in feedforward postural adjustments...The results suggests that these changes can be retained for six months despite the cessation of training. Together with existing clinical trials that support the efficacy of training of isolated voluntary contractions (O'Sullivan et al 1997, Stuge et al 2004), the present findings suggest that improvements in motor control may be a possible mechanism underlying the clinical improvements in individuals with LBP, but future randomized controlled trials are needed to confirm these findings.
>
> Tsao & Hodges 2008.

Clinically, we find that not all patients need to begin their training with a focus on TrA. Careful assessment is required to determine if the impaired ability to recruit TrA (or other deep muscles) appropriately is the true primary impairment or if it is secondary; that is, the result of another driving impairment (e.g. a dominant IO, thoracic impairment, emotional barrier, etc.) that, once treated, allows the nervous system to use the deep muscles appropriately. Assessment is also required to determine the specific deficits in the deep muscle system and a cue must be found that coactivates all of the deep muscles synergistically (find the 'chord cue'). This still qualifies as isolation training in that activation of the deep muscle system is isolated from the superficial muscle system. This chapter will cover how to find the 'chord cue' for the deep muscle system and then train both the deep and superficial muscle systems to build the foundation for a new neural network, and a new strategy that will be a key component for moving into functional tasks (Chapter 12).

Posture and movement training

Training new strategies for meaningful postures and movement begins as early in the treatment program as possible. As soon as there is any letting go of the non-optimal strategies, component pieces of new postural and movement strategies can be taught. For example, as the unilateral butt-gripper described above learns to release their piriformis/ischiococcygeus (Release and Align – Chapter 10), they are taught a new way to support their pelvis and hips

(Connect), as well as how to sit symmetrically and equally on the ischial tuberosities with the femoral heads centered (Move – Chapter 12) (see Fig. 11.2C). This will facilitate optimal alignment in the pelvis and a centered hip joint, and often relieves groin and/or posterior pelvic girdle pain in sitting. It is not necessary to correct all components of the posture or movement task right away; starting with two or three key alignment points or control points is enough to begin training a new strategy. Chapter 12 will provide further specifics on how to train new strategies for posture and movement.

Role of supports: sacroiliac belts and taping

A sacroiliac belt can be a useful adjunct for external support of the LPH complex at this time in the therapeutic process. Although it is not exactly known how the various belts or tape work, or whether one belt is better than another, it is known that the stiffness of the SIJ is enhanced when a generic belt is worn just below the ASISs (Damen et al 2002a,b). There are many sacroiliac belts on the market and most will be effective in providing some degree of compression (Vleeming et al 1992a). However, patients often require more or less compression than a general belt can supply and often it is difficult to specify the location of the compression (bilateral anterior, bilateral posterior, unilateral anterior, and/or unilateral posterior) with a general belt. This led to the development of the Com-Pressor, a patented belt that allows compression to be applied specifically to different aspects of the pelvic girdle (Lee DG 2002) (Fig. 11.4A).

The Com-Pressor SI belt is used in conjunction with 'waking up' and training the deep muscle system and training a new strategy for posture and movement, and is thought to provide both mechanical support and proprioceptive input to remind the brain which muscle(s) need facilitation. How does it do this? The Com-Pressor supports the pelvis through the tension of very strong elastic straps. The straps are attached to an underlying body belt (Fig. 11.4B) that should be applied directly against the skin around the pelvis. If the need is to compress the SIJs, the belt should be worn just below the ASISs (Damen et al 2002b), and if the need is to compress the pubic symphysis it should be worn just above the greater trochanters of the femurs (Vleeming et al 1992a). The location of the strap(s) is variable and depends on the specific needs of the

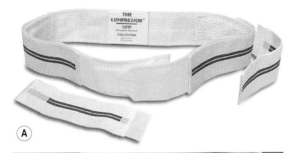

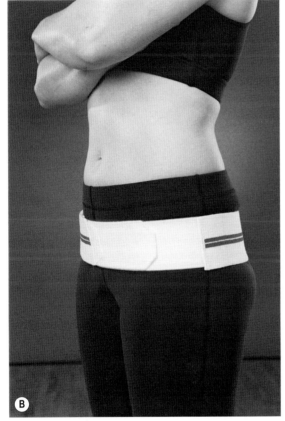

Fig. 11.4 • (A) The Com-Pressor, a patented belt that allows compression to be applied specifically to different aspects of the pelvic girdle (Lee DG 2002). (B) The Com-Pressor belt applied with a compression strap supporting the right anterior and left posterior aspect of the pelvis. The location of the straps is determined by the results of the ASLR test (Chapter 8).

patient determined by the active straight leg raise test (Chapter 8). The straps can be overlapped (doubled up) to increase the amount of compression at any location. Initially, the belt should support the pelvis whenever the patient is vertical (i.e. standing, sitting, or during any activity of daily living). As function returns, the patient should wean off the belt by

reducing the amount of compression (loosen the tension in the straps) and finally removing the belt altogether for short periods of time (begin with 30 minutes). Ultimately, they should be able to eliminate the need for any external support.

Further details on how this belt is specifically applied and integrated into the treatment program can be found in the case reports in Chapter 9 (see Videos CD11, JG9, JG12 🖱). The pelvis can also be taped for support (Chapter 12, see Video 12.13 🖱). The principles for applying tape are identical to those for using the Com-Pressor SI belt.

Finding the best position to start training the deep muscle system of the abdominal canister

The assessment of the muscles of the abdominal wall is done in the supine, or crook lying (knees over a bolster), position as this is a way to easily standardize position, assess symmetry, and be able to fully observe the entire abdominal wall for substitution strategies during assessment (Chapter 8). However, supine or crook lying is not often the best place to teach patients how to recruit the deep muscles. Sapsford et al (2001) investigated the effect of lumbopelvic position on abdominal muscle recruitment during a 'hollowing' maneuver (a task that aimed to recruit primarily TrA and IO) and a bracing maneuver (a task that aimed to co-contract all of the abdominal muscles). The neutral and extended lumbopelvic positions were found to produce the greatest increase in TrA activity. When the pelvis was tilted posteriorly and the lumbar spine flexed, the EO muscle had the greatest increase in activity with both the hollowing and bracing maneuvers. Although the study was performed with a small number of subjects, the findings are consistent with what we observe in the clinical setting. That is, a neutral LPH alignment is the best position to facilitate learning to recruit the deep muscles. Notably, a common substitution strategy for load transfer in patients with lumbopelvic disability and pain is butt-gripping (see Fig. 11.1) or chest-gripping (abdominal bracing) (Fig. 11.5A,B). These patterns of activation both result in a posterior pelvic tilt, a flexed lumbar spine, and often a non-centered, braced hip joint, and usually patients cannot 'let go' and neutralize these joints in the supine, or crook lying, position.

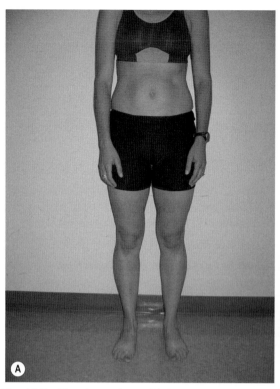
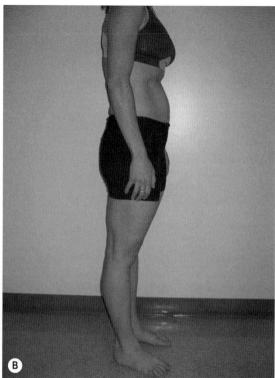

Fig. 11.5 • The chest-gripper. (A) From the front, note the drawing in of the upper abdominal wall and the widening/protrusion of the lower abdominal wall. (B) From the side, the impact of this strategy on the abdominal profile is clearly seen.

Attempting to isolate the deep muscles (TrA, pelvic floor, psoas, deep fibers of multifidus) without first correcting the lumbopelvic position can often lead to frustration for both the therapist and the patient. Therefore, it is key to first release all barriers (Chapter 10), so that the ability to passively obtain a neutral LPH alignment is now available to the patient. Then, training of the deep system is begun in a position (sidelying, prone, crook lying, supine) where the patient is best able to maintain a neutral LPH. In our experience, patients with LPH disability and pain often have the most difficulty maintaining a neutral LPH in supine or crook lying, especially those that butt-grip or chest-grip; sidelying and prone are usually the best positions to train the deep system for these patients.

There are two ways to teach a patient how to attain their best position for a neutral LPH and subsequently train the deep muscle system:

1. position the patient passively into a neutral LPH alignment and then teach the patient how to perform and check self-positioning at home (see sidelying or prone lying below); or

2. use an active movement task *without excessive superficial muscle activity*, especially in the erector spinae and superficial multifidus muscles, to find a neutral LPH alignment (see crook lying roll up/down below). Teach the patient how to check alignment in this position.

It has been our clinical experience that, by addressing neutral LPH alignment first, the cues for recruitment and isolation of the deep muscles are more effective and efficient. Usually both passive positioning for practice, as well as active movements to learn how to find neutral LPH, are included in a patient's program; however, initially they may be separate practices performed in two different positions.

For example, a patient, who in crook lying rests with the pelvis tilted posteriorly and the lumbar spine flexed, may be given the crook lying roll up/down practice to learn how to find neutral LPH alignment as they release the superficial muscles of the trunk and hip (previously learned, see Chapter 10). The patient's position will improve with practice and with the concurrent release techniques being performed by themselves and the therapist (Chapter 10). However, if the patient cannot fully attain neutral LPH even with this practice and treatment (i.e. remains in some low lumbar flexion and posterior pelvic tilt but to a less degree), the addition of cues to recruit the deep muscle system in this position will still bias recruitment of the EO (superficial muscle system). For this patient, recruitment and isolation of the deep muscle system is taught in a different position. The alternate position chosen is the one where the patient can easily find neutral, and thus will have the easiest time recruiting the deep muscles. Sidelying and prone are the most common alternate positions for patients who have difficulty moving out of posterior pelvic tilt (see below).

Note that all ranges and positions of LPH movement are required for function, and that optimal control of the deep system is required during all functional ranges. Thus, during progression of the program, tasks are used that involve using the deep system while moving in and out of LPH neutral (see Chapter 12). However, in the initial stages of teaching the brain how to 'find,' or 'wake up,' and then confidently isolate the deep system, neutral LPH alignment is used to facilitate success and build the neural networks.

It should be noted that there are other benefits and effects of neutral LPH practice. Notably, by using active movements to retrain neutral, the patient becomes aware of where they tend to live in their body and how to move in and out of this place. This creates new options for movement, increases the variety of movement strategies, and reinforces the movement training that is to come (Chapter 12).

Neutral lumbopelvic–hip position: passive positioning sidelying

Patient and therapist position. The patient is sidelying facing the therapist with their knees bent. Stand facing the patient with your body at the level of the patient's lumbar spine. With your cranial hand, palpate the lumbar curve. Identify levels of excessive flexion or extension or whether the entire lumbar spine is generally flexed/extended. Note the position of the pelvis; the butt-gripper often lies with the pelvis rotated or 'tucked under,' such that the greater trochanter is excessively compressed. Note the

resting tone of muscles of the superficial system (ES, sMF, EO, IO, hip muscles) in this position (Video MQ17 📱).

Correction technique. If the pelvis is rotated and 'tucked under,' derotate it to a neutral position so that the weight is evenly distributed along the lateral femur and the entire lateral aspect of the pelvis (Fig. 11.6A,B). Recheck the lumbar curve and correct the intersegmental position by flexing/extending the patient's legs (Fig. 11.6C). When a gentle, even, lumbar lordosis is achieved, place the legs on the plinth at that position. Note any change in the resting tone of the muscles of the superficial system and the position of the feet relative to the rest of the body. The neutral lumbopelvic posture often results when the soles of the feet lie in the same plane as the trunk. Instruct the patient how to find this position at home. The idea of pretending to lie against a wall with the soles of the feet and the back both touching the wall is a helpful cue. Have the patient palpate the lumbar spinal curve in their habitual sidelying position and in the new position. Ensure that the patient can find the neutral position without your assistance. Sidelying will not be the best position for those who have a narrow waist compared to their hips, but for most others it is a good place to start training the deep muscle system.

Neutral lumbopelvic–hip position: passive positioning prone

Patient and therapist position. Have the patient assume a prone lying position and stand at the patient's side. Note the lumbar curve and identify any segmental levels of excessive flexion or extension. Palpate the femoral heads and note any anterior displacement (Fig. 11.7). The pelvis should be in neutral alignment, there should be an even lumbar curve, and the femoral heads should be centered. Note the resting tone of the muscles of the superficial system (ES, sMF, EO, IO, hip muscles) in this position and compare to the tone noted in the sidelying position.

Correction technique. Use verbal and tactile cues to see if the patient can reduce any hypertonicity anywhere in the LPH complex and assess the response. If the patient is more relaxed in this position and the LPH complex can attain a neutral position, then this position is chosen for subsequent training of the deep muscle system. This position

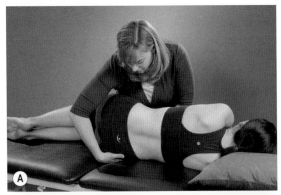

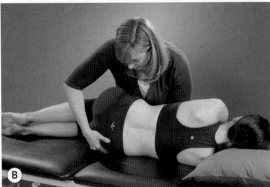

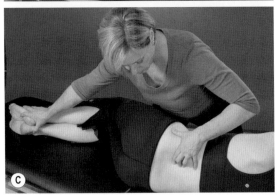

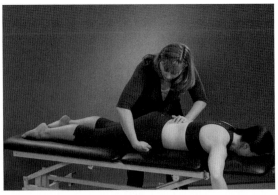

Fig. 11.7 • Neutral lumbopelvic–hip position: passive positioning prone. In this illustration the therapist is checking the lumbar lordosis and the position of the right femoral head. The lumbar curve should be even and the femoral head centered if this position is to be used for isolation training of the deep muscle system.

Neutral lumbopelvic–hip position: active movement practice – crook lying roll up/down

Patient and therapist position. The patient is supine with their hips and knees comfortably flexed. Stand at the patient's side. Slide one hand under the lumbar spine, spreading the fingers to allow palpation of several interspinous spaces. Make note of the resting position of each lumbar segment. Observe the rib cage and look for a 'lifted sternum' or space under the lower thoracic spine (Fig. 11.8). While in this position, use your fingers to give tactile feedback as you educate the patient about the goal of the active movement practice: 'Your low back is very flat/the curve is uneven here, this is where we need to change the curve.' In order to help learn the movement practice, the patient's hands are placed on the upper and lower sternum, and the therapist's hands are placed so that one hand palpates at one hip, and the other hand palpates in the lower abdomen (Fig. 11.9A). During the active roll up/down, and in subsequent repetitions of the movement, the therapist's hands will move to palpate, and facilitate, at several key 'points of control,' depending on the correction needed for optimal movement execution.

Correction technique – verbal and manual cues. The patient is asked to posteriorly tilt the pelvis, or flatten/flex the lumbar spine to the plinth, then to push through the feet and lift the hips off the plinth up to the level of the lower thoracic spine,

Fig. 11.6 • Neutral lumbopelvic–hip position: passive positioning sidelying. (A) The butt-gripper habitually rests with the pelvis rotated under, such that excessive force is placed on the greater trochanter. This posture also causes flexion of the lumbar spine. (B) Initial correction technique to attain a neutral LPH posture. (C) Fine tuning of the neutral LPH position ensuring a gentle, even lordosis is achieved at all levels of the lumbar spine.

is often best for strong chest-grippers and athletes with high levels of superficial abdominal muscle development, as the cue to 'let go and relax the abdominals' is reinforced by the sensation of the skin against the floor/plinth.

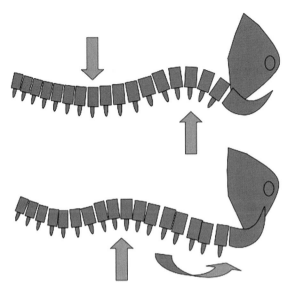

Fig. 11.8 • Neutral lumbopelvic–hip position: active movement practice – crook lying roll up/down. Top: the position of the thoracolumbar segments and the pelvis in an ideal neutral position. Bottom: the result of a posterior pelvic tilt; the lumbar lordosis often shifts to the thoracolumbar region. These figures were drawn by Dr. Paul Hodges and are reproduced with his permission.

rolling the spine gently into a 'C' (Fig. 11.9B). The height of the lift depends on the patient's ability to maintain a flexed spine. Lifting is not permitted beyond the point where spinal extension and/or activity in the erector spinae muscles occur. Next, ask the patient to sequentially lie the spine back down on the plinth, starting from the rib cage. The thorax is kept heavy on the plinth to maintain the thoracic kyphosis, and the vertebrae are unrolled one segment at a time. Once the lumbar spine is flat on the plinth, ask the patient to 'let the tailbone float or fall to the bed' or 'let the pelvis roll forward' and *allow* a small curve in the low back to occur (Fig. 11.9C). Observe and palpate where the lordosis occurs, watch for a sternal lift (thoracic extension), and feel for excessive segmental lordosis (e.g. L3). The goal is a gentle, even, lumbar lordosis shared by all lumbar segments. Have the patient repeat the movement several times, each time using your hands and cues to improve the end 'released' position. Do not let the patient force the spine into lumbar extension. This active movement will cause a strong contraction of the thoracic erector spinae or superficial multifidus and will inhibit recruitment of the deep muscles as well as potentially increase

back pain due to excessive compression. See Box 11.2 for key points of hand control and additional verbal and visual cues for use during this task.

Ideal response. As the roll up portion of this task is performed, the extensors of the thorax and lumbar spine should relax and segmental flexion should occur from L5–S1 up to the lower thorax. At the end of the roll down component, the thorax should remain in a flexed position as the lumbar spine passively falls into a lordosis. The anterior and posterior hip muscles should be relatively relaxed and the pelvis neutral with the femoral heads centered. If the patient has now achieved a neutral LPH position and the superficial muscle system is relaxed, they can use this position for training the deep muscle system.

Other considerations. If the patient cannot relax the buttocks, try supporting the legs at the knees with a bolster and perform the roll up/down task through a smaller range of motion.

The criteria for deciding which of the above positions is the best to use for 'waking up' the deep muscle system are:

1. which position facilitates the best LPH neutral alignment; as well as
2. which position facilitates the most relaxation in the superficial muscles, especially those superficial muscles used in the patient's current non-optimal strategy.

'Waking up' and building the neural network for the deep muscle system of the abdominal canister

Building a new neural network for optimal coordination of the deep and superficial muscle systems begins with restoring optimal breathing patterns (restore the multitasking function of the diaphragm (Chapter 4)), and then teaching the patient to isolate and maintain a tonic contraction of the deep muscles separate from the superficial muscles, and to integrate this with their breathing. This is, in part, artificial as in normal function the deep muscles work in conjunction with the superficial. However, although both muscle systems work together in functional movements, the central nervous system appears to control the deep muscle system independently of the superficial system (Chapter 4). In LPH disability and pain this independent control is lost, and, in

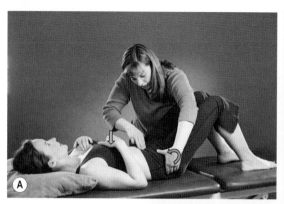
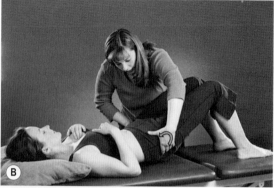
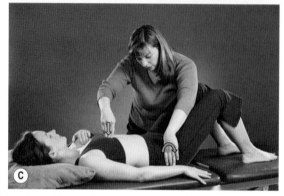

Fig. 11.9 • Neutral lumbopelvic–hip position: active movement practice – crook lying roll up/down. (A) The patient palpates the sternum to self-cue a heavy, relaxed thorax (vertical arrow) during the movement. No lifting of the sternum is permitted. The therapist palpates at the lower abdomen to cue a gentle drawing in of the lower abdomen and around the hip to facilitate a posterior tilt (curved arrow) of the pelvis and flexion of the lumbar spine. (B) The hips and pelvis are lifted off the plinth (arrow) to continue the flexion movement into the upper lumbar and lower thoracic levels. The hips are lifted only to the point that spinal flexion can be maintained; in this example the lift is stopped at the thoracolumbar junction. (C) Release into lumbar lordosis. The therapist provides gentle posterior pressure on the lower sternum (vertical arrow) to prevent thoracolumbar extension as the pelvis falls forward into an anterior tilt. The therapist's left hand is providing a cue to release the anterior hip as well as drawing the pelvis anteriorly and inferiorly (curved arrow). On subsequent repetitions of the task the therapist can palpate the lumbar spine to facilitate the lordosis and ensure that the superficial multifidus and erector spinae remain relaxed during the roll up and at the final 'release' into neutral lordosis.

Box 11.2

Crook lying roll up/down task

Key points of control for hands:

- Fingers can provide tactile cues at the levels that need to 'lengthen' into a lordosis – glide your fingers along the spinous processes in a vertical line.
- Hand on sternum to prevent lifting of chest – keep 'heavy.'
- Hands in hip creases to facilitate 'folding' of hips and 'opening' of pelvis (anterior tilt).
- Use small 'wiggles' (gentle rotation) of the rib cage, pelvis, and/or hips to facilitate decreased superficial muscle contraction and rigidity.

Verbal/visual cues:

- 'Relax your buttocks, and let your sitz bones go wide as the tailbone falls to the bed.'
- 'Let your hips go heavy as they sink to the bed.'
- 'Let your low back lengthen as you let your pelvis fall forward.'
- 'Imagine a line between the bottom of the sternum to the pubic bone; the line should get longer during the release phase; the length comes from the pubic bone falling forward, while the sternum point stays still.'
- 'Keep the chest heavy, relax the back.'

order to address the change in motor control, the deep muscle system should be trained separately. As previously noted, new evidence highlights that this approach of training the deep system separately creates the desired changes in motor control of these muscles during function (automatic trunk control during perturbation) (Tsao & Hodges 2007, 2008). Recent studies also show that the underlying mechanisms for changes in TrA control involve reorganization of the motor cortex (changed brain maps) in patients with low back pain (Tsao et al 2008) and that these maps are changed by training (Tsao & Hodges 2007, 2008).

The diaphragm

The diaphragm has multiple functions, including maintaining respiration while contributing to increased intra-abdominal pressure for trunk control (Chapter 4). Altered breathing patterns are commonly seen in patients with LPH disability with or without pain, resulting in compromised efficiency of both respiration and trunk control. Retraining optimal breathing patterns achieves several goals simultaneously. Firstly, there is improved function of the diaphragm. Secondly, unwanted excessive superficial muscle activity in both the trunk and hip can be reduced. Breathing practice also facilitates general relaxation and may help address cognitive or emotional barriers. Finally, as respiration is a primary drive for survival, the need for trunk control will be a secondary priority to breathing. By first retraining breathing, the stage is set for retraining the rest of the deep muscle system and then coordinating both the deep and superficial muscle systems with the breath. This way a new neural network is created that includes optimal breathing patterns into all tasks trained.

Three-dimensional movement of the rib cage and abdomen occurs during optimal diaphragmatic breathing (Detroyer 1989, Lee et al 2010). In patients with LPH disability with or without pain, the most common movement lost is lateral and posterolateral costal expansion. Consequently, either excessive excursion of the abdomen, or the upper chest, occurs (Video 11.1 📱). Several factors can contribute to the loss of lateral/posterolateral expansion. These include, but are not limited to, joint restrictions in the thorax (spinal or costal), hypertonicity of the thoracic portions of the erector spinae, serratus posterior inferior, and/or oblique

abdominal muscles, and excessive recruitment of these superficial muscles during the respiratory cycle. Changes in spinal alignment in the sagittal plane (slumped versus extended postures) also affect the three-dimensional shape and movement of the ribcage (Lee et al 2010); thus neutralizing spinal alignment as described above is important in retraining breathing. Any articular restrictions and/or muscular hypertonicity should have been noted during the objective assessment. Abdominal muscle recruitment during respiration should also be assessed (described below). If the abdominal muscles are recruited during inspiration, rib cage expansion will be restricted to the apical region (Video 11.1 📱). Expiration in the supine position during relaxed breathing should be a passive event, with no activity in the superficial abdominal muscles. It is crucial that the clinician identifies and corrects these patterns prior to teaching isolation of TrA. An isolated contraction of TrA cannot occur if excessive abdominal muscle activity persists; furthermore, using this pattern during progressions of the program prevents the optimal strategy for recruitment of the muscles of the abdominal wall (inappropriate timing occurs).

Observation and facilitation of lateral costal expansion

Patient and therapist position. The patient is in crook lying, or supine, in a neutral LPH position with the abdomen and lower rib cage exposed. Stand at the patient's side. Before placing your hands on the patient, first observe the chest, lateral rib cage, and abdomen over several inspiratory and expiratory phases. Look for movement in the upper chest (apical breathing), the lateral lower rib cage (lateral costal expansion), and the abdomen (upper and lower abdomen). Note the area where most movement occurs. Next, place your hands on the lateral aspect of the lower rib cage to monitor movement. Check for the amount of movement and the symmetry between the left and right sides. Make note of any expiratory abdominal activation. Keep your hands on the lateral aspect of the lower rib cage and give the patient an image to redirect their inspiration (Fig. 11.10A). If posterolateral excursion is the most restricted movement, move your hands more posteriorly on the rib cage. For a unilateral restriction, stand on the same side as the restriction. Place one hand posteriorly under the rib cage, and the other on the anterior rib cage at the same level (Fig. 11.10B).

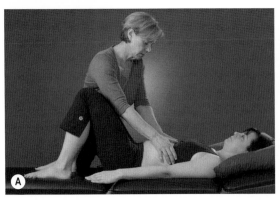
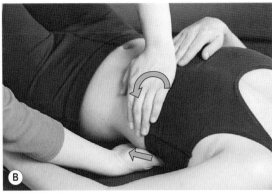

Fig. 11.10 • The diaphragm. (A) Observation and facilitation of lateral costal expansion in supine. The therapist's hands provide awareness of where the patient needs to redirect inspiration. Further facilitation can be added with rib springing. (B) Hand position for correcting a unilateral restriction of costal expansion. On inspiration draw the posterior ribs laterally (bottom arrow); on expiration provide a posterolateral pressure to the anterior thorax (top arrow).

Correction technique – verbal and manual cues. 'As you breathe in, imagine bringing the air into my hands.' 'Imagine your ribs are like an umbrella, and when you breathe in the bottom of the umbrella is opening up.' 'With each breath open your ribs into my hands.' With both hands, apply a slow, gentle, inward pressure at the end of expiration and release this pressure slightly after the start of the inspiration phase (recoil technique or rib springing). Allow your hands to follow the rib cage opening and then apply the gentle pressure again at the end of expiration. With the unilateral restriction, provide gentle pressure into the erector spinae and draw the ribs laterally with the posterior hand as you cue opening into your hand with inspiration. As the patient exhales, apply a posterior pressure to simulate a 'heavy' feeling with your anterior hand (to facilitate thoracic flexion).

For muscle activity on expiration: 'As you breathe out, let the air fall out of you and relax your stomach.' 'Imagine I am slowly pulling the air out of you.' 'Sigh as you breathe out – ahhhhh.' 'Let your chest and sternum go heavy to the floor as you exhale.' 'Let your rib cage sink into my hand(s) as you breathe out.' Gently wiggle the rib cage a small amount to release the muscle holding as the patient breathes out.

Progressions/other considerations. The patient should practice focused breathing pattern training two to three times a day, using both normal and deeper breaths, for several minutes. The patient uses their own hands on the sides of the rib cage to provide self-feedback. Alternately, a resistive exercise band (e.g. Thera-Band®) can be used around the lower rib cage for proprioceptive feedback (Fig. 11.11); use the lowest resistance of band to allow flexibility

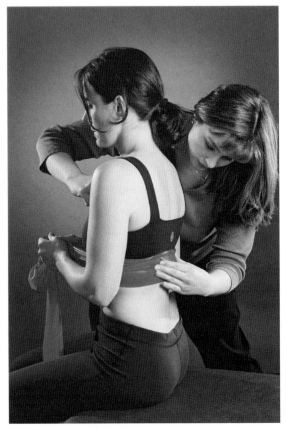

Fig. 11.11 • Home practice for facilitation of posterolateral costal expansion. A resistive exercise band can be used for proprioceptive feedback laterally and posterolaterally. With every breath in, the patient thinks of opening the rib cage into the band. In this example the therapist cues the patient to open the ribs posteriorly.

and rib cage expansion. This technique is especially helpful for patients with decreased posterolateral expansion, excessive erector spinae activity, and excessive thoracolumbar extension. Alternate positions should be assessed, as optimal breathing patterns may be easier for patients to perform in different positions. To encourage posterolateral costal expansion, the 'prayer' position can be used (see Fig. 10.27B). The patient kneels with the elbows bent on the floor, the hips resting back over the heels, and the head resting. This flexed spinal position 'opens' the posterior rib cage and helps release excessive erector spinae tone, while inhibiting excessive lower abdominal breathing. For patients with a large abdomen, breathing practice in supine is often uncomfortable; moving to the sidelying position allows for greater ease and success. To encourage the transfer of the new breathing pattern into a more automatic strategy, have the patient 'check-in' on their pattern at different points throughout the day, in different postures, and during different activities (sitting, standing, walking, etc.).

Posterolateral costal expansion and erector spinae release

Patient and therapist position. The patient is supine with the legs straight or in crook lying (whichever is more comfortable for the patient). Stand at the patient's side. Scoop your hands bilaterally underneath the trunk and rib cage and palpate for hypertonic areas in the thoracic erector spinae muscles. Start at L2 and the thoracolumbar junction and move up into the middle/upper thoracic spine to find the most hypertonic area. If there is primarily a unilateral restriction, use the unilateral hand position as shown in Figure 11.10B.

Correction technique – verbal and manual cues. While using the breathing techniques described above, provide a deep sinking pressure into the hypertonic muscles as the patient exhales and then add the following verbal cue: 'Imagine that your back is an ink blot that has been dropped on the floor. Imagine that with every exhale the ink blot is spreading on the floor and getting bigger and bigger.' As the patient exhales, apply pressure to the trigger point in the muscles with your finger pads as you use the whole hand to draw the rib cage laterally, as if opening the posterior rib cage. If using the unilateral hand position, use posterior pressure with your anterior hand to simulate the 'heavy' feeling as the patient exhales.

Other deep muscles of the abdominal canister

The assessment of other deep muscles of the abdominal canister (the pelvic floor, transversus abdominis, and the deep fibers of multifidus) involves, in part, an analysis of the muscle's response to certain verbal cues known to activate the muscle in a healthy individual (Chapter 4) as well as analysis during automatic tasks (Chapter 8). For the patient with LPH disability with or without pain, these cues alone are often inadequate to facilitate recruitment of the desired muscles, resulting in:

- no activation of one or more of the deep muscles; and/or
- asymmetrical activation (in timing or amount of response) of one or more of the deep muscles; and/or
- phasic activity in one or more of the deep muscles; and/or
- proper activation but an inability to maintain proper diaphragmatic breathing during the contraction; and/or
- any of the above combined with a pattern of excessive superficial muscle activity.

These non-optimal activation patterns are evident during palpation, observation, and ultrasound imaging (Chapter 8). All deficiencies in the deep muscle system need to be addressed; however, as there is often impairment in more than one of the muscles of the deep system, the clinician needs to decide which muscle to 'wake up' first (note cue) before integrating its response with the others (chord cue). Clinically, we have found that, if all of the hypertonic superficial muscles have been released (or relatively released), the pattern of manual compression that maximally changes the ease of the ASLR test (Chapter 8) indicates which of the deep muscles should be trained first. There should also be an associated deficit in this muscle in response to a verbal cue to contract (delayed or absent response). Note that the best pattern of compression at any time reflects the *net vectors* required to balance the forces across the pelvis; when you use this information with the other findings (which muscles are hypertonic, which muscles are poorly recruited, which joints are stiff), a complete picture emerges that enables the identification of the primary deep muscle impairments (which muscle(s) to train first). It is important that the ASLR test and the effect of manual

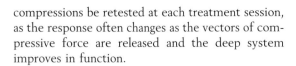

compressions be retested at each treatment session, as the response often changes as the vectors of compressive force are released and the deep system improves in function.

General guidelines for training the muscles of the deep system

There are some general guidelines that apply to training any of the muscles of the deep system (Box 11.3). They include:

- The goal is a symmetrical contraction and co-contraction of the deep muscles (transversus abdominis, the pelvic floor, and the deep fibers of multifidus), while maintaining an optimal breathing pattern.
- Encourage a *minimal* contraction, that is, 10–15% of MVC (maximal voluntary contraction). Often simply asking the patient to perform *less* of a contraction can produce the desired result.
- There should be no activity in the superficial muscle system.
- There should be no spinal or pelvic movement with the contraction.
- Encourage the patient to contract the muscle as S-L-O-W-L-Y as possible; speaking your cues slowly and providing slow tactile cues will facilitate the proper speed of contraction. This is a key modification whenever a phasic response is present, or if activity in the superficial muscle system is observed.
- Choose the position that best relaxes the superficial muscles, facilitates an optimal

Box 11.3

Guidelines for training the deep muscle system

- The goal is a symmetrical contraction and co-contraction of the deep muscles.
- Encourage a *minimal* contraction.
- There should be no activity in the superficial muscle system.
- There should be no spinal or pelvic movement with the contraction.
- Encourage the patient to contract the muscle as S-L-O-W-L-Y as possible.
- Choose the best neutral LPH position.
- Use images and mental intent instead of movement.
- 'Think' or 'intend' instead of 'do'.

breathing pattern, and facilitates a neutral LPH position.

- Use images and mental intent instead of movement to rewire the neural network; 'think' or 'intend' instead of 'do.'

The pelvic floor

Evidence suggests that activation of the abdominal muscles should accompany contraction of the pelvic floor muscles and vice versa (Chapter 4). Although this may be true in healthy individuals, in patients with LPH disability with or without pain/incontinence an associated co-contraction between TrA and the pelvic floor does not always occur. Even if TrA responds optimally with a cue to contract the pelvic floor, this does not guarantee that a proper contraction of the pelvic floor has occurred. Building a new neural network for the deep muscles of the abdominal canister requires finding cues and images that result in a co-contraction of all the deep muscles. If the assessment suggests that the pelvic floor is non-responsive, asymmetrical, and/or delayed in its activation, then specific training is required. Note that hypertonicity of the pelvic floor may be a cause for inappropriate recruitment; an internal pelvic floor assessment and treatment (specific release) may be required in these cases prior to training the correct activation patterns of the pelvic floor.

In both transverse and parasagittal abdominal views of the bladder, contraction of the pelvic floor muscles results in a slow indentation and encroachment of the bladder wall (see Figs 8.86A–C, 8.87A–C, Videos 8.8, 8.9). In the perineal view, contraction of the pelvic floor results in a cranioventral lift of the anorectal angle towards the bladder neck (see Fig. 8.89B, Video 8.10). When the contraction is absent, or a Valsalva response is observed with ultrasound imaging (see Fig. 8.89C, Videos 8.11, 8.14), the patient is given different cues to try to facilitate a proper response on the screen (see below) (Video LC19).

To retrain the tonic function of the pelvic floor muscles, it is important that the patient understands that although the final goal is to be able to do three sets of 10 second contractions, repeated 10 times, the duration and number of contractions performed correctly may vary on a given day. This information allows the patient to self-progress the training protocol. Certain subgroups of patients with stress urinary incontinence may need to couple the protocols for training the tonic holding ability of the pelvic floor muscles with those for strength training and hypertrophy (endurance deficit – see Video 11.2a,b 🖰) (Bø et al 1990) as well as for timing ('the Knack'). The approach presented here is designed to address the impairment in motor control and synergy of the pelvic floor muscles in conjunction with the other muscles of the deep system.

Ultrasound imaging can be used in conjunction with abdominal wall palpation and observation to assess the function of the pelvic floor muscles. Common clinical patterns of abnormal response are described below with facilitation and correction cues.

Ultrasound image – no indentation of the bladder, no lift observed

The bladder shape does not change at the posteroinferior aspect and there is no cranioventral motion on the parasagittal view (see Fig. 8.87B) or the perineal view (Fig. 8.89A). Some movement may be evident during the breathing cycle, but there is no change when the patient thinks of squeezing the urethra, lifting the vagina/testicles, or drawing the anus towards the back of the pubic bone.

Palpation of abdominal wall. There is usually no change in the abdominal wall tension. The fingers can sink into the softness of the abdomen.

Observation. There may be concurrent breath holding with the effort to recruit the pelvic floor or superficial abdominal muscle activity on expiration, but usually no other activity in the superficial abdominal muscles is evident during an attempt to perform a contraction.

Correction technique – verbal cues. In this case, the patient does not have an intact neural pathway between *thinking* about a contraction and performing the contraction. In order to obtain a contraction, different cues are used and the response is noted on ultrasound. Verbal cue examples:

- 'Instead of thinking of squeezing, imagine that you are lifting a tampon.'
- For men: 'Imagine that you are slowly walking into a cold lake, and the water is starting to come up between your inner thighs...'
- 'Connect a string between your pubic bone and your tailbone, then between your right and left sitz bones, now draw the string up into the center like a drawstring.'
- Alternately, cues for transversus abdominis or deep fibers of multifidus (listed below) can be tried to see if they can facilitate a co-contraction.

- If incorrect breathing patterns are noted then it is essential to teach correct diaphragmatic breathing; restoring the function of the pelvic floor muscles is closely linked with the function of the diaphragm and its effects on intra-abdominal pressure.

An absent response may also result from nerve damage (pudendal nerve and nerves to levator ani from S3 and S4), insufficiency in the fascial connections of the pelvic floor muscles (Chapter 3), or hypertonicity of the pelvic floor muscles. Keep in mind that, due to the limitations of ultrasound, when no movement is observed it is possible that a small response has occurred (i.e. there is muscle activity), but the amount of activity is insufficient to result in architectural changes measurable by ultrasound. In this situation an internal pelvic floor exam will be more sensitive for assessing pelvic floor activity. However, our clinical opinion is that, if there is no visible response on ultrasound, it is an insufficient response that needs to be addressed. If no response is observed after the above cues and corrections in breathing pattern have been tried, biofeedback tools such as 'The Pelvic Floor Educator™' (www.neenhealth.com) can be used (Fig. 11.12). These tools provide sensory and proprioceptive feedback, and allow the patient to practice contractions with the assurance that they are performing the correct activation. Pelvic floor function can then be re-assessed with ultrasound imaging in 1–2 weeks. If there is still no response, a referral to a therapist specializing in pelvic floor dysfunction and manual assessment of the floor is recommended.

Ultrasound image – no indentation of the bladder, caudodorsal movement (Valsalva) observed

In the transverse abdominal view, the descent of the dorsal aspect of the bladder will be observed as the Valsalva occurs (Fig. 11.13A,B Video 11.3a 🖰).

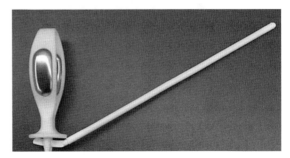

Fig. 11.12 • The Pelvic Floor Educator™ (www.neenhealth. com).

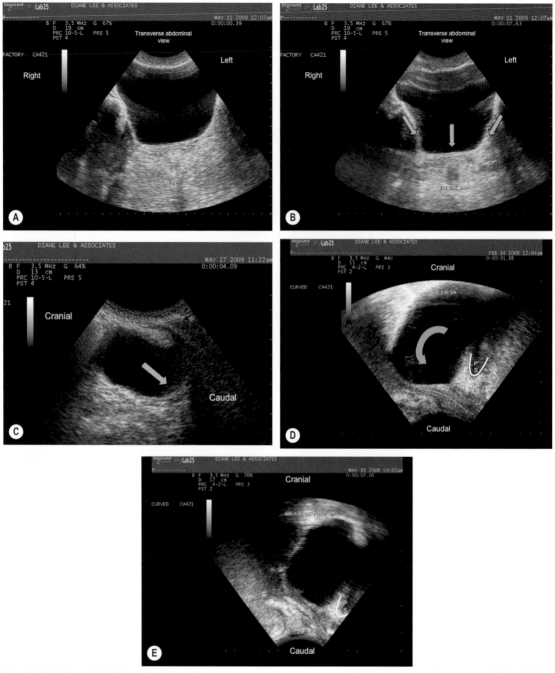

Fig. 11.13 • The pelvic floor: ultrasound image – no indentation of the bladder, caudodorsal movement (Valsalva) observed. A Valsalva maneuver results in a deformation of the bladder shape and a caudodorsal shift. (A) Transverse view, bladder at rest. (B) Transverse view, same bladder during a Valsalva maneuver (see Video 11.3a 🖱). (C) Parasagittal view, different bladder during a Valsalva (see Video 11.3b 🖱). (D) Perineal view. This woman has marked laxity of her pelvic floor structure (cystocele, enterocele, rectocele). Note the level of her bladder compared to her pubic symphysis (PS) during the Valsalva maneuver (see Video 11.3c 🖱). (E) Perineal view. This illustration is of the same woman during a Valsalva maneuver after reconstructive surgery to restore the anatomy of her pelvic floor (see Video 11.3d 🖱). The video clips dramatically illustrate the difference pre- and postoperatively.

In the parasagittal view, the bladder may move caudodorsally (Fig. 11.13C, Video 11.3b 🖱). The best view to observe this non-optimal strategy is the perineal view; the descent of the pelvic structures is clearly seen in relationship to a fixed bony point, the pubic symphysis. Video 8.11 🖱 demonstrates a Valsalva maneuver in a nulliparous woman with no SUI and healthy fascial restraints. Figure 11.13D and Video 11.3c 🖱 demonstrate a Valsalva maneuver in a multiparous woman with SUI and marked laxity of the fascial structures. Figure 11.13E and Video 11.3d 🖱 demonstrate a Valsalva maneuver in this same woman after reconstructive surgery for her pelvic floor.

Palpation of abdominal wall. A bulge and/or bracing tension occurs particularly in the suprapubic region; the bulge may develop slowly or quickly.

Observation. Activity in the superficial abdominal muscles is often seen, especially in the internal and external oblique muscles. Flexion of the rib cage may occur if there is no co-contraction of the thoracic portions of the erector spinae muscle to counteract the flexion moment of the oblique abdominals. The abdomen may bulge with concurrent narrowing of the rib cage (see Fig. 11.5A,B).

Correction technique – verbal cues. The goal in this scenario is to reduce the superficial muscle activity that is causing the Valsalva maneuver (Chapter 10) (a non-optimal response to the cue to perform a submaximal pelvic floor contraction), and then train a proper lift of the pelvic floor muscles. Draw the patient's attention to the screen, and point out the movement and deformation of the bladder shape that occurs when a contraction is attempted. Cue proper breathing with a special focus on abdominal relaxation during exhalation. Palpate the inner thighs bilaterally to focus the patient's attention away from the abdomen. The same cues can be used, with some modifications. Verbal cue examples:

- 'Imagine a tension that is coming up from your inner thighs into the front of your pelvic floor and then lifting your pelvic floor.'
- 'Really focus low down in your pelvic floor, now imagine slowly and gently lifting a tampon.'
- When a Valsalva is present, it is essential to encourage a S-L-O-W-E-R contraction – 'This time contract at 10% of the speed of the last contraction' – as well as a L-I-G-H-T-E-R contraction – 'This time I want you to think of contracting only 10% of the last contraction.'

- Alternately, try cues for transversus abdominis or the deep fibers of multifidus.

After the first session, the patient will often go home with an image to practice that ensures no Valsalva but produces only minimal or no lift. The patient is taught to palpate bilaterally in the abdomen (just medial to the ASISs) to ensure that no abdominal bulge is felt as this occurs with the Valsalva. At subsequent training sessions, the lift component can then be effectively trained.

Ultrasound image – indentation and lift of the bladder, followed by a Valsalva

An ideal response of the bladder wall is observed, but then quickly followed by a caudodorsal movement of the bladder (Videos 11.4a,b 🖱). The Valsalva may also occur slowly as the patient attempts to maintain a tonic contraction.

Palpation of abdominal wall. A tension in the abdominal wall consistent with a TrA contraction is followed by a bulge and/or bracing.

Observation. A small flattening, or hollowing, of the lower abdominal wall is followed by activity in the superficial abdominal muscles, especially in the internal and external oblique muscles. Flexion of the rib cage may occur if there is no co-contraction of the thoracic portions of the erector spinae muscle to counteract the flexion moment of the oblique abdominals. A bulge in the lower abdomen is usually present; there may be concurrent narrowing of the rib cage.

Correction technique. This response is best corrected by cues that focus on decreasing the speed and effort of the contraction (see verbal cues as above). The correct neural pathway exists but is over-ridden by the incorrect Valsalva. It is very effective to have the patient observe the screen and to learn to stop the contraction before the Valsalva occurs and pushes the bladder caudodorsally. Before the patient goes home to practice, it is important to have them try several contractions without watching the screen while stopping before the Valsalva. This ensures the rewiring of the neural pathway and learning of the internal sensation of the correct activation pattern. It is also important to assess how long the patient can hold a contraction before a Valsalva starts to occur. Note the number of seconds for which the isolated contraction is maintained. Teach the patient to palpate the abdominal wall to monitor for bulging; the patient is instructed to practice holding the correct contraction as long as possible without the Valsalva occurring.

Ultrasound image – indentation and lift of the bladder, slow release of contraction when attempting to increase the duration of hold (decreased endurance)

An ideal response of the bladder wall is observed but it then slowly returns to its rest position even though the patient believes they are maintaining the contraction (Video 11.2a,b 🖱).

Palpation of abdominal wall. A tension in the abdominal wall consistent with a TrA contraction occurs but slowly releases as the patient attempts to maintain the contraction.

Observation. A small flattening, or hollowing, of the lower abdominal wall occurs but releases as the patient attempts to maintain the contraction.

Correction technique. Often the patient *thinks* that they are maintaining a contraction but it is evident from the ultrasound image and palpation of the abdominal wall that the contraction is no longer continuing. The key in this case is to make the patient aware of when the contraction is truly occurring and the point at which it starts to let go. Teaching the patient to palpate the abdomen while watching the screen, and then repeating contractions without watching the screen, will internalize and reaffirm the new awareness.

Ultrasound image – asymmetrical activation

An asymmetrical activation (Fig. 11.14, Video 11.5 🖱) is usually corrected by having the patient direct extra focus and attention to the side of the abnormal response. However, if there are neural or myofascial impairments underlying the asymmetry (hypertonicity, nerve damage, loss of fascial integrity, etc.), then retraining of symmetrical function is facilitated by referral to a therapist who specializes in internal palpation and treatment of the pelvic floor.

Transversus abdominis (TrA)

Patient and therapist position

The initial position chosen for training TrA depends on the patient's ability to achieve a neutral LPH alignment; the options are sidelying, prone, supine, or crook lying. Ultimately, the patient needs to be able to activate TrA in all positions including vertical ones (Videos CD12 and 12.14 🖱), but to begin the most supportive position that optimizes success is chosen.

Correction technique – verbal and manual cues

Several verbal cues can help to facilitate a contraction of TrA that is isolated from the superficial muscle system (Video 11.6 🖱). If coactivation of the pelvic floor and TrA exists (Chapter 8), then using a pelvic floor cue (urethral squeeze, vaginal/testicular lift, or drawing the anus to the back of the pubic bone) to elicit a response in TrA is a good place to start. However, for many postpartum women, activating the pelvic floor does not automatically evoke a response in TrA and an additional cue/image is needed. To specifically focus on activating and restoring symmetry between the left and right TrA ('waking up' and rewiring a new neural network), try the following cues:

- 'Breathe in, breathe out, then don't breathe as you slowly, gently draw your lower abdomen away from my fingers (or hand).' (Fig. 11.15A).
- 'Imagine that there is a slow tension coming up from the inner thighs into the front of your pelvic floor, then extend that tension up into my fingers in your lower abdomen' (Fig. 11.15B, Video 11.7 🖱).
- 'Imagine a guy wire that connects the inside of your hip bones (ASISs), then slowly and gently draw them together.'
- 'Imagine your pelvis is like an open book and your hip bones are its covers. Gently think about a force that would close the book covers.' When one TrA is delayed or absent have them think about closing just one book cover.

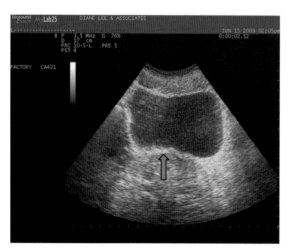

Fig. 11.14 • The pelvic floor: ultrasound image – asymmetrical activation (see Video 11.5 🖱).

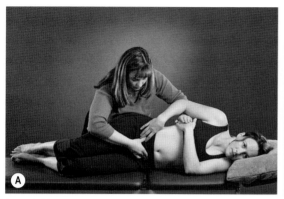
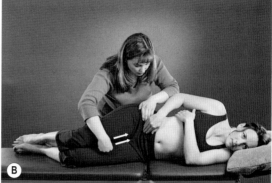

Fig. 11.15 • Facilitation of transversus abdominis isolation, sidelying position. (A) In this example, the patient palpates for lateral costal expansion with the left hand and TrA contraction with the right hand; the therapist similarly palpates and provides manual facilitation. Note that patients often have more awareness of the lower abdomen lifting from the bottom side (in this case, the left side); for patients with an asymmetrical TrA contraction, sidelying *on the side of poor activation* can facilitate more symmetrical recruitment. (B) In this example, the patient palpates for lateral costal expansion with the left hand and for TrA contraction with the right hand. The therapist palpates the right TrA for evidence of an ideal contraction while the caudal hand provides gentle sinking pressure into the inner thighs bilaterally. While sliding the fingers up the thighs a short distance (arrows), give the cue, 'Imagine tension coming up from my fingers in your inner thighs, moving up into the front of your pelvic floor.' The image can be extended up to the lower abdomen if necessary.

- 'Imagine drawing your stomach away from your pubic bone.' 'Very lightly and slowly think of lifting up in your pelvic floor' (women can imagine lifting the vagina, whereas men can imagine doing a small lift of the testes).
- 'Imagine a sling or hammock that runs from the pubic bone to the right and left hip bones (ASISs), slowly and gently create tension in the sling to lift up your lower stomach.'

Provide a sinking pressure into the abdomen and tension the TrA fascial layer by drawing your fingers superolaterally (in a 'v') to provide a sensory cue as you give the verbal cues slowly and gently. Tactile pressure can also be given just above the pubic bone or with the hand cupping the abdomen; sink into the tissue slowly to encourage a slow, tonic contraction instead of a fast, phasic response. If there is excessive upper abdominal activity, the patient can continue to palpate at the ASIS points while the therapist provides gentle tactile pressure bilaterally into the upper medial thighs to take the focus away from the stomach. The patient is then encouraged to imagine the contraction starting lower than the abdomen.

Ideal and abnormal responses

A slow development of gentle tensioning under the fingers should be felt (like tensioning a sheet, no bulging). It should be remembered that only a 10–15% contraction of this muscle is required. If the patient uses too much effort or performs a fast contraction, a bulge into the fingers will be felt, pushing the fingers away from the abdomen; this is the internal oblique (IO) muscle and is a normal or expected response as effort increases. A similar IO bulge can often be felt with a cough or with lifting the head from the floor. During an isolated TrA contraction there should be no movement of the pelvis or spine, and little movement in the upper abdomen. Rectus abdominis (RA) and the oblique abdominals should remain relaxed. If the rib cage is depressed and drawn in, this is a sign of external oblique (EO) activation. Perform a small 'wiggle' of the rib cage by pushing it gently laterally; if there is a lot of resistance to your pressure, this means that overactive superficial muscles are bracing the rib cage and an isolated TrA contraction has not been achieved. The rib cage should still move easily in response to the lateral pressure in the presence of an isolated TrA contraction.

The common abnormal responses are described here and categorized according to patterns seen with ultrasound imaging (UI). The reader should note that UI is an adjunct to palpation and observation and is not an essential tool for teaching activation of the TrA; however, it is often a useful tool for providing feedback to patients and objective assessment of dysfunction.

Ultrasound image – no TrA recruitment, no substitution with IO

Imaging. On the UI image, the following is seen (Fig. 8.81C, Video 11.8 🖰):

- No widening (change in thickness) of the TrA muscle layer.
- No corseting of TrA laterally or lateral slide of the medial fascia of TrA.
- No change in thickness in the IO muscle layer.

Palpation. On palpation, the following is felt:

- the lower abdomen remains soft and no tensioning or contraction is felt just medial to the ASIS; or
- a tensioning in the superficial fascia is palpated rather than a deep tension. This can occur due to a contraction of the EO muscle and the resultant tension in the EO fascia that occurs over the palpation point. The ultrasound image confirms that TrA is not active. There may be no change in EO observed on the ultrasound image, as the correlation between activity in the EO and change in the thickness of the muscle on the ultrasound screen is poor (Hodges et al 2003a). Activity in the EO can be palpated at the lower rib attachments of the muscle (Fig. 11.16). If no spinal movement occurs but the EO is active, there will be palpable activity in the erector spinae muscles. The rib cage wiggle test will be restricted.

Observation. On observation, the following is noted: if TrA does not contract there will be no flattening or drawing in of the lower abdomen; however, there may be substitution patterns that are not observable from the ultrasound image. The possible scenarios include:

- EO contraction – movement of the abdominal wall is initiated from the upper abdomen and activity in the EO muscle fibers at their rib cage attachments will be observed. There may also be a horizontal skin crease in the abdomen just above the umbilicus (Fig. 11.17A,B), as well as an increase in the lateral diameter of the lower abdominal wall (widening at the waist). Lateral costal expansion will be reduced along with the passive ribcage wiggle (Video 11.9 🖰). If the erector spinae muscles remain relaxed,

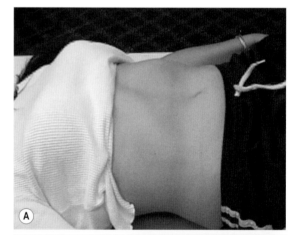

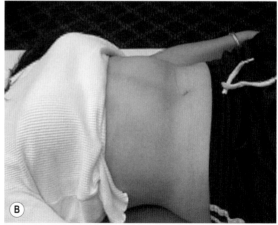

Fig. 11.17 • Substitution response from EO during a cue to isolate a contraction of TrA. (A) Abdominal wall at rest. (B) Abdominal wall profile resulting from activation of the EO. Note the narrowing of the infrasternal angle, the horizontal skin crease just above the umbilicus, and the widening of the lower abdomen.

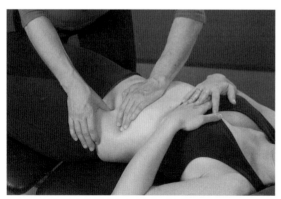

Fig. 11.16 • Facilitation of transversus adominis. In this illustration the therapist is palpating the left TrA (note the depth of this palpation) and simultaneously palpating the upper abdominal wall checking for any substitution from either EO or IO (note that the depth of this palpation is less than that for TrA).

there will be thoracolumbar flexion and narrowing of the infrasternal angle.

- Breath holding – the upper abdomen will move superiorly and pull in (Video 11.10 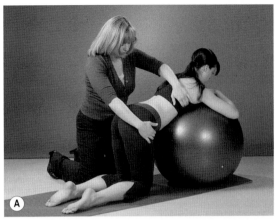); the rib cage will flare and may lift if there is a concurrent contraction of the erector spinae.

Correction technique. Several techniques/cues can be used to 'wake up' TrA and facilitate a symmetrical, synergistic contraction.

- Change patient position: if there is no activity in TrA or any other abdominal muscle on cuing, choose a position that will provide more gravity pull on the abdomen such as sidelying, prone, four-point kneeling (or kneeling over a ball), or supported standing (Fig. 11.18A,B). The increased sensory and proprioceptive input is often sufficient to produce the desired response. If the response is primarily in the EO (EO dominant pattern), make sure that the patient is positioned in neutral LPH alignment. Sidelying and prone are good positions for allowing relaxation of the abdominal wall when EO is dominant.

- For EO dominance: check for EO activity on expiration. Add the cue, 'Breathe in, breathe out, *now really relax your stomach*, do not breathe, and gently think of lifting your lower abdomen away from your hand (or another image).' Use verbal cues that draw focus away from the abdomen; for example, think of the pelvic floor, tension coming up from the inner thighs, or a multifidus (deep fibers) contraction.

- For no abdominal muscle activity: try the verbal cues listed above, starting first with those that use palpation, and focus on the lower abdomen to increase awareness of the area.

Ultrasound image – no TrA, substitution with IO with or without EO and RA

Imaging. On the UI image, the following is seen:

- The IO layer increases in thickness with a fast, phasic response or with a slow, gradual increase (Fig. 11.19A). No increase in thickness of the TrA layer is seen underneath, no lateral glide of the fascia is observed, and there is no corseting of the TrA layer laterally. Due to the lack of fascial tension from TrA, a downward bulge (into the abdomen) at the medial edge of the IO will often be observed. When the patient is asked to do the contraction slowly, the same pattern will be evident but occurs more slowly. In Video 11.11a 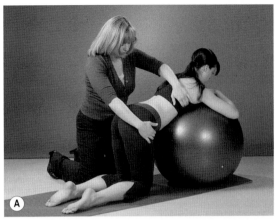, the IO contracts

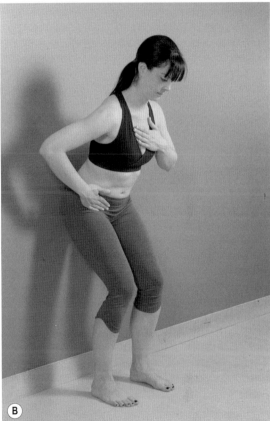

Fig. 11.18 • Facilitation of transversus abdominis, alternate positions. (A) If the patient can attain a neutral LPH position in four-point kneeling, this can be an alternate position to train an isolated contraction of TrA. (B) The supported standing position in neutral LPH is another good place to train TrA.

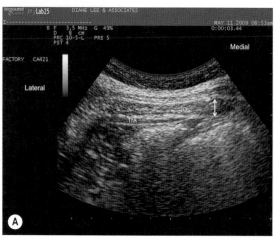
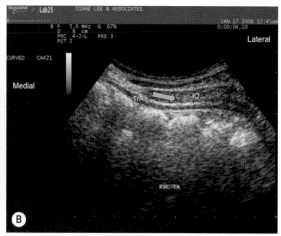

Fig. 11.19 • Transversus abdominis: ultrasound image – no TrA, substitution with IO with or without EO and RA. (A) Note the bulging of IO medially with no TrA response. (B) On occasion, the internal oblique will actually slide laterally over the non-active TrA (arrow).

first (note the downward bulge medially as it broadens), TrA then contracts slightly (note the lateral corseting and broadening), and then TrA relaxes and IO continues to contract. On occasion the IO will actually slide laterally over the top of the inactive TrA (Fig. 11.19B, Video 11.11b🖱).

Palpation. On palpation, the following is felt:

- A fast bulge or slow pressure/bulge (rather than a tensioning) can be felt medial to the ASIS (Video 11.12 🖱).

In order to determine if EO or RA is also being recruited with the IO, palpate along the lower rib cage (below the eighth rib) (see Fig. 11.16, Video 11.9 🖱) and inferior to the sternum.

Observation. On observation, the following is noted:

- Bilateral contraction of only the IO will result in flaring (widening) of the infrasternal angle; in lean individuals, the upper anterior fibers may be palpable and visible as an oblique band running superomedially from the anterior iliac crest to the ribs. If both the IO and EO are active, rib cage bracing and decreased lateral costal expansion will be observed along with lower abdominal bulging.
- RA activity will result in thoracolumbar flexion and/or a posterior pelvic tilt.
- Co-contraction of the erector spinae muscles will reduce the amount of thoracolumbar flexion observed, but will result in trunk rigidity and a restricted 'rib cage wiggle.'

- If the dysfunctional substitution pattern is primarily unilateral, a lateral shift in the rib cage will occur with the contraction (Fig. 11.20).

Correction technique. Several techniques/cues can be used to 'wake up' TrA and facilitate a symmetrical, synergistic contraction. In conjunction with releasing and downtraining IO/EO/RA (Chapter 10):

- Change patient position: choose a position that best facilitates relaxation of the trunk. This may be supine/crook lying (as long as the pelvis is not posteriorly tilted) or prone lying. If the erector spinae is being recruited along with the superficial

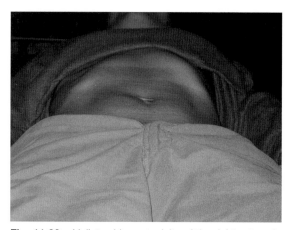

Fig. 11.20 • Unilateral hypertonicity of the right external oblique. Note the lateral shift and asymmetry of the rib cage.

abdominal muscles, a pillow can be placed under the stomach in prone to encourage further relaxation.

- Start with verbal and tactile cues that draw focus away from the abdomen (activating the pelvic floor, tension coming up from the inner thighs (Video 11.7), contracting multifidus (deep fibers)).

- Check for superficial abdominal activity on expiration. Add the cue, 'Breathe in, breathe out, *now really relax your stomach*, don't breathe, and gently think of lifting in your pelvic floor.'

Ultrasound image – TrA contracting but not in isolation

When TrA comes on first, followed by IO and the other abdominals (may occur quickly or more gradually), this indicates that proper timing of the muscles is occurring; however, the recruitment of the superficial muscle system is happening too early and needs to be eliminated to get an isolated TrA contraction.

Imaging. On the UI image, the following is seen (Fig. 11.21A, Video 11.13):

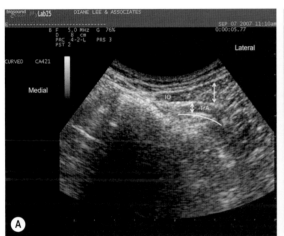
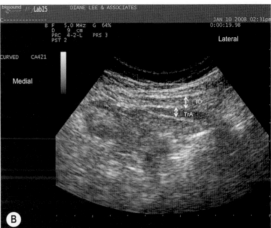
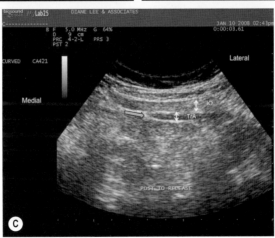

Fig. 11.21 • Transversus abdominis: ultrasound image – TrA contracting but not in isolation. (A) TrA first and then IO. Note the shape of the medial end of IO; it is conical, not bulbous as in Figure 11.19A. (B) Concurrent contraction of TrA and IO. Note the lack of lateral slide of TrA beneath the IO. (C) TrA first and then IO. This is the same patient as in (B) immediately after release of the IO (12 minutes as noted by the time on the images). Observe this in real time online in Video 11.14a,b . These two video clips demonstrate the importance of releasing any hypertonicity in the superficial muscle system prior to isolation training of the deep system.

- The TrA layer increases in thickness and moves laterally, drawing the medial fascial connection laterally. This is followed by an increase in thickness in the IO layer. There is less internal bulging and less fascial blurring of the medial portion of IO (as compared to an IO contraction without an underlying TA) due to the pretensioning of the underlying fascia by the TrA contraction.

Palpation. On palpation, the following is felt:

- A deep tensioning followed by a fast or slow bulge can be felt medial to the ASIS. It is easy to miss the initial deep tension if the IO contracts quickly.

In order to determine whether EO or RA is also being recruited with the IO, palpate along the lower rib cage (below the eighth rib, Fig. 11.22, Video 11.9 🖱) and inferior to the sternum.

Observation. On observation, the following is noted:

- The lower abdomen will gently flatten, or hollow, followed by signs of superficial abdominal muscle activity (described in sections above).

Correction technique. Several techniques/cues can be used to facilitate a symmetrical, synergistic contraction.

- Encourage a slower contraction; start with 50% of current speed, then 50% of the new speed, and so on.
- Encourage a lighter contraction; start with 50% of current effort, then 50% of the new effort, and so on. Remind the patient that only 10–15%

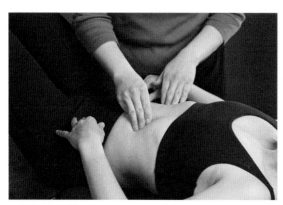

Fig. 11.22 • Palpation points for transversus abdominis and external oblique. The patient is palpating medial and inferior to the ASISs bilaterally to feel a contraction of the TrA; the therapist palpates for substitution by the EO as the muscle comes off its attachment at the anterior surfaces of the lower ribs.

of MVC is required and that they should be *imagining* a contraction rather than *doing* a contraction.

- If decreasing the speed and effort still result in superficial muscle activity, try changing the patient's position such that the superficial muscles are more relaxed.
- Direct the patient's attention to the ultrasound screen. Ask the patient to stop the contraction before movement in the superficial muscle layers (notably IO) occurs. Once this is mastered, have the patient perform the contraction without looking at the screen so that the new skill is internalized.

When the TrA and IO (with or without EO and RA) activate together, this indicates that there is incorrect timing and no separation of control of the deep and superficial muscle systems.

Imaging. On the UI image, the following is seen:

- The TrA layer increases in thickness and moves laterally, drawing the medial fascial connection laterally, but there is a concurrent increase in thickness in the IO layer (see Fig. 11.21B, Video 11.14a 🖱). Often there is less lateral slide of the TrA layer than usually observed with an isolated TrA contraction, and blurring of the medial fascia connections can occur depending on the amount of contraction in the TrA. The lateral corseting occurs but there is concurrent inward movement of both the TrA and IO layers. Figure 11.21C and Video 11.14b 🖱 show the change in the recruitment pattern of TrA and IO in this same patient immediately after a release of the internal oblique (Chapter 10). Although there is still some activation of the IO, it is now occurring after the contraction of TrA.

Palpation. On palpation, the following is felt:

- A fast or slow pressure/bulge can be felt medial to the ASIS. In this scenario, palpation cannot identify whether there is TrA activity underneath, or not, as the bulge dominates the palpation findings.
- In order to determine whether EO or RA are also being recruited with the IO, palpate along the lower rib cage (below the eighth rib, Fig. 11.22) and inferior to the sternum.

Observation. On observation, the following is noted:

- The signs of superficial abdominal muscle activity will be evident and depend on which superficial muscles are activated (see above).

Correction technique. Several techniques/cues can be used to facilitate a symmetrical isolated contraction.

- Use manual release or other techniques to dampen the activity of the superficial muscle system (Chapter 10) prior to another attempt at training the deep muscle system.
- Change the patient's position to one that maximizes relaxation of the abdominal wall.
- Encourage a slower contraction; start with 50% of current speed, then 50% of the new speed, and so on.
- Encourage a lighter contraction; start with 50% of current effort, then 50% of the new effort, and so on. Remind the patient that only 10–15% of MVC is required and that they should be *imagining* a contraction rather than *doing* a contraction.
- Start with verbal and tactile cues that draw focus away from the abdomen (activating the pelvic floor, tension coming up from the inner thighs, contracting deep fibers of multifidus (see below)).
- Check for superficial abdominal activity on expiration. Add the cue, 'Breathe in, breathe out, *now really relax your stomach*, don't breathe, and gently think of lifting in your pelvic floor.'

Ultrasound image – asymmetrical patterns

Asymmetrical activation of the left and right TrA is a very common clinical presentation and is often associated with asymmetrical activation of the deep fibers of multifidus and/or the pelvic floor. Any of the above scenarios can occur asymmetrically, with one side producing an ideal response and the other side producing one of the abnormal responses, or with both sides showing abnormal but different responses. Correction of asymmetry will require a combination of the above facilitation techniques (chord cues). Successful correction of the asymmetry is often achieved by simply adding a small increase in patient focus and attention to the dysfunctional side when the activation is attempted. Some chord cues used to address asymmetry in the deep muscle system will be addressed later under co-contraction training.

Ultrasound image – hypertonicty

On occasion, increased activation of TrA will be observed via ultrasound imaging, and is often linked to the respiratory cycle (i.e. at rest TrA is broadened and corseted and its activity increases further

with expiration). To restore optimal recruitment of TrA, it is often necessary to treat the thorax and reduce the neural drive to TrA as opposed to 'waking it up.' Recall from Chapter 3 that TrA is supplied by the ventral rami from T6–L1. Clinically, it appears that optimal function of TrA is linked to optimal function of the thorax, a topic outside the scope of this book (www.discoverphysio.ca).

Deep fibers of multifidus

Patient and therapist position

Choose the position where the patient can attain the best neutral LPH alignment with the superficial muscles relaxed, especially the erector spinae, the deep hip external rotators, and the ischiococcygeus. Prone lying is a useful position for comparing right/left recruitment symmetry, but is not often the easiest position for patients to first practice 'waking up' their multifidus. Sidelying is a useful position for most patients as it allows easy palpation of the muscle and relaxation into the neutral LPH posture. The supine and crook lying positions can also be beneficial for some patients.

Palpate multifidus just lateral to the spinous processes of the lumbar spine, or sacrum, bilaterally at the level of atrophy. The muscle must be palpated close to the spine to monitor the deep fibers; in the lower lumbar and sacral segments the lateral muscle bulk consists of the more superficial fibers. Teach the patient how to find the dysfunctional segment ('Feel for the soft part of the muscle') and how to sink into the muscle with the fingers (Fig. 11.23).

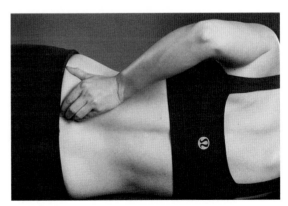

Fig. 11.23 • Facilitation of the deep fibers of multifidus. The patient is in a neutral LPH position in sidelying and palpating the appropriate level of the deep fibers of multifidus; they are ready to begin the isolation training.

Correction technique – verbal and manual cues

Several verbal cues can help to facilitate a contraction of the deep fibers of multifidus (dMF). Images that create the idea of the vertebra/spine being 'suspended' appear to be most effective for facilitating a contraction of the deep fibers of multifidus (Video 11.15 🖱). Various descriptions can be used, but the common theme is that the spine is a central pole that needs to be suspended by tension wires from both sides. The tension in the wires needs to be equal on the right and left sides; if there is loss of activity in one side of the deep multifidus, it can be described as a loss of the connection in the wire, allowing rotation and collapse of the spine on that side. The image of energy coming up vertically along the wires to support the spine helps to create the sense of 'suspension.' In each case, the deep multifidus is palpated at the dysfunctional level; this is where the 'guy wires' attach. The inferior attachment, or starting point, of the wire can vary; the image ultimately chosen is the one that produces the best response in the deep multifidus. The timing of the tactile pressure from the therapist's hands creates the sensation to match the image and provides feedback as to how quickly the muscle should be contracted. The fingers should sink into the multifidus and provide a cranial pressure to encourage a 'lifted' or 'suspended' feeling. The inferior attachment of the wire can be just medial to the ASISs (Fig. 11.24A), superior to the pubic bone, or from a connection to the inner thighs up through the pelvic floor (Fig. 11.24B); the sequence of tactile feedback is from the anterior palpation point first, then up into the multifidus palpation point.

- 'Imagine a guy wire that runs from the back of your pubic bone to this spot in your spine' – apply gentle pressure to provide a tactile cue as to where 'this spot' is. 'Connect along the wire and then gently think of suspending or lifting this vertebra up towards your head.'

- 'Imagine a guy wire that runs from your groin, or inner thigh, to this spot in your spine' – apply gentle pressure to provide a tactile cue as to where 'this spot' is. 'Connect along the wire and then gently think of suspending or lifting this vertebra up towards your head.'

- For the fibers at the level of S1 – 'Imagine there is a guy wire connecting these two bones of your pelvis (palpate the PSISs) and imagine a force that would draw them together.'

- Alternately, try cues for transversus abdominis or the pelvic floor and see if this evokes a co-contraction response in the deep fibers of multifidus.

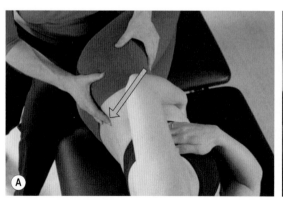 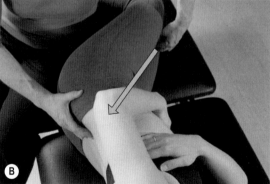

Fig. 11.24 • Facilitation of the deep fibers of multifidus. Describe the image to the patient: 'Imagine that there is a tension wire, or string, that is going to suspend your spine. We are going to connect the wire from the front of your body, up and in through your body diagonally to my fingers in your spine. Breathe in, breathe out, now slowly connect a wire from this finger here (give pressure at anterior palpation point) to this finger here (give pressure into multifidus).' Options for anterior connection points include: (A) the therapist sinks the fingers and thumb just medial to the ASIS on each side, while the patient imagines a wire ascending diagonally and medially from the ASIS to the left side of the vertebra being palpated. This image can also be bilateral. (B) The therapist uses pressure into the inner thighs bilaterally to cue a wire starting in the pelvic floor.

Ideal and abnormal responses

A slow development of firmness in the muscle (Fig. 11.25) will be felt as a deep swelling and indentation of the pads of the palpating fingers. A fast contraction is indicative of activation of the superficial multifidus and/or lumbar erector spinae; the fingers will be quickly pushed off the body. A fast generation of superficial tension can also be felt if the thoracic erector spinae are contracting. The common tendon of the erector spinae muscle overlies the lumbar multifidus (see Fig. 3.48), and activity in the muscle will change tension in the tendon, especially in individuals where this muscle is well developed. It is important to teach the patient how easy it is to push the fingers into the muscle when it is relaxed ('feels like a mushy banana'), as compared to when the deep fibers of multifidus contract ('feel how it is firmer and harder to sink your fingers into the muscle'). There should be no pelvic or spinal motion observed, and no activity in the superficial abdominal or hip musculature. A co-contraction of TrA is acceptable and desired.

The common abnormal responses that occur are described here and categorized according to patterns seen with ultrasound imaging. The reader should note that UI is an adjunct to palpation and observation and is not an essential tool for assessing or training the deep muscle system; in fact, although UI is commonly used in research studies, clinically we find that palpation and observation are more sensitive for training than ultrasound imaging. Recall from Chapter 8 that on occasion there is hypertonicity in the dMF, which prevents the muscle from being recruited appropriately during function or in response to a verbal cue. Release of the dMF precedes training; IMS is a useful tool for this.

Ultrasound image – no recruitment of the deep or superficial fibers of multifidus

Imaging. On the UI image, the following is seen (see Fig. 8.91B):

- No change in the thickness of the muscle layers is seen on ultrasound.

Palpation. On palpation, the following is felt:

- The muscle remains soft and no tension is felt in the multifidus.
- Alternately, rapid tension in the superficial layers may be felt from the tensioning of the long tendons of the thoracic erector spinae muscles.
- Palpation of the abdomen may reveal a TrA contraction or the TrA may remain inactive.
- Activity is felt in any muscles being used in substitution (e.g. the oblique abdominals).

Observation. On observation, the following is noted:

- Breath holding is commonly observed, as well as posterior tilting of the pelvis or segmental lumbar flexion as the patient attempts to 'push' the muscle into the therapist's fingers. Abdominal bracing may also be evident.
- If the thoracic erector spinae muscles are active, the tone will be evident up into their origins in the thoracic spine, either symmetrically or asymmetrically, and spinal extension will occur unless there is co-contraction of the abdominals.

Correction technique. Several facilitation techniques can be tried.

- Try a variety of images until one is found that enables the patient to 'find' the muscle. If lumbar flexion is occurring, use cues that emphasize a 'suspended' or 'lifted' feeling rather than 'make the muscle swell.'
- Check the posterior pelvic floor (ischiococcygeus) and posterior hip for hypertonicity; if there is butt-gripping it will inhibit activation of the multifidus. Change the patient's position, or use release techniques, to decrease the tone prior to facilitating a multifidus contraction.
- If the thoracic erector spinae are active, choose a position that will maximize relaxation of these muscles, such as prone lying.
- Check the breathing pattern and ensure there are no periods of breath holding. Use the exhalation phase to encourage relaxation of the erector spinae muscles.

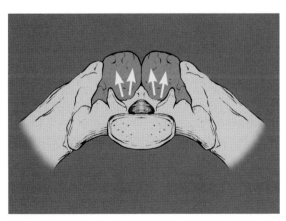

Fig. 11.25 • At the level of the lumbosacral junction, when the deep fibers of multifidus contract they broaden (swell) posteriorly thus increasing the tension in the overlying thoracolumbar fascia. This contraction feels like an increase in tension of the fascia as well as an increase in the firmness of the muscle itself.

Ultrasound image – no recruitment of the deep fibers of multifidus, activity in the superficial layers

Imaging. On the UI image, the following is seen:

- No change in the width of the muscle layers in the deep layers of multifidus. An increase in width of the superficial layers is observed, often a fast, phasic response.

Palpation. On palpation, the following is felt:

- The fingers will be rapidly pushed out from the muscle, without any palpation of deep tension prior to the rapid contraction.
- Alternately, a fast contraction in the multifidus fibers lateral to the palpation point will be felt while the medial palpation point (deep fibers) stays soft and inactive.

Observation. On observation, the following is noted:

- If the superficial multifidus is active without concurrent abdominal activity then an increase in the lumbar lordosis will be evident. No change in the lumbar curve will occur if there is concurrent abdominal bracing.

Correction technique. Several facilitation techniques can be tried.

- Use manual release or other techniques (Chapter 10) to decrease the tone and sensitivity in the superficial fibers prior to another attempt at training the deep layers.
- Try a variety of images until one is found that enables the patient to 'find' the muscle. Avoid images that encourage an extension movement (e.g. 'Pretend you are arching your back but don't actually move it') as these feed into the predisposition to recruit the superficial fibers.
- Check the breathing pattern and ensure there are no periods of breath holding. Use the exhalation phase to encourage relaxation of the erector spinae and superficial multifidus.
- Change the patient's position to one where there is best relaxation of the superficial multifidus. A pillow under the abdomen is often effective.

Ultrasound image – concurrent phasic contraction of the deep and superficial fibers of multifidus

Imaging. On the UI image, the following is seen:

- A change in thickness of the superficial and deep layers occurs simultaneously in a fast, phasic response (Videos 8.18, 8.19).

Palpation. On palpation, the following is felt:

- The fingers will be rapidly pushed out from the muscle, without any palpation of deep tension prior to the rapid contraction.

Observation. On observation, the following is noted:

- If the multifidus is active without concurrent abdominal activity then an increase in the lumbar lordosis will be evident. No change in the lumbar curve will occur if there is concurrent abdominal bracing.

Correction technique. Several facilitation techniques can be tried.

- Use manual or other techniques to decrease the tone and sensitivity in the superficial fibers prior to another attempt at isolating the deep layers.
- Encourage a much slower contraction, with much less effort. Often, by repeatedly reducing speed and effort, the pattern of activation can be altered such that the tension develops primarily in the deep layers of multifidus first. Use the ultrasound and manual cuing to teach the patient the point at which to stop the contraction (before the large bulge occurs).
- Try a variety of images until one is found that enables the patient to 'find' the muscle. Avoid images that encourage an extension movement (e.g. 'Pretend you are arching your back but don't actually move it') as these feed into the predisposition to recruit the superficial fibers.
- Check the breathing pattern and ensure there are no periods of breath holding. Use the exhalation phase to encourage relaxation of the erector spinae and superficial multifidus.

Ultrasound image – deep then superficial fibers of multifidus (correct timing but not isolated)

This is an acceptable recruitment pattern; however, the contraction of the superficial multifidus should be downtrained so that it is not excessive or phasic. The ultrasound image, palpation, and observation will be similar to that described above for the concurrent contraction of deep and superficial; however, the deep contraction can be observed on ultrasound and palpated prior to being overlaid with the superficial contraction. Cues for decreasing speed and effort are effective for reducing the activity in the superficial multifidus, and thus bias the contraction to occur primarily in the deep layers.

Finding the 'chord cue' – coactivation of the deep muscle system of the abdominal canister

It is not uncommon to find asymmetries of activation simultaneously in multiple muscles of the deep system. The deep fibers of multifidus on one side may be poorly recruited in conjunction with excessive superficial multifidus activity on the ipsilateral or contralateral side. This may occur despite having released the superficial multifidus; in this case it is still the brain's preference to activate the superficial multifidus first. The left and right TrA may not co-contract simultaneously with either an absent or optimal response occurring on one side and a delayed or substitution response from IO or EO on the other. The pelvic floor may activate asymmetrically and not occur with a symmetrical response in one or both TrAs. In the same patient, the left TrA and the right dMF may be inhibited or absent, in another the left TrA and the left dMF may be inhibited or absent and the pelvic floor may not activate well at all! The combinations of recruitment patterns are numerous. In these situations, restoring coactivation requires a combination of the above facilitation techniques for all the deep muscles; we call this finding, or striking, the 'chord cue.'

Ultimately, the goal for response to a verbal cue in a symmetrical posture or task is a symmetrical co-contraction of the deep muscle system (the pelvic floor, transversus abdominis, and the deep fibers of multifidus) with normal breathing patterns (normal modulation of the diaphragm) and minimal effort.

Clinical examples for developing a chord cue for the deep system muscles

Unilateral activation of TrA or dMF

If the patient presents with an asymmetrical contraction (left TrA activates before the right TrA or the left dMF contracts and not the right dMF), the verbal cues and images can be altered such that more focus is directed towards the dysfunctional side. For example, to activate more of the left TrA, have the patient think about 'closing only the left book cover' (draw the left ASIS towards the midline). To activate the left dMF and relax the left sMF have them first think of 'letting your back relax and letting the bones of your back fall

towards the table,' and then 'imagine a guy wire running from the left groin through your pelvis to the left side of this vertebra of your low back (give them tactile feedback at the side and level of the inhibited multifidus) and gently connect along the line and then suspend the vertebra towards your head.'

In some cases, a bilateral contraction is cued first, and then the patient is instructed to think 'a little bit more' about the side of the poor response ('Think of drawing the left ASIS farther to the center,' 'Close the left book cover,' 'Create more tension in the guy wire to the right side of your low back'). In other cases, the best result is produced when only the dysfunctional side is cued ('Just think of pulling in the left side of your tummy,' 'Draw only the left ASIS to the center,' 'Create a guy wire that only connects to the right side of your low back'). Although the patient is *thinking* of a unilateral contraction, a bilateral contraction is produced and palpated by the therapist. Usually this cuing needs to be progressed to a bilateral cuing as the superficial muscles on the dysfunctional side become less active and the isolated deep muscle system contraction more precise (Video JG11).

Unilateral activation of TrA and dMF

If there are asymmetries in *both* the front and back of the canister (TrA and dMF), combine the previously found 'note' cues. They will have already established the neural network to activate each muscle (find the note); the next step is to combine them. The image of the guy wire for isolation of deep multifidus often results in a co-contraction of TrA and dMF. If it does not, have them activate the specific dMF with the guy wire suspend cue and then activate TrA either through a pelvic floor or an abdominal can (Videos LC15, MQ17). Diagonal lines or guy wires are also useful cues for asymmetrical activation of both TrA and dMF (Video 11.16). Instruct this patient to 'think of connecting a wire from your right ASIS to the left low back where my finger is' (Fig. 11.26). When the ASLR test, performed after the release of the superficial muscle system, indicates that asymmetrical compression is most beneficial, asymmetrical cues such as these often restore co-contraction of the deep muscle system quickly (without needing to practice the 'note' cues).

Pelvic floor and TrA and dMF

For restoring coactivation of the pelvic floor with TrA try this cue: 'Imagine a guy wire from your anus to the back of your pubic bone and gently connect

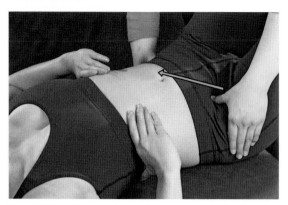

Fig. 11.26 • Cuing for correcting asymmetries in the deep muscle system. The therapist provides deepening pressure at the palpation points as the verbal cue is given. In this example, the left thumb palpates the TrA and the right hand (under the trunk) palpates the deep fibers of multifidus. The arrow indicates the direction of the diagonal suspension wire cue. The patient palpates the rib cage bilaterally to self-cue a proper breathing pattern while the contraction is held.

along this line. Maintain that gentle connection and now connect along a line between your hip bones (ASISs), or close the book covers.' The cues can be more focused to one side if necessary. To add on dMF, simply have them connect to their PF and continue that connection from the back of the pubic bone through their pelvis to the level of the inhibited multifidus, then close the book covers for TrA.

Reinforcing the newly developed neural network for coactivation of the deep muscle system

Once a successful chord cue/combined image for coactivating the deep muscle system has been identified, the patient is encouraged to work towards increasing the duration of the tonic co-contraction while maintaining normal breathing (Video MQ17 🖱). It is important that the patient is taught how to recognize when the deep muscle system stops working and they have reverted back to their old patterns of activation. We use a load effort task analysis to educate the patient for this. By now you have found the best supported position for the isolation training practice (sidelying, prone, supine, or crook lying), as well as the most effective chord cue for coactivation of the deep muscle system. First, have them 'think of nothing' and note the effort it takes to begin to lift their knee if sidelying (Fig. 11.27A), bend their

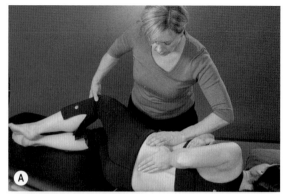

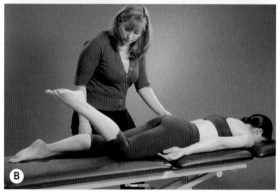

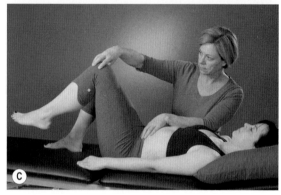

Fig. 11.27 • Reinforcing the newly developed neural network for coactivation of the deep muscle system. Release, Align, Connect, and Move = RACM. From the best supported neutral LPH position, have the patient think of nothing specific and then apply a load by (A) lifting the knee if in sidelying, (B) bending the knee if prone, and (C) lifting the foot if crook lying. Then have them use their previously found cues/images for release, align, and connect, and then repeat the same task and note the difference in the effort required to perform the task as well as any changes in their pain experience (this is called load effort task analysis). The second strategy should require less effort and produce less pain if it is more optimal.

knee if prone (Fig. 11.27B), or extend their hip if prone (Video MQ17 🖱), lift their foot if crook lying (Fig. 11.27C), or lift their leg if supine (Video 11.16 🖱). Then, have them use the better strategy involving the deep muscle pre-contraction and then repeat the task (i.e. RACM = Release, Align, Connect, and Move, Video CD10 🖱). Ask them if they notice any difference in the effort required to perform the lift as well as any difference in their pain between the two strategies. Both the patient and the therapist should be able to easily observe the effort difference when the better strategy is used. Resistance can be given to the lower extremity to reinforce the difference in strength that is achieved with the two different strategies (Fig. 11.28A,B) (Videos LC16, MQ17 🖱). This demonstration is often very effective in convincing a patient that there is value in this training.

Instruct the patient to watch for any change in effort during their home practice by using the load effort task analysis periodically. As the new neural network becomes a default strategy (more automatic), they will be able to perceive when the deep muscle system is no longer working without using this test. That is, they will have developed an inner sense of when they revert back to the non-optimal strategy. Patients should be taught to monitor and progress their own program on a day-to-day basis, working towards three sets of 10 repetitions of 10-second holds with 2-minute rests between sets (Tsao & Hodges 2007). The duration and number of contractions at each practice session are varied depending on how accurate the performance of

the skill is at that time. Remind the patient that more practice sessions in a day, with smaller numbers of repetitions (e.g. 5-second holds, five repetitions, 10 times a day), is more effective at retraining the skill than one session of large numbers of repetitions (e.g. 5-second holds, 50 repetitions, once a day). As the skill of coactivating the deep muscle system is mastered in supported positions, more upright positions and tasks are added to the program. Be sure to explain that these are preliminary training sessions that ultimately will be incorporated into tasks that have meaning for them. We find that our committed patients who diligently follow this protocol are able to move to more upright functional tasks within 7–10 days.

Coordinating the deep and superficial muscle systems

Coordination of the deep and superficial muscle systems is essential for functional movement. This section will cover the training to promote further development of the neural network moving towards the restoration of optimal strategies for multiple tasks (Chapter 12). At this stage of rehabilitation, the goal is to integrate the co-contraction of the deep muscle system into tasks that also require activation of the superficial muscle system.

Tasks can be designed to challenge control of flexion, extension, or rotation through the lumbar spine, pelvis, and hips depending on the direction that the limbs are moved or the direction of the application

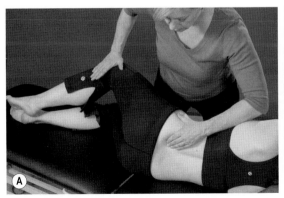
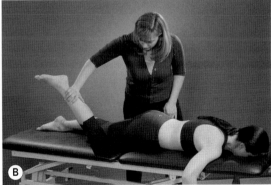

Fig. 11.28 • Confirming the best strategy. To reinforce that the second strategy is truly the best one, apply resistance to external rotation/abduction of the hip if (A) sidelying or to flexion of the bent knee if (B) prone and compare the relative strength with the two different strategies (thinking of nothing and then RACM). The difference in strength (performance) between the two strategies is often significant and reassuring to both the patient and the therapist that the image/cues are helping to creating a new, more optimal, neural network for function.

of external forces (weights, resistive exercise bands, pulleys). Upright positions and movement of the limbs require activation of the superficial muscles and thus the connected myofascial slings. For each progression, focus should be first on *movement control*; in patients with LPH disability with or without pain, it is often essential to master dissociation of hip movement from trunk movement. Focus is on attaining proximal control first, and then adding the rest of the limb in functional patterns. As movement control is mastered, training can be progressed to *resisted movements* to strengthen the muscles in functional patterns. It is important to identify the direction of loss of control and the area of loss of control (sacroiliac joints versus lumbar spine joints), so that the program can be specific and not involve so many tasks that patient compliance is unlikely.

When the superficial muscle system is activated in a coordinated, properly timed manner with a pre-contraction of the deep muscle system, the resultant movements will be performed with optimal alignment and fluidity of movement (beautiful movements). Palpation of the poorly controlled segment will reveal maintained control (e.g. no unlocking of the hemipelvis, no loss of femoral head centering, no lumbar segmental hinging). Observation of the relative positions of the limbs in relation to the trunk, and of the thorax in relation to the pelvis, will reveal maintained alignment of all joints in the kinetic chain such that the entire body is positioned to share and transmit forces equally. This overall body alignment is sustained by balanced length, strength, and timing in both the deep and superficial muscle systems. Observation of the *quality* of task performance during activities on unstable surfaces with expected, or unexpected, challenges to balance will reveal control of postural equilibrium without long periods of excessive superficial muscle activation (minimal bracing) and trunk rigidity.

It is critical that, for each new task or movement practice, the therapist palpates the segment(s)/region where failed load transfer was identified on assessment. This will reveal whether or not the deep muscle system is continuing to function in the new movement and/or loading environment. Palpation points include:

- For the pelvic girdle, the innominate and the sacrum are palpated on the affected side to ensure that anterior rotation of the innominate (or unlocking of the hemipelvis) does not occur with limb loading (see Fig. 8.18).

- For the lumbar spine, the articular pillars or interspinous spaces are palpated to check for loss of control in the relevant direction (flexion, extension, rotation, or hinging) (see Fig. 8.24D).
- For the hip, the innominate and the greater trochanter of the femur are palpated to check for anterior displacement of the femoral head or loss of rotational control (see Fig. 8.19B).

As tasks are added that include full limb movement, each joint in the kinetic chain should be observed/palpated for control of the optimal axis of movement and joint position. The position of the thorax in relation to the pelvis is monitored for alterations in the anteroposterior (sagittal), lateral (coronal), and rotational (transverse) planes (see Fig. 8.31B). The femoral head should remain seated (centered in the acetabulum) without loss of control into internal/external rotation, abduction/adduction, flexion or extension (see Fig. 8.30C, Video 11.17). The knee should not excessively rotate or abduct/adduct (fall into a valgus or varus position); the foot should not excessively supinate or pronate (Fig. 8.21). In closed kinetic chain tasks, the knee should stay aligned such that mid-patella tracks over the second toe (Fig. 8.20). By correcting deviations of alignment with tactile cues, imagery, and/or proprioceptive input (e.g. via resistive exercise bands, tape, or other tools), the appropriate components of the deep and superficial muscle systems, as well as the myofascial slings of the lower extremity, will be activated for total body movement control and flow.

When adding the superficial muscle system of the abdominal canister and the myofascial slings of the lower extremity to the deep muscle system, the discerning clinician may ask, 'How much is too much superficial muscle and myofascial sling activity?' It is evident that there needs to be enough activity to control the imposed forces. However, excessive activity is best avoided as it creates too much compression through the joints and often restricts mobility. Thus, the clinician needs to be able to identify when the added muscle activity crosses over from 'just enough' to 'too much.' Each patient will present with a specific pattern of superficial muscle hyperactivity; this pattern will have been identified during the assessment tests and the dominant muscles released as part of the treatment program. By specifically palpating and observing these muscles during task progressions, the clinician will get an idea of how much activity is present; comparing for symmetry of activation between affected and non-affected sides is often revealing. The patient can be taught how to monitor the specific muscles and pattern of substitution for their home practice.

Checkpoints for optimal strategy – avoiding rigidity

Throughout the rehabilitation process our goal is to restore optimal strategies for function and performance, to reduce rigid, bracing strategies and develop ones that promote fluidity of movement with underlying control. When training new strategies for the patient with LPH disability with or without pain, watch for excessive activity in the superficial muscle system and the connected myofascial sling systems as this will reduce rib cage mobility, lateral costal expansion, spinal mobility, and hip mobility. The following are techniques to use at any time during movement practice and training to monitor for excessive muscle activation; they are called 'checkpoints for rigidity' (Box 11.4 Video 12.17).

Rib cage wiggle

Place your hands bilaterally on the lateral aspect of the rib cage (Video LC13). With one hand, apply a gentle lateral translation force in one direction followed by an opposite lateral translation force with the other hand. Repeat several oscillatory translations to the left and right, and note the amount of resistance to the applied force. There should be a symmetrical amount of lateral movement with only a small amount of force. A loss of this lateral joint play is an indication of a restriction of movement and overactivation of the superficial muscle system.

Breathing pattern

Observe the rib cage during respiration. If there is excessive superficial muscle activity, there will be a non-optimal pattern of rib cage expansion, bilaterally or unilaterally. Often there is minimal lateral costal expansion and excessive upper rib cage expansion or abdominal movement. (Video 11.1).

> ### Box 11.4
>
> #### Checkpoints for rigidity
> - Rib cage 'wiggle.'
> - Breathing pattern.
> - Internal/external rotation of the hip.
> - Toe 'wiggle.'

Internal/external rotation of the hip

A decrease in the range of internal or external rotation of the hip can be an indication of excessive muscle activity overly compressing the hip joint. When the deep muscle system is coactivated, there should be no change in the ease of hip rotation. Thus, in many tasks, hip rotation can be used to ensure that the superficial muscles of the hip are not being overly recruited. This test can be easily performed in supine, crook lying, sitting, supported standing, and other functional positions. The therapist lightly grasps the patient's lower thigh and attempts to move the hip passively into internal rotation and then external rotation with a gentle force. Alternately, the patient can perform a 'self-check' by attempting to actively move the hips into internal and external rotation; we call this the 'chicken-dance,' named for a song of the same name.

Toe wiggle

As the program progresses to an upright, weight bearing position, alignment of the lower extremity and activation of the myofascial slings of the lower extremity must be considered. Gripping the toes into flexion indicates an imbalance in the myofascial slings of the lower leg; ask the patient to 'keep the toes relaxed' and to 'wiggle the toes' between repetitions to correct and avoid rigidity of the foot.

General principles for coordinating the deep and superficial muscle systems (Box 11.5)

- Release, Align, Connect, and Move (RACM) – the patient uses previously found images/cues to relax/release/remove the habitual old strategy (Chapter 10), finds their neutral LPH alignment, and then coactivates the deep muscle system using their previously found 'chord cue' (Chapter 11) as the starting point for each task practice.
- Initially the patient may need to relax the 'chord cue' for co-contraction of the deep muscle system after each contraction; however, the goal is to encourage a maintained deep muscle system co-contraction as long as the old non-optimal substitution strategies are not observed.
  The number of repetitions possible with one RACM will increase as control improves.
- Initially focus on low load and control of movement.

357

Box 11.5

General principles for coordinating the deep and superficial muscle systems

- Release, Align, Connect, and Move (RACM).
- Maintain the chord cue connection focusing on low load and movement control.
- Build endurance up to three sets of 10, 10-second holds.
- Watch for signs of loss of segmental/joint control and excessive superficial muscle activity; use the checkpoints for optimal strategy.
- Progress from stable to unstable surfaces.
- Build exercises on components taken from the meaningful task.

- Aim for high repetitions to build endurance (massed practice is an essential component for rewiring neural networks). Start with only as many repetitions as the patient can perform with an effective deep and superficial muscle system activation and control of the movement (sometimes as few as three to five repetitions), and progress to three sets of 10 repetitions with 2 minutes of rest between sets.
- Avoid fast ballistic movements in early stages; use only for relevant, meaningful task training.
- Palpate and monitor the deep muscle system recruitment where necessary, and joint motion control (lumbar segment, SIJ, PS, hip) during the task, especially when adding a new progression. Ensure that the deep muscle system does not turn off and that there are no signs of loss of control (previously found in the assessment).
- Check for excessive superficial muscle system activity by monitoring the breathing pattern (should continue to see lateral costal and abdominal expansion) and by monitoring for bracing/rigidity (see *Checkpoints for optimal strategy – avoiding rigidity*).
- Use the manual and verbal cues for facilitating the maintenance of neutral LPH if loss of control/position occurs *during task practice.*
- Progress from stable to unstable surfaces to increase proprioceptive input, challenge, and provide unexpected perturbations.
- Incorporate a deep muscle system co-contraction into daily functional activities (meaningful tasks) as early and as often as possible; break down

functional tasks into component movements and use separate components for task practice.
- Focus on co-contraction and control of position instead of single muscle strengthening.
- If high-load and high-speed activities are required for work or sport, add these at the end stages of rehabilitation and ensure that low-load, slow-speed control is present for the same movement pattern first. High-speed/high-load activities should be only one part of the patient's program; low-load tasks should be continued concurrently to ensure the ongoing development of optimal strategies for all tasks.

Coordinating the deep and superficial muscle systems

The goal for all of the task practice in this section is to develop and train (endurance and strength) an optimal strategy for coordinating the deep and superficial muscle systems with the LPH in neutral. The principles for this training are highlighted in Box 11.5. To ensure maintenance of neutral LPH, note the spinal curves (including any relevant segments that tend to lose control) as well as the thoracopelvic, intrapelvic, and hip positions throughout the task. The movements should be slow and controlled in both the concentric and eccentric phases of movement.

Two types of task can be used: those that control dissociation of the arm from the trunk, and those that control dissociation of the leg from the trunk. This practice builds on the foundation laid during training for coactivation of the deep muscle system and is preparatory for the next stage of rehabilitation – building new strategies for meaningful tasks, function, and performance (Chapter 12). Note that not all of the following tasks are used for each patient. Often only one progression is used while simultaneously training more total body strategies (Chapter 12). A general guideline is to use the base position (side-lying, prone, supine, or crook lying) in which the patient was most successful at achieving the chord cue, and then use arm or leg movements/loading to add a further challenge.

Palpation of the poorly controlled joints noted during the assessment will reveal whether or not control is maintained throughout the task. Observation of the orientation between the pelvis and the rib cage will reveal whether or not an optimal strategy for activation of the superficial muscle system is occurring. Adding verbal cues/images for the superficial muscle system is useful to help keep optimal align-ment and control. For thoracopelvic control during these tasks, the following cues can be used:

- If there is extension and right rotation of the thorax, use the following cue: 'Keep the bottom of your rib cage on the right side connected to the left ASIS throughout the task.'

- If there is flexion and rotation of the thorax to the right, cue by saying: 'Imagine that there is a line going from your left bottom rib at the back to your right hip (or PSIS); keep tension in that line throughout the task.'

- If the pelvis is rotating left, ask the patient to: 'Imagine that there is a pin going through your right ASIS that is holding the right side of your pelvis down on the bed and keeping it still while you move your leg.'

These cues are added *after* the initial chord cue that resulted in co-contraction of the deep muscle system and are emphasized *during* movement of the arm or leg so that continued activation of the appropriate myofascial sling occurs during increased limb loading.

Trunk and arm dissociation – supine or crook lying

Patient position. Crook lying in a neutral LPH posi-tion on a flat surface. Arms are flexed to 90° so that the hands are vertically over the shoulder joints.

Instruction. Cue the image that facilitates a co-contraction of the deep muscle system. Palpate transversus abdominis and multifidus at the dysfunc-tional level(s), ensuring that recruitment occurs with this cue. Ask the patient to keep breathing and maintain neutral LPH while performing various arm movements:

(a) Triceps press (extension control) (Fig. 11.29): bend the elbows and bring the hands towards the head. The elbows are then straightened (triceps press movement). The shoulders should not flex or extend; movement occurs only at the elbow joints.

(b) Overhead flexion (extension control): keep the arms straight while elevating the arms through flexion. The patient will require adequate length in the latissimus dorsi muscles to perform this progression with good control of the lumbar lordosis. The task can also be started with the arms at the sides instead of at 90° flexion.

(c) One arm fly (rotation control): keep the arm straight while lowering the arm through

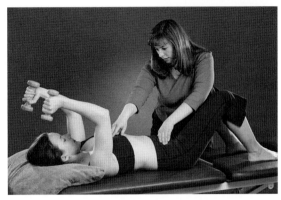

Fig. 11.29 • Coordinating the deep and superficial muscle systems: trunk and arm dissociation – supine or crook lying triceps press (extension control). The therapist palpates for the recruitment and tonic contraction of the transversus abdominis while providing gentle pressure on the sternum to cue maintenance of the thoracic kyphosis and to prevent loss of neutral into thoracolumbar extension.

horizontal abduction one arm at a time. Palpate the dysfunctional area (lumbar spine, sacroiliac joints) to ensure no loss of control of the neutral position.

Progressions/other considerations. Progress to lying on a half roll or other unsupported surface.

Hand weights can be added to increase the chal-lenge to the spine while concurrently strengthening the arm muscles.

Trunk and leg dissociation – crook lying

Several authors have described various leg loading tasks and their progressions (Hall & Brody 1999, Richardson et al 1999, Sahrmann 2001). Some spe-cific and modified examples that we find useful for patients with LPH disability with or without pain are presented here.

Patient position. Crook lying in neutral LPH on a flat surface.

Instruction. Cue the image that facilitates a co-contraction of the deep muscle system. Palpate TrA and dMF at the dysfunctional level(s), ensuring that recruitment occurs with your cue. Ask the patient to keep breathing and maintain the LPH neu-tral position while performing various leg move-ments. Should the femoral head lose its centered position relative to the acetabulum during any of these tasks, the patient is not ready to progress to leg dissociation at this time. Instead they will require training for 'waking up' and building a better strategy for the deep muscle system of the hip joint (see below). Subsequently, the following can be introduced.

(a) Heel slides (extension/rotation and flexion/rotation control): ensure that the feet can slide on the surface easily (have the patient wear socks). Ask the patient to slowly slide one heel away from the trunk, straightening the leg as far as possible without losing control of the neutral LPH position. Palpate the segment(s) of poor control to ensure that no rotation occurs in the lumbar spine or pelvis. This phase of the task challenges extension and rotation control; the return of the leg back to the flexed position challenges flexion and rotation control. The easiest position from which to start the slide is the crook lying position; to increase the challenge have the patient start the slide with the leg straight. The task can also be changed from a single leg slide to alternating slides (from moving one leg at a time to moving both legs at the same time, one sliding down while the other slides up).

(b) Bent knee fall out (rotation control) (Videos JG12, JG13): from the crook lying position one knee is slowly taken to the side so that the hip abducts and externally rotates (Fig. 11.30A). The other leg stays stationary. Careful observation and palpation of the femoral head is necessary to ensure that the patient is not butt-gripping and pushing the femoral head anteriorly. Palpate at the ASISs or in the interspinous spaces of the lumbar spine for rotation control. To progress the task, straighten the non-moving leg.

(c) Heel 'drops' from 90° (extension control): to attain the starting position, the patient requires 90° of hip flexion with a centered femoral head. The patient initially cues their release, align, and connect images for the deep muscle system and then flexes their hips to 90° such that the knees are vertically over the hip joints. Check the lumbar lordosis to ensure the lumbopelvis has remained in neutral. Ensure the patient continues to breathe and instruct them to slowly lower one foot, keeping the knee flexed, until the foot is placed on the plinth/floor (or until the LPH control is lost) (Fig. 11.30B). The foot is then lifted from the plinth/floor and returned to 90° hip flexion. The task can be progressed by having the patient extend the knee as the foot is lowered (increase the lever arm). This is a useful precursor to any task that involves lifting one foot off the ground in supine or sitting, as well as for training coordination of psoas and the deep muscles of the abdominal canister for control of hip centering (see below for 'waking up' and building a better strategy for the deep muscle system of the hip).

Progressions/other considerations. Progress to lying on a half roll or other unsupported surface. Initially

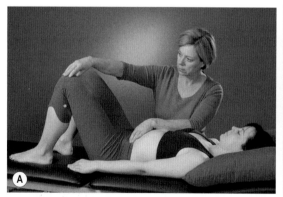 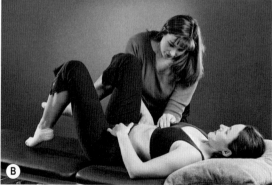

Fig. 11.30 • Coordinating the deep and superficial muscle systems: trunk and leg dissociation. (A) Crook lying bent knee fall out (rotation control). The therapist palpates either the lumbar interspinous spaces or the pelvic girdle to ensure that neutral is maintained (no rotation occurs) as the knee is slowly taken laterally (abduction and external rotation of the hip). (B) Crook lying heel drops from 90°. In this illustration the therapist is palpating the TrA and dMF on the right side; the patient is palpating the left TrA and the sternum. As the foot is lowered towards the table the tendency will be to lose the neutral LPH position and move into anterior pelvic tilt and lumbar extension. The hand on the sternum helps to prevent thoracolumbar extension.

the patient will only be able to move the leg through a small range of motion. As control improves, the leg can move through a larger range of motion. It is important to teach the patient what it feels like when they lose control so that the task can be monitored and progressed at home. Remind the patient to use the load effort task analysis during the practice to ensure they are using an optimal strategy. Check for excessive bracing or rigidity of the rib cage (rib cage wiggle and monitor lateral costal expansion breathing) and hip joints (IR/ER) during the practice. Lifting the weight of the leg off the floor and lowering the leg into a fully extended position are high-level tasks, especially in those patients with muscular legs. Also, supine, or crook lying, progressions are high level for patients with pelvic girdle disability and/or pain as this is the most challenging position to control the pelvis. In these cases, tasks in more upright positions such as sitting and supported standing can be added to the program before the higher progressions of leg loading in supine are achieved (Chapter 12).

Trunk and leg dissociation – sidelying

Patient position. Sidelying in neutral LPH on a flat surface.

Instruction. Cue the image that facilitates co-contraction of the deep muscle system and palpate TrA and dMF to provide feedback and check recruitment. Ask the patient to keep breathing and maintain the LPH neutral position while performing various leg movements. Should the femoral head lose its centered position relative to the acetabulum, the patient is not ready to progress to leg dissociation tasks at this time. Instead they will require training for 'waking up' and building a better strategy for the deep muscle system of the hip joint (see below). Subsequently, these tasks can be introduced.

Clam shell (rotation control): ensure that the patient's ankles remain together and instruct the patient to lift the top knee towards the ceiling. Palpate the segment(s) of poor control to ensure that no rotation occurs in the lumbar spine or pelvis. Only the femur should move during this task; the lumbar spine and pelvis should remain in neutral (Fig. 11.31A).

Progressions/other considerations. The task can be progressed by having the patient maintain the lift of the top knee and then lift the foot of the same leg (increase the lever arm) (Fig. 11.31B). The hip should remain abducted/externally rotated with

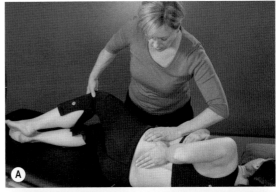

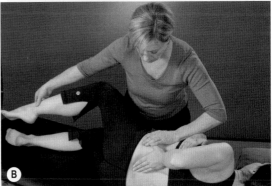

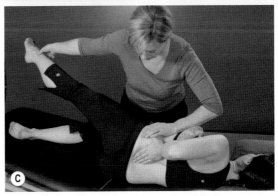

Fig. 11.31 • Coordinating the deep and superficial muscle systems: trunk and leg dissociation – sidelying. (A) Clamshell. In this illustration the patient is palpating their dMF and the therapist is monitoring the pelvis as they RACM into a left clamshell (lift the top knee without losing the neutral LPH position). Clinically, the therapist would palpate the joint/segment of poor control noted in the assessment of this task to ensure an optimal strategy was chosen and trained. (B) Once the patient can perform three sets of 10, 10-second holds of this task, further challenge can be added by having them lift the foot of the same leg without lowering the knee. (C) Subsequently, an additional challenge would be to have them extend the top leg while maintaining neutral LPH in the abducted/externally rotated position. This is a high-level task, especially when repeated 30 times.

the knee higher than the ankle. The lumbopelvis should remain neutral throughout the practice. A further progression would be to have the patient extend the abducted/externally rotated hip from this position (Fig. 11.31C). The leg should then flex, the ankles should approximate, and the knee then lowers to return to the starting position. As control improves, the leg can move through a larger range of motion. It is important to teach the patient what it feels like when they lose control so that the task can be monitored and progressed at home. Remind the patient to use the load effort task analysis during the practice to ensure they are using an optimal strategy. Check for excessive bracing or rigidity of the rib cage (rib cage wiggle) and monitor lateral costal expansion breathing.

Trunk and leg dissociation – prone

Patient position. Prone lying in neutral LPH on a flat surface. Pillows or towels under the abdomen or thorax can be used to obtain the correct alignment.

Instruction. Cue the image that facilitates co-contraction of the deep muscle system and palpate TrA and dMF to provide feedback and check recruitment. Ask the patient to bend one knee to 90° flexion, lifting the foot and then lowering it to the table (Fig. 11.32A,B). Repeat on the other side.

Progressions/other considerations. Palpate the lumbar segment(s) of poor control to ensure that no rotation occurs in the lumbar spine, then palpate the SIJs to ensure no unlocking of the pelvis occurs. Careful observation and palpation of the femoral

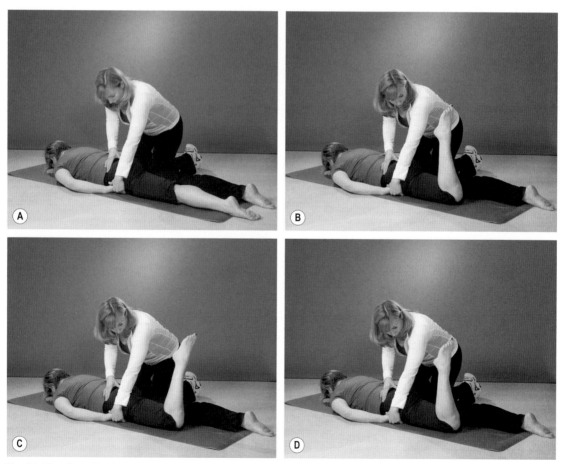

Fig. 11.32 • Coordinating the deep and superficial muscle systems: trunk and leg dissociation – prone. (A) In this illustration the patient is palpating their left femoral head and the therapist is monitoring the pelvis. (B) The patient bends the ipsilateral knee after imaging their release and connect cues. The femoral head should remain centered and the SIJ controlled throughout the task. Once sagittal plane motion is controlled, introduce a rotation challenge by having the patient (C) externally and (D) internally rotate the femur.

head is necessary to ensure that the patient is not losing control of the hip during this practice. The task can be progressed by having the patient:

(a) externally rotate the hip while maintaining intrapelvic control and a centered femoral head (Fig. 11.32C);

(b) internally rotate the hip while maintaining intrapelvic control and a centered femoral head (Fig. 11.32D);

(c) extend the hip with the knee extended (Fig. 11.33A–C). This is a useful precursor to any exercise that involves moving the entire leg into extension off the ground and requires good LPH control.

'Waking up' and building the neural network for coordinating the deep and superficial muscle systems of the hip joint

Building a new neural network for optimal coordination of the muscles of the hip begins with teaching the patient a strategy that prepares the hip for loading. To the authors' knowledge, it is not known which hip muscles should coactivate prior to the onset of motion; however, it is believed that an optimal neuromuscular strategy will result in a centered femoral head for all tasks performed. When a cue is given that results in a contraction of psoas, which is isolated from the superficial hip flexors and adductors, most patients with failed load transfer through the hip are able to perform trunk and leg dissociation tasks with an optimal strategy (centered femoral head). This is not to say that other, deeper, muscles such the obturators or gemelli do not co-contract; this is still a matter of speculation. The key point is to ensure that the resultant strategy keeps the femoral head centered and allows the hip to move in the desired direction(s).

Clinically, we have found that, if all of the hypertonic superficial muscles of the hip have been released (or relatively released), the 'hip cue' can be easily added to the lumbopelvic 'chord cue' and subsequent training for trunk and leg dissociation can begin.

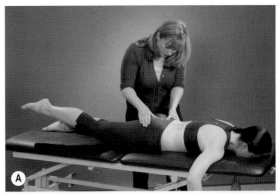

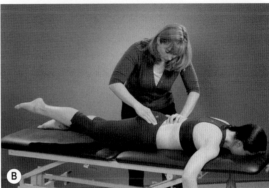

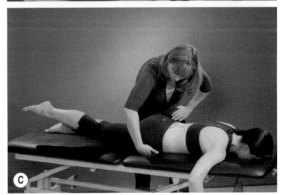

Fig. 11.33 • Coordinating the deep and superficial muscle systems: trunk and leg dissociation – prone. (A) Prone hip extension task. This is a progression from the prone knee bend task. In this illustration, the therapist is ensuring that the strategy chosen is optimal for the left SIJ (no unlocking). (B) In this illustration, the therapist is monitoring the right SIJ and the various segments of the lumbar spine. (C) Here, the therapist is monitoring the right femoral head position. Optimally, the femoral head should remain centered, the SIJs should not unlock, and the pelvis and the lumbar spine should not rotate or tilt/flex/extend/sideflex during this task.

Finding the optimal 'hip cue'

Patient and therapist position

Choose the position where the patient can attain the best neutral LPH position with the superficial muscles of the hip relaxed, especially the tensor fascia latae, rectus femoris, sartorius, and short adductors. A common best position for this is crook lying with feet supported over a bolster or with one foot (Fig. 11.34A), or both feet, supported on a wall. Palpate psoas with one hand and the dominant superficial hip muscles with the other. Alternately, monitor the femoral head position in the groin. If the best neutral position is sidelying or prone, palpate the femoral head with one hand and the dominant superficial hip muscles with the other. Teach the patient how to palpate either psoas or the femoral head in the chosen neutral position.

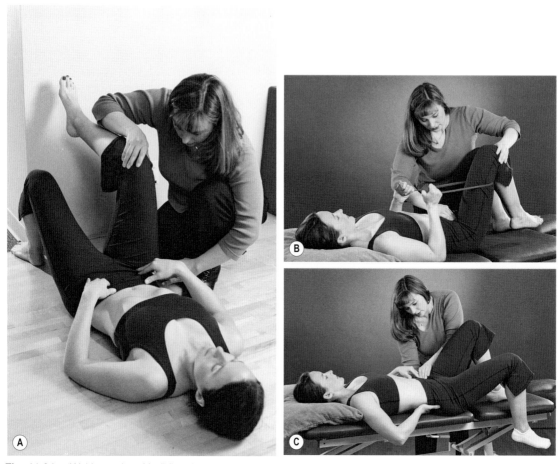

Fig. 11.34 • 'Waking up' and building the neural network for coordinating the deep and superficial muscles of the hip joint. (A) Finding the best hip cue. In this illustration, the patient is palpating the anterior groin while the therapist palpates tensor fascia latae, rectus femoris, and sartorius laterally. The patient's left hand is palpating TrA. Several verbal cues are tried (see text) and the load effort task analysis is used to confirm the best cue/strategy for optimal recruitment of the hip flexors. (B) A resistive exercise band is a useful assist and decreases the amount of load. In this example the therapist is palpating TrA bilaterally to monitor the activation of the deep muscle system during the task. The femoral head can also be monitored to ensure an optimal strategy. (C) Progression – in this example, the patient is palpating the left TrA and right multifidus to ensure co-contraction while the therapist monitors lumbopelvic alignment. As the leg moves into the outer range, the superficial hip flexors will activate to some degree, but this activity should not result in rigidity of the hip joint.

Correction technique – verbal and manual cues

Several verbal cues and images can facilitate a contraction of the psoas. The load effort task analysis will confirm whether the cue chosen facilitates a better strategy for loading through the hip in that reduced effort will be required to move the leg with the best cue.

- 'Imagine a guy wire from the end of the greater trochanter (palpate this spot so their brain feels where it is) through the neck of the femur to a place deep in the center of your pelvis. Connect along this wire thinking of gently compressing the femur into the hip socket.'

- 'Imagine a guy wire from the inside of your groin (region of the lesser trochanter) running through your pelvis to the middle of your low back. Connect along this wire thinking of gently suspending the vertebra after connecting the hip.' This guy wire can also begin at the end of the femur.

- 'Imagine your leg is like a Barbie doll's leg that someone is attempting to pull off. Gently resist this longitudinal force.'

Ideal and abnormal responses

If you are able to palpate psoas, you should feel a slow development of firmness in the muscle and no response from the dominant superficial hip muscles. This contraction is also visible with ultrasound imaging (Video 8.20 🖰). Have the patient maintain the 'hip cue,' add-on their 'chord cue' for the lumbopelvis, and then lift the foot (if crook lying) (Video 11.18a,b 🖰), knee (if sidelying), or bend the knee (if prone). In some cases, using the 'chord cue' for the lumbopelvis is required first, and then the 'hip cue' (Video 11.19 🖰). The lumbopelvis should remain in the neutral position, the femoral head should remain centered, and a difference in effort to perform this task should be noted by both the patient and the therapist.

Trunk and leg dissociation – hip joint control progressions

Patient position. Crook lying in neutral LPH with the foot supported on a wall, with the hip flexed approximately 70–80°.

Instruction. Cue the image that facilitates a co-contraction of the deep muscle system of the lumbopelvis and combine it with the cue found to facilitate an optimal strategy for loading the hip (new combined chord cue). Ask the patient to keep breathing and to slowly lift the foot off the wall (Fig. 11.34A). Ankle plantarflexion (heel lift) can be used as an assist to get the foot off the wall. Palpate the lumbopelvis and the femoral head and ensure the strategy is optimal for maintaining a neutral lumbopelvis and centered femoral head. The task is progressed by moving the patient farther away from the wall, thus increasing the level arm. If load assist is required (e.g. patients with long or muscular legs), a piece of high-resistance Thera-Band™ can be used to partially support the leg during these progressions (Fig. 11.34B). Finally, the task is performed over the edge of a table so that the foot can be lowered past the level of the table and the hip can move into full extension (Fig. 11.34C).

Progressions/other considerations. Progress to lying on a half roll or other unsupported surface. Initially the patient will only be able to move the leg through a small range of motion. As control improves, the leg can move through a larger range of motion. It is important to teach the patient what it feels like when they lose control (load effort task analysis) so that the task can be monitored and progressed at home. Be sure to check for rigidity of the rib cage and hip, and to monitor lateral costal expansion breathing to prevent excessive activation of the superficial muscles. Lifting the weight of the leg off the floor and lowering the leg into a fully extended position are high level, especially in those patients with muscular legs. In these cases, tasks in more upright positions such as sitting and supported standing can be added to the program (Chapter 12) before the higher progressions of leg loading in supine are achieved.

When to refer for prolotherapy

Prolotherapy (Cusi et al 2010, Dorman 1994, 1997) is indicated when there has been a loss of integrity of the articular system restraints (articular system impairment) and the neural and myofascial systems cannot provide sufficient compression to compensate and control the joint under load. When the myofascial and neural systems are functioning well, co-contraction of the muscles of the deep system should compress the joint, increase its stiffness, and reduce the neutral zone of motion to zero. If the healthy myofascial and neural systems are unable to control motion in the neutral zone, it is unlikely that conservative treatment will be successful; this is the primary indication for prolotherapy (Video 11.20).

Prolotherapy involves injecting the capsule and/or ligaments of the impaired joint with an irritant solution that subsequently creates an inflammatory reaction. Fibroblasts then migrate into the inflamed tissue and produce collagen, which increases the stiffness of the capsule/ligament. Typically, the capsule/ligaments are injected every 2–6 weeks, and the treatment is repeated for three to six sessions. The role of the therapist during this process is to ensure that the joint is supported with an external support or tape to prevent excessive shearing of the joint and to ensure that optimal alignment is maintained. As prolotherapy is often painful, the therapist should be prepared to provide emotional support during this process. Once the myofascial and neural systems can affect the neutral zone of motion (the joint glide can be reduced with a co-contraction of the deep muscle system), recovery of the articular system restraints has reached a point where appropriate motor control and movement training can now be implemented.

Summary – where are we at and what's left?

By now the patient should be able to:

1. release their old strategies using cues/images/tools taught from Chapter 10 (release and align);
2. find a neutral LPH alignment in either crook lying, supine, sidelying, or prone lying;
3. connect to the deep muscle system for the abdominal canister and hip (connect); and then
4. integrate the deep and superficial muscle systems using either arm or leg loading (maintaining neutral LPH) dissociated from any trunk or pelvic movement (move).

New neural networks have formed and it is time to take this into function, to make it all meaningful, and to really change how the patient lives in their body. Without these first foundational steps, the next part of the program is extremely difficult and sometimes impossible. Functional movement training will reinforce the new neural networks and build more. Here we go – onto the last chapter and the last piece of the program, the piece that pulls it all together and hopefully leads to the resolution of the Clinical Puzzle!

Training new strategies for posture and movement

12

Linda-Joy Lee

CHAPTER CONTENTS

Introduction 367
Advanced assessment 368
  Finding the driver for the whole body . . 368
  Whole body meaningful task analysis . . 373
  Center of mass over base of support
  (body centering test) 378
Tools and techniques to facilitate new
strategies 379
  Increase awareness 379
  Celebrate success 381
  Transform task analysis into training
  activities 381
  General principles for designing
  movement building blocks 383
  Key points of control to cue and
  facilitate optimal strategies 387
Training strategies for static tasks 389
  Standing posture 390
  Sitting posture 391
  Task-specific postures 395
Training strategies for dynamic tasks –
functional and sport-specific 396
  Essential progressions for function 397
Summary 405

Introduction

The ultimate goal of treatment, based on The Integrated Systems Model, is to change strategies for function and performance; that is, to change the way patients live, move, and experience their bodies. This is quite a different perspective from one that aims to 'fix the patient,' in that the responsibility for making change lies with the patient. Using a combination of manual tools, teaching skills, and personal knowledge, the therapist creates the options and opportunities for the patient to learn and train new strategies for function and performance. The final decision to choose the new strategies on a daily basis resides with the patient, as only they can create and maintain a different experience of their body. Teaching new strategies for function and performance relies heavily on the capacity of the nervous system for change (the art and science of neuroplasticity), which gives human beings amazing potential for transformation in both physical and emotional realms. It is less about increasing strength of specific muscles, or increasing cardiovascular endurance, although both strength and cardiovascular capacity change and improve in the process of a graduated return to work and sports program. However, strength, power, endurance, and cardiovascular capacity serve meaningful goals best if they are developed with optimal patterns of movement. This speaks to the importance of training quality of movement versus quantity of movement. But how do we help our patients change how they perform habitual, automatic, and well-established postural and movement strategies?

The general principles underlying how to facilitate change were discussed in Chapter 9 (see *Treatment principles for an integrated evidence-based program*). It is essential to remove as many barriers as possible and delete old neural networks, which creates an open canvas to design new strategies for posture and movement (specific techniques were described in Chapter 10). In any one treatment session, the best time to train new strategies is immediately after barriers have been addressed. Thus, when planning time allocation

DOI: 10.1016/B978-0-443-06963-5.00012-2

for treatment, allow at least 10–15 minutes to train *and practice* new postural and movement strategies (i.e. minimum of 15 repetitions for each training task) after manual and other release techniques have been used. Otherwise the window of opportunity created by removing barriers is missed. Manual treatment effects will be most lasting and sustained if new networks are immediately trained by providing the verbal cues and encouragement, manual feedback and facilitation, and appropriate environment to alter all inputs to the body-self neuromatrix (see Fig. 7.9). Providing the patient with a new experience of their body creates new positive beliefs and emotions, which will change central pain drivers. Empowering the patient with a sense of control over their body will reduce threat, fear, and change stress-related outputs. All of these factors will feed back into the neuromatrix and provide better physiology for healing, and even more gains. Designating focused training time (where the therapist provides 1:1 feedback and cuing for optimal performance of the task) thus consolidates new maps and builds precision and confidence, so that the patient can continue to use the new networks as they walk out of the treatment session and go about the rest of their day.

Recall from Chapter 4 and Chapter 7 that our definition of 'optimal strategy for function and performance' is broad and encompasses both quantitative and qualitative features of human movement; that is, optimal strategies are painfree, energy efficient, support stability of the spine and pelvis, highly robust, and enable all outcomes relevant to the patient's goals and values. Optimal strategies also create an experience of 'flow,' 'ease,' and 'grace.' Many of our patients experience their bodies as a source of frustration, pain, and despair; we aim to change this experience to one of freedom and ease, and full enjoyment of their bodies.

Part of the process of creating new strategies for function is to address any deficits in the deep muscle system, and to use specific training tasks to start coordinating the deep and superficial muscles; this was covered in Chapter 11. The intent of this chapter is to further develop strategy and meaningful task analysis (advanced assessment) and to provide specific principles and techniques to train new postural and movement strategies for functional tasks that require integrated total body movement. It is essential to explain to the patient that the aim of their home program is to practice the building blocks and use the new neural networks, which are component skills necessary to learn a new strategy for function and performance. Thus, these building blocks are concurrently incorporated into all activities of daily life, and most importantly into their meaningful tasks. This is quite different to having a routine of exercises that exists as a separate activity that is then forgotten during other activities. Successful training of new strategies for function and performance requires awareness and mindful practice, until the new strategies are fully integrated and become a part of the person in the middle of the puzzle.

Recall from Chapter 11, by now the patient should be able to:

1. release their old strategies using cues/images/tools taught from Chapter 10 (release and align);
2. find a neutral LPH alignment in either crook lying, supine, sidelying, or prone lying;
3. connect to the deep muscle system for the abdominal canister and hip (connect); and then
4. integrate the deep and superficial muscle systems using either arm or leg loading (maintaining neutral LPH) dissociated from any trunk or pelvic movement (move).

The stage is set to integrate these new neural networks into meaningful tasks. Before we discuss the specific techniques and examples of functional progressions, we need to consider some additional assessment tools.

Advanced assessment

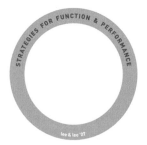

Finding the driver for the whole body

Any functional task, whether it be sustained postural positions or dynamic activities, requires integration of all regions of the body. When a patient presents with lumbar, pelvic girdle, and/or hip pain, along with functional limitations, the clinician must determine whether the driving cause for the pain experience and loss of function is intrinsic or extrinsic to the lumbopelvic–hip (LPH) complex. In order to make this decision, it is often not sufficient to only assess function of the LPH complex during functional tasks (as described in Chapter 8). The therapist must also determine if failed load transfer (FLT = non-optimal alignment, biomechanics, and/or control required for the given task) exists in other parts of the body and then assess the interactions between the LPH complex and these other areas of FLT (that may be painful or painfree). This is an essential process that enables the therapist to determine how all areas of the body are linking and interacting with each other during total body function. By considering the connections between all parts of the body, the patient's injury history and pain experience can be better reasoned and explained. Especially in cases of insidious onset pain, this integrated understanding of the synergies (and dyssynergies) in the body (and body–mind interactions) can help explain and answer the question: 'What caused my low back/foot/shoulder/hip pain?' Analyzing the interactions between areas of the body also reveals:

- which impairments are relevant to the current clinical presentation and which are not;
- which are compensatory (and whose treatment will, therefore, not result in full resolution of the problem);
- which are non-optimal but appropriate for the phase of tissue healing or level of tissue irritability (for example to unload painful structures); and
- which are driving the LPH dysfunction (and therefore the underlying cause).

Note that because human beings are continually changing entities, the driver can change during the process of recovery (see case reports Julie G and Louise, Chapter 9 🖱).

The principles for 'finding the driver' were described in detail in Chapter 8 (see Fig. 8.1 and Box 8.1) and illustrated in the case reports in Chapter 9. Specific assessment techniques for other regions of the body are beyond the scope of this text; however, what follows is a review of the principles for 'finding the driver' in The Integrated Systems Model, in relation to total body function, as these same principles are required for more complex task analysis. Furthermore, from the perspective of facilitating change in movement behavior, treating 'the driver' is the 'way in' and the key to creating new neural networks.

The patient's story provides insight into:

- the underlying mechanisms for the current pain experience (see Chapter 7);

- the functional positions and movements that are meaningful to the patient (meaningful tasks) because of how they relate to their pain experience or because they are performance limitations; and
- problems in other systems such as urogynecological, respiratory, or postural equilibrium (balance).

Note that the primary driver(s) for the whole body strategy will relate to all of these problems. That is, treating the key driver(s) should positively impact all problems; if it does not, then there are other underlying impairments that are concurrent drivers that need to be addressed.

The objective examination is then tailored to use the key screening tests for strategy analysis (OLS, squat, prone knee bend (PKB), etc.) that are most related to the meaningful tasks. As noted in Chapter 8, the strategy analysis tests previously described do not encompass all of the possible screening tests for automatic strategy analysis. Specific strategy tests are designed based on details revealed in the patient's story. For each relevant screening task:

1. Identify all areas of FLT in the kinetic chain – assess for non-optimal alignment, biomechanics, and/or control (areas assessed are based on hypotheses generated from the story and are usually several areas between head to toe):

    (a) in relevant posture (standing posture, seated posture, simulated work or sport posture; and/or

    (b) during relevant movement task (forward bending, one leg standing, prone knee bend, etc.) (Fig. 12.1A–D).

2. Assess the level of commitment to the current strategy:

    (a) first in standing, and then in positions related to the meaningful task. Attempt to manually correct the alignment in the area of failed load transfer (use cues to release if needed), and determine which region of the body is more resistant to correction (pelvis/hips, thorax, foot). Often the area(s) that are the most resistant to correction are the area(s) of the current primary driver(s) and will need release and training of a new strategy for restoration of optimal function (see case report Louise, Chapter 9, Video LL14, Video 12.1); 🖱

    (b) if you are unable to correct an area of failed load transfer, this indicates that the area

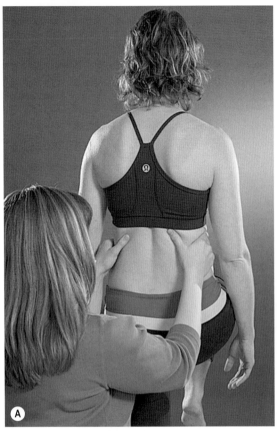 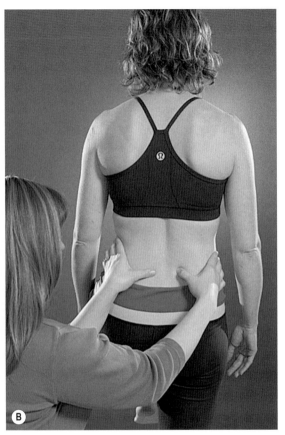

Fig. 12.1 • Advanced assessment – identifying areas of failed load transfer (FLT). (A) In this illustration the therapist is palpating a thoracic ring as the patient stands on one leg and notes the presence or absence of failed load transfer *specifically* at this ring (i.e. no translation or rotation of this ring should occur during this task). (B) Here, the therapist is palpating L4 during the same task and again notes the presence/absence of FLT at L4–5.

Continued

needs further assessment to determine why; further assessment will direct what to release (Chapter 10) and then the task can be reassessed to determine how this area relates to the pain experience and total body strategy.

3. Establish *relative timing* between areas of FLT; that is, determine which joint(s) exhibit FLT at the earliest point in the task as this joint is likely to be the primary driver (Fig. 12.2A,B, Video 12.2a,b 🖰).

4. Use verbal cues and manual correction(s) to provide better biomechanics at the areas of FLT (one at a time) and assess the impact of the correction on:

   (a) ROM (range of motion) (Videos 12.3a,b, LC26 🖰);

   (b) strength output on resisted tests (Videos 12.4, MQ5 🖰);

   (c) FLT at other joints in the chain (compare foot to pelvis, thorax to pelvis, neck to pelvis, etc.) (Videos 12.5,12.6, LL14 🖰);

   (d) pain experience during the task (Video 12.7 🖰);

   (e) effort to move/experience of the patient in ease of movement (Videos 12.8, JG22 🖰); and the

   (f) function of other systems such as respiratory, urogynecological, and balance.

When the driver is corrected, it will have the greatest positive impact on all of these outcomes; correcting the driver should create improved or optimal load transfer in the other regions that previously demonstrated FLT.

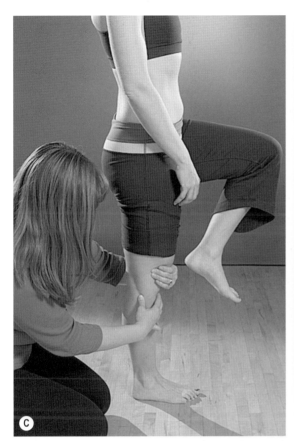
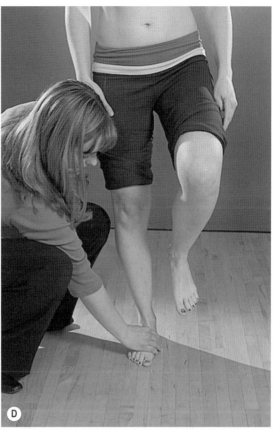

Fig. 12.1 – cont'd • (C) During one leg standing the femur should remain 'stacked' over the tibia and in this illustration the therapist is palpating the tibiofemoral joint to observe the presence or absence of FLT during this task (no translation or rotation of the joint should occur). (D) Non-optimal strategies for load transfer through the foot are a common precursor to low back and pelvic girdle pain and impairment. The therapist is palpating for maintenance of the optimal pyramid of the foot and, if the foot 'fails,' notes specifically which joint/part of the foot requires further assessment.

To some, this method of using biomechanical outcomes (i.e. FLT of joints) may appear to imply a purely biomechanical approach that is relevant only for mechanical pain. However, as noted in Chapter 9 and illustrated by the case reports, non-optimal strategies relate to both mechanical and non-mechanical pain presentations, and treatment based on The Integrated Systems Model is effective for patients with pain driven by multiple mechanisms, in both acute and chronic states. This is because the approach addresses cognitive and emotional features of the meaningful task, as well as mechanical features, and how they relate to the person in the middle of the puzzle. There are multiple ways to facilitate correction of the area of FLT, as broadly ranged from cuing the release of the posterior hip muscles, or giving a mental image of floating the ninth thoracic ring, to cuing a positive (joy) versus a negative (anger) emotional state and imagining different contextual environments (cycling in a training ride versus during a race).

Furthermore, consider the discussion on stability and performance from Chapter 4. The observation of biomechanical outcomes and FLT is related to the goal of stability during tasks (maintenance of the desired trajectory despite kinetic, kinematic, and control disturbances (Hodges & Cholewicki 2007)), but there are several other outcomes that are noted in task analysis. Assessment of function and performance must include other measurable parameters such as speed and accuracy, as well as those that reflect quality of movement. These subjective features allow an observer to state that one performance looks 'better' than another, and yet both may be achieved with the same speed and accuracy. We can intuitively know that one motor control strategy has more 'flow' or

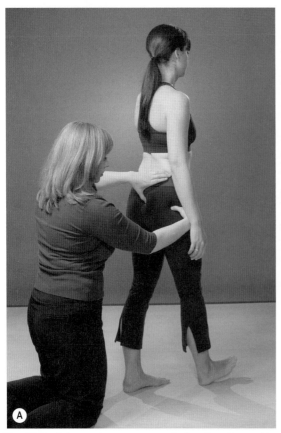
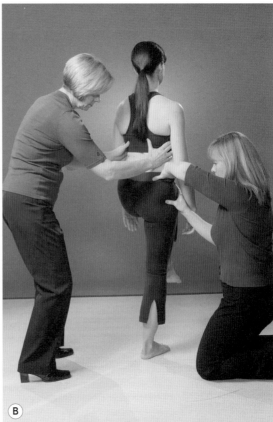

Fig. 12.2 • Advanced assessment – finding the primary driver. When multiple joints/regions fail to transfer load optimally, it is imperative to find the primary driver (the one that has the biggest impact on the others) *for the meaningful task being assessed.* (A) In this illustration the meaningful task is a step forward. The therapist is monitoring the right sacroiliac joint (SIJ) with her left hand (left thumb monitors the right inferior lateral angle of the sacrum and fingers/hand the right innominate) and the right hand monitors the femur (hip). As the patient steps forward the therapist notes which joint (SIJ versus hip) demonstrates failed load transfer (FLT) first (i.e. fails to transfer load with optimal biomechanics and strategy). (B) Here two therapists are working together to identify the primary driver for FLT at the SIJ during a right one leg standing task. The therapist on the left is monitoring a thoracic ring while the therapist on the right is monitoring both the SIJ (through the right innominate) and the right hip. It is very common for all three regions to fail; the first one to do so is identified as the primary driver. Manual or verbal cues for correction are then applied to the primary driver and the impact of this correction on all joints being assessed is noted.

'ease' or 'grace,' or that it evokes a different emotion when we observe it, but science is not yet able to measure these qualitative aspects of optimal function and performance that allow us to call it 'beautiful movement' (Fig. 12.3).

In the method described above (p. 376) to 'find the driver,' the relationship of correcting FLT and these qualitative aspects relates to outputs such as reduced muscle activation to accomplish the same task (more efficient) and increased strength output (b), but most strongly to item (e), the *effort to move* and the *experience* of the patient. In advanced task analysis and consideration of total body function

and performance, both objective biomechanical outcomes as well as the subjective and qualitative components of the total body strategy are evaluated. This requires creating an awareness in the patient and drawing their attention to 'how the task feels' with and without different cues and manual corrections, as well as pre- and post-treatment to the key driver (see case reports Chapter 9, Mike, Video MQ5, Louise, Video LL18 🖱). Although difficult to test objectively, it is our experience that when you find the *best* correction of the driver, the new strategy that this facilitates also minimizes metabolic costs and thus maximizes efficiency and synergy of all

Fig. 12.3 • Advanced assessment – finding the primary driver. Beautiful movement requires more than optimal biomechanics.

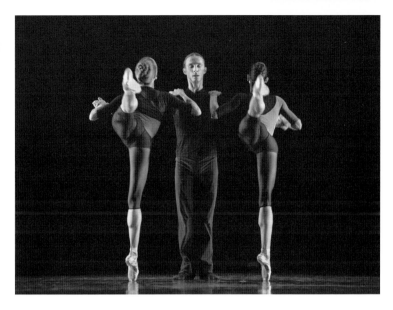

systems. Patients are amazed by the ease they feel in their body, and the increased energy and reduction in fatigue levels they experience. Thus, when working through the kinetic chain and providing manual and verbal input to facilitate better strategies (via addressing regions of FLT), you will know you have found the driver when the patient says, 'that feels great, can you just walk around with me?' If these techniques are then applied to simulating the patient's meaningful task, the response to correcting the driver will simply be 'Wow!'

So what is involved in meaningful task analysis?

Whole body meaningful task analysis

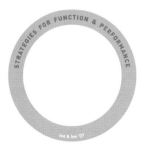

Once a hypothesis is made about where the driver is, the next step is to test this hypothesis in a task that most closely resembles the meaningful task. Depending on the complexity of the task, this step may be as simple as adding load to the whole body screening task already assessed (for example as would be case for the deadlift analysis above, see Video 12.3a 🖱). Often the meaningful task is more complex than the whole body screening task in multiple aspects and the aim in meaningful task analysis is to simulate as many components and aspects as possible. Although from a therapist's perspective it may seem redundant to test more complex tasks (more joints to control, higher loads, less base of support, less predictability, etc.), when loss of control or non-optimal movement have been observed in easier but related tasks, meaningful task analysis is an essential part of the early assessment for several reasons. Firstly, if you have truly identified the driver, correcting the driver will positively impact the strategy used for the aggravating and goal-related tasks, providing further confirmation and support for your hypothesis. Correcting the driver should also positively impact all features of a multisystem presentation; for example, if a patient with pelvic girdle pain has coexisting complaints of stress urinary incontinence and/or difficulty breathing in certain tasks, correcting the driver should improve these symptoms, or improve impairments related to these symptoms as well (e.g. the ability to contract the pelvic floor muscles). If correcting the driver makes these symptoms worse, this suggests that you are correcting a compensatory component and that the driver may lie in one of the other systems. Thus, meaningful task analysis provides further information for testing your hypothesis (confirmation or rejection, Chapter 9).

Secondly, meaningful task analysis impacts the patient's experience and perception of the therapist's understanding of their problem. It helps patients understand how their experience of the problem and your evaluation of the driving cause for the problem are related. This is important for the patient's 'buy in,' confidence in the health professional, and compliance to the treatment program. Also, although it may be obvious to the therapist that the ability to transfer load during one leg standing (OLS) is relevant to being able to run, this may not be obvious to the patient. A step forward task will have more meaning to the patient's goal of running (see case report Chapter 9, Louise, Video LL14 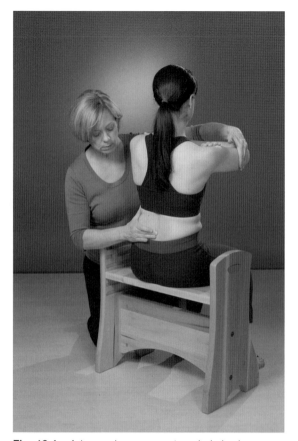). Note that if the patient exhibits FLT in several areas during OLS, it is highly likely that the same areas will be found during a step forward task, as the tasks are closely related in terms of the ability to transfer vertical loads through the LPH complex. However, when gait is more closely simulated (allowing thoracopelvic rotation, and movement through the hip, knee, and foot for the whole stance phase from heel strike to toe off), the more differences there are in the biomechanical requirements of the two tasks (step forward versus gait). It is, therefore, also possible that the key impairments driving the patient's pain and disability will not be evident until the meaningful task is more closely replicated. This may be due to mechanical, cognitive, emotional, or contextual factors. For example, if a patient's story involves low back pain, or difficulty with tasks involving using their arms in a forward bent posture, using forward bending as a screening test alone may not reveal the key driver. However, using arm movements that replicate the specific aggravating movement in range, load, and direction (pushing, pulling, elevating the arms into flexion) while in the forward bent posture will be much more specific and thus more likely to reveal the relevant area of FLT (note the similarities and differences in the task characteristics and key drivers in Videos 12.3a and 12.5). Combining resisted arm movements with relevant postures provides specific information about the level and direction of the poorly controlled segment (Fig. 12.4, see case report Laura, Chapter 9, Video LC12).

Thus, more complex task analysis may reveal other areas of FLT that are actually most relevant to the patient presentation, or may be required to elicit a painful response and thus is most meaningful to the patient. For example, a performer from the Cirque du Soleil reported that his pain was provoked only when he repetitively moved his legs over his body in multiple directions during a sustained one-arm handstand. This activity required lateral bending of his trunk. In standing, an area of loss of control was noted during lateral bending of the trunk, but no pain

Fig. 12.4 • Advanced assessment – whole body meaningful task assessment. In the seated position, load can be applied through the elevated arms to challenge and assess control specifically, in this illustration, at L4–5. The direction of the load can be varied (flexion, extension, rotation) and the segmental response noted. This test is indicated if the patient reports difficulty with arm loading in the seated position (narrative reasoning and hypothesis development). If the segment fails to function optimally when loaded (note the specific direction), then this finding has confirmed your hypothesis that L4–5 is a primary driver for their meaningful task (deductive logic). If, however, L4–5 remains controlled no matter how the trunk is loaded through the arms, then L4–5 is *not* the primary driver for this meaningful task – go look elsewhere!

was provoked, and he did not report any difficulty with the lateral bending task in standing. Without assessing the aggravating task, it would be a weak hypothesis that the area of FLT observed during lateral bending was related to his symptoms. However, the same control deficit was amplified, and more obvious, when he performed the aggravating task, lateral bending of his lower body while sustaining a one-arm handstand. Not only could the area of FLT be linked to his symptomatic task, but the process now had meaning for the performer and this had relevance for his ability to commit to the recovery process (Video 12.9 🖱).

In situations where cardiovascular or neuromuscular fatigue are contributors to change in strategy from an optimal to non-optimal/pain relevant strategy, it may be necessary to ask the patient to load or challenge the system in the appropriate way prior to the assessment. For example, if a runner does not experience problems until 45 minutes into a run, the primary driver may be easier to observe if you assess the patient soon after they have done a 45-minute run to compare their strategy from a rested start point and at a more fatigued point.

A patient's meaning perspective and psychosocial features can also impact the strategy chosen for a task (see Chapters 5, 7). If the meaning perspective (beliefs, expectations, motivations, attitudes; see Chapter 9) or emotional context is a significant contributor to the non-optimal strategy, it is essential to try to replicate these dimensions in meaningful task analysis. Again, this is a situation where meaningful task analysis provides key information and should be performed in the first one or two appointments.

Finally, assessing strategies during tasks that closely simulate meaningful tasks provides a basis for designing a treatment program tailored specifically to the patient. This is further discussed later in this chapter. Although is it usually not possible to simulate every aspect (biomechanical, environmental, social, emotional) of the goal-related functional task, a creative approach to this challenge can often simulate the key aspects. The more specific the information elicited from the patient about aggravating activities and tasks that they have difficulty performing, the easier it will be to identify which features are key to replicate. For example, if a patient says, 'I can't do yoga right now because of my injury,' a good question to ask would be, 'Are there any specific poses that you have tried but found difficulty performing more than the others?' The task-specific analysis would then focus on those specific poses (Fig. 12.5). If a patient says, 'I can't run,' questions that inquire about:

(a) which part of the gait cycle is painful/difficult;
(b) if running uphill or downhill is more difficult; and
(c) how long they can run before having trouble;

are key for facilitating task simulation. Asking these questions often leads the patient to reflect on, and realize, subtleties related to context or environment that are relevant.

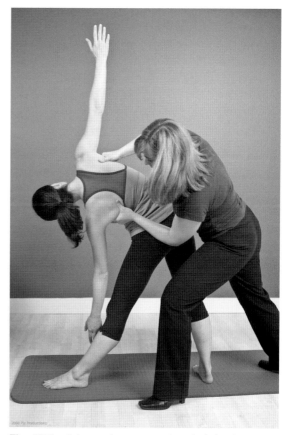

Fig. 12.5 • Advanced assessment – whole body meaningful task assessment. This patient reported that in her yoga practice performing the triangle pose was more difficult to the left (not painful). Here, the therapist is monitoring a thoracic ring during this meaningful task; however, she could also monitor the response of any segment in the lumbar spine, or joint in the pelvis or lower extremity, and use the principles previously described and illustrated to determine the various segment/regions of failed load transfer (FLT) and, by noting the timing of FLT for each, determine the primary driver for this meaningful task involving the whole body.

Sometimes, patients cannot identify consistent features related to mechanical stressors that aggravate their pain. For example, a patient may report pain with sitting at work, but note that 'some days it is fine, other days it is not.' This is an indication to ask further questions around context, such as, 'Do you notice it more when you are working on specific projects that require more focus or concentration?' It is not uncommon for people to adopt different motor control strategies for the very same task (sitting at a desk), depending on the amount of mental focus or environmental stress involved.

Once the key biomechanical, psychosocial, and contextual features of the meaningful task are identified, the task is broken down into component blocks and the components that simulate those key features are used. Appropriate space for movement, as well as equipment such as treadmills, wind trainers (Fig. 12.6A–C), steps, and exercise mats, are useful tools to facilitate meaningful task analysis. Visualization and imagery can be used to simulate different environments and contexts. For example, an elite mountain bike racer presented with low back pain only experienced during races. He was painfree

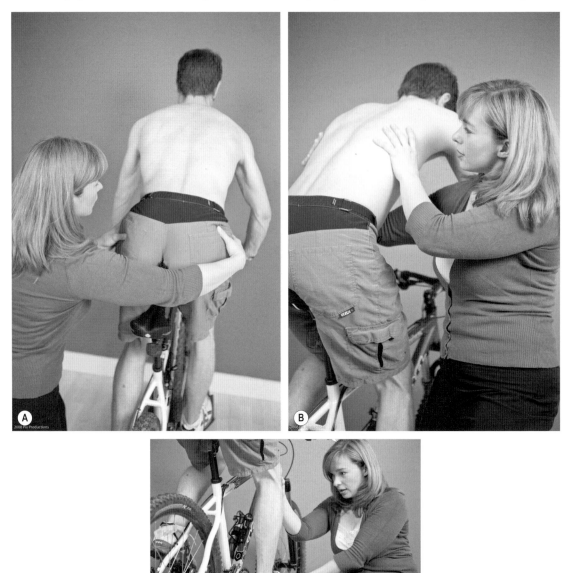

Fig. 12.6 • Advanced assessment – whole body meaningful task assessment. This mountain biker (who also runs) complained of persistent low back pain that was aggravated by cycling and not running. To determine the primary driver for this whole body task, several areas require assessment of the strategy he uses during his meaningful task, cycling on *his* bike. Here, the therapist is monitoring his (A) hips, (B) thorax, and (C) knee and foot, specifically paying attention to regional/segmental position, mobility, and control as well as activation of the superficial muscle systems for synergy.

during training rides, even if they were much longer in duration than his races. Screening tests of simple tasks revealed his areas of failed load transfer and a hypothesis of the source of his problem was made. An assessment on the wind trainer revealed some loss of control; however, this was more evident when he was talked through a race scenario and his strategy changed as he mentally focused as though racing. Correction of the driver was then performed while he was on the wind trainer, while in 'race mindset,' and he then was able to experience in his body the impact that altering his strategy could have on his mountain bike racing task, both in terms of:

1. decreased tension in the muscles of his low back (related to his pain); and in

2. the sense of decreased effort and increased power in his legs (related to his function and performance).

Identical to the analysis of base screening tasks as described above, specific features of the driving FLT problem are identified during meaningful task analysis, both *intrinsic* (Fig. 12.7A) and *extrinsic* (Fig. 12.7B) to the LPH region. This often requires that the therapist moves with the patient, and care must be taken to use gentle and specific enough handling to feel and assess without altering the patient's pattern or postural equilibrium. Recall that identification of FLT and non-optimal strategies in the body will include identification of areas and joints with:

1. poor control (including the specific direction(s));

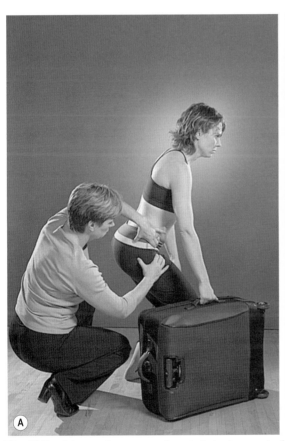
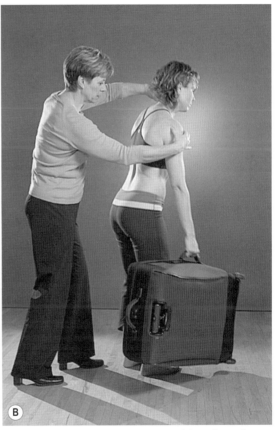

Fig. 12.7 • Advanced assessment – whole body meaningful task assessment. Lifting a heavy weight unilaterally (i.e. suitcase) requires an optimal strategy for function of all joints/regions of the body. (A) The task should begin with an optimal squat; here the therapist is monitoring the right hip (through the femur) and the right sacroiliac joint (through the innominate) prior to the load being applied, as failed load transfer is often manifested at the initiation of the task. (B) For this task, control is also required in the cervical spine and glenohumeral joint (and every other joint to the toes!) and non-optimal strategies for control of these joints can create excessive stress and ultimately pain in regions far distant to the primary driver. The victim cries the loudest, the criminal is quiet and often discreet – seek him out!

2. restricted mobility (including the identification of any overactive/dominant superficial muscles or slings of muscles);

3. inactive/inappropriately recruited muscles.

The findings from the whole body meaningful task analysis are compared to the findings from the less specific screening tasks and other assessment findings, as well as related to the patient's problem and story (performance goal and/or pain experience) (Videos 12.10, 12.11 🖱).

Center of mass over base of support (body centering test)

An accurate sense of where the center of mass (COM) is located relative to the base of support (BOS) is essential to maintaining postural equilibrium in all situations and is relevant for all populations and purposes, from preventing falls to maximizing athletic performance. The perception of where the COM is centered (in all directions/planes) over the BOS is referred to as the 'sense of body center.' The sense of body center can be assessed in both static and dynamic tasks. In standing posture, stand directly behind the patient and center yourself behind the center of their pelvis (sacrum). Place one hand on each innominate. Imagine a

vertical line running through the center of the sacrum and consider this the reference point for their COM (just anterior to S2). Note the position of this COM reference line and the mid-point between the patient's feet. Is the pelvis centered between the two feet in the coronal plane? Use small movements of the pelvis forward, backward, and laterally, then allow the patient to return to their usual posture, to determine where the pelvis rests habitually relative to the center point between the feet (BOS). Note any concurrent IPT and/or transverse plane rotation of the pelvis (Videos 12.12, LL9, see case report Louise, Chapter 9, Videos LC1, LC2 🖱). To get a measure of the patient's dynamic sense of body center, ask them to perform a lunge to the side, forward, or back; note that any angle or direction of movement can be used, depending on the meaningful task. A side lunge is often assessed first to obtain a measure of any right to left difference. The therapist demonstrates the task and instructs the patient to try to land with their trunk centered and equally supported between their two feet. The therapist then observes where the body aligns relative to the feet and whether the trunk is centered between the two feet (Fig. 12.8A,B, see case report Louise, Chapter 9, Video LL10 🖱). If the patient performs this task well, both to the right and to the left, then repeat the test with the eyes

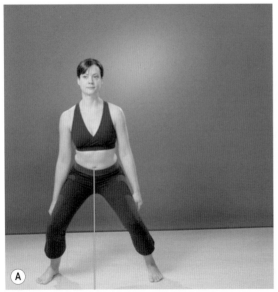
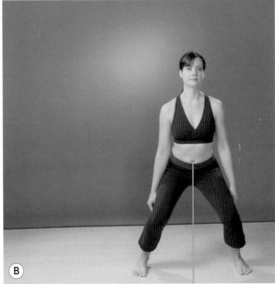

Fig. 12.8 • Advanced assessment – centre of mass over base of support (body centering test). Side lunge. (A) When this individual side lunges to their right, note where her body aligns in relation to the feet (to the right). (B) Conversely, when this same individual side lunges to her left she is much better able to find a centered position for her body over her base of support.

closed to determine how much the visual system is contributing to the accuracy in the task.

Many patients have an altered sense of body center, and it can be said that their 'virtual body' (their current representation of when and where their COM is centered over their BOS) is not aligned to their real body, in that where they think is center is clearly not. An inaccurate sense of body center is commonly observed in patients, and can contribute to:

1. the uneven distribution of loads;
2. altered joint forces (shear, torsion, compression, change in joint axis);
3. an inability to accurately recover from an unexpected perturbation and maintain a desired path of movement;
4. falls;
5. a predisposition of certain joints to injury/re-injury;
6. poor movement efficiency; and
7. non-optimal performance.

Thus, the sense of body center is important to assess at some point in the course of the rehabilitation process, especially when considering return to work or sport. In some cases, the patient's story will indicate that testing the sense of body center should be included in the initial assessment. For example, dancers often report that they have difficulty keeping their center while doing turns, whereas other patients use the term feeling 'off centered' during certain functional tasks, always falling to one side, or that they always 'overcorrect' in one direction during certain movements (forehand versus backhand). These story features all suggest an altered and incorrect sense of body center. Training techniques to align the virtual body and real body sense of center will be described later in this chapter (see *Lunges and variations*).

Tools and techniques to facilitate new strategies

Increase awareness

As discussed in detail in Chapter 9 (*Treatment principles for an integrated evidence-based program, Train a new strategy based on meaningful tasks*) and reviewed in Chapter 11 (*Principles for training new strategies for function and performance*), 'intense focus' and 'paying close attention' are key requirements to turn on the control system for plasticity

and to form new brain maps that persist long term. It is also known that 'sensory input determines the form of cortical reorganization' and that 'perceptual learning and cortical plasticity are specific to attended sensory features' (Moucha & Kilgard 2006). Together, increasing attention, interoception, and sensory input during posture and movement training constitute increasing awareness. There are multiple tools that can be used to increase awareness. Changing the location and timing of tactile input (manual facilitation), together with verbal cues and encouragement, can make significant changes in the strategy used for task performance. Determine the key points of control for manual facilitation of a better strategy, and then teach the patient how to self-monitor (Figs 12.9A–C, 12.10A–C). The specific verbal and manual cues that are most effective will have already been determined (Chapters 10, 11). A common thread during all posture and movement training is that the patient should have one 'release and align' cue as well as a 'connect' cue (specific to the deep chord and/or the superficial sling) during functional movement progressions (see case report Chapter 9, Laura, Video LC16, Louise, LL17 🖱). This reinforces the brain maps through repetition of the cues that address the key driving impairments for their problem.

Other tools can be incorporated into movement training to increase afferent input, such as Thera-Band (Fig. 12.11A,B), balls (Fig. 12.12), and belting or taping (see Figs. 9.4B, 9.5, Video 12.13 🖱). Feedback on performance can be enhanced with biofeedback tools such as rotational discs (Video 12.14 🖱), ultrasound imaging (Chapter 10), mirrors, and surface electromyography (EMG). Showing patients their non-optimal strategy visually through photos and video, followed by showing them a new strategy, can also increase awareness and demonstrate visually the potential available for change. Asking them to sense the effort or feeling in their body (interoception) as they move with the old strategy compared to the new strategy also strengthens an inner awareness (Videos 12.15, 12.16 🖱). If they have a good strategy moving in one direction or loading on one leg, then mirrors and cues to focus on the internal feel of what happens in this 'good' reference strategy can be used to train a better strategy in other directions and loading on the other leg. This type of training likely takes advantage of mirror neurons in the brain, and is facilitated by performing alternating movements on the optimal and then non-optimal sides.

Similarly, visualization and imagery activates specific patterns in the brain and can be added to enhance formation and long-term maintenance of new brain maps. If there is access to video footage of, for example, athletes performing the same tasks well and at a high level, have your patient imagine that they are performing the same tasks while watching the videos. When physical and technical training regimes are kept constant between groups, this type of video imagery has been shown to significantly improve performance and accuracy in groups using video imagery compared to groups who merely watched the videos without imagery or had no exposure to video performances (Orlick 2008). Even in situations where no video footage is available for patients, having the patient perform several sessions a day where they spend a few minutes imagining

themselves doing the things they want to do, without pain, and with freedom, power, and ease, can significantly impact their recovery process. In his book, *In pursuit of excellence*, Terry Orlick describes this imagery process:

> Your ultimate objective is to re-experience or pre-experience ideal performances using the senses that you use in real performances. When perfecting performance skills through your imagery, try to call up the feeling, not something merely visual. The more vivid and accurate the feeling, and the more effectively that you perform within that image, the greater your chances of replicating the image in the real situation. With daily practice, your imagery skills will improve immensely, and your imagined performances will feel real, in the same way that your nighttime dreams feel real.

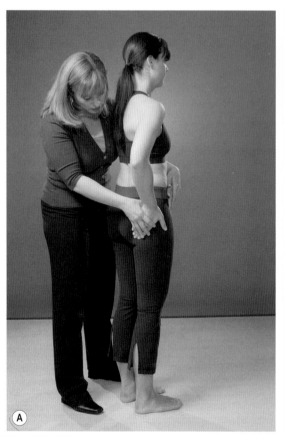 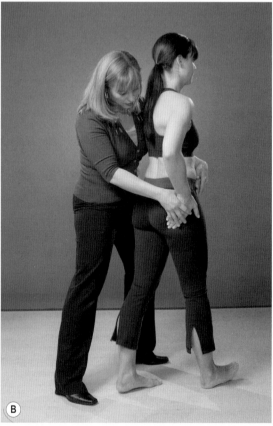

Fig. 12.9 • Tools and techniques to facilitate new strategies – increase awareness. (A) In this step forward task, the therapist is teaching the patient how to monitor femoral head position as well as activation of the superficial muscles of the hip (anterior and posterior). Tactile and verbal cues (including imagery and visualization) are used in the starting position to ensure release of the old strategy. The patient then remembers their best 'connect cue,' ensuring that this does not elicit an increase in activation of the superficial hip muscles (release and connect) and then (B) moves into the step forward task. The muscles and femoral head position are monitored continuously throughout the task, particularly as the load increases.

Continued

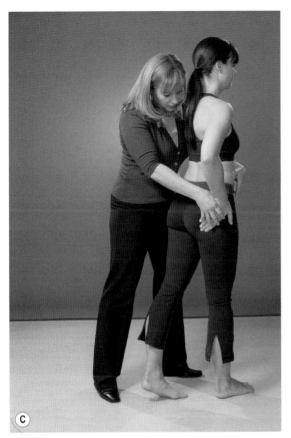

Fig. 12.9 – cont'd • (C) In the final stages of this task, the right leg is fully loaded (left heel is lifting) and the hip is fully extended. This is often a challenging phase for this task and it is imperative that the patient be shown how to monitor their own strategy for performance.

Note the focus on getting connected to the *feeling* that optimal movement creates in the body, and consider how this relates to Melzack's body-self neuromatrix and the pain experience (Chapter 7), and how it could impact emotional and cognitive barriers to new strategies. Connecting to this inner feeling is all about increasing awareness. Whether the patient's goal is to return to running, to lift and carry their baby without pain, or to win an Olympic gold medal, increasing awareness can have powerful effects on facilitating optimal strategies for function and performance (Box 12.1).

Celebrate success

Attention, reward, and novelty are known to enhance plasticity by increasing the release of specific neurotransmitters such as dopamine and acetylcholine (Mahncke et al 2006). Positive feedback could be considered a form of 'reward' that enhances neuromodulatory function. It also increases confidence. Interestingly, we have found that patients respond better when given verbal cues such as, 'Yes, you've got it, that's the right pattern' instead of 'No, don't do that, that's wrong.' When a patient is not exhibiting the optimal strategy, it is better to say, 'Stop, let's try something different,' rather than telling them repeatedly that they are doing it wrong. It is up to you as the therapist to design the training task to be at the appropriate level for successful completion. Although it is important to teach patients what not to do (e.g. 'Your goal is to control the joints of your pelvis without gripping your right buttock, so if you feel your right buttock gripping it is time to stop and rest'), this is more effective as an explanation *before* they practice the task rather than giving negative cues *during* the movement training.

Furthermore, successful execution of the new strategy should be celebrated by highlighting to the patient the many different benefits of the new strategy and the improved performance they are achieving in the rehabilitation process. In comparing the old and new strategies, have the patient note:

- decreased pain;
- decreased effort to move;
- increased strength/power;
- increased ROM;
- and/or increased ease/feeling of 'flow' of movement experienced when using the better strategy.

Transform task analysis into training activities

Therapists often want to know, 'What are the best exercises to give patients with a poorly controlled SIJ, pubic symphysis pain, recurrent hamstring strains, … etc.' Although there are some common features and 'exercises' between rehabilitation programs, it will be evident to the reader that in The Integrated Systems Model we believe that the best program will be custom tailored for each patient, based on the underlying driving impairments. A tailored program minimizes the number of different tasks, which enhances compliance while maximizing results. Each training task is targeted and has a specific reason for being prescribed.

The treatment techniques and principles outlined thus far in Chapters 10 and 11 have set the stage for training more complex posture and movement tasks.

A combination of techniques and approaches (e.g. education to address beliefs and emotional barriers, manual and dry needling techniques) have been used to remove the non-optimal strategy. Training has been given to reinforce 'letting go' of the old strategy; that is, the patient has been practicing and acquiring the motor skills of how to use certain muscles less, decrease tone, and maintain the gains from the dry needling and/or manual therapy techniques (*self-release with awareness, stretch with awareness*). Training to wake up specific parts of the deep muscle system has been practiced with the aim of increasing precision, confidence, and ease of recruitment of the deep system 'chord,' and integrated into a few relevant exercises that involve trunk–leg dissociation or trunk–arm dissociation, and coordination of the deep and superficial muscles. These key neuromuscular control skills, how to release specific patterns of muscle activity, and how to recruit others (RACM – Release, Align, Connect, and Move), are now used in functional progressions that are most related to the meaningful task(s). Specific muscle release exercises are progressed to 'sling release,' where the patient practices the skill of releasing multiple muscles simultaneously, in a position or posture that is related to their meaningful task. This is

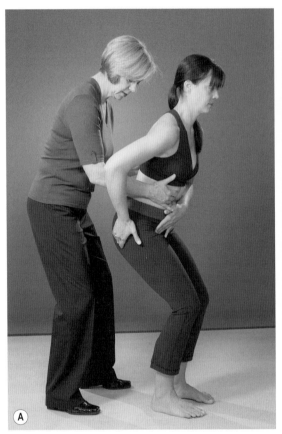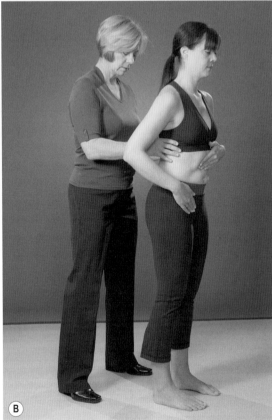

Fig. 12.10 • Tools and techniques to facilitate new strategies – increase awareness. (A) In this task (squat), the patient is palpating the posterior buttock and anterior hip fold to provide tactile cues for herself to release both anterior and posterior hip muscles and to ensure an optimal strategy for hip flexion during the squat (feel the hip fold). Simultaneously, the therapist is providing verbal and tactile cues for the superficial abdominal and back muscles to ensure there is no 'gripping,' or overactivation, of these muscles. (B) As the patient's awareness improves, less tactile input is required in one region (e.g. here she is no longer using a tactile cue for her posterior hip muscles but still requires a tactile cue for the anterior hip muscles to ensure an optimal strategy for movement and control of the hip) and she takes over the tactile cue for the anterior abdominal wall. The therapist is now only monitoring the thorax and superficial back muscles as

Continued

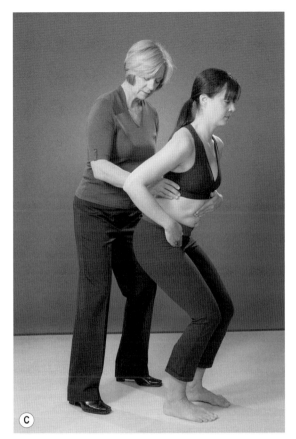

Fig. 12.10 – cont'd • (C) she initiates and then performs the squat task. Ultimately, the therapist uses fewer tactile and verbal cues and the patient takes all control for the chosen strategy.

described below in the section *Training strategies for dynamic tasks – functional and sport-specific*.

The initial trunk–leg or trunk–arm dissociation exercises are replaced by more complex movements; the most effective way to return the patient to their meaningful task(s) is to creatively break down complex functional, work, or sport movements into component parts. These movement building blocks then have meaning for the patient, and allow them to experience success in goal-related tasks, while training the nervous and musculoskeletal systems to recruit and load in a task-specific manner.

General principles for designing movement building blocks

The principles outlined in Chapter 11 under *Coordinating the deep and superficial muscle systems* and summarized in Box 11.5 hold true for task practice

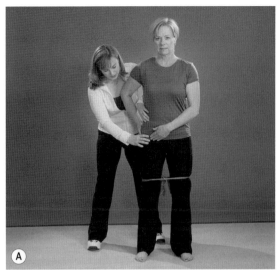

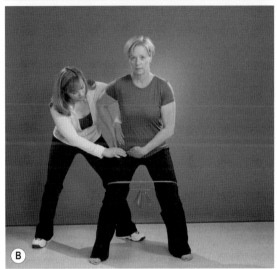

Fig. 12.11 • Tools and techniques to facilitate new strategies – increase awareness. Thera-Band can be used to increase sensory input and improve awareness while performing many tasks. (A) In the standing position, Thera-Band is tied around the distal femurs and the patient is instructed to gently resist the adduction force induced by the Thera-Band. While monitoring key points (sacroiliac joint, hip, specific muscles) the patient then thinks of the release and connect cues and then moves (B) into the task (squat) while maintaining optimal alignment of the lower extremity.

that progresses into meaningful task movement building blocks. The deep system chord is coordinated with the superficial muscles by layering tactile and verbal imagery cues to connect and recruit specific superficial muscles (if necessary) while moving in the movement building block patterns

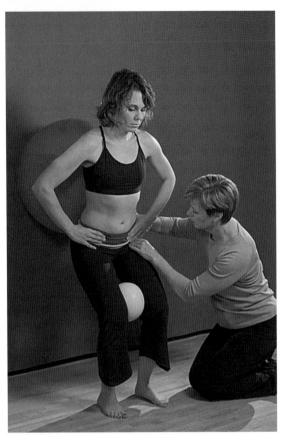

Fig. 12.12 • Tools and techniques to facilitate new strategies – increase awareness. A small ball placed in the inner, upper thigh can also be used to increase sensory input and improve awareness particularly for the individual whose legs drift into external rotation as they squat.

(Fig. 12.13A,B). When the superficial muscles are activated in a coordinated manner, synergistic with the deep muscles, the resultant movements will be performed with optimal alignment and fluidity of movement. Palpation of the poorly controlled segment will reveal maintained control of the neutral zone, while allowing the necessary movement related to the task. The alignment and muscle activity around all the joints of the kinetic chain will facilitate sharing of loads and smooth transfer of forces. This overall body alignment is sustained by balanced length, strength, and timing in the superficial sling systems.

For each new training task that is designed and attempted, the therapist uses the *checkpoints for rigidity* (Box 11.4, Video 12.17) to determine whether the task can be performed without excessive use of the superficial muscles. Loads are added as needed to replicate the meaningful task, or when

---

Box 12.1

Increasing awareness

With verbal and tactile cues, help the patient focus their attention on the quality of movement during meaningful tasks:

First – using the old, non-optimal strategy; and

Then – using the new strategy (initially facilitated by the therapist).

Use language such as:

'I'd like you to pay attention to how this feels in your body – the level of effort, the areas of ease, and any areas of tension of holding or resistance to the movement.'

Experiment with different language and verbal cues, along with different areas of sensory input, to see which combination facilitates the best strategy

Encourage the patient to 'remember what this new strategy feels like in your body, so that you can come back to and create this pattern again.'

---

there are specific strength deficits related to the myofascial system. Proprioceptive challenges (e.g. wobble boards) can add unpredictability to the task, which often enhances automatic patterning of the new strategy, but is also essential if the meaningful task involves a context with unpredictable perturbations (Fig. 12.14). Using eyes-closed to reduce visual input also enhances use of proprioceptive information and automatic recruitment. Visualization can be used to simulate different levels of threat or different emotional contexts to assess and train strategies. Task characteristics such as speed and ballistic movements are usually progressions at the end stages of the program. In general, progressing from tasks that maintain neutral spine to tasks that require contralateral thoracopelvic dissociation, or moving into flexion/extension of the spine, requires greater levels of control and skill.

How many exercises?

It is important that the total number of different tasks in the program remains small (five to seven), which requires replacing previous building blocks with more advanced training tasks rather than continuing to add to the list at each subsequent session. This is to balance the need for practice with time demands, and also to maintain novelty, interest, and focus during the training sessions, thereby enhancing neuroplasticity.

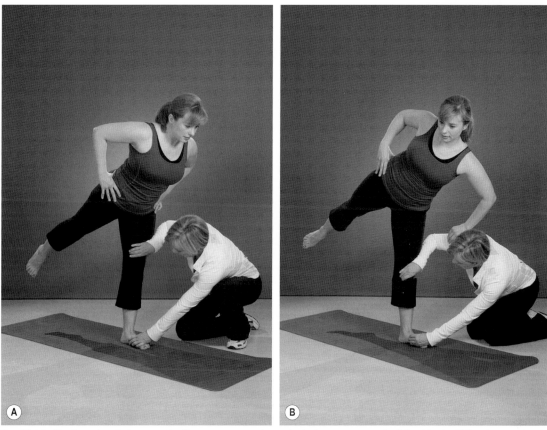

Fig. 12.13 • Tools and techniques to facilitate new strategies – designing movement building blocks. When integrating the lower extremity to the lumbopelvic–hip (LPH) in functional tasks, impairments within the myofascial slings become apparent (insufficient activation and/or insufficient lengthening). Tactile and verbal cues are used as the patient performs the meaningful task to facilitate synergy of these myofascial slings. Here, the patient is performing the initial phase of an arabesque. She has applied her release and connect cues for the LPH region and now the therapist is cuing her (through touch, words, and images) to (A) connect a line between the medial aspect of the foot and the inner thigh to facilitate activation of the adductors and lower leg muscles and collectively support a medial neuromyofascial sling as she moves into the task. This cue would be used if, during this task, insufficient activation was noted in any part of this neuromyofascial sling. (B) From this position, the patient is now attempting to rotate the trunk on the weight bearing limb (dissociate the lower extremity from the trunk) and the therapist is monitoring the knee and foot as well as providing support and release cues as necessary to ensure optimal biomechanics and strategy, i.e. beautiful movement!

How many repetitions?

A minimum of five to seven repetitions should be successfully demonstrated in the clinic (i.e. with the optimal strategy); this qualifies the training task as an appropriate level (not too difficult). Beyond this, facilitate patient self-efficacy by giving the patient control over progressing the number of repetitions; the goal is 20–30 repetitions easily and with little mental effort but guided by the movement having the right internal feel. Teach the patient to watch for their non-optimal strategy (usually evident by gripping in a specific area) and to monitor the checkpoints for rigidity and effort to move (load effort task analysis). When they can no longer complete the task with good quality, they know that, for that given training session on that specific day, they have fatigued the relevant system(s) and done enough. Remind them that for a variety of reasons the total number of repetitions attained in each training session may vary; what is important is that overall there is a progression towards a higher number of repetitions.

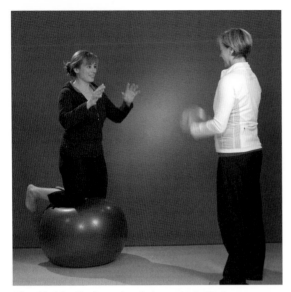

Fig. 12.14 • Tools and techniques to facilitate new strategies – designing movement building blocks. Create fun and challenging ways to automate new strategies as skills improve.

When choosing new tasks to add, if the patient is unable to control more than two to three repetitions in the task-related direction of poor control, use movement into the direction of good control to promote confidence and success and alternate with two to three repetitions in the direction of poor control (Video 12.18 🖱). Gradually increase the repetitions in the direction of poor control until the whole set of repetitions is performed in the meaningful direction.

Facilitating automatic patterns

Adding a proprioceptive challenge to the meaningful task (e.g. rocker boards) is one way to facilitate automation of the new strategy. We have found that encouraging the patient to internalize the 'feeling' of the optimal strategy (be aware of their interoception), rather than to 'think' about how to perform the optimal strategy (staying cognitive about the task), is a powerful method for automation of optimal strategies for function and performance. Once they are aware of how the optimal strategy feels, they can find it again anytime during daily activities. Having the patient close their eyes during movement tasks and focus on 'the feel' enhances reliance on sensory input and internalizes the feeling, while also preparing the patient for contexts where less visual information is available (e.g. skiing in poor visibility).

When to go on-field

In some cases, in order to make the final gains and full integration back into sport activities or work activities, doing sessions on-field is necessary. For example, a patient who was a recreational ice hockey player found that he could control his L5/S1 spondylolisthesis and alleviate his first toe numbness after a program of treatment that taught him how to release his poor strategy (unilateral butt-gripping and thorax-gripping), to connect to the deep fibers of multifidus, and then integrate this cue into his work postures and daily activities (RACM). However, he felt he did not know how to integrate these skills into skating and into a game situation where he could not pay as much attention to his body. Thus, an on-ice session was provided, which not only reinforced all of the key neural maps he had previously practiced, but also trained new components related to applying these skills while skating and shooting. During the first on-ice session it was apparent that he returned immediately to his old strategy (butt-gripping and chest-gripping). However, after one session of manual cues and integration of his skills into the on-ice environment, he was able to release the old, and use a new, strategy that increased his agility and performance. This enabled him to play hockey with only an occasional recurrence of his symptoms. Excellent gains can be made by using all of the previously discussed skills in the on-field environment, or other real-life contexts (Video 12.19 🖱).

This chapter will describe a variety of options for progressing exercises, but it is essential to note that these are some common examples, not an exhaustive list, and that in clinical practice many advanced exercises evolve from the specific task analysis.

Some meaningful tasks require more creativity to simulate; keep an open mind and you may be surprised at what you can do. For example, it may seem impossible to simulate the task of skydiving without an airplane and a parachute. However, by exploring the position, body forces, and movements during the skydiving activity that the patient found aggravating, the key components could be simulated (Video 12.20a 🖱). At this point in Amanda's rehabilitation, the load induced by the simulated task was too high for her to control, and thus a different building block exercise was designed to train the correct strategy. Although this training task, 'wall landing' (Video 12.20b 🖱), looks nothing like skydiving, because it was derived from the simulation activity, in the patient's mind it was completely relevant to her meaningful task.

Key points of control to cue and facilitate optimal strategies

If the non-optimal strategy, and the barriers to a new strategy, have been effectively addressed (Chapter 10) and new neural networks developed (Chapter 11), then gentle manual pressure and tactile feedback at key points of control in the body will be sufficient to 'remind' and 'reinforce' the new optimal strategies for posture and movement. Multiple combinations of therapist and patient hand positions are possible (e.g. Figs 12.9, 12.10, 12.11, 12.13). When initially training the patient to self-monitor it is best for the therapist to overlay their hands on top of the patient's hands to guide and provide feedback during the learning phase (Fig. 12.9). Then, as the patient learns what they should feel, and monitor, with their own hands, the therapist can move their hands to check and facilitate better alignment or control in other areas (Fig. 12.10). Commonly used key points of control for integrating optimal strategies for function of the LPH region include:

1. the pubic symphysis and manubriosternal junction – teach the patient that these points should be vertically aligned and that this indicates that the pelvis is aligned under the thorax (Fig. 12.15A,B);
2. the upper or lower sternum, depending on where the spinal curves and control needs to be facilitated. Inferior or superior pressure is applied anteriorly on the sternum, or on the posterior thorax, to anteriorly rotate/flex the thorax, posteriorly rotate/extend the thorax, or decompress and lengthen the thorax (Fig. 12.16A,B);

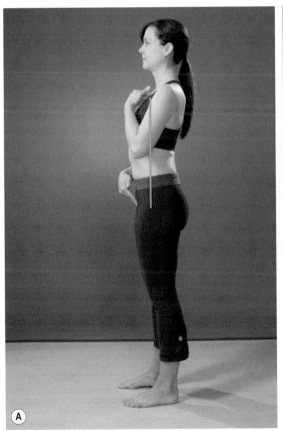
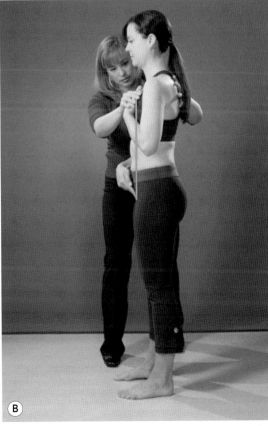

Fig. 12.15 • Tools and techniques to facilitate new strategies – key points of control to cue and facilitate optimal strategies. (A) Note the non-optimal alignment of the thorax over the pelvis as determined by two key points of control – the manubriosternal junction and the pubic symphysis. (B) With verbal and tactile cues, the therapist shows the patient how to find a better alignment and strategy.

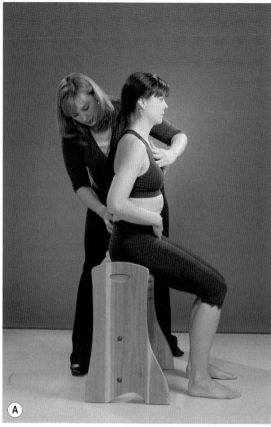

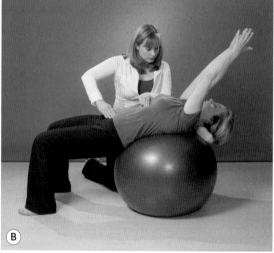

Fig. 12.16 • Tools and techniques to facilitate new strategies – key points of control to cue and facilitate optimal strategies. (A) In sitting, the therapist is providing a tactile cue through the upper sternum and monitoring the response of this cue on both spinal and pelvic alignment and strategy. The patient notes, both through their interoception (internal feeling) and kinesthetic sense (their hands), the effect of the tactile and verbal cues. (B) In this task, the therapist is monitoring the lower sternum and the pubic symphysis to ensure that optimal alignment is maintained between the thorax and pelvis as the arms are taken overhead.

3. the anterolateral or posterolateral lower ribcage to draw the thorax as a whole posteriorly, anteriorly, or vertically (Fig. 12.10B,C);

4. a combination of points around the hip including the mid-inguinal ligament, along the hip crease, under the medial aspect of the ischial tuberosity, around the greater trochanter, or the iliac crest and hip crease; determine whether unilateral compared to bilateral palpation creates the best strategy (Figs 12.7, 12.9, 12.10, 12.11, 12.12);

5. the interspinous spaces, or along the articular pillar of the lumbar spine (either multiple or single segments), to cue imagery for specific control or manually create the feeling of 'lengthening' and 'suspension,' or to facilitate an increase or decrease in lumbar lordosis as needed (can be applied to any area of the spine) (Fig. 12.17);

6. the muscle belly of specific muscles that need to decrease or increase their activity; these specific muscles may change or remain the same as more complex tasks are assessed and added as training exercises (Fig. 12.18).

When training any task, it is the therapist's goal to discover a specific verbal cue, or image, in combination with a specific key point of manual control that creates the best facilitation of the desired new strategy for that task. Different examples of verbal cues have been used in Chapters 10 and 11 and further cues will be given in examples below, but note that imagery will vary patient to patient and will be influenced by

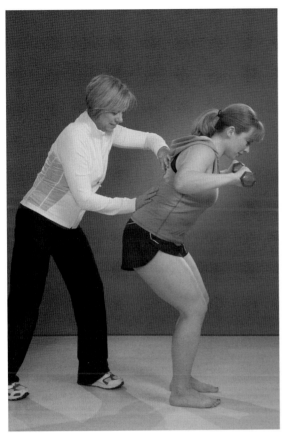

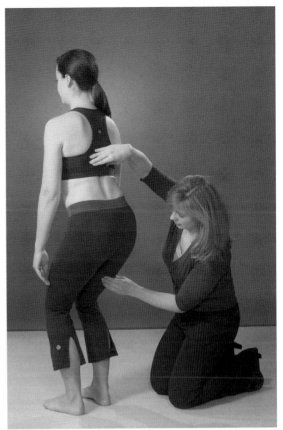

Fig. 12.17 • Tools and techniques to facilitate new strategies – key points of control to cue and facilitate optimal strategies. In this loaded squat task, the therapist is monitoring both the thorax and lumbar spine to ensure that the strategy chosen transfers load evenly throughout the task and can also provide segmental and regional tactile and verbal cues when necessary (e.g. 'Think of suspending your L4 vertebra, open the rings of your thorax, soften your chest at the upper sternum').

Fig. 12.18 • Tools and techniques to facilitate new strategies – key points of control to cue and facilitate optimal strategies. Tactile and verbal cues are also used to increase or decrease activation of specific muscles; the specific muscle then becomes a key point of control for either connect or release. This figure illustrates the therapist monitoring the erector spinae and hamstrings during a squat task in an individual who is a habitual 'back-gripper.' She is cuing a release of the erector spinae and a connection of the hamstrings (in addition to the deep system chord cue) to balance and distribute forces throughout the entire neuromyofacial sling.

culture and other contexts. Thus, it is essential that the therapist be willing to try different verbal cues until they find what works for each individual.

Training strategies for static tasks

Recall from Chapter 4 that there are very few truly static tasks in daily function. 'Static' postures require movement and 'give' in the system for breathing and dampening potential perturbations. Excessive co-contraction of the trunk muscles (i.e. excessive stiffness) will negatively impact other systems such as

postural equilibrium (balance) and respiratory function. Thus, a patient may have ideal alignment but a detrimental, non-optimal strategy to attain that alignment. While teaching your patient the optimal alignment for load transfer in different postures, be mindful that both alignment and the strategy they use to attain and maintain that alignment need to be assessed, cued, and corrected. The *checkpoints for rigidity* are key indicators in any posture to determine if there is excessive superficial muscle activity.

Furthermore, rather than thinking of posture as one position to always maintain (i.e. have one option), it is best to think of standing and sitting postures as places to begin from, move in and out of, and return to. That is, the aim of restoring optimal alignment and neutral spine in postural training is to restore options. In general, patients who have pain and disability related to sustained postures maintain one type of posture and tend not to sit in other postures (i.e. have loss of options) (Dankaerts et al 2006). Indeed, teaching optimal postural strategies likely decreases pain by decreasing strain and compression on irritable tissues and improving distribution of loads throughout the spine. It is also highly probable that postural training provides a vehicle for new movement options and for using different strategies throughout the duration of a sustained task.

Neutral spine can be defined as the alignment where the 'normal' spinal curves are present and the thorax is centered over the pelvis. When training neutral spine in a relevant task (sitting, standing, four-point kneeling, etc.), the same spinal orientation is desired: gradual, even curves with a neutral pelvic tilt (ASISs and pubic symphysis in the same coronal plane), lumbar lordosis, thoracic kyphosis, and cervical lordosis. In each region, any increase or decrease in the curve, as well as specific segmental levels of abnormal curvature, are noted. A common presentation is excessive lordosis in the upper lumbar levels, the thoracolumbar junction, and lower thoracic spine, whereas the lower lumbar spine has a loss of lordosis (i.e. L4–L5 and L5–S1 levels remain flexed) with a posterior pelvic tilt (see Fig. 5.6). The patient with a spondylolisthesis often has a decreased lordosis, or flexed segments, above and below the level of excessive anterior translation. To train optimal alignment *and* strategy, the key points of control, as described above, are used along with specific segmental manual and verbal cues in the areas determined by assessment. The reader is by now familiar with the term RACM, Release, Align, Connect, and then Move; in correcting postural tasks the focus is on the first three of these components, release, align, and connect. Alternately, patients can think of 'release and reposition,' which reminds them to 'let go' of the old strategy and find a new alignment with a new strategy.

Standing posture

In general it is difficult to correct spinal curves unless the pelvis is aligned under the thorax. Correction of standing posture thus begins with teaching the

patient how to self-assess the relationship between the manubriosternal junction and the pubic symphysis. The common pattern of an anterior pelvic sway is corrected by using cues that help the patient 'bring the pelvis back underneath the ribcage' or 'bring the pelvis back over the feet' (see Fig. 12.15A,B). If one femoral head is translated anteriorly, use cues directed at that specific hip and evaluate the impact of correcting the hip position on any transverse plane rotation of the pelvis and/or IPT. Try a variety of verbal and tactile cues until the best combination of cues is found. The aim is to facilitate the following:

- release of butt-gripping as the pelvis moves backwards under the thorax;
- centering of the femoral heads (the pelvis also simultaneously becomes more vertical over the femurs);
- restoration of a neutral (slight anterior) pelvic tilt and gentle even lumbar lordosis;
- correction of any transverse plane rotation of the pelvic girdle and any IPT;
- alignment of the MS and PS points vertically, neutral rotation of the thorax and pelvic girdle, and alignment of the head vertically over the thorax without flattening of the cervical lordosis.

Another component important to correct in standing posture is where the patient's center of mass (COM) is aligned over their base of support (BOS). As the key barriers to optimal alignment and strategy will have been released, it should be relatively easy to correct the COM over BOS and to teach the patient how to find this position themselves. Use the innominates bilaterally to guide the patient into the correct alignment of COM over BOS. Using a mirror in this task to teach the patient where they are aligning their pelvis over their feet is often useful. Dynamic retraining of COM over BOS is integrated once squats and lunges are able to be successfully completed (described below).

Once the thorax–pelvis–feet sagittal alignment and the COM over BOS have been addressed, there may be small areas or specific segments requiring correction to restore optimal spinal curvatures. These are detailed further in the section on *Sitting posture, Step 2 – setting the spinal position* below. Depending on the stage in the rehabilitation process, these cues may be added immediately, or in a following session, once the patient has had the opportunity to practice and integrate the first postural correction components.

In general it should not feel difficult or 'hard work' for the patient to attain this improved postural alignment as long as the barriers to this new posture have been addressed (Chapter 10). If the patient reports that the new posture is effortful, assess for specific neuromyofascial or articular vectors that are still presenting barriers and release them. This is essential to ensure that an optimal strategy is used to attain optimal alignment. Once the key manual and verbal/imagery cues have been determined, teach the patient to self-palpate and self-correct, with less and less manual assistance on each repetition, so that they are confident in being able to perform the postural training independently several times a day.

Sitting posture

Many patients with LPH disability with or without pain report difficulty with tasks involving sustained sitting. Thus, it is an important task to assess to determine how their strategy and postural alignment for/in sitting is related to their presenting problem (Chapter 8). It is common for the position of the pelvis and femoral heads in sitting to be related to how they move from standing to sitting (i.e. how they squat to sit down). For example, if during moving from standing to sitting, a strategy of gripping the right hip creates anterior translation of the femoral head, this often results in a left IPT and a left transverse plane rotation of the pelvis, along with an anterior femoral head, all noted in the seated posture (see Fig. 8.32B). Correction of the lumbar and thoracic curves cannot be performed until the twist in the pelvic base and hips is addressed. Thus, correction of sitting strategy usually involves teaching the patient how to assess and correct their position once seated, as well as teaching them how to move from standing into sitting (see *Squat* below). This section will discuss correcting and training strategy in sitting.

Step 1 – setting the optimal pyramid base

Patient and therapist position. The patient sits on a chair or plinth. The therapist stands or kneels beside the patient on the same side as the 'butt-gripping' hip. Place one hand under the ischial tuberosity, and the other hand along the top of the iliac crest.

Correction technique – verbal and manual cues. Teach the patient how to palpate the anterior aspect of the femoral heads and check for equal 'grooves' in the hip fold bilaterally to self-check femoral head position (Fig. 12.19A). Instruct the patient to slightly lean away from you, taking the weight off the affected buttock. Now, lift and pull the ischial

tuberosity laterally and posteriorly, and apply a gentle medial counter-force to the iliac crest as the patient slowly returns the buttock back down to the chair (Fig. 12.19B,C). Use the cue, 'As you lower your buttock, think of letting the sitz bone on this side go wide and open behind you, and let the front of your hip relax and fold.' In the new position, the patient should recheck the position of the femoral heads anteriorly for equal grooves, and will often feel more equal weight distribution between the two ischial tuberosities (Fig. 12.19D). The optimal pyramid base provides a wide, stable platform for correcting alignment of the rest of the spine.

Ideal response. In the new position, the pelvis should not be rotated in the transverse plane and the iliac crests should be level. Compared to the initial sitting position (pre-correction), sideflexion and rotation curves in the lumbar spine are often less pronounced or completely corrected. The anterior and posterior hip muscles on the affected side are softer and more equal in tone to those of the other hip, and the femoral head seats more posteriorly in the acetabulum (there will be a deeper crease in the anterior hip).

Progressions/other considerations. The patient can be taught how to 'set the pyramid base' independently for training functional activities in sitting. The patient's ipsilateral hand is used to pull the ischial tuberosity 'out and back' as the weight is shifted and replaced. The patient may need to perform a few repetitions of this movement to get an equal placement of the ischial tuberosities. *Self-release with awareness* practice for the relevant LPH muscles should be concurrently performed, with the eventual goal that the patient can assume the 'wide pyramid base' position without needing manual self-correction. Patients with limited hip flexion should initially sit on a higher chair or stool for this exercise so that the pelvis can move anteriorly over the femoral heads into a neutral tilt position.

Step 2 – setting the spinal position

Patient and therapist position. The patient sits on a chair or a ball, with an optimal pyramid base (see above). If the patient has limited hip flexion either unilaterally or bilaterally, increase the height of the sitting surface so that the pelvis is able to move anteriorly over the femurs (to allow the creation of a neutral lordosis in the lumbar spine). The therapist stands or kneels beside the patient. Hand placement will depend on which levels of the spine need correction (see *Key points of control to cue and facilitate optimal strategies* above, Figs 12.16, 12.17). As the verbal cues are given, the therapist uses the key points of control to create the ideal curvatures and impart the feeling and awareness of the correct alignment to the patient. To facilitate increased thoracic kyphosis, the hand on the sternum creates an inferior and posterior pressure (Fig. 12.20A). To decrease an excessive kyphosis, the hands lift and gently traction the rib cage from the sides or give a superior and slightly anterior pressure at the levels of excessive curve. To correct a flat lumbar spine, the fingers push gently anterior and superior, creating a 'lifting' sensation and gentle lordosis (Fig. 12.20A). For an excessive lumbar lordosis at one or two segments, focus on facilitating a lordosis at levels above or below that are flexed, and then 'lengthening' or 'stretching' the curve at the hyperextended segment(s) by spreading the fingers and applying a vertical pressure. Correct

the thoracic curve first, then the lumbar curve, and finally the head/cervical position.

Correction technique – verbal cues. For areas of decreased thoracic kyphosis (usually accompanied by excessive erector spinae activity, e.g. back-gripping):

- 'Let the chest sink' or 'Go heavy under my hand.'
- 'As your chest sinks, imagine your back opening between your shoulder blades.'
- 'Imagine that the distance from your sternum to your belly button is decreasing as you let the chest go heavy.'

For areas of increased thoracic kyphosis:

- 'Imagine a string attached to your back (palpate at level of increased curve); the string is gently being pulled up to heaven.'

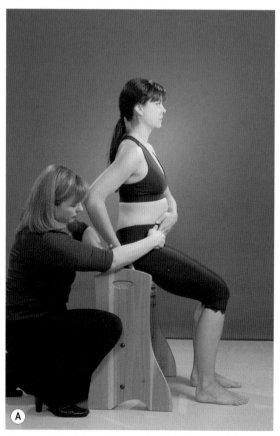 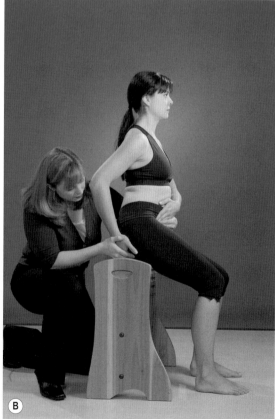

Fig. 12.19 • Training strategies for static tasks – sitting posture. (A) For training an optimal strategy for sitting, the patient is first taught where to monitor the femoral head anteriorly and where to find the ischial tuberosity (sitz bone). (B) Subsequently, they unload the non-optimal side and pull the ischium 'out and back,' while imaging an opening of the sitz bones (release of the posterior hip and buttock muscles) and folding of the hip (centering of the femoral head).

Continued

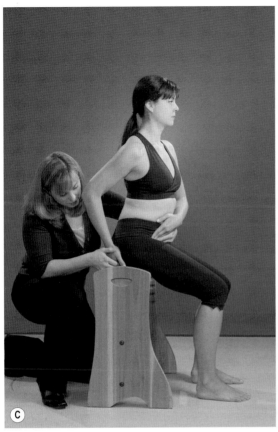
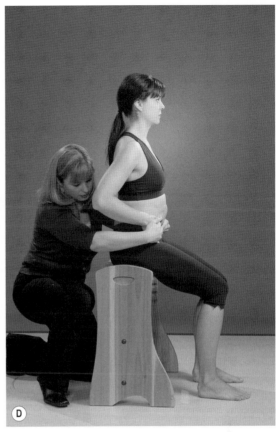

Fig. 12.19 – cont'd • (C) Maintaining this release, they return to the sitting position and (D) recheck their femoral head position on both the left and right sides. They should feel seated and symmetrical.

- 'Let the space between your vertebrae slightly increase, as if floating the vertebra one millimeter above the other.'
- 'Imagine that your sternum is being gently lifted.'

For a decreased lumbar lordosis (flexed lumbar spine):

- 'Imagine a string attached to your tailbone, and someone else is gently pulling the string up to heaven.'
- 'Grow tall from the tailbone.'
- 'Let your pelvis fall forward as you lengthen and create space in your spine from my fingers.'
- 'Imagine that your pelvis is a bowl, and that it is tipping forward as you let your sitz bones go wide.'
- 'Let your buttocks go wide, let your hips fold.'
- 'Allow the ball to roll underneath you as the pelvis rocks forward.'

For an increased lumbar lordosis (hyperextended lumbar spine at one or several levels):

- 'Relax and let your back round out, then as you grow tall, think of lengthening your low back.'
- 'Rather than arching your back, think of the spine being long and tall, with a gentle even curve.'

Ideal response. The creation of the lumbar lordosis should be a 'release' into an optimal curve, not a forced effort with contraction of the erector spinae. As sitting is an upright position, there will be some tone in the erector spinae and superficial multifidus, but it should be symmetrical and not excessive. Rigidity between the thorax and pelvis (inability to dissociate the thorax from the pelvis) is a sign of excessive erector spinae activity (palpate for tone and check lateral mobility of the rib cage – see 'rib cage wiggle,' Chapter 11). Once the thoracic curve has been corrected, the sternal hand should not move superiorly or anteriorly as the lumbar lordosis is facilitated (i.e. the thoracic kyphosis should be maintained while the lumbar lordosis is created). The goal is to create a gentle, even kyphosis in the thoracic

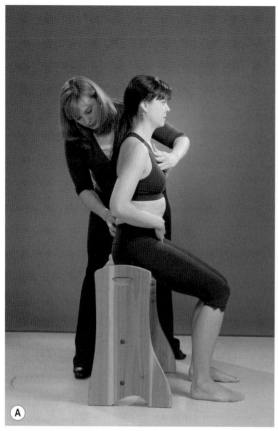
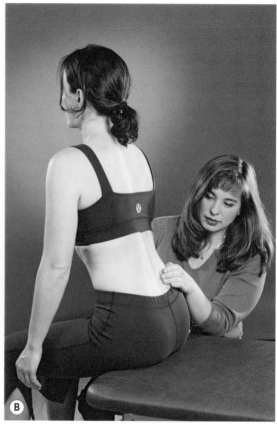

Fig. 12.20 • Training strategies for static tasks – sitting posture. (A) Therapist and patient position for setting the spinal position in neutral spine sitting posture. (B) Training dissociation of spinal flexion and hip flexion is important for developing an optimal strategy for moving from sitting to standing.

spine, a gentle, even lordosis in the lumbar spine, and a gentle lordosis in the cervical spine; palpate and observe to ensure that one or two segments do not remain excessively flexed or extended. The patient's weight should be centered equally over the ischial tuberosities (the optimal pyramid base), the pubic symphysis and the ASISs should be in the same plane, and the manubriosternal symphysis should be vertically in line with the pubic symphysis. If the rib cage is shifted anterior or posterior to the pelvis (i.e. the manubriosternal symphysis is anterior or posterior to the pubic symphysis), use these two points as patient palpation points for learning and correcting thoracopelvic alignment. The therapist uses a combination of the above points of control to maintain correct thoracic position as the pelvis is brought under the rib cage or to maintain the optimal pyramid base as the thorax is moved into alignment over the pelvis.

Progressions/other considerations. The breath can be used to facilitate the proper curves. 'Breathe deeply and allow the air to fill the space':

- between your shoulder blades (if midthorax is lordotic);
- beneath your sternum (if midthorax is kyphotic);
- between your lowest ribs:
  ○ posteriorly (if lordotic);
  ○ anteriorly (if kyphotic).

If there are any rotation/side flexion curves present, it is usually necessary to correct the sagittal curves first, and to decrease any back-gripping strategy, before rotation/sideflexion curves can be corrected. The presence of these curves is an indication to include an assessment of the thorax, as the thorax is the key center for rotation in the trunk. Note that rotation and lateral bending asymmetries will correlate with neuromyofascial imbalances in the superficial trunk muscles, especially those linking the thorax and pelvis. Scapular position and the muscle balance relationships of the scapulothoracic muscles and scapulocervical muscles can also impact thoraco-pelvic alignment. Although assessment and treatment of the thorax is beyond the scope of this text, there are some simple correction techniques, which provide a good starting point.

Correction techniques include:

- bilaterally palpating the rib cage (laterally at the mid-axillary line) at the levels of rotation/sideflexion and manually correcting the asymmetry while providing gentle traction through the thorax (this allows the patient to relax). This is known as correcting the 'thoracic ring' (Lee & Lee 2008b);
- taping or manually supporting the scapula to assist in spinal/costal position correction. A 'dumped' scapula (depressed and downwardly rotated) can contribute to lateral bending of the thoracic and lumbar spines to the same side;
- verbal cuing such as 'open the rib cage in the front on the right side' and 'imagine the space between your rib cage and pelvis on the right side increasing or lengthening' to provide the patient with images to self-correct the asymmetry;
- retraining of lateral costal expansion breathing (see Chapter 11) unilaterally to release tone in muscles contributing to the asymmetrical spinal position. Lateral costal expansion and breathing patterns will be asymmetrical.

Once a neutral spine position has been facilitated, ask the patient to maintain the new position and breathe normally. Observe what happens to the spinal position with breathing (apical breathing often causes excessive thoracolumbar (T11–12–L1) extension); use re-education of the breathing pattern (Chapter 11) to integrate breathing with postural control. Note that small deviations of trunk and lower limb position will occur in sync with the breathing cycle (see Chapter 4), but these should not be excessive or result in high levels of global muscle activity and postural rigidity. Check internal and external rotation mobility of the hips; if the patient is unable to move the hips actively or allow passive rotation this is an indication of excessive global muscle activity and 'butt-gripping' (see checkpoints for rigidity).

If it is important for the patient's meaningful task to train dissociation of spinal flexion and hip flexion, a 'sitting forward lean' from an optimal sitting posture can be practiced as a progression. The patient uses the appropriate cues to find optimal alignment and strategy in sitting (release, align, connect), and then palpates the anterior hip crease bilaterally. Instruct the patient to hinge at the hips to bring the trunk forward over the hips while keeping the spine neutral (move) (Fig. 12.20B). Only allow movement through a range of motion where there is no loss of neutral spine. Start with small amounts of movement and progress to larger ranges. This task can be progressed to standing ('waiter's bow' (Sahrmann 2001)).

A 'pelvic rock' can also be used to train neutral LPH. The patient sits on a ball or chair, and is taught to roll the pelvis into an anterior tilt, then a posterior tilt, and then resume a 'comfortable position halfway between the two positions.' Care must be taken with this kind of exercise if given without specific manual or verbal cues. In a population with lumbopelvic dysfunction (whether painful or painfree), the 'comfortable' position will be one that avoids restrictions and moves into areas of already excessive movement or poor control. It cannot be assumed that this is true neutral spine. It is essential that the therapist performs segmental palpation and observation of substitution patterns while giving this task. However, with specific corrections, the pelvic rock can be a useful method for teaching thoracopelvic movement dissociation and can facilitate awareness of where the center of gravity falls in relation to the sitz bones. In a posterior pelvic tilt the patient can be made aware that the center of gravity falls behind the sitz bones, and in an anterior pelvic tilt the patient can be made aware that the center of gravity falls in front of the sitz bones. The goal is that the center of gravity falls in line with the sitz bones, and this awareness can be used as a self-check for the patient when practicing the exercise independently.

Task-specific postures

The principles and techniques to train new postural alignment and strategies in standing and sitting can be applied to any posture required for work- or sport-related tasks, both sustained and dynamic. For dynamic tasks, if the starting postural alignment and/or strategy is non-optimal, the initiation of movement and following movement patterns will be non-optimal. Thus, training new strategies for postural alignment is imperative for breaking complex tasks down into movement building blocks. For example, for golfers it is essential to assess the strategy and alignment in the posture of 'addressing the ball.' At this point, there should be no pelvic rotation in the transverse plane, or IPT, and both femoral heads should be centered. The trunk should flex from the hips symmetrically. Note that the 'waiter's bow' mentioned above could be a good movement building block for this meaningful task if the patient was unable to move to the golf simulation immediately. However, if the meaningful task (address the ball) can be simulated and the patient is able to perform the task, treatment efficacy will be far better if task-specific training is used rather than the waiter's bow.

In rowing, although one single posture is not sustained during the task, the base posture is sitting. Simulation of this specific seated position is required to train optimal strategies in the meaningful task. As in sitting in a chair, both hips should be symmetrical and centered in the acetabulum and the pelvis in neutral rotation without an IPT left or right. Any asymmetry in the pelvic base and hips will impact rotational alignment and control throughout the stroke (Video 12.15). Four-point kneeling and prone over a ball are useful positions to train optimal postural strategies for jobs that require crawling or sports such as swimming (Fig. 12.21). Training neutral spine in these positions also requires dissociation of trunk–hip movement, and thus are useful base movement block training tasks for activities that require control of the joints of the LPH complex while allowing hip motion to occur (Chapter 11,

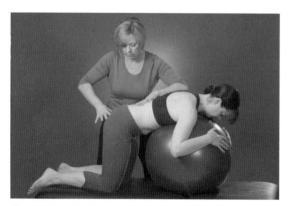

Fig. 12.21 • Training strategies for static tasks – prone over ball. The ball is a useful tool for supporting the thorax in a neutral spine position during training of an optimal strategy in the lumbopelvic–hip region for four-point kneeling tasks. Here, the therapist is providing a tactile cue to release the ischiococcygeus (a verbal cue could also be used, i.e. 'let the sitz bones go wide') and monitoring the lumbar spine to ensure a gentle even curve is present.

Video 12.18). If squats or other upright tasks are too challenging, then four-point kneeling or prone/kneeling over a ball can be used.

As discussed previously, in all postural retraining it is imperative to bring the patient's attention and awareness to how the new postural strategy feels in their body, compared to the old strategy. This trains interoception and creates positive reinforcement, helps to realign the virtual body and the real body, and reinforces that the patient is responsible for 'finding' the new place in their body during daily activities.

Training strategies for dynamic tasks – functional and sport-specific

At this point in the program, the therapist should have identified:

- which key sensory and verbal cues are most effective to remind the patient where and how to release the old strategy;
- which key images create best segmental control for the joints of interest (connect cues);
- which key points of control best facilitate optimal alignment and strategy for meaningful postures;
- which self-cues (palpation and imagery) (performed by the patient) create best strategies for release, connecting to the deep system, and aligning the joints of the relevant kinetic chain in meaningful postures; and
- the key characteristics of the meaningful tasks that need to be simulated in training (level of predictability, load, endurance, speed, agility, relaxed power, etc.).

Collectively, this information provides the therapist with the tools needed to facilitate optimal strategies during meaningful task simulation and training. As noted earlier, training more complex movement tasks, starting with the component parts of the meaningful tasks, is begun as early as possible in the treatment program. What follows is a description of some commonly used training tasks; these are meant to illustrate the previously discussed principles and are not intended as an exhaustive list. The reader is encouraged to creatively consider and design key training tasks from the patient's meaningful goals rather than use recipes and standard 'exercise programs.'

Essential progressions for function

Given that everyone needs to be able to sit, stand, and walk, tasks in upright positions are added as early as possible in the treatment program, even if it is as simple as starting component pieces of postural training (for both strategy and alignment). Standing posture (described above) is the starting place for upright tasks. In general, squats are added early in the program to train synergistic activation of the deep and superficial muscles as well as to provide stimulus for hypertrophy and endurance if needed for meaningful tasks. Squats are also used to teach patients how to initiate an optimal sitting posture. As illustrated in many ways throughout this text, often people with LPH dysfunction exhibit failed load transfer (FLT) at one or several areas in the kinetic chain when standing on one leg (OLS test, Chapter 8). Thus, progressing training tasks from bilateral weight bearing to unilateral weight bearing is the next essential step in order to train optimal strategies for walking and running. Combinations of lunges, step forward and step back, and dynamic COM over BOS retraining can be used to achieve these goals.

Squats

Task instructions

Patient position. Have the patient stand in optimal alignment with the new strategy for posture (cue appropriate release, align, and connect as necessary). When correcting strategy and position in the standing position, it is important to use all of the 'checkpoints for global rigidity' from the rib cage to the toes.

Exercise instruction. Demonstrate the squat movement, highlighting that the task is initiated by moving the hips backwards and simultaneously leaning the trunk forward. Body weight should stay centered over the feet (not anterior on the toes or posterior on the heels, medial or lateral; the optimal triangle of the foot should be maintained) and the spine should maintain neutral. If the patient flexes or extends the spine during the squat, use the key points of control at the MS and PS to cue, 'Keep these points the same distance apart.' The therapist can palpate the relevant joints that failed to transfer load (FLT) to ensure there is no loss of control or optimal joint axis; alternately specific muscles are palpated to cue release or recruitment as required (see Fig. 12.10). During the return to starting position, watch for, and correct, any 'butt-gripping' as the hips extend.

Task considerations

If free standing squats are too difficult for the patient, they can be performed against a wall or using a ball on the wall. Ensure that the pattern of hip flexion and trunk forward lean can occur. A ball should support the lumbar lordosis and should not restrict the movement of the thorax into a neutral kyphosis. As the squat occurs, the lumbar lordosis should be maintained and the hips should move posteriorly under the ball (see Fig. 12.12).

The depth of the squat is varied depending on the control of the movement, but is not usually progressed to lower than 90° knee flexion (unless sport or work demands require it). In deep squatting, the lumbar spine will flex and the pelvis will posteriorly tilt at the end of range but there should be no intrapelvic torsion or unlocking of the hemipelvis on either side.

During the initial introduction of the squatting task, a resistive exercise band can be tied around the lower thigh to provide increased proprioception; this also helps to facilitate the posterior fibers of gluteus medius. The patient is asked to maintain pressure against the band at the knee with a 5% effort during the task. There should be no visible external rotation movement of the hip or change in alignment of the knee and foot; however, an increase in the activity of the posterior fibers of gluteus medius will be palpated (see Fig. 12.11). The task is progressed by *removing* the band and having the patient maintain the control and activity in the gluteus medius. Alternately, a small ball in the upper inner thigh can be used when control is lost into external rotation (see Fig. 12.12).

The patient's arm position depends on where tactile feedback is required for correct task performance. Initially, the multifidus and transversus abdominis may need to be palpated. Alternately, palpation at the hip can facilitate folding anteriorly and maintenance of the axis for hip movement. As the movement pattern becomes more automatic, arm position will depend on what meaningful task needs to be simulated and may be integrated with thorax rotation.

Progressions

Remember that any progression is designed with the meaningful task in mind. To integrate foot control, the squat can be progressed to a 'sling squat'; the patient squats, then lifts both heels to stand on the balls of the feet (Fig. 12.22A,B), then straightens

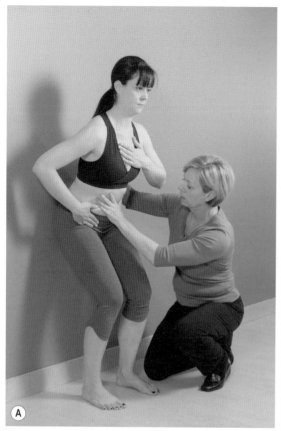 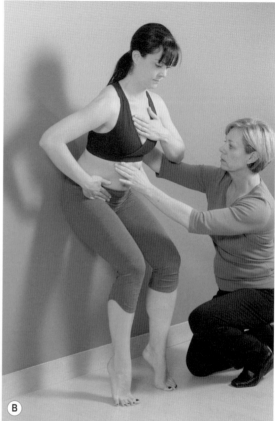

Fig. 12.22 • Training strategies for dynamic tasks, functional and sport-specific – sling squat. A sling squat is a progression of the squat task and requires coordination and control of multiple joints of the lower kinetic chain. (A) The patient is monitoring her key points of control, manubriosternal junction and right hip. She tends to grip with her erector spinae and posteriorly tilt her thorax (back-grip) so the therapist is monitoring the posterior back muscles, the anterior lower thorax, and abdominal wall as she moves into the squat position. (B) Sling squat – from the squat position the patient is instructed to plantarflex the ankles and rise onto the balls of both feet without losing any alignment/ position or control of the rest of the kinetic chain.

the knees and hips to come up to standing while remaining on the toes, then lowers the heels to return to the starting position. This task can be performed in reverse to challenge eccentric control.

Split squats are an intermediate progression to lunges, which require unilateral weight bearing. This is an excellent way to train hip control for a centered femoral head and patterning of the deep and superficial hip muscles while the hips are in different ranges of motion. Thera-Band resistance can be added to challenge rotational control (Fig. 12.23A–C). Contralateral arm swing and rotation of the thorax on the pelvis can be added as a building block for training contralateral thoracopelvic rotation required for gait (see below).

Step forward, step back, backwards walking

These tasks simulate components of the gait cycle in a progressive manner. However, depending on what phase of the gait cycle is problematic for the patient (meaningful task), different components of these training blocks may be selectively prescribed. The patient palpates the key muscles to focus on to either release and/or connect (adductors, fascicle of the external oblique, deep multifidus, posterior fibers of gluteus medius, transversus abdominis, etc.). Initially, work on weight shift from front to back in stride standing. Progress to unilateral weight bearing by lifting the back foot from the ground at the end of the weight shift forward, while checking and cuing control in the key areas. Then a step back is performed and the front foot is lifted from the ground at the end of the weight shift backwards. As confidence and optimal patterning are gained during the unilateral loading phase, practicing stepping forward from standing posture (swing phase) (see Fig. 12.9A,B) and stepping backwards is added. Backwards walking is a useful way to train and solidify new strategies and break out of old habits, as it is a novel task that the central nervous system is not used to performing. Arm swings are added as less tactile feedback is required. The size of the steps is gradually increased to a functional stride length. In the first stages of this training, the goal is to maintain a neutral spine as weight is transferred forward and back, but as the exercise progresses to become more like gait, contralateral thoracopelvic rotation is added and facilitated (Fig. 12.24A,B).

Often as functional progressions are added, new non-optimal vectors of force in connected myofascial slings become apparent; for example, during step forward progressions, the patient may report tension in the posterior leg that is creating a barrier and preventing an optimal strategy during the heel strike phase. At this point, the training should be paused and the barriers released (Fig. 12.25A–D). The impact of the release is then re-assessed during the heel strike phase of the step forward task. Thus, the manual interventions evolve along with the training program to facilitate a new strategy for the meaningful task.

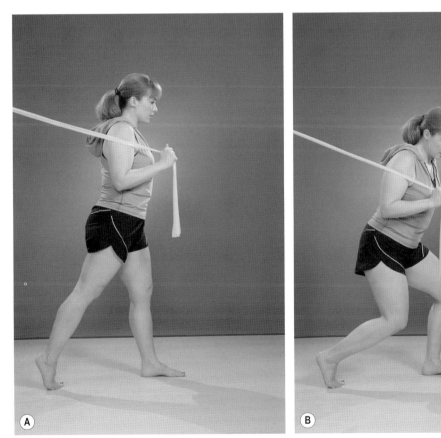

Fig. 12.23 • Training strategies for dynamic tasks, functional and sport-specific – split squat with rotation control. (A) This task begins in the stride position. Ensure that the whole body begins in optimal alignment. Release and connect cues are used to prepare for movement. (B) Here, the individual has lost thoracopelvic rotation control as she moves into the split squat (note the right rotation of her thorax).

Continued

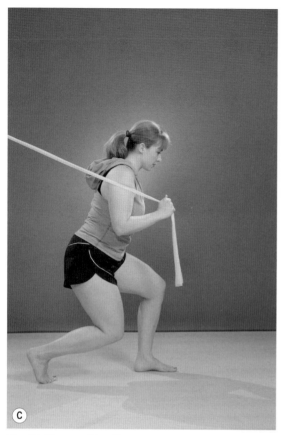

Fig. 12.23 – cont'd • (C) This is much better – well done LJ!

Lunges and variations

Task instructions

Patient position. Have the patient stand with optimal postural strategy and palpate the muscles that need attention for release or connect to facilitate optimal performance. Palpate the area of failed load transfer (sacrum and innominate, lumbar spine, hip, etc.), and then use different palpation points as needed to facilitate the best strategy for function and performance.

Task instruction. Instruct the patient to step forward with one foot, landing heel first, allowing the heel of the back foot to come off the ground so that weight bearing is performed through the ball of the back foot. Ask the patient to bend both knees so that the body drops between the legs, while keeping the weight equally distributed. The front knee should be vertically in line with the ankle joint as the knee bends. Provide a verbal cue for folding of both hips and maintenance of the neutral lumbopelvic curve as

the hips flex. To return to the starting position, the hips and knees extend as the patient pushes backwards off the heel of the front foot and brings the legs back together into a neutral standing posture.

Task progressions and other considerations

The depth of the lunge can be varied depending on the patient's control. Watch for any lateral tilting or excessive rotation of the pelvis. During the step forward, observe the stationary leg (the back leg). Failed load transfer at the sacroiliac joint (unlocking) and decreased gluteus medius activation in the back leg are common causes for compensatory hip strategies in the other leg such as hip hiking (lateral pelvic tilt) and pelvic rotation because of the 'unstable' base for movement. Tie a resistive exercise band around the lower thigh to provide increased sensory input during the initial introduction of this task. The patient's arm position depends on where tactile feedback is required for correct exercise performance. As the movement pattern becomes more automatic, use less tactile feedback and have the patient swing the arms while moving the legs. During forward and diagonal lunges use the arms in a contralateral swing pattern, and facilitate contralateral thoracopelvic rotation.

Progressions depend on the patient's requirements for function. These include a lunge with one knee lift progressing to walking lunges. The basic lunge is performed to the point where the body drops between the two legs. Now, instead of pushing back off the front leg to return the legs together, the body moves forward onto the front leg while lifting the back knee and hip forward into flexion (unilateral weight bearing on the front leg). This end position resembles the one leg standing test and is held for a few seconds to challenge control of balance. To return to the start position, a step backwards is performed by the non-weight bearing leg. The task is then performed on the other side. A further progression is to remove the final step backwards and link alternating 'lunge knee lifts' together so that the patient moves forward with each lunge. These are now 'walking lunges.' Using brief 'holds,' where the patient stops with the knee lifted in between several walking lunges, adds proprioceptive challenge to the movement practice, and allows opportunity for the therapist to monitor checkpoints for rigidity.

Backwards lunges – one leg moves into extension to land on the ball of the foot so that the squatting motion is performed in the same position as the forward squat, but the initiation of the task requires

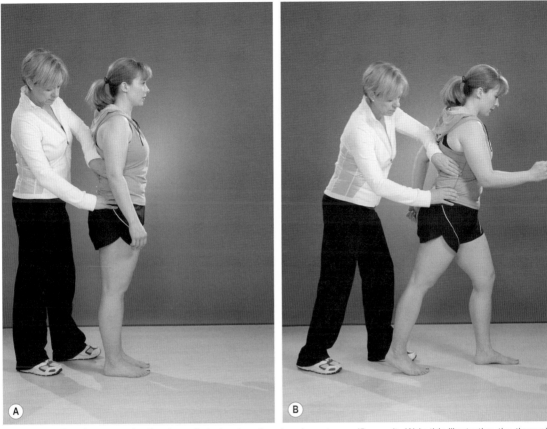

Fig. 12.24 • Training strategies for dynamic tasks, functional and sport-specific – gait. (A) In this illustration the therapist is providing a tactile and verbal cue aimed at releasing overactivation of the superficial muscles of the abdominal canister to allow thoracopelvic dissociation during gait. (B) 'Think of opening the space between your lower rib cage and pelvis as you step forward.' Remember to celebrate their success with positive reinforcement.

different muscle patterning. Backward lunges are useful for training eccentric gluteus maximus control in one leg standing.

Side or diagonal lunges – the stepping leg moves in a side step, and a squat is performed so that the body weight is equal between the legs. Alternately, the stepping leg moves in a forward and diagonal line or a backward and diagonal line. Correct the body position when the foot lands to teach the patient how to land with the weight already equally distributed between both feet; this retraining helps to correct and facilitate better awareness of 'sense of body center,' and to align the virtual body center with the real body center, which is often altered in patients with lumbopelvic–hip dysfunction (see case report Louise, Chapter 9, Video LL19 🖱). The body center awareness training can be performed at different speeds to increase automatic reactions. Using mirrors to help the patient realize where their body is in relation to where they *think* it is, can be a useful tool.

Lunge against a resistive exercise band – a piece of resistive exercise band is secured behind the patient at shoulder level. The patient stands while holding the band with one hand at the ipsilateral shoulder (elbow is bent). With a focus on their release, align, connect cues, the patient then moves into a dynamic lunge against the unilateral resistance of the band. The lunge can be performed on the leg ipsilateral or contralateral to the arm holding the band. In both cases a rotational force is imparted to the trunk. The patient is instructed to keep the spine in neutral throughout the performance of the movement.

Lunge with trunk rotation – this task integrates incongruent rotation between the thorax and the pelvis during movement of the full kinetic chain. The patient performs a lunge with the lower

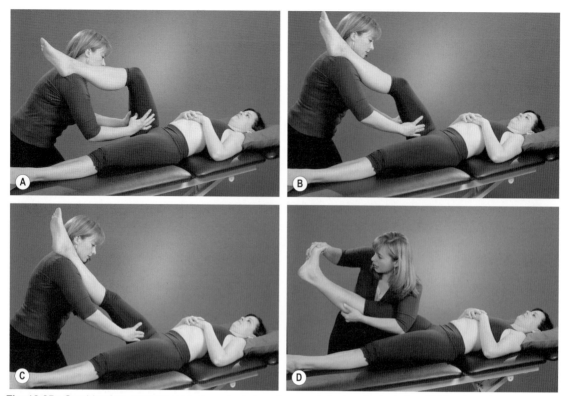

Fig. 12.25 • Combined neuromyofascial release technique for a posterior longitudinal sling. (A) The therapist is monitoring the tone in the hamstrings and cuing a release with awareness. (B) As the tone dampens, the knee is taken into further extension while the therapist applies a myofascial stretch to the intramuscular tissue, if necessary. (C) The goal is to achieve full knee extension with sufficient hip flexion for heel strike. (D) The 'sling stretch' is completed by lengthening the gastrocnemius/soleus and structures of the sole of the foot/toes.

extremity, while simultaneously rotating the trunk against a resistive exercise band. For lunges with the right leg, the band is secured above and anterior to the right shoulder. The left arm holds the band in elevation across the body. The patient is instructed to step forward and lunge with the right foot, then straighten the right leg and lift the left hip and knee into flexion to move into a lunge with the left leg. As the right leg is straightened, the left arm draws the band down across the body in the direction of the left hip (extension and abduction diagonal) and the thorax is rotated to the left. Note that the overall direction of body motion is forwards (as per walking lunges) so that gait patterns are simulated.

Other progressions

Clearly, there are multiple tasks that can be used to train the integrated function of the deep and superficial muscles of the body to serve optimal

performance in meaningful tasks. Step up and step down tasks (Fig. 12.26) would be added if the patient goals involved performance in stair climbing or descending, or hiking activities. One leg squats can be used to further load and challenge unilateral control, and should be performed with the same pattern as bilateral squats (hip flexion, trunk forward lean) (Fig. 12.27). Thera-Band can be used if specific muscle training such as eccentric hamstring training is required based on specific impairments.

As rotation and rotational control are key components of most functional tasks, screening of the thorax (Lee & Lee 2008b) is often required in order to fully return patients to optimal function and performance. Any training task that involves movement of one extremity while maintaining neutral spine creates a rotational challenge to the thorax and LPH complex, and early training tasks were introduced in Chapter 11. Progressions to upright rotational tasks should be designed with the specific meaningful task

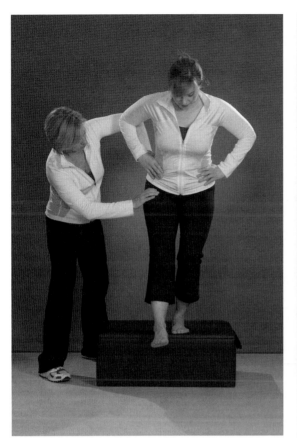

Fig. 12.26 • Training strategies for dynamic tasks, functional and sport-specific – step up/step down. This is a meaningful task for anyone who presents with aggravating complaints during ascending or descending stairs. The patient and therapist monitor relevant key points of control for regions of failed load transfer, and engage appropriate release and connect cues prior to moving either down or up the step.

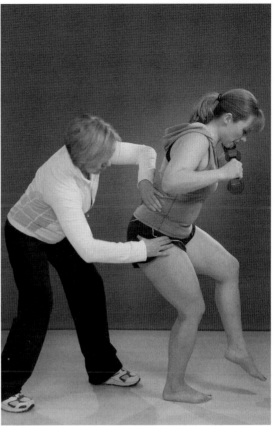

Fig. 12.27 • Training strategies for dynamic tasks, functional and sport-specific – one leg squat. In this loaded one leg squat the therapist is monitoring the right sacroiliac joint and the right hip joint to ensure an optimal strategy is maintained throughout the task.

in mind. Resisted pulley activities in diagonal patterns integrate trunk rotation with the upper extremity. Alternately, as shown in Figure 12.28A,B, a ball on the wall can be used to train rotational control and thoracopelvic dissociation from below. Equipment such as the BOSU® can facilitate speed and agility training, as well as create proprioceptive challenges for automatic patterning (Fig. 12.29). Lunges can be performed as alternating plyometric jumps if power and speed are required. For sports that require the ability to quickly change direction at speed, different drills and patterns can be designed such as figure eights and zigzag practice. During speed training, have the patient pause at different times during the training sequences to perform quick manual screens at the checkpoints for rigidity (hip IR/ER, ribcage wiggle, etc.) and ensure that strategies are not moving into excessive stiffness and bracing. This can be done in many different activities and simulations.

Building blocks for runners

Hopefully, by now the reader is aware that the training program for each patient is highly individual. However, there are some common patterns. For example, if a runner complains of difficulty (e.g. loss of power) or pain during the push off phase of gait, the therapist should assess whether the patient can:

1. lengthen the anterior myofascial sling of the hip and lower extremity;

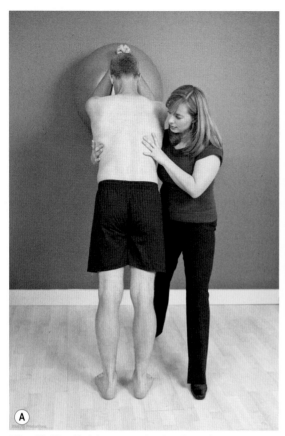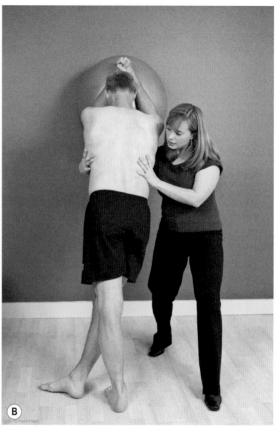

Fig. 12.28 • Training strategies for dynamic tasks, functional and sport-specific – upright rotation tasks. This is an excellent task for learning to dissociate rotation of the lumbopelvis and lower extremity from the thorax. (A) Starting position. (B) Here, the therapist is monitoring the thoracopelvic dissociation.

2. maintain control of the hemipelvis (no unlocking of the SIJ) and a centered femoral head during hip extension (requires synergistic activation of the deep and superficial muscles);

3. dissociate the thorax and pelvis to allow contralateral rotation; and

4. push off through a supinated foot pyramid through the first ray.

If this is the meaningful task for a patient, initial training to coordinate the deep and superficial muscles of the trunk and hip would include trunk–leg dissociation in prone, starting with prone knee bend (Fig. 11.32A–D) and prone hip extension tasks (Fig. 11.33A–C). Progression of the training may then be to release and align the femoral head in a lunge position. This requires multiple portions of the anterior sling to lengthen (Fig. 12.30), which may be performed as release with awareness in the

functional task position or as a separate technique. If there are specific myofascial barriers to address, foam rollers and release balls can be used to target these vectors (Fig. 12.31A–C). To practice and cue the specific relevant phase of gait (in this case midstance to push off), feedback and manual cues are given to encourage appropriate patterning (Fig. 12.32A–D). Training progressions, including slow walking lunges that progress from keeping the thorax and pelvis neutral to adding contralateral thoracopelvic rotation, can be added to the program (Video 12.21). As the patient practices interoception and awareness in each training task, they are advised to try to create that feeling and connection in their body when they are running. Unless running actually provokes pain, patients are allowed to continue their normal running regime, but the aim is that their strategy is continually altered during the progression of the rehabilitation program.

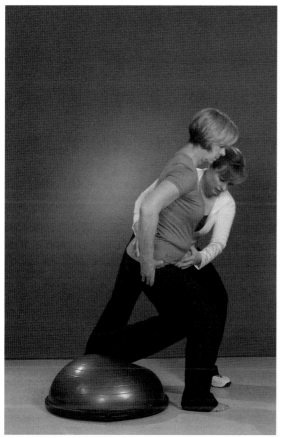

Fig. 12.29 • Training strategies for dynamic tasks, functional and sport-specific – step down using a BOSU®. Wow, what can I say – awesome technique Diane!! Yeah, well it took a lot of coaching; this was tough.

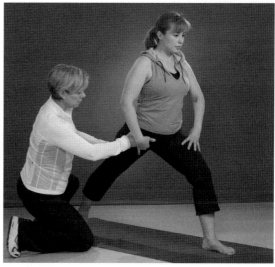

Fig. 12.30 • Training strategies for dynamic tasks, functional and sport-specific – building blocks for runners – release with awareness in a functional position – lunge. In this lunge the therapist is using tactile, verbal, and imagery cues to facilitate release, with control, of an anterior myofascial sling that was preventing full hip extension with an optimal axis for femoral motion.

Summary

Diane Lee & Linda-Joy Lee

So, this is the end of chapter 12 and the fourth edition of *The Pelvic Girdle*. What is different about this edition? We have illustrated how clinicians gain knowledge through their practice, experiences, and consideration of the available research evidence. We have introduced a new model, The Integrated Systems Model, which has evolved from our combined clinical practice, consideration of the available evidence, and personal life experiences. We use this model as a framework for organizing all of our knowledge (propositional, non-propositional, and personal) and apply it to every patient, each of whom presents with a unique Clinical Puzzle. The multiple online cases, and clinical examples, illustrate the uniqueness of each person/case

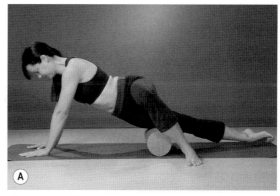

Fig. 12.31 • Training strategies for dynamic tasks, functional and sport-specific – building blocks for runners. Foam rollers are useful tools to target specific vectors that are myofascial barriers to achieving an optimal strategy for the task. (A) In this illustration, the patient is using a foam roller to assist release of the anterior thigh musculature.

Continued

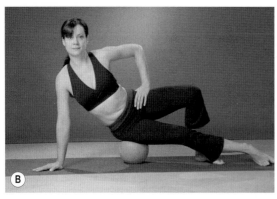

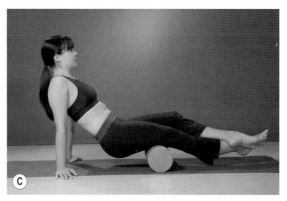

Fig. 12.31 – cont'd • (B) It is common for the muscles of the posterior hip to be hypertonic and myofascially restricted concurrently with the anterior thigh. Here, she is using a body-rolling ball to facilitate release of the posterior hip. (C) If there are intramuscular adhesions in the hamstrings, they will require release before optimal recruitment can be restored. Foam rollers can assist in this task.

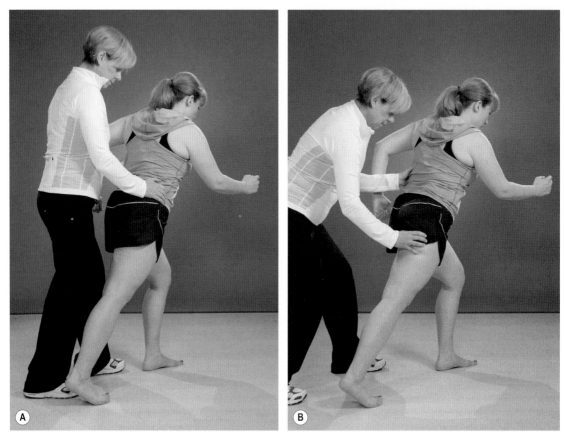

Fig. 12.32 • Training strategies for dynamic tasks, functional and sport-specific – building blocks for runners. (A) Training optimal strategies for push off. Here, the therapist is monitoring the thorax and the pelvis and reminding the patient of their relevant release and connect cues for the specific regions of failed load transfer for this task. (B) Tactile and verbal cues for the left abdominal wall and ischiococcygeus, for example 'Open your rib cage and let your breath move into my hand as you let your right sitz bone go wide.'

Continued

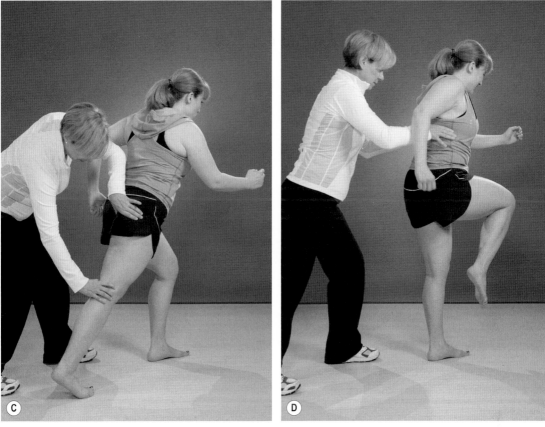

Fig. 12.32 – cont'd • (C) Tactile and verbal cues for the right medial hamstring and ischiococcygeus, for example 'Let your right sitz bone go wide and then imagine and connect along a guy wire from the back of your knee here (poke the appropriate spot) to your sitz bone, remembering to keep that sitz bone wide.' (D) You've released, aligned, connected, now MOVE!!!

and how effective treatment requires a multimodal approach, which considers all three dimensions of the patient's experience: sensorial (what they feel in their bodies), cognitive (what they think is happening to them), and emotional (how they feel about what is happening). Each dimension can be a barrier or a facilitator to their recovery and each must be addressed in the treatment program if the puzzle is to be solved. Specific tests for detecting and treating relevant impairments in each system (articular, neural, myofascial, visceral), including the clinical reasoning (critical thinking, hypothesis development, and reflective practice) necessary to support the most likely and lovely hypotheses to explain the individual experience, have been described.

According to the definition of Sackett et al (2000), we strongly feel that The Integrated Systems Model is an evidence-based approach. It is centred around the patient's values (thoughts, feelings, expectations) and integrates the practitioner's expertise (clinical reasoning and skills) with the available research evidence into decision making for appropriate assessment and therapeutic interventions. Treatment principles are consistent with evidence from neuroscience that explains how to best facilitate change and optimize neuroplasticity – key components include *Release* (the primary barrier(s)), *Align* (correct posture/position for load/change postural strategies), *Connect* (rewire the brain for a new neuromuscular strategy) and *Move* (choose postural tasks and movements (or building blocks towards movements) according to the patient's meaningful task). In our experience, there are no recipes, prediction rules, or guidelines for patients presenting with lumbopelvic–hip disability with or without pain, and we feel that a multimodel approach will always be more effective for long-term success. Although temporary improvement in function and/or pain may be gained by using one component of the therapeutic intervention (release or align or connect or move) (or one treatment modality), it is the long-term solution that is sought by the patient. We strive to empower our patients to understand what is driving their disability or pain experience, to be aware of the contexts or situations that facilitate their poor strategies, and to team how they can change those strategies and move towards ones that are more optimal for their bodies (Empower through Knowledge, Movement, and Awareness). In this way, we hope that they can Move better, Feel better, and Be better!

Please join us online at www.discoverphysio.ca to follow our journey, attend some courses, and participate in the online education we offer. Above all, have fun with this approach, be creative and reflective in your clinical practice, and *DISCOVER PHYSIO!!*

References

Abe, I., Haranda, Y., Oinuma, K., et al., 2000. Acetabular labrum: abnormal findings at MR imaging in asymptomatic hips. Radiology 216 (2), 576.

Abitbol, M.M., 1995. Energy storage in the vertebral column. In: Vleeming, A., Mooney, V., Dorman, T., Snijders, C. (Eds.), Second interdisciplinary world congress on low back pain: the integrated function of the lumbar spine and sacroiliac joint, Part 1. San Diego, California, p. 257.

Abitbol, M.M., 1997. Quadrupedalism, bipedalism, and human pregnancy. In: Vleeming, A., Mooney, V., Dorman, T., Snijders, C., Stoeckart, R. (Eds.), Movement, stability and low back pain. Churchill Livingstone, Edinburgh, p. 395.

Abrams, P., Cardozo, L., Fall, M., et al., 2002. The standardization of terminology of lower urinary tract function: report from the standardization sub-committee of the International Continence Society. Neurourol. Urodyn. 21, 167.

Acland, R.D., 2004. Acland's DVD atlas of human anatomy. DVD 3: The trunk. Lippincott Williams & Wilkins, Baltimore.

Adams, J.C., 1973. Outline of orthopaedics, seventh ed. Churchill Livingstone, Edinburgh.

Adams, M.A., McMillan, D.W., Green, T.P., et al., 1996. Sustained loading generates stress concentrations in lumbar intervertebral discs. Spine 21, 434.

Albee, F.H., 1909. A study of the anatomy and the clinical importance of the sacroiliac joint. J. Am. Med. Assoc. 53, 1273.

Albert, H., Godskesen, M., Westergaard, J., 2000. Evaluation of clinical tests used in classification procedures in pregnancy-related pelvic joint pain. Eur. Spine J 9, 161.

Albert, H.B., Godskesen, M., Westergaard, J.G., 2002. Incidence of four syndromes of pregnancy-related pelvic joint pain. Spine 27, 2831.

Allen, R.E., Hosker, G.L., Smith, A.R.B., Warrell, D.W., 1990. Pelvic floor damage and childbirth: a neurophysiological study. Br. J. Obstet. Gynaecol. 97, 770.

Anda, S., Svenningsen, S., Dale, L.G., et al., 1986. The acetabular sector angle of the adult hip determined by computed tomography. Acta Radiol. Diagn. 27 (4), 443.

Andersson, E.A., Grundstrom, H., Thorstensson, A., 2002. Diverging intramuscular activity patterns in back and abdominal muscles during trunk rotation. Spine 27 (6), E152.

Andersson, E., Oddsson, L., Grundstrom, H., et al., 1995. The role of the psoas and iliacus muscles for stability and movement of the lumbar spine, pelvis and hip. Scand. J. Med. Sci. Sports 5 (1), 10.

Arab, M.A., Abdollahi, I., Joghataei, M.T., et al., 2009. A Inter- and intra-examiner reliability of single and composites of selected motion palpation and pain provocation tests for sacroiliac joint. Man. Ther. 14, 213.

Arendt-Nielsen, L., Graven-Nielsen, T., Svarrer, H., et al., 1996. The influence of low back pain on muscle activity and coordination during gait: a clinical and experimental study. Pain 64 (2), 231.

Aruin, A.S., Latash, M.L., 1995. Directional specificity of postural muscles in feed-forward postural reactions during fast voluntary arm movements. Exp. Brain Res. 103 (2), 323.

Ashton-Miller, J.A., DeLancey, J.O.L., 2007. Functional anatomy of the female pelvic floor. Ann. N. Y. Acad. Sci. 1101, 266.

Ashton-Miller, J.A., DeLancey, J.O.L., 2009. On the biomechanics of vaginal birth and common sequelae. Annu. Rev. Biomed. Eng. 11, 163.

Ashton-Miller, J.A., Howard, D., DeLancey, J.O.L., 2001. The functional anatomy of the female pelvic floor and stress continence control system. Scand. J. Urol. Nephrol. Suppl. 207, 1–7.

Askar, O.M., 1977. Surgical anatomy of the aponeurotic expansions of the anterior abdominal wall. Ann. R. Coll. Surg. Engl. 59, 313.

Assendelft, W.J., Morton, S.C., Yu, E.I., et al., 2003. Spinal manipulative therapy for low back pain: a meta-analysis of effectiveness relative to other therapies. Ann. Intern. Med. 138, 871–881.

Austin, A.B., Souza, R.B., Meyer, J.L., et al., 2008. Identification of abnormal hip motion associated with acetabular labral pathology.

J. Orthop. Sports Phys. Ther. 38 (9), 558.

Axer, H., von Keyserlingk, D.G., Prescher, A., 2000. Collagen fibers in linea alba and rectus sheaths. II. Variability and biomechancial aspects. J. Surg. Res. 96, 239.

Axer, H., von Keyserlingk, D.G., Prescher, A., 2001. Collagen fibers in linea alba and rectus sheaths. I. General scheme and morphological aspects. J. Surg. Res. 96, 127–134.

Barbic, M., Kralj, B., Cor, A., 2003. Compliance of the bladder neck supporting structures: importance of activity pattern of levator ani muscle and content of elastic fibers of endopelvic fascia. Neurourol. Urodyn. 22, 269.

Barker, P.J., 2005. Applied anatomy and biomechanics of the lumbar fascia: implications for segmental control. PhD thesis. University of Melbourne, Australia.

Barker, P.J., Briggs, C.A., 1999. Attachments of the posterior layer of the lumbar fascia. Spine 24 (17), 1757.

Barker, P.J., Briggs, C.A., 2007. Anatomy and biomechanics of the lumbar fasciae: implication for lumbopelvic control and clinical practice. In: Vleeming, A., Mooney, V., Stoeckart, R. (Eds.), Movement, stability and lumbopelvic pain, second ed. Elsevier, Edinburgh, p. 63.

Barker, P.J., Briggs, C.A., Bogeski, G., 2004. Tensile transmission across the lumbar fasciae in unembalmed cadavers: effects of tension to various muscular attachments. Spine 29 (2), 129.

Barker, P.J., Guggenheimer, K.T., Grkovic, I., et al., 2006. Effects of tensioning the lumbar fascia on segmental stiffness during flexion and extension. Spine 31 (4), 397.

Barral, J.P., 1993. Urogenital manipulation. Eastland Press, Seattle.

Basmajian, J.V., Deluca, C.J., 1985. Muscles alive: their functions revealed by electromyography. Williams & Wilkins, Baltimore.

Beales, D.J., O'Sullivan, P.B., Briffa, N.K., 2008. Motor control patterns during active straight leg raise in pain-free subjects. Spine 34 (1), E1.

Beattie, P., Nelson, R., 2006. Clinical prediction rules: what are they and what do they tell us? Aust. J. Physiother. 52 (3), 157.

Belenkii, V., Gurfinkel, V.S., Paltsev, Y., 1967. Elements of control of voluntary movements. Biofizika 12, 135.

Bellamy, N., Park, W., Rooney, P.J., 1983. What do we know about the sacroiliac joint? Semin. Arthritis Rheum. 12, 282.

Bergmark, A., 1989. Stability of the lumbar spine. A study in mechanical engineering. Acta Orthop. Scand. 230 (60), 20.

Bernard, T.N., Kirkaldy-Willis, W.H., 1987. Recognizing specific characteristics of nonspecific low back pain. Clin. Orthop. 217, 266.

Bø, K., 2003. Pelvic floor muscle strength and response to pelvic floor muscle training for stress urinary incontinence. Neurourol. Urodyn. 22, 654.

Bø, K., Borgen, J.S., 2001. Prevalence of stress and urge urinary incontinence in elite athletes and controls. Med. Sci. Sports Exerc. 33 (11), 1797.

Bø, K., Hagen, R.H., Dvarstein, B., et al., 1990. Pelvic floor muscle exercise for the treatment of female stress urinary incontinence: III Effects of two different degrees of pelvic floor muscle exercises. Neurourol. Urodyn. 9, 489.

Bø, K., Lilleas, F., Talseth, T., 2001. Dynamic MRI of the pelvic floor muscles in an upright sitting position. Neurourol. Urodyn. 20, 167.

Bø, K., Stein, R., 1994. Needle EMG registration of striated urethral wall and pelvic floor muscle activity patterns during cough, Valsalva, abdominal, hip adductor, and gluteal muscles contractions in nulliparous healthy females. Neurourol. Urodyn. 13, 35.

Bogduk, N.L.T., 1983. The innervation of the lumbar spine. Spine 8, 286.

Bogduk, N.L.T., 1997. Clinical anatomy of the lumbar spine and sacrum, third ed. Churchill Livingstone, New York.

Bogduk, N., Pearcy, M., Hadfield, G., 1992. Anatomy and biomechanics of psoas major. Clin. Biomech. 7, 109–119.

Boissonault, J.S., Blaschak, M.J., 1988. Incidence of diastasis recti abdominis during the childbearing year. Phys. Ther. 68 (7), 1082.

Boissonnault, W.G. (Ed.), 1995. Examination in physical therapy practice: screening for medical disease. Churchill Livingstone, New York.

Bonica, J.J., 1953. The management of pain. Lea & Febiger, Philadelphia.

Bouisset, S., Zattara, M., 1981. A sequence of postural adjustments precedes voluntary movement. Neurosci. Lett. 22, 263.

Bowen, V., Cassidy, J.D., 1981. Macroscopic and microscopic anatomy of the sacroiliac joint from embryonic life until the eighth decade. Spine 6, 620.

Boxer, S., Jones, S., 1997. Intra-rater reliability of rectus abdominis diastasis measurement using dial calipers. Aust. J. Physiother. 43 (2), 109.

Bradlay, K.C., 1985. The posterior primary rami of segmental nerves. In: Glasgow, E.F., Twomey, L.T., Scull, E.R., Kleynhans, A.M. (Eds.), Aspects of manipulative therapy, second ed. Churchill Livingstone, Melbourne, p. 59.

Brooke, R., 1924. The sacro-iliac joint. J. Anat. 58, 299.

Brooke, R., 1930. The pelvic joints during and after parturition and pregnancy. The Practitioner, London, p. 307.

Brown, S.H.M., McGill, S.M., 2009. Transmission of muscularly generated force and stiffness between layers of the rat abdominal wall. Spine 34 (2), E70.

Brukner, P., Khan, K., 2007. Clinical sports medicine, second ed. McGraw-Hill, Sydney, Australia.

Bump, R.C., Hurt, G.W., Fantl, J.A., et al., 1991. Assessment of Kegal pelvic muscle exercise performance after brief verbal instruction. Am. J. Obstet. Gynecol. 165, 322.

Burnett, S., Della Roca, G., Prather, H., et al., 2006. Clinical presentation of patients with tears of the acetabular labrum. J. Bone Joint Surg. Am. 88 (7), 1448.

Butler, D.S., 2000. The sensitive nervous system. NOI Group Publications, Adelaide, Australia.

Butler, D.S., Moseley, G.L., 2003. Explain pain. NOI Group Publications, Adelaide, Australia.

Buyruk, H.M., Guler-Uysal, F., Lotgering, F.K., 2002. The prognostic value of asymmetric laxity of the sacroiliac joints in pregnancy-related pelvic pain. Spine 27 (24), 2820.

Buyruk, H.M., Snijders, C.J., Vleeming, A., et al., 1995b. The measurements of sacroiliac joint stiffness with colour Doppler imaging: a study on healthy subjects. Eur. J. Radiol. 21, 117.

Buyruk, H.M., Stam, H.J., Snijders, C.J., et al., 1995a. The use of colour Doppler imaging for the assessment of sacroiliac joint stiffness: a study on embalmed human pelvises. Eur. J. Radiol. 21, 112.

Buyruk, H.M., Stam, H.J., Snijders, C.J., 1999. Measurement of sacroiliac joint stiffness in peripartum pelvic pain patients with Doppler imaging of vibrations (DIV). Eur. J. Obstet. Gynecol. Reprod. Biol. 83 (2), 159.

Cannon, W.B., Rosenblueth, A., 1949. The supersensitivity of denervated structures: a law of denervation. Macmillan, New York.

Carey, T.S., Garrett, J.M., Jackman, A., Hadler, N., 1999. Recurrence and care seeking after acute back pain: results of a long-term follow-up study. North Carolina Back Pain Project. Med. Care 37 (2), 17.

Carmichael, J.P., 1987. Inter- and intra-examiner reliability of palpation for sacroiliac joint dysfunction. Journal of Manipulative Physical Therapy 10 (4), 164.

Chamberlain, W.E., 1930. The symphysis pubis in the Roentgen examination of the sacroiliac joint. AJR. Am. J. Roentgenol. 24, 621.

Cholewicki, J., Crisco, J., Oxland, T.R., et al., 1996. Effect of posture and structure on three-dimensional coupled rotations in the lumbar spine. A biomechanical analysis. Spine 21 (21), 2421.

Cholewicki, J., McGill, S.M., 1996. Mechanical stability of the in vivo lumbar spine: implications for injury and chronic low back pain. Clin Biomech. 11, 1–15.

Cholewicki, J., McGill, S.M., Norman, R. W., 1991. Lumbar spine loading during the lifting of extremely heavy weights. Med. Sci. Sports Exerc. 23, 1179.

Cholewicki, J., Panjabi, M.M., Khachatryan, A., 1997. Stabilizing function of trunk flexor-extensor muscles around a neutral spine posture. Spine 22 (19), 2207.

Cholewicki, J., Van Vliet, J.J., 2002. Relative contribution of trunk muscles to the stability of the lumbar spine during isometric exertions. Clin. Biomech. (Bristol, Avon) 17, 99.

Chow, D.H.K., Luk, D.K., Leong, J.C.Y., et al., 1989. Torsional stability of the lumbosacral junctions. Significance of the iliolumbar ligament. Spine 1989 (14), 611.

Cleland, J.A., Noteboom, T.A., Whitman, J.M., et al., 2008. A primer on selected aspects of evidence-based practice relating to questions of treatment, Part 1: asking questions, finding evidence, and determining validity. J. Orthop. Sports Phys. Ther. 38 (8), 476.

Cochrane, A.L., 1972. Effectiveness and efficiency. Random reflections on health services. Nuffield Provincial Hospitals Trust, London. Reprinted in 1989 in association with the BMJ, Reprinted in 1999 for Nuffield Trust by the Royal Society of Medicine Press, London (ISBN 1-85315-394-X).

Colachis, S.C., Worden, R.E., Bechtol, C.O., et al., 1963. Movement of the sacroiliac joint in the adult male: a preliminary report. Arch. Phys. Med. Rehabil. 44, 490.

Coldron, Y., Stokes, M.J., Newham, D.J., et al., 2008. Postpartum characteristics of rectus abdominis on ultrasound imaging. Man. Ther. 13, 112.

Constantinou, C.E., Govan, D.E., 1982. Spatial distribution and timing of transmitted and reflexly generated urethral pressures in healthy women. J. Urol. 127, 964.

Cook, C., 2008. Potential pitfalls of clinical prediction rules. Journal of Manual and Manipulative Therapy 16 (2), 69.

Coste, J., Paolaggi, J.B., Spira, A., 1992. Classification of nonspecific low back pain, I: psychological involvement in low back pain. Spine 17, 1028.

Cowan, S.M., Schache, A.G., Brukner, P., et al., 2004. Delayed onset of transversus abdominis in long-standing groin pain. Med. Sci. Sports Exerc. 36 (12), 2042.

Cresswell, A., 1993. Responses of intra-abdominal pressure and abdominal muscle activity during dynamic loading in man. Eur. J. Appl. Physiol. 66, 315.

Cresswell, A., Grundstrom, H., Thorstensson, A., 1992. Observations on intra-abdominal pressure and patterns of abdominal intra-muscular activity in man. Acta Physiol. Scand. 144, 409.

Crisco, J.J., Panjabi, M.M., 1991. The intersegmental and multisegmental muscles of the lumbar spine: a biomechanical model comparing lateral stabilizing potential. Spine 16 (7), 793.

Crisco, J.J., Panjabi, M.M., 1992. Euler stability of the human ligamentous lumbar spine. Part 1: theory. Clin. Biomech. 7, 19.

Crisco, J.J., Panjabi, M.M., Yamamoto, I., Oxland, T.R., 1992. Euler stability of the human ligamentous lumbar spine: Part II experiment. Clin. Biomech. (Briston, Avon) 7, 27.

Crock, H.V., 1980. An atlas of the arterial supply of the head and neck of the femur in man. Clin. Orthop. Relat. Res. 152, 17.

Cundiff, G.W., 2004. The pathophysiology of stress urinary incontinence: a historical perspective. Rev. Urol. 6 (Suppl 3), S10.

Cundiff, G.W., Fenner, D., 2004. Evaluation and treatment of women with rectocele: focus on associated defecatory and sexual dysfunction. Obstet. Gynecol. 104 (6), 1403.

Cusi, M., Saunders, J., Hungerford, B., et al., 2010. The use of prolotherapy in the sacroiliac joint. Br. J. Sports Med. 44 (2), 100.

Cyriax, J., 1954. Textbook of orthopaedic medicine. Cassell, London.

Damen, L., Buyruk, H.M., Guler-Uysal, F., 2001. Pelvic pain during pregnancy is associated with asymmetric laxity of the sacroiliac joints. Acta Obstet. Gynecol. Scand. 80, 1019.

Damen, L., Mens, J.M.A., Snijders, C.J., 2002a. The mechanical effects of a pelvic belt in patients with pregnancy-related pelvic pain. PhD thesis, Erasmus University, Rotterdam, The Netherlands.

Damen, L., Spoor, C.W., Snijders, C.J., 2002b. Does a pelvic belt influence sacroiliac joint laxity? Clin. Biomech. (Bristol, Avon) 17 (7), 495.

Damen, L., Stijnen, T., Roebroeck, M.E., et al., 2002c. Reliability of sacroiliac joint laxity measurement with Doppler imaging of vibrations. Ultrasound Med. Biol. 28, 407.

Dangaria, T., Naesh, O., 1998. Changes in cross-sectional area of psoas major muscle in unilateral sciatic caused by disc herniation. Spine 23 (8), 928.

Dankaerts, W., O'sullivan, P., Burnett, A., Straker, L., 2006. Difference in sitting postures are associated with nonspecific chronic low back pain disorders when patients are subclassified. Spine 31 (6), 698.

Danneels, L.A., Vanderstraeten, G.G., Cambier, D.C., et al., 2000. Imaging of trunk muscles in chronic low back pain patients and healthy control subjects. Eur. Spine J. 9, 266.

Dar, G., Khamis, S., Peleg, S., et al., 2008. Sacroiliac joint fusion and the implications for manual therapy diagnosis and treatment. Man. Ther. 13, 155.

David, M., 2005. The slow down diet: eating for pleasure, energy and weight loss. Healing Arts Press, Vermont, USA.

de Groot, M., Pool-Goudzwaard, A.L., Spoor, C.W., 2008. The active straight leg raising test (ASLR) in pregnant women: differences in muscle activity and force between patients and healthy subjects. Man. Ther. 13 (1), 68.

Deindl, F.M., Vodusek, D.B., Hesse, U., et al., 1993. Activity patterns of pubococcygeal muscles in nulliparous continent women. Br. J. Urol. 72, 46.

Deindl, F.M., Vodusek, D.B., Hesse, U., 1994. Pelvic floor activity patterns: comparison of nulliparous continent and parous urinary stress incontinent women. A kinesiological EMG study. Br. J. Urol. 73, 413.

DeLancey, J.O.L., 1994. Structural support of the urethra as it relates to stress urinary incontinence: the hammock hypothesis. Am. J. Obstet. Gynecol. 170 (6), 1713.

DeLancey, J.O.L., 2002. Fascial and muscular abnormalities in women with urethral hypermobility and anterior vaginal wall prolapse. Am. J. Obstet. Gynecol. 187 (1), 93.

DeLancey, J.O.L., 2005. The hidden epidemic of pelvic floor dysfunction: achievable goals for improved prevention and treatment. Am. J. Obstet. Gynecol. 192, 1488.

DeLancey, J.O.L., Kearney, Q., Chou, et al., 2003. The appearance of levator ani muscle abnormalities in magnetic resonance images after vaginal delivery. Obstet. Gynecol. 101 (1), 46.

DeLancey, J.O.L., Morgan, D.M., Fenner, D.E., et al., 2007. Comparison of levator ani muscle defects and function in women with and without pelvic organ prolapse. Obstet. Gynecol. 109, 295.

Delitto, A., Erhard, R.E., Bowling, R.W., 1995. A treatment-based classification approach to low back syndrome: identifying and staging patients for conservative treatment. Phys. Ther. 75, 470.

DeRosa, C., 2001. Functional anatomy of the lumbar spine and sacroiliac joint. In: Proceedings from the 4th Interdisciplinary World Congress on Low Back and Pelvic Pain, Montreal, Canada.

DeTroyer, A.D., 1989. The mechanism of the inspiratory expansion of the rib cage. J. Lab. Clin. Med. 114 (2), 97.

Dietz, H.P., Clarke, B., 2005. Prevalence of rectocele in young nulliparous women. Aust. N. Z. J. Obstet. Gynaecol. 45 (5), 391.

Dietz, H.P., Korda, A., 2005. Which bowel symptoms are most strongly associated with a true rectocele? Aust. N. Z. J. Obstet. Gynaecol. 45 (6), 505.

Dietz, H.P., Lanzarone, V., 2005. Levator trauma after vaginal delivery. Obstet. Gynecol. 106 (4), 707.

Dietz, H.P., Shek, C., 2007. Levator avulsion and grading of pelvic floor muscle strength. Int. Urogynecol. J. Pelvic Floor Dysfunct. Nov 13 – epub ahead of print.

Dietz, H.P., Shek, C., 2008. Validity and reproducibility of the digital detection of levator trauma. Int. Urogynecol. J. Pelvic Floor Dysfunct. 19 (8), 1097.

Dietz, H.P., Simpson, J.M., 2007. Does delayed child-bearing increase the risk of levator injury in labour. Aust. N. Z. J. Obstet. Gynaecol. 47 (6), 491.

Dietz, H.P., Steensma, 2005. Posterior compartment prolapse on two-dimension and three-dimensional pelvic floor ultrasound: the distinction between true rectocele, perineal hypermobility and enterocele. Ultrasound Obstet. Gynecol. 26, 73.

Dietz, H.P., Steensma, A.B., 2006. The prevalence of major abnormalities of the levator ani in urogynaecological patients. Br. J. Obstet. Gynaecol. 113, 225.

Dietz, H.P., Steensma, A.B., 2006. The role of childbirth in the aetiology of rectocele. Br. J. Obstet. Gynaecol. 113, 264.

Dietz, H.P., Hyland, G., Hay-Smith, J., 2006. The assessment of levator trauma: a comparison between palpation and 4D pelvis floor ultrasound. Neurourol. Urodyn. 25, 424.

Dijkstra, P.F., Vleeming, A., Stoeckart, R., 1989. Complex motion tomography of the sacroiliac joint. An anatomical and roentgenological study. Rofo 150 (6), 635.

Doidge, N., 2007. The brain that changes itself. Stories of personal triumph from the frontiers of brain science. Penguin Books, New York.

Dommerholt, J., Myoral del Moral, O., Gröbli, C., 2006. Trigger point dry needling. Journal of Manual and Manipulative Therapy 14 (4), E70.

DonTigny, R.L., 1985. Function and pathomechanics of the sacroiliac joint: a review. Phys. Ther. 65, 35.

DonTigny, R.L., 1990. Anterior dysfunction of the sacroiliac joint as a major factor in the etiology of idiopathic low back pain syndrome. Phys. Ther. 70, 250.

DonTigny, R.L., 1997. Mechanics and treatment of the sacroiliac joint. In: Vleeming, A., Mooney, V., Dorman, T., Snijders, C., Stoeckart, R. (Eds.), Movement, stability and low back pain. Churchill Livingstone, Edinburgh, p. 461.

Dorman, T., 1994. Failure of self bracing at the sacroiliac joint: the slipping clutch syndrome. J. Orthop. Med. 16, 49.

Dorman, T., 1997. Pelvic mechanics and prolotherapy. In: Vleeming, A., Mooney, V., Dorman, T., Snijders, C., Stoeckart, R. (Eds.), Movement, stability and low back pain. Churchill Livingstone, Edinburgh, p. 501.

Dreyfuss, P., Michaelsen, M., Pauza, D., McLarty, J., Bogduk, N., 1996. The value of history and physical examination in diagnosing sacroiliac joint pain. Spine 21, 2594.

Edwards, I., Jones, M.A., 2007. Clinical reasoning and expert practice. In: Jensen, G.M., Gwyer, J., Hack, L.M., Shepard, K.F. (Eds.), Expertise in

physical therapy practice, second ed
Saunders Elsevier, St Louis.

Egund, N., Olsson, T.H., Schmid, H.,
1978. Movements in the sacro-iliac
joints demonstrated with Roentgen
stereophotogrammetry. Acta Radiol.
19, 833.

Encyclopœdia Britannica, 1981. Fifteenth
ed. vol. 7. William Benton, Chicago.

Ericsson, K.A., Smith, 1991. Towards a
general theory of expertise: prospects
and limits. Cambridge University
Press, New York.

Fabry, G., 1997. Normal and abnormal
torsional development of the lower
extremities. Acta Orthop. Belg.
63 (4), 229.

Faflia, C.P., Prassopoulos, P.K.,
Daskalogiannaki, M.E., et al., 1998.
Variations in the appearance of the
normal sacroiliac joint on pelvic CT.
Clin. Radiol. 53 (10), 742.

Falvey, E.C., Franklyn-Miller, A.,
McCrory, P.R., 2009. The groin
triangle: a patho-anatomical approach
to the diagnosis of chronic groin pain
in athletes. Br. J. Sports Med.
43, 213.

Fantl, J.A., Newman, D.K., Colling, J.,
et al., 1996. Managing acute and
chronic urinary incontinence. clinical
practice guideline, no. 2. US
Department of Health and Human
Services, Rockville, MD.

Farfan, H.F., 1973. Mechanical disorders
of the low back. Lea & Febiger,
Philadelphia.

Farfan, H.F., 1978. The biomechanical
advantage of lordosis and hip
extension for upright activity. Spine
3, 336.

Flynn, T., Fritz, J., Whitman, J., et al.,
2002. A clinical prediction rule for
classifying patients with low back pain
who demonstrate short term
improvement with spinal
manipulation. Spine 27, 2835.

Fortin, J.D., Dwyer, A., West, S., Pier, J.,
1994a. Sacroiliac joint pain referral
patterns upon application of a new
injection/arthrography technique. I:
Asymptomatic volunteers. Spine
19 (13), 1475.

Fortin, J.D., Dwyer, A., Aprill, C., et al.,
1994b. Sacroiliac joint pain referral
patterns. II: Clinical evaluation. Spine
19 (13), 1483.

Fortin, J.D., Kissling, R.O., O'Connor,
B.L., Vilensky, J.A., 1999. Sacroiliac
joint innervation and pain. Am. J.
Orthop. 28 (12), 687.

Freeman, M.A.R., Wyke, B.D., 1967.
The innervation of the knee joint: an
anatomical and histological study in
the cat. J. Anat. 101, 505.

Fritz, J.M., 2009. Clinical prediction
rules in physical therapy: coming of
age? J. Orthop. Sports Phys. Ther.
39 (3), 159.

Fritz, J.M., Childs, J.D., Flynn, T.W.,
2005. Pragmatic application of a
clinical prediction rule in primary care
to identify patients with low back
pain with a good prognosis following a
brief spinal manipulation
intervention. BMC Fam. Pract. 6, 29.

Fritz, J.M., Cleland, J.A., Childs, J.D.,
2007. Subgrouping patients with
low back pain: evolution of a
classification approach to physical
therapy. J. Orthop. Sports Phys.
Ther. 37 (6), 290.

Fryette, H.H., 1954. Principles of
osteopathic technique. American
Academy of Osteopathy, Colorado.

Gamble, J.G., Simmons, S.C.,
Freedman, M., 1986. The symphysis
pubis. Anatomic and pathologic
considerations. Clin. Orthop. Relat.
Res. (203), 261.

Gandevia, S.C., 1992. Some central
and peripheral factors affecting
human motorneuronal output in
neuromuscular fatigue. Sports Med.
13 (2), 93.

Ganz, R., Parvizi, J., Beck, M., et al.,
2003. Femoroacetabular
impingement: a cause for
osteoarthritis of the hip. Clin.
Orthop. Relat. Res. 417, 112.

Gerlach, U.J., Lierse, W., 1992.
Functional construction of the
sacroiliac ligamentous apparatus.
Acta Anat. (Basel) 144, 97.

Gibbons, S., Comerford, M.,
Emerson, P., 2002. Rehabilitation
of the stability function of psoas
major. Orthopaedic Division Review
Jan/Feb, 9.

Gifford, L., 1998. Pain, the tissues and
the nervous system: a conceptual
model. Physiotherapy 84 (1), 27.

Gill, N.W., Teyhen, D.S., Lee, I.E., 2007.
Improved contraction of the
transversus abdominis immediately
following spinal manipulation: a case
study using real-time ultrasound
imaging. Man. Ther. 12 (3), 280–285.

Gilmore, J., 1998. Groin pain in
the soccer athlete: fact, fiction
and treatment. Clin. Sports Med.
17, 787.

Gilmore, K.L., 1986. Biomechanics of
the lumbar motion segment. In:
Grieve, G.P. (Ed.), Modern manual
therapy of the vertebral column.
Churchill Livingstone, Edinburgh,
p. 103.

Gladwell, M.B., 2005. The power of
thinking without thinking. Little,
Brown and Company, New York.

Goldthwait, J.E., Osgood, R.B., 1905.
A consideration of the pelvic
articulations from an anatomical,
pathological and clinical standpoint.
Boston Medical and Surgical Journal
152, 593.

Gombatto, S.P., Collins, D.R.,
Sahrmann, S.A., Engsberg, J.R., Van
Dillen, L.R., 2007. Patterns of lumbar
region movement during trunk lateral
bending in 2 subgroups of people with
low back pain. Phys. Ther. 87 (4),
441.

Goodall, J., 1979. Life and death at
Gombe. National Geographic
155 (5), 59.

Gracovetsky, S., 1997. Linking the spinal
engine with the legs: a theory of
human gait. In: Vleeming, A.,
Mooney, V., Dorman, T.,
Snijders, C., Stoeckart, R. (Eds.),
Movement, stability and low back
pain. Churchill Livingstone,
Edinburgh, p. 243.

Gracovetsky, S., Farfan, H.F., 1986. The
optimum spine. Spine 11, 543.

Gracovetsky, S., Farfan, H.F., Lamy, C.,
1981. The mechanism of the lumbar
spine. Spine 6, 249.

Gracovetsky, S., Farfan, H., Helluer, C.,
1985. The abdominal mechanism.
Spine 10, 317.

Gräßel, D., Prescher, A., Fitzek, S., von
Keyserlingk, D.G., Axer, H., 2005.
Anisotropy of human linea alba: a
biomechanical study. J. Surg. Res.
124, 118.

Greenman, P.E., 1990. Clinical aspects of
sacroiliac function in walking. Journal
of Manual Medicine 5, 125.

Greenman, P.E., 1997. Clinical aspects of
the sacroiliac joint in walking. In:
Vleeming, A., Mooney, V.,
Dorman, T., Snijders, C.,
Stoeckart, R. (Eds.), Movement,
stability and low back pain. Churchill
Livingstone, Edinburgh, p. 235.

Grenier, S.G., McGill, S.M., 2007.
Quantification of lumbar stability by
using 2 different abdominal activation
strategies. Arch. Phys. Med. Rehabil.
88, 54.

Grieve, G.P., 1981. Common vertebral joint problems. Churchill Livingstone, Edinburgh.

Grieve, G.P., 1986. Modern manual therapy of the vertebral column. Churchill Livingstone, Edinburgh.

Grob, K.R., Neuhuber, W.L., Kissling, R.O., 1995. Innervation of the sacroiliac joint of the human. Z. Rheumatol. 54, 117.

Gunn, C.C., 1996. The Gunn approach to the treatment of chronic pain. Intramuscular stimulation for myofascial pain of radicolopathic origin. Churchill Livingstone, New York.

Gutke, A., Ostgaard, H.C., Oberg, B., 2007. Predicting persistent pregnancy-related lumbopelvic pain. In: Proceedings from the Sixth Interdisciplinary World Congress on Low Back and Pelvic Pain, 6.

Guyatt, G., Cairns, J., Churchill, D., et al., 1992. ['Evidence-Based Medicine Working Group'] Evidence-based medicine. A new approach to teaching the practice of medicine. J. Am. Med. Assoc. 268, 2420.

Hagen, R., 1974. Pelvic girdle relaxation from an orthopaedic point of view. Acta Orthop. Scand. 45, 550.

Hall, C.M., Brody, L.T., 1999. Therapeutic exercise – moving toward function. Lippincott/Williams & Wilkins, Philadelphia.

Hanson, P., Sonesson, B., 1994. The anatomy of the iliolumbar ligament. Arch. Phys. Med. Rehabil. 75, 1245.

Hebb, D.O., 1949. The organization of behavior: a neuropsychological theory. John Wiley & Sons, New York.

Herzog, W., Read, L., Conway, P.J.W., Shaw, L.D., McEwen, M.C., 1989. Reliability of motion palpation procedures to detect sacroiliac joint fixations. Journal of Manipulative and Physical Therapy 12 (2), 86.

Hewitt, J.D., Glisson, R.R., Guilak, F., Parker Vail, T., 2002. The mechanical properties of the human hip capsule ligaments. J. Arthroplasty 17 (1), 82.

Hides, J.A., Richardson, C.A., Jull, G.A., 1995a. Magnetic resonance imaging and ultrasonography of the lumbar multifidus muscle; comparison of two different modalities. Spine 20 (1), 54.

Hides, J.A., Richardson, C.A., Jull, G.A., 1996. Multifidus recovery is not automatic following resolution of acute first episode low back pain. Spine 21 (23), 2763.

Hides, J.A., Stokes, M.J., Saide, M., Jull, G.A., Cooper, D.H., 1994. Evidence of lumbar multifidus muscles wasting ipsilateral to symptoms in patients with acute/subacute low back pain. Spine 19 (2), 165.

Hides, J., Gilmore, C., Stanton, W., Bohlscheid, E., 2008. Multifidus size and symmetry among chronic LBP and healthy asymptomatic subjects. Man. Ther. 13 (1), 43.

Higgs, J., 2004. Educational theory and principles related to learning clinical reasoning. In: Jones, M.A., Rivett, D.A. (Eds.), Clinical reasoning for manual therapists. Elsevier, Edinburgh.

Higgs J Jones, M., 2000. Clinical reasoning in the health professions. In: Higgs, J., Jones, M.P. (Eds.), Clinical reasoning in the health professions, second ed. Butterworth-Heinemann, Oxford, p. 3.

Higgs, J., Titchen, A., 1995. Propositional, professional and personal knowledge in clinical reasoning. In: Higgs, J., Jones, M. (Eds.), Clinical reasoning in the health professions, second ed. Butterworth-Heinemann, Oxford, p. 129.

Hilton, P.S.L, Stanton, 1983. Urethral pressure measurement by micro-transducer: the results in symptom-free women and in those with genuine stress incontinence. Br. J. Obstet. Gynaecol. 90, 919.

Hodges, P.W., 1997. Feedforward contraction of transversus abdominis is not influenced by the direction of arm movement. Exp. Brain Res. 114, 362.

Hodges, P.W., 2001. Changes in motor planning of feedforward postural responses of the trunk muscles in low back pain. Exp. Brain Res. 141, 261.

Hodges, P.W., 2003. Neuromechanical control of the spine. PhD thesis, Karolinska Institutet, Stockholm, Sweden.

Hodges, P.W., 2005. Why do exercise interventions work for low back pain? In: Proceedings of the Second International Conference on Movement Dysfunction, Pain & Performance: Evidence & Effect. Edinburgh.

Hodges, P.W., Butler, J.E., McKenzie, D.K., Gandevia, S.C., 1997. Contraction of the human diaphragm during rapid postural adjustments. J. Physiol. 505 (2), 539.

Hodges, P.W., Cholewicki, J.J., 2007. Functional control of the spine. In: Vleeming, A., Mooney, V., Stoeckart, R. (Eds.), Movement, stability and lumbopelvic pain, second ed. churchill Livingstone, Edinburgh, p. 489.

Hodges, P.W., Cresswell, A.G., Daggfeldt, K., et al., 2000. Three dimensional preparatory trunk motion precedes asymmetrical upper limb movement. Gait Posture 11, 92.

Hodges, P.W., Cresswell, A.G., Daggfeldt, K., Thorstensson, A., 2001a. In vivo measurement of the effect of intra-abdominal pressure on the human spine. J. Biomech. 34, 347.

Hodges, P.W., Cresswell, A.G., Thorstensson, A., 1999. Preparatory trunk motion accompanies rapid upper limb movement. Exp. Brain Res. 124, 69.

Hodges, P.W., Cresswell, A.G., Thorstensson, A., 2001b. Perturbed upper limb movements cause short-latency postural responses in trunk muscles. Exp. Brain Res. 138, 243.

Hodges, P.W., Eriksson, A.E.M., Shirley, D., Gandevia, S.C., 2005. Intra-abdominal pressure increases stiffness of the lumbar spine. J. Biomech. 38, 1873.

Hodges, P.W., Ferreira, P.H., Ferreira, M.L., 2009. Lumbar spine: treatment of instability and disorders of movement control. In: Magee, D.J., Zachazewski, J.E., Quillen, W.S. (Eds.), Pathology and intervention in musculoskeletal rehabilitation. Saunders Elsevier, St Louis, p. 389.

Hodges, P.W., Gandevia, S.C., 2000a. Changes in intra-abdominal pressure during postural and respiratory activation of the human diaphragm. J. Appl. Physiol. 89, 967.

Hodges, P.W., Gandevia, S.C., 2000b. Activation of the human diaphragm during a repetitive postural task. J. Physiol. 522 (1), 165.

Hodges, P.W., Heinjnen, I., Gandevia, S.C., 2001c. Postural activity of the diaphragm is reduced in humans when respiratory demand increases. J. Physiol. 537 (3), 999.

Hodges, P.W., Holm, A.K., Hansson, T., et al., 2006. Rapid atrophy of the lumbar multifidus follows experimental disc or nerve root injury. Spine 31 (25), 2926.

Hodges, P.W., Kaigle Holm, A., Holm, S., et al., 2003a. Intervertebral stiffness of the spine is increased by evoked contraction of transversus abdominis and the diaphragm: in vivo porcine studies. Spine 28 (23), 2594.

Hodges, P.W., Moseley, G.L., 2003. Pain and motor control of the lumbopelvic region: effect and possible mechanisms. J. Electromyogr. Kinesiol. 13, 361.

Hodges, P.W., Moseley, G.L., Bagrielsson, A., 2003b. Experimental muscle pain changes feedforward postural responses of the trunk muscles. Exp. Brain Res. 151, 262.

Hodges, P.W., Richardson, C.A., 1996. Inefficient muscular stabilization of the lumbar spine associated with low back pain: a motor control evaluation of transversus abdominis. Spine 21 (22), 2640.

Hodges, P.W., Richardson, C.A., 1997. Contraction of the abdominal muscles associated with movement of the lower limb. Phys. Ther. 77, 132.

Hodges, P.W., Sapsford, R., Pengel, L.H.M., 2007. Postural and respiratory functions of the pelvic floor muscles. Neurourol. Urodyn. 26 (3), 362.

Howard, D., Miller, J.M., DeLancey, J.O.L., et al., 2000. Differential effects of cough, Valsalva, and continence status on vesical neck movement. Obstet. Gynecol. 95 (4), 535.

Hungerford, B., Gilleard, W., Hodges, P., 2003. Evidence of altered lumbopelvic muscle recruitment in the presence of sacroiliac joint pain. Spine 28 (14), 1593.

Hungerford, B., Gilleard, W., Lee, D., 2004. Alteration of pelvic bone motion determined in subjects with posterior pelvic pain using skin markers. Clin. Biomech. (Bristol, Avon) (19), 456.

Hungerford, B., Gilleard, W., Moran, M., et al., 2007. Evaluation of the reliability of therapists to palpate intra-pelvic motion using the stork test on the support side. J. Phys. Ther. 87 (7), 879.

Hunt, D., Clohisy, J., Prather, H., 2007. Acetabular labral tears of the hip in women. Phys. Med. Rehabil. Clin. N. Am. 18, 497.

Indahl, A., Kaigle, A.M., Reikeras, O., et al., 1997. Interaction between the porcine lumbar intervertebral disc, zygapophysial joints, and paraspinal muscles. Spine 22 (24), 2834.

Indahl, A., Kaigle, A., Reikeras, O., et al., 1995. Electromyographic response of the porcine multifidus musculature after nerve stimulation. Spine 20 (24), 2652.

Indahl, A., Kaigle, A., Reikeras, O., et al., 1999. Sacroiliac joint involvement in activation of the porcine spinal and gluteal musculature. J. Spinal Disord. 12 (4), 325.

Inman, V.T., Ralston, H.J., Todd, F., 1981. Human walking. Williams & Wilkins, Baltimore.

Intolo, P., Milosavljevic, S., Baxter, D.G., et al., 2009. The effect of age on lumbar range of motion: a systematic review. Man. Ther. 14 (6), 596.

Jacob, H.A.C., Kissling, R.O., 1995. The mobility of the sacroiliac joints in healthy volunteers between 20 and 50 years of age. Clin. Biomech. (Bristol, Avon) 10 (7), 352.

Janda, V., 1978. Muscles, central nervous motor regulation and back problems. In: Korr, I. (Ed.), The neurobiologic mechanisms in manipulative therapy. Plenum Press, London, p. 27.

Janda, V., 1986. Muscle weakness and inhibition (pseudoparesis) in back pain syndromes. In: Grieve, G.P. (Ed.), Modern manual therapy of the vertebral column. Churchill Livingstone, Edinburgh, p. 197.

Jarcho, J., 1929. Value of Walcher position in contracted pelvis with special reference to its effect on true conjugate diameter. Surg. Gynecol. Obstet. 49, 854.

Jensen, G.M., Gwyer, J., Hack, L.M., Shepard, K.F., 2007. Expertise in physical therapy practice, second ed. Saunders, St Louis.

Jones, M.A., Rivett, D., 2004. Introduction to clinical reasoning. In: Jones, M.A., Rivett, D.A. (Eds.), Clinical reasoning for manual therapists. Elsevier, Edinburgh, p. 3.

Kaigle, A.M., Wessberg, P., Hansson, T.H., 1998. Muscular and kinematic behavior of the lumbar spine during flexion-extension. J. Spinal Disord. 11 (2), 163.

Kampen, W.U., Tillmann, B., 1998. Age-related changes in the articular cartilage of human sacroiliac joint. Anat. Embryol. (Berlin) 198 (6), 505.

Kang, C.H., Shin, M.J., Kim, S.M., et al., 2007. MRI of paraspinal muscles in lumbar degenerative kyphosis patients and control patients with

chronic low back pain. Clin. Radiol. 62 (5), 479.

Kang, Y.M., Choi, W.S., Pickar, J.G., 2002. Electrophysiologic evidence for an intersegmental reflex pathway between lumbar paraspinal tissues. Spine 27 (3), E56.

Kapandji, I.A., 1970. The physiology of the joints II: the lower limb, second ed. Churchill Livingstone, Edinburgh.

Kapandji, I.A., 1974. The physiology of the joints III: the trunk and vertebral column, second ed. Churchill Livingstone, Edinburgh.

Kassarjian, A., Brisson, M., Palmer, W.E., 2007. Femoroacetabular impingement. Eur. J. Radiol. 63, 29.

Kavcic, N., Grenier, S., McGill, S.M., 2004. Determining the stabilizing role of individual torso muscles during rehabilitation exercises. Spine 29 (11), 1254.

Keagy, R.D., Brumlik, J., 1966. Direct electromyography of the psoas major muscle in man. J. Bone Joint Surg. 48A, 1377.

Kendall, F.P., Kendall McCreary, E., Provance, P.G., 1993. Muscles testing and function, fourth ed. Williams & Wilkins, Baltimore.

Kerry, R., 2009. Clinical reasoning in combined movement theory. In: McCarthy, C. (Ed.), Combined movement theory: rational mobilization and manipulation of the vertebral column. Elsevier (in press).

Kerry, R., Maddocks, M., Mumford, S., 2008. Philosophy of science and physiotherapy: an insight into practice. Physiother. Theory Pract. 24 (6), 1.

Kirkaldy-Willis, W.H. (Ed.), 1983. Managing low back pain. Churchill Livingstone, New York.

Kirkaldy-Willis, W.H., Hill, R.J., 1979. A more precise diagnosis for low back pain. Spine 4, 102.

Kirkaldy-Willis, W.H., Wedge, J.H., Yong-Hing, K., et al., 1978. Pathology and pathogenesis of lumbar spondylosis and stenosis. Spine 3, 319.

Kjaer, P., Bendix, T., Sorensen, J.S., et al., 2007. Are MRI-defined fat infiltrations in the multifidus muscles associated with low back pain? BCM Med. 5, 2.

Knox, 2002. The functional anatomy of the thoracolumbar fascia and associated muscles and ligaments.

Masters Thesis. Unviersity of Otago, Dunedin, New Zealand.

Koes, B.W., van Tulder, M.W., Ostelo, R., et al., 2001. Clinical guidelines for the management of low back pain in primary care: an international comparison. Spine 26, 2504.

Kristiansson, P., 1997. S-Relaxin and pelvic pain in pregnant women. In: Vleeming, A., Mooney, V., Dorman, T., Snijders, C., Stoeckart, R. (Eds.), Movement, stability and low back pain. Churchill Livingstone, Edinburgh, p. 421.

Kunduracioglu, B., Yilmaz, C., Yorubulut, M., Kudas, S., 2007. Magnetic resonance findings of osteitis pubis. J. Magn. Reson. Imaging 25, 535.

Laslett, M., Aprill, C.H., McDonald, B., et al., 2005. Diagnosis of sacroiliac joint pain: validity of individual provocation tests and composites of tests. Man. Ther. 10, 207.

Laslett, M., Williams, W., 1994. The reliability of selected pain provocation tests for sacroiliac joint pathology. Spine 19 (11), 1243.

Lavignolle, B., Vital, J.M., Senegas, J., et al., 1983. An approach to the functional anatomy of the sacroiliac joints in vivo. Anat. Clin. 5, 169.

Lawrence, J.S., Bremner, J.M., Bier, F., 1966. Osteoarthrosis: prevalence in the population and relationship between symptoms and X-ray changes. Ann. Rheum. Dis. 25, 1.

Lawson, T.L., Foley, W.D., Carrera, G.F., Berland, L.L., 1982. The sacroiliac joints: anatomic, plain roentgenographic, and computed tomographic analysis. J. Comput. Assist. Tomogr. 6 (2), 307.

Leboeuf-Yde, C., Lauritsen, J.M., Lauritzen, T., 1997. Why has the search for causes of low back pain largely been inconclusive? Spine 22 (8), 877.

Lee, D.G., 1992. Intra-articular versus extra-articular dysfunction of the sacroiliac joint – a method of differentiation. In: IFOMT Proceedings, 5th international conference. Vail, Colorado, p. 69.

Lee, D.G., 1993. Biomechanics of the thorax: a clinical model of in vivo function. Journal of Manual and Manipulative Therapy 1, 13.

Lee, D.G., 1999. The pelvic girdle, second ed. Churchill Livingstone, Edinburgh.

Lee, D.G., 2002. The Com-Pressor. Available online at: www.dianelee.ca or www.optp.com.

Lee, D.G., 2003. The thorax – an integrated approach. Diane G. Lee Physiotherapist Corporation, Surrey, Canada. Available online at: www.dianelee.ca. www.discoverphysio.ca.

Lee, D.G., 2004. The pelvic girdle, third ed. Churchill Livingstone, Edinburgh.

Lee, D.G., 2006. Foreword. In: Morris, C.E. (Ed.), Low back syndromes. Integrated clinical management. McGraw-Hill, New York, p. xvii.

Lee, D.G., 2007a. The evolution of myths and facts regarding function and dysfunction of the pelvic girdle. In: Vleeming, A., Mooney, V., Stoeckart, R. (Eds.), Movement, stability and lumbopelvic pain: integration of research and therapy, second ed. Churchill Livinstone, Edinburgh.

Lee, D.G., 2007b. Clinical expertise in evidence-based practice for pelvic girdle pain – show me the patient!. In: Proceedings from the Sixth Interdisciplinary World Congress on Low Back and Pelvic Pain, Barcelona, November, p. 27.

Lee, D.G., Lee, L.J., 2004a. An integrated approach to the assessment and treatment of the lumbopelvic-hip region. Available online at www.discoverphysio.ca. www.dianelee.ca.

Lee, D.G., Lee, L.J., 2004b. Stress urinary incontinence – a consequence of failed load transfer through the pelvis? In: Proceedings from the 5th Interdisciplinary World Congress on Low Back and Pelvic Pain, Melbourne, Australia, p. 138.

Lee, D.G., Lee, L.J., 2006. Postpartum health for moms – restoring form and function after pregnancy. Available online at www.discoverphysio.ca.

Lee, D.G., Lee, L.J., 2007. Bridging the gap: the role of the pelvic floor in musculoskeletal and urogynecological function. In: Proceedings of the World Physical Therapy Conference, Vancouver, Canada.

Lee, D.G., Lee, L.J., 2008a. Integrated, multimodal approach to the treatment of pelvic girdle pain and dysfunction. In: Magee, D.J.,

Zachazewski, J.E., Quillen, W.S. (Eds.), Pathology and intervention in musculoskeletal rehabilitation. Elsevier, Saunders, p. 473.

Lee, D.G., Lee, L.J., McLaughlin, L.M., 2008a. Stability, continence and breathing: the role of fascia following pregnancy and delivery. Journal of Bodywork and Movement Therapies 12, 333.

Lee, D.G., Vleeming, A., 1998. Impaired load transfer through the pelvic girdle – a new model of altered neutral zone function. In: Proceedings from the 3rd Interdisciplinary World Congress on Low Back and Pelvic Pain. Vienna, Austria.

Lee, D.G., Vleeming, A., 2004. The management of pelvic joint pain and dysfunction. In: Boyling, J.D., Jull, G. (Eds.), Grieve's modern manual therapy. The vertebral column, third ed. Elsevier, Churchill Livingstone, p. 495.

Lee, D.G., Vleeming, A., 2007. An integrated therapeutic approach to the treatment of pelvic girdle pain. In: Vleeming, A., Mooney, V., Stoeckart, R. (Eds.), Movement, stability and lumbopelvic pain, second ed. Elsevier, Edinburgh, p. 621.

Lee, L.J., 2003. Restoring force closure/ motor control of the thorax. In: Lee, D. (Ed.), The thorax – an integrated approach. Available online at www.dianelee.ca.

Lee, L.J., Chang, A.T., Coppieters, M. W., Hodges, P.W., 2010. Changes in sitting posture induce multiplanar changes in chest wall shape and motion with breathing. Respir. Physiol. Neurobiol. 170 (3), 236.

Lee, L.J., Coppieters, M.W., Hodges, P.W., 2009. Anticipatory postural adjustments to arm movement reveal complex control of paraspinal muscles in the thorax. J. Electromyogr. Kinesiol. 19 (1), 46.

Lee, L.J., Lee, D.L., 2008b. Integrated, multimodal approach to the thoracic spine and ribs. In: Magee, D.J., Zachazewski, J.E., Quillen, W.S. (Eds.), Pathology and intervention in musculoskeletal rehabilitation. Saunders, Elsevier, p. 306.

Lee, M.W.L., McPhee, R.W., Stringer, M.D., 2008b. An evidence-based approach to human dermatomes. Clin. Anat. 21, 363.

Leffler, K.S., Thompson, J.R., Cundiff, G.W., et al., 2001. Attachment of the rectovaginal septum to the pelvic sidewall. Am. J. Obstet. Gynecol. 185 (1), 41.

Leong, J.C.Y., Luk, D.K., Chow, D.H.K., Woo, C.W., 1987. The biomechanical functions of the iliolumbar ligament in maintaining stability of the lumbosacral junction. Spine 12, 669.

Lesher, J.M., Dreyfuss, P., Hager, N., 2008. Hip joint pain referral patterns: a descriptive study. Pain Med. 9 (1), 22.

Levin, S.M., 1997. A different approach to the mechanics of the human pelvis: tensegrity. In: Vleeming, A., Mooney, V., Dorman, T., Snijders, C., Stoeckart, R. (Eds.), Movement, stability and low back pain. Churchill Livingstone, Edinburgh, p. 157.

Loeser, J.D., Treede, R., 2008. The Kyoto protocol of IASP basic pain terminology. Pain 137, 477.

Lovejoy, C.O., 2007. Evolution of the human lumbopelvic region and its relationship to some clinical deficits of the spine and pelvis. In: Vleeming, A., Mooney, V., Stoeckart, R. (Eds.), Movement, stability and lumbopelvic pain, second ed. Churchill Livingstone, Edinburgh, p. 141.

Lovett, R.W., 1903. A contribution to the study of the mechanics of the spine. Am. J. Anat. 2, 457.

Lucas, D., Bresler, B., 1961. Stability of the ligamentous spine. In: Technical report no. 40. Biomechanics Laboratory, University of California, San Francisco.

Luk, K.D.K., Ho, H.C., Leong, J.C.Y., 1986. The iliolumbar ligament: a study of its anatomy, development and clinical significance. J. Bone Joint Surg. 68B, 197.

Lund, P.J., Drupinski, E.A., Brooks, W.J., 1996. Ultrasound evaluation of sacroiliac motion in normal volunteers. Acad. Radiol. 3, 192.

Lynch, F.W., 1920. The pelvic articulations during pregnancy, labor, and the puerperium. Surg. Gynecol. Obstet. 30, 575.

MacConaill, M.A., Basmajian, J.V., 1977. Muscles and movements; a basis for human kinesiology, second ed. Krieger, New York.

MacDonald, D.A., Moseley, G.L., Hodges, P.W., 2006. The lumbar multifidus: does the evidence support clinical beliefs? Man. Ther. 11 (4), 254.

MacDonald, D., Moseley, G.L., Hodges, P.W., 2009. Why do some patients keep hurting their back? Evidence of ongoing back muscle dysfunction during remission from recurrent back pain. Pain 142 (3), 183.

MacDonald, G.R., Hunt, T.E., 1951. Sacro-iliac joint observations on the gross and histological changes in the various age groups. Can. Med. Assoc. J. 66, 157.

MacIntosh, J.E., Bogduk, N., 1991. The attachments of the lumbar erector spinae. Spine 16 (7), 783.

MacNab, I., 1977. Backache. Williams & Wilkins, Baltimore.

Magee, D.J., Zachazewski, J.E., Quillen, W.S., 2007. Scientific foundations and principles of practice in musculoskeletal rehabilitation. Saunders Elsevier, St Louis.

Magee, D.J., Zachazewski, J.E., Quillen, W.S., 2009. Pathology and intervention in musculoskeletal rehabilitation. Saunders Elsevier, St Louis.

Magora, A., Schwartz, A., 1976. Relation between the low back pain syndrome and x-ray findings 1. Degenerative osteoarthritis. Scand. J. Rehabil. Med. 8, 115.

Magnusson, M.L., Aleksiev, A., Wilder, D.G., et al., 1996. Unexpected load and asymmetric posture as etiologic factors in low back pain. European Spine Society – the AcroMed Prize for Spinal Research 1995. Eur. Spine J. 5 (1), 23.

Mahncke, H.W., Bronstone, A., Merzinich, M.M., 2006. Brain plasticity and functional losses in the aged: scientific bases for a novel intervention. Prog. Brain Res. 157, 81.

Maigne, J.Y., 1997. Lateral dynamic X-rays in the sitting position and coccygeal discography in common coccydynia. In: Vleeming, A., Mooney, V., Dorman, T., Snijders, C., Stoeckart, R. (Eds.), Movement, stability and low back pain. Churchill Livingstone, Edinburgh, p. 385.

Maigne, J.Y., Aivaliklis, A., Pfefer, F., 1996. Results of sacroiliac joint double block and value of sacroiliac pain provocation tests in 54 patients with low back pain. Spine 21, 1889.

Marin Valladolid, J.A., Saudedo Ortiz, J. A., Orozco, C.F., et al., 2004. Variation of intraabdominal pressure caused by abdominoplasty in healthy women. Rev. Gastroenterol. Mex. 69 (3), 156.

Marnach, M.L., Ramin, K.D., Ramsey, P.S., et al., 2003. Characterization of the relationship between joint laxity and maternal hormones in pregnancy. Obstet. Gynecol. 101 (2), 331.

Masani, K., Sin, V.W., Vette, A.H., et al., 2009. Postural reactions of the trunk muscles to multi-directional perturbations in sitting. Clin. Biomech. (Bristol, Avon) 24 (2), 176.

Mason, J.B., 2001. Acetabular labrum tears. Diagnosis and treatment. Clin. Sports Med. 20, 779.

McCarthy, J., Nable, P., Alusio, F.V., et al., 2003. Anatomy, pathologic features and treatment of acetabular labral tears. Clin. Orthop. Relat. Res. 403, 38.

McGill, S., 2002. Low back disorders – evidence-based prevention and rehabilitation. Human Kinetics, Canada.

McGill, S.M., Cholewicki, J.J., 2001. Biomechanical basis for stability: an explanation to enhance clinical utility. J. Orthop. Sports Phys. Ther. 31, 96.

McGill, S.M., Stuart, M., 2004. Linking latest knowledge of injury mechanisms and spine function to the prevention of low back disorders. J. Electromyogr. Kinesiol. 14 (1), 43.

McGill, S.M., Grenier, S., Kavcic, N., et al., 2003. Coordination of muscle activity to assure stability of the lumbar spine. J. Electromyogr. Kinesiol. 13, 353.

McKenzie, R.A., 1981. The lumbar spine: mechanical diagnosis and therapy. Spinal Publications, Wellington, New Zealand.

McLain, R.F., Pickar, J.G., 1998. Mechanoreceptor endings in human thoracic and lumbar facet joints. Spine 23 (2), 168.

McLauchlan, G.J., Gardner, D.L., 2002. Sacral and iliac articular cartilage thickness and cellularity: relationship to subchondral bone end-plate thickness and cencellous bone density. Rheumatology 41, 375.

McLaughlin, L.M., 2008. The role of focused manipulation in back pain. Presented at: North American Institute of Orthopaedic Manipulative Therapy Symposium on Spinal Manipulation, Portland, OR.

McNeill, A.R., 1997. Elasticity in human and animal backs. In: Vleeming, A., Mooney, V., Dorman, T., Snijders, C., Stoeckart, R. (Eds.), Movement, stability and low back pain. Churchill Livingstone, Edinburgh, p. 227.

Meijne, W., van Neerbos, K., Aufdemkampe, G., et al., 1999. Intraexaminer and interexaminer reliability of the Gillet test. J. Manipulative Physiol. Ther. 22 (1), 4.

Meisenbach, R.O., 1911. Sacro-iliac relaxation; with analysis of eighty-four cases. Surg. Gynecol. Obstet. 12, 411.

Melzack, R., 2001. Pain and the neuromatrix in the brain. J. Dent. Educ. 65 (12), 1378.

Melzack, R., 2005. Evolution of the neuromatrix theory of pain. The Prithvi Raj Lecture: Presented at the third World Congress of World Institute of Pain, Barcelona, 2004. Pain Pract. 5 (2), 85.

Melzack, R., Wall, P.D., 1965. Pain mechanisms: a new theory. Science 150, 971.

Mens, J.M.A., Vleeming, A., Snijders, C.J., Koes, B.J., Stam, H.J., 2001. Reliability and validity of the active straight leg raise test in posterior pelvic pain since pregnancy. Spine 26 (10), 1167.

Mens, J.M.A., Vleeming, A., Snijders, C.J., Stam, H.J., Ginai, A.Z., 1999. The active straight leg raising test and mobility of the pelvic joints. Eur. Spine J. 8, 468.

Mens, J.M., Vleeming, A., Snijders, C.J., Koes, B.W., Stam, H.J., 2002. Validity of the active straight leg raise test for measuring disease severity in patients with posterior pelvic pain after pregnancy. Spine 27 (2), 196.

Merskey, H., Bogduk, N. (Eds.), 1994. Classification of chronic pain: descriptions of chronic pain syndromes and definitions of pain terms, second ed. Prepared by the Task Force on Taxonomy of the International Association for the Study of Pain. IASP Press, Seattle, USA.

Merzenich, M., Wright, B., Jenkins, W., et al., 1996. Cortical plasticity underlying perceptual, motor, and cognitive skill development: implications for neurorehabilitation. Cold Spring Harb. Symp. Quant. Biol. 61, 1–8.

Meyer, G.H., 1878. Der Mechanismus der Symphysis sacroiliaca. Archiv für Anatomie und Physiologie 1, 1.

Mezirow, J., 1990. Fostering critical reflection in adulthood: a guide to transformative and emancipator learning. Jossey-Bass, San Francisco.

Miller, J.A.A., Schultz, A.B., Andersson, G.B.J., 1987. Load-displacement behavior of sacro-iliac joints. J. Orthop. Res. 5, 92.

Miller, W.R., Rollnick, S., 2002. Motivational interviewing: preparing people for change, second ed. Guilford Press, New York.

Mixter, W.J., Barr, J.S., 1934. Rupture of intervertebral disc with involvement of the spinal cord. N. Engl. J. Med. 211, 210.

Mok, N.W., Brauer, S.G., Hodges, P.W., 2007. Failure to use movement in postural strategies leads to increased spinal displacement in low back pain. Spine 32 (19), E537.

Mørkved, S., Salvesen, K.A., Bø, K., et al., 2004. Pelvic floor muscle strength and thickness in continent and incontinent nulliparous pregnant women. Int. Urogynecol. J. Pelvic Floor Dysfunct. 15, 384.

Morris, D.M., Taub, E., Mark, V.W., 2006. Constraint-induced movement therapy: characterizing the intervention protocol. Eura. Medicophys. 42 (3), 257.

Moseley, G.L., 2002. Combined physiotherapy and education is efficacious for chronic low back pain. Aust. J. Physiother. 48, 297.

Moseley, G.L., 2003a. A pain neuromatrix approach to patients with chronic pain. Man. Ther. 8 (3), 130.

Moseley, G.L., 2003b. Unraveling the barriers to reconceptualization of the problem in chronic pain: the actual and perceived ability of patients and health professionals to understand the neurophysiology. J. Pain 4 (4), 184.

Moseley, G.L., 2007a. Motor control in chronic pain: new idea for effective intervention. In: Vleeming, A., Mooney, V., Stoeckart, R. (Eds.), Movement, stability and lumbopelvic pain, second ed. Elsevier, Edinburgh, p. 513.

Moseley, G.L., 2007b. Reconceptualising pain according to modern pain science. Phys. Ther. Rev. 12, 169.

Moseley, G.L., Hodges, P.W., 2004. Are the changes in postural control associated with low back pain caused by pain interference? Clin. J. Pain 21 (4), 323.

Moseley, G.L., Hodges, P.W., 2005. Chronic pain and motor control. In: Jull, G., Boyling, J. (Eds.), Grieve's modern manual therapy. The vertebral column. Churchill Livingstone, Edinburgh, p. 215.

Moseley, G.L., Hodges, P.W., Gandevia, S.C., 2002. Deep and superficial fibers of the lumbar multifidus muscle are differentially active during voluntary arm movements. Spine 27 (2), E29.

Moseley, G.L., Hodges, P.W., Gandevia, S.C., 2003. External perturbation of the trunk in standing humans differentially activates components of the medial back muscles. J. Physiol. 547 (2), 581.

Moucha, R., Kilgard, M.P., 2006. Cortical plasticity and rehabilitation. Prog. Brain Res. 157, 111.

Myers, T.W., 2001. Anatomy trains. Churchill Livingstone, Edinburgh.

Nachemson, A., 1999. Back pain; delimiting the problem in the next millennium. Int. J. Law Psychiatry 22 (5-6), 473.

Nelson, H., Jurmain, R., 1985. Introduction to physical anthropology, third ed. West Publishing, St Paul.

Neumann, P., Gill, V., 2002. Pelvic floor and abdominal muscle interaction: EMG activity and intra-abdmominal pressure. Int. Urogynecol. J. 13, 125.

Nygaard, I.E., Thompson, F.L., Svengalis, S.L., et al., 1994. Urinary incontinence in elite nulliparous athletes. Obstet. Gynecol. 84 (2), 183.

Orlick, T., 2008. In pursuit of excellence, fourth ed. Human Kinetics, Champaign, IL.

O'Sullivan, P., 2000. Lumbar segmental "instability": clinical presentation and specific stabilizing exercise management. Man. Ther. 5 (1), 2.

O'Sullivan, P., 2005. Diagnosis and classification of chronic low back pain disorders: maladaptive movement and motor control impairments as underlying mechanism. Man. Ther. 10 (4), 242.

O'Sullivan, P.B., Beales, D., Beetham, J. A., et al., 2002. Altered motor control strategies in subjects with sacroiliac joint pain during the active straight leg raise test. Spine 27 (1), E1.

O'Sullivan, P., Beales, D., 2007. Diagnosis and classification of pelvic girdle pain disorders – Part 1: a mechanism based approach within a biopsychosocial framework. Man. Ther. 12, 86.

Ostgaard, H.C., 1997. Lumbar back and posterior pelvic pain in pregnancy. In: Vleeming, A., Mooney, V., Dorman, T., Snijders, C., Stoeckart, R. (Eds.), Movement, stability and low back pain. Churchill Livingstone, Edinburgh, p. 411.

Ostgaard, H.C., 2007. What is pelvic girdle pain? In: Vleeming, A., Mooney, V., Stoeckart, R. (Eds.), Movement, stability and lumbopelvic pain, second ed. Elsevier, Edinburgh, p. 353.

Ostgaard, H.C., Andersson, G.B.J., Karisson, K., 1991. Prevalence of back pain in pregnancy. Spine 16, 49.

Ostgaard, H.C., Andersson, 1992. Postpartum low back pain. Spine 17 (1), 53.

Ostgaard, H.C., Zetherstrom, G., Roos-Hansson, E., 1994. The posterior pelvic pain provocation test in pregnant women. Eur. Spine J. 3, 258.

Panjabi, M.M., 1992a. The stabilizing system of the spine. Part I: function, dysfunction, adaptation, and enhancement. J. Spinal Disord. 5 (4), 383.

Panjabi, M.M., 1992b. The stabilizing system of the spine. Part II. Neutral zone and instability hypothesis. J. Spinal Disord. 5 (4), 390.

Panjabi, M.M., 2006. A hypothesis of chronic back pain: ligament subfailure injuries lead to muscle control dysfunction. Eur. Spine J. 15, 668.

Paris, S., 2000. A history of manipulative therapy through the ages and up to the current controversy in the United States Journal of Manual and Manipulative Therapy 8, 2.

Paterson, I., 1957. The torn acetabular labrum: a block to reduction of a dislocated hip. J. Bone Joint Surg. Br. 39, 306.

Pearcy, M., Tibrewal, S.B., 1984. Axial rotation and lateral bending in the normal lumbar spine measured by three-dimensional radiography. Spine 9, 582.

Pearson, N., 2007. Understand pain, live well again. Available online at www. lifeisnow.ca.

Pel, J.J.M., Spoor, C.W., Pool-Goudzwaard, A.L., et al., 2008. Biomechanical analysis of reducing sacroiliac joint shear load by optimization of pelvic muscle and ligament forces. Ann. Biomed. Eng. 36 (3), 415.

Peng, Q., Jones, R., Constantinou, C.E., 2006. 2D Ultrasound image processing in identifying responses of urogenital structures to pelvic floor muscle activity. Ann. Biomed. Eng. 34 (3), 477.

Peng, Q., Jones, R., Shishido, K., et al., 2007. Ultrasound evaluation of dynamic responses of female pelvic floor muscles. Ultrasound Med. Biol. 33 (3), 342.

Pengel, L.H., Herbert, R.D., Maher, C. G., et al., 2003. Acute low back pain: systematic review of its prognosis. Br. Med. J. 327, 323.

Peschers, U.M., Ganger, G., Schaer, G. N., et al., 2001. Bladder neck mobility in continent nulliparous women. Br. J. Obstet. Gynaecol. 108, 320.

Pettman, E., 2006. Manipulative thrust techniques: an evidence-based approach. Aphema Publishing, Abbotsford, Canada.

Pettman, E., 2007. A history of manipulative therapy. Journal of Manual and Manipulative Therapy 15 (3), 165.

Pickar, J.G., 2002. Neurophysiological effects of spinal manipulation. Spine 2 (5), 357.

Pickering, M., Jones, J.F.X., 2002. The diaphragm: two physiological muscles in one. J. Anat. 201, 305.

Pitkin, H.C., Pheasant, H.C., 1936. Sacroarthrogenetic telalagia II. A study of sacral mobility. J. Bone Joint Surg. 18, 365.

Pool-Goudzwaard, A., Hoek van Dijke, G., Mulder, P., et al., 2003. The iliolumbar ligament: its influence on stability of the sacroiliac joint.

Clin. Biomech. (Bristol, Avon) 18 (2), 99.

Pool-Goudzwaard, A., Hoek van Dijke, G., van Gurp, M., et al., 2004. Contribution of pelvic floor muscles to stiffness of the pelvic ring. Clin. Biomech. (Bristol, Avon) 19, 564.

Pool-Goudzwaard, A., Kleinrensink, G., Snijders, C.J., et al., 2001. The sacroiliac part of the iliolumbar ligament. J. Anat. 199, 457.

Pool-Goudzwaard, A., Slieker ten Hove, M.C., Vierhout, M.E., et al., 2005. Relations between pregnancy-related low back pain, pelvic floor activity and pelvic floor dysfunction. Int. Urogynecol. J. Pelvic Floor Dysfunct. 16 (6), 468.

Popper, K., 1980. The logic of scientific discovery, fourth ed. Routledge, London.

Porterfield, J.A., DeRosa, C., 1998. Mechanical low back pain. Perspective in functional anatomy. W B Saunders, Philadelphia.

Potter, N.A., Rothstein, J., 1985. Intertester reliability for selected clinical tests of the sacroiliac joint. Phys. Ther. 65 (11), 1671.

Primal Pictures, 2003. Interactive pelvis and perineum. Available online at www.primalpictures.com.

Puhakka, K.B., Melsen, F., Jurik, A.G., et al., 2004. MR imaging of the normal sacroiliac joint with correlation to histology. Skeletal Radiol. 33, 15.

Radebold, A., Cholewicki, J., Panjabi, M. M., et al., 2000. Muscle response pattern to sudden trunk loading in healthy individuals and in patients with chronic low back pain. Spine 25 (8), 947.

Radebold, A., Cholewicki, J., Polzhofer, G.K., et al., 2001. Impaired postural control of the lumbar spine is associated with delayed muscle response times in patients with chronic idiopathic low back pain. Spine 26 (7), 724.

Rath, A.M., Attali, P., Dumas, J.L., et al., 1996. The abdominal linea alba: an anatomo-radiologic and biomechanical study. Surg. Radiol. Anat. 18, 281.

Reeves, N.P., Cholewicki, J., Milner, T. E., 2005. Muscle reflex classification of low-back pain. J. Electromyogr. Kinesiol. 15 (1), 53.

Reeves, N.P., Everding, V.Q., Cholewicki, J., Morrisette, D.C.,

2006. The effects of trunk stiffness on postural control during unstable seated balance. Exp. Brain Res. 174 (4), 694.

Reeves, N.P., Narendra, K.S., Cholewicki, J., 2007. Spine stability: the six blind men and the elephant. Clin. Biomech. (Bristol, Avon) 22 (3), 266.

Reikeras, O., Bjerkrein, I., Kolbenstvedt, A., 1983. Anteversion of the acetabulum and femoral neck in normals and in patients with osteoarthritis of the hip. Acta Orthop. Scand. 54 (1), 18.

Reilly, J., Yong-Hing, K., MacKay, R.W., et al., 1978. Pathological anatomy of the lumbar spine. In: Helfet, A.J., Gruebel-Lee, D.M. (Eds.), Disorders of the lumbar spine. J B Lippincott, Philadelphia.

Resnick, D., Niwayama, G., Goergen, T. G., 1975. Degenerative disease of the sacroiliac joint. J. Invest. Radiol. 10, 608.

Retzky, S.S., Rogers, R.M., 1995. Urinary incontinence in women. Clin. Symp. 47 (3), 2.

Richardson, C.A., Jull, G.A., Hodges, P. W., Hides, J.A., 1999. Therapeutic exercise for spinal segmental stabilization in low back pain – scientific basis and clinical approach. Churchill Livingstone, Edinburgh.

Richardson, C.A., Snijders, C.J., Hides, J.A., et al., 2002. The relationship between the transversely oriented abdominal muscles, sacroiliac joint mechanics and low back pain. Spine 27 (4), 399.

Riddle, D.L., 1998. Classification and low back pain: a review of the literature and critical analysis of selected systems. Phys. Ther. 78, 708.

Rivett, D.A., Jones, M.A., 2004. Improving clinical reasoning in manual therapy. In: Jones, M.A., Rivett, D. (Eds.), Clinical reasoning for manual therapists. Elsevier, Edinburgh, p. 403.

Rizk, N.N., 1980. A new description of the anterior abdominal wall in man and mammals. J. Anat. 131, 373.

Robinson, H.S., Brox, J.I., Robinson, R., et al., 2007. The reliability of selected motion- and pain provocation tests for the sacroiliac joint. Man. Ther. 12 (1), 72.

Robinson, P., Barron, D.A., Parsons, W., et al., 2004. Adductor-related groin pain in athletes: correlation of MR imaging with clinical findings. Skeletal Radiol. 33, 451.

Rodman, P.S., McHenry, M., 1980. Bioenergetics and the origin of hominid bipedalism. Am. J. Phys. Anthropol. 52, 103.

Rodriguez, C., Miguel, A., Lima, H., Heinrichs, K., 2001. Osteitis pubis sydrome in the professional soccer athlete: a case report. J. Athl. Train. 36, 437.

Rohen, J.W., Yokochi, C., 1983. Color atlas of anatomy, a photographic study of the human body. F K Schattauer, Stuttgart/Igaku-Shoin, Tokyo.

Romer, A.S., 1959. A shorter version of the vertebrate body. W B Saunders, Philadelphia.

Rost, C.C., Jacqueline, J., Kaiser, A., et al., 2004. Pelvic pain during pregnancy, a descriptive study of sign and symptoms of 870 patients in primary care. Spine 29 (22), 2567.

Rothman, R.H., Simeone, F.A., 1975. Spine, vol. IV. W B Saunders, London.

Rousseau, M.A., Bradford, D.S., Hadi, T. M., Pedersen, K.L., Lotz, J.C., 2006. The instant axis of rotation influences facet forces at L5-S1 during flexion/ extension and lateral bending. Eur. Spine J. 15 (3), 299.

Rowinski, M.J., 1985. Afferent neurobiology of the joint. In: Gould, J.A., Davies, J.D. (Eds.), Orthopaedic and sports physical therapy. C V Mosby, St Louis, p. 50.

Sackett, D.L., Straus, S., Richardson, W.S., Rosenberg, R.B., 2000. Evidence-based medicine. How to practice and teach EBM. Elsevier Science, New York.

Sahrmann, S., 2001. Diagnosis and treatment of movement impaired syndromes. Mosby, St Louis.

Sahrmann, S.A., 1988. Diagnosis by the physical therapist – a prerequisite for treatment. Phys. Ther. 68 (11), 1703.

Sakamoto, N., Yamashita, T., Minaki, Y., et al., 1999. Mechanoreceptors in the sacroiliac joint. Trans. Orthop. Res. Soc. 24, 988.

Sapsford, R.R., Hodges, P.W., 2001. Contraction of the pelvic floor muscles during abdominal maneuvers. Arch. Phys. Med. Rehabil. 82, 1081.

Sapsford, R.R., Hodges, P.W., Richardson, C.A., et al., 2001. Co-activation of the abdominal and pelvic floor muscles during voluntary exercises. Neurourol. Urodyn. 20, 31.

Sapsford, R.R., Richardson, C.A., Maher, C.F., et al., 2008. Pelvic floor muscle activity in different sitting postures in continent and incontinent women. Arch. Phys. Med. Rehabil. 89, 1741.

Sashin, D., 1930. A critical analysis of the anatomy and the pathologic changes of the sacro-iliac joints. J. Bone Joint Surg. 12, 891.

Saunders, S., Rath, D., Hodges, P., 2004a. Postural and respiratory activation of the trunk muscles changes with mode and speed of locomotion. Gait Posture 20, 280.

Saunders, S.W., Coppieters, M., Magarey, M., Hodges, P.W., 2004b. Low back pain and associated changes in abdominal muscle activation during human locomotion. In: Australian conference of science and medicine in sport: hot topics from the red centre. Sports Medicine, Alice Springs, Australia.

Saunders, S., Schache, A., Rath, D., et al., 2005. Changes in three dimensional lumbo-pelvic kinematics and trunk muscle activity with speed and mode of locomotion. Clin. Biomech. 20, 784.

Schleip, R., 2008. The nature of fascia: latest news from connective tissue research. DVD available at wwwinfo@fasciaresearchcom.

Schleip, R., Klingler, W., Lehmann-Horn, F., 2005. Active fascial contractility: fascia may be able to contract in a smooth muscle-like manner and thereby influence musculoskeletal dynamics. Med. Hypotheses 65 (2), 273.

Schunke, G.B., 1938. The anatomy and development of the sacro-iliac joint in man. Anat. Rec. 72, 313.

Schwarzer, A.C., Aprill, C.N., Bogduk, N., 1995. The sacroiliac joint in chronic low back pain. Spine 20, 31.

Shacklock, M., 2005. Clinical neurodynamics. Elsevier, Edinburgh.

Shah, J.P., Phillips, T.M., Danoff, J.V., Gerber, L.H., 2005. An in vivo micro-analytical technique for measuring the local biochemical milieu of human skeletal muscle. J. Appl. Physiol. 99, 1980.

Shibata, Y., Shirai, Y., Miyamoto, M., 2002. The aging process in the sacroiliac joint: helical computed tomography analysis. J. Orthop. Sci. 7 (1), 12.

Shindle, M.K., Ranawat, A.S., Kelly, B. T., 2006. Diagnosis and management of traumatic and atraumatic hip instability in the athletic patient. Clin. Sports Med. 25, 309.

Siebenrock, K.A., Schoeniger, R., Ganz, R., 2003. Anerior femoro-acetabular impingement due to acetabular retroversion. Treatment with periacetabular osteotomy. J. Bone Joint Surg. Am. 85–A (2), 278.

Simons, D.G., Travell, J.G., Simons, L.S., 1999. Travell and Simons' myofascial pain and dysfunction: the trigger point manual, vol. 1, second ed. Williams & Wilkins, Baltimore, MD.

Simons, D.G., Dommerholt, J., 2006. Myofascial trigger points and myofascial pain syndrome: a critical review of recent literature. Journal of Manual and Manipulative Therapy 14 (4), E124.

Singleton, M.C., LeVeau, B.F., 1975. The hip joint: structure, stability, and stress. Phys. Ther. 55, 957.

Sjodahl, J., Kvist, J., Gutke, A., Oberg, B., 2009. The postural response of the pelvic floor muscles during limb movements: a methodological electromyography study in parous women without lumbopelvic pain. Clin. Biomech. (Bristol, Avon) 24 (2), 183.

Smidt, G.L., 1995. Sacroiliac kinematics for reciprocal straddle positions. In: Vleeming, A., Mooney, V., Dorman, T., Snijders, C. (Eds.), Second interdisciplinary world congress on low back pain: the integrated function of the lumbar spine and sacroiliac joint, part 2. San Diego, California, p. 695.

Smith, M.D., Coppieters, M.W., Hodges, P.W., 2007a. Postural activity of the pelvic floor muscles is delayed during rapid arm movements in women with stress urinary incontinence. Int. Urogynecol. J. Pelvic Floor Dysfunct. 18 (8), 901.

Smith, M.D., Coppieters, M.W., Hodges, P.W., 2007b. Postural response of the pelvic floor and abdominal muscles in women with and without incontinence. Neurourol. Urodyn. 26 (3), 377.

Smith, M.D., Russell, A., Hodges, P.W., 2006. Disorders of breathing and continence have a stronger association with back pain than obesity and physical activity. Aust. J. Physiother. 52, 11.

Smith, M.D., Russell, A., Hodges, P.W., 2008. Is there a relationship between parity, pregnancy, back pain and incontinence? Int. Urogynecol. J. Pelvic Floor Dysfunct. 19 (2), 205.

Snijders, C.J., Vleeming, A., Stoeckart, R., 1993a. Transfer of lumbosacral load to iliac bones and legs. 1: Biomechanics of self-bracing of the sacroiliac joints and its significance for treatment and exercise. Clin. Biomech. (Bristol, Avon) 8, 285.

Snijders, C.J., Vleeming, A., Stoeckart, R., 1993b. Transfer of lumbosacral load to iliac bones and legs. 2: Loading of the sacroiliac joints when lifting in a stooped posture. Clin. Biomech. (Bristol, Avon) 8, 295.

Soderberg, G.L., Barr, J.O., 1983. Muscular function in chronic low-back dysfunction. Spine 8, 79–85.

Solonen, K.A., 1957. The sacro-iliac joint in the light of anatomical roentgenological and clinical studies. Acta Orthop. Scand. Suppl. 26.

Spitznagle, T.M., Leong, F.C., Van Dillen, 2007. Prevalence of diastasis recti abdominis in a urogynecological patient population. Int. Urogynecol. J. Pelvic Floor Dysfunct. 18 (3), 321.

Standring, S., 2008. Gray's anatomy, fortieth ed. Elsevier, Edinburgh.

Stein, P.L., Rowe, B.M., 1982. Physical anthropology, third ed. McGraw-Hill, New York.

Stokes, I.A.F., 1986. Three-dimensional biplanar radiography of the lumbar spine. In: Grieve, G.P. (Ed.), Modern manual therapy of the vertebral column. Churchill Livingstone, Edinburgh, p. 576.

Stuge, B., Lærum, E., Kirkesola, G., Vøllestad, N., 2004. The efficacy of a treatment program focusing on specific stabilizing exercises for pelvic girdle pain after pregnancy. Spine 29 (4), 351.

Sturesson, B., 1999. Load and movement of the sacroiliac joint. PhD thesis. Lund University, Sweden.

Sturesson, B., Selvik, G., Uden, A., 1989. Movements of the sacroiliac joints: a Roentgen stereophotogrammetric analysis. Spine 14 (2), 162.

Sturesson, B., Uden, A., Vleeming, A., 2000. A radiosteriometric analysis of movements of the sacroiliac joints during the standing hip flexion test. Spine 25 (3), 364.

Sunderland, S., 1978. Traumatized nerves, roots and ganglia: musculo-skeletal factors and neuropathological consequences. In: Korr, (Ed.), The neurobiologic mechanisms in manipulative therapy. Plenum Press, London, p. 137.

Sung, P.S., Kang, Y., Pickar, J.G., 2005. Effect of spinal manipulation duration on low threshold mechanoreceptors in lumbar paraspinal muscles: a preliminary report. Spine 30 (1), 115.

Swindler, D.R., Wood, C.D., 1982. An atlas of primate gross anatomy: baboon, chimpanzee, and man. Robert E Krieger, Florida.

Tanzer, M., Noiseux, N., 2004. Osseous abnormalities and early osteoarthritis: the role of hip impingement. Clin. Orthop. Relat. Res. 170.

Taylor, J.R., Twomey, L.T., 1986. Age changes in lumbar zygapophyseal joints: observations on structure and function. Spine 11 (7), 739.

Taylor, J.T., Twomey, L.T., 1992. Structure and function of lumbar zygapophyseal (facet) joints: a review. J. Orthop. Med. 14 (3), 71.

Taylor, J.T., Twomey, L.T., Corker, M., 1990. Bone and soft tissue injuries in post-mortem lumbar spines. Paraplegia 28, 119.

Thind, P., Lose, G., Jorgensen, L., et al., 1991. Urethral pressure increment preceding and following bladder pressure elevation during stress episode in healthy and stress incontinent women. Neurourol. Urodyn. 10, 177.

Thompson, J.A., O'sullivan, P.B., Briffa, N.K., et al., 2006. Altered muscle activation patterns in symptomatic women during pelvic floor muscle contraction and Valsalva manoeuvre. Neurourol. Urodyn. 25, 268.

Tonnis, D., Heinecke, A., 1999. Decreased acetabular anterversion and femur neck antetorsion cause pain and arthrosis. 1: statistics and clinical sequelae. Z. Orthop. Ihre Grenzgeb. 137 (2), 153.

Toranto, I.R., 1988. Resolution of back pain with the wide abdominal rectus plication abdominoplasty. Plast. Reconstr. Surge. 81 (5), 777.

Torgerson, W.R., Dotter, W.E., 1976. Comparative roentgenographic study of the asymptomatic and symptomatic lumbar spine. J. Bone Joint Surg. 58A, 850.

Torry, M.R., Schenker, M.L., Martin, H.D., et al., 2006. Neuromuscular hip biomechanics and pathology in the athlete. Clin. Sports Med. 25, 179.

Trotter, M., 1937. Accessory sacro-iliac articulations. Am. J. Phys. Anthropol. 22, 247.

Tsao, H., Hodges, P.W., 2007. Immediate changes in feedforward postural adjustments following voluntary motor training. Exp. Brain Res. 181 (4), 537.

Tsao, H., Hodges, P.W., 2008. Persistence of improvements in postural strategies following motor control training in people with recurrent low back pain. J. Electromyogr. Kinesiol. 18 (4), 559.

Tsao, H., Galea, M.P., Hodges, P.W., 2008. Reorganization of the motor cortex is associated with postural control deficits in recurrent low back pain. Brain 131 (8), 2161.

Tuttle, R.H. (Ed.), 1975. Primate functional morphology. Mouton, The Hague.

Twomey, L.T., Taylor, J.R., 1985. A quantitative study of the role of the posterior vertebral elements in sagittal movements of the lumbar vertebral column. In: Glasgow, E.F., Twomey, L.T., Scull, E.R., Kleynhans, A.M. (Eds.), Aspects of manipulative therapy, second ed. Churchill Livingstone, Melbourne, p. 34.

Twomey, L.T., Taylor, J.R., Taylor, M.M., 1989. Unsuspected damage to lumbar zygapophyseal (facet) joints after motor-vehicle accidents. Med. J. Aust. 151, 210.

Uhtoff, H.K., 1993. Prenatal development of the iliolumbar ligament. J. Bone Joint Surg. Br. 75, 93.

Urquhart, D.M., Barker, P.J., Hodges, P.W., et al., 2005. Regional morphology of transversus abdominis, and obliquus internus and externus abdominis. Clin. Biomech. (Bristol, Avon) 20 (3), 233.

Urquhart, D.M., Hodges, P.W., 2007. Clinical anatomy of the anterolateral abdominal muscles. In: Vleeming, A., Mooney, V., Stoeckart, R. (Eds.), Movement, stability and lumbopelvic pain, second ed. Elsevier, Edinburgh, p. 75.

van Dieen, J.H., 2007. Low-back pain and motor behavior: contingent adaptations, a common goal. In: Proceedings from the Sixth Interdisciplinary World Congress on Low Back and Pelvic Pain. Barcelona, November 7–10, p. 3.

van Dieen, J.H., Cholewicki, J., Radebold, A., 2003a. Trunk muscle recruitment patterns in patients with low back pain enhance the stability of the lumbar spine. Spine 28, 834.

van Dieen, J.H., de Looze, M.P., 1999. Directionality of anticipatory activation of trunk muscles in a lifting task depends on load knowledge. Exp. Brain Res. 128, 397.

van Dieen, J.H., Selen, L.P.J., Cholewicki, J., 2003b. Trunk muscle activation in low-back pain patients, an analysis of the literature. J. Electromyogr. Kinesiol. 13, 333.

van Wingerden, J.P., Vleeming, A., Snijders, C.J., et al., 1993. A functional-anatomical approach to the spine-pelvis mechanism: interaction between the biceps femoris muscle and the sacrotuberous ligament. Eur. Spine J. 2, 140.

van Wingerden, J.P., Vleeming, A., Buyruk, H.M., et al., 2004. Stabilization of the sacroiliac joint in vivo: verification of muscular contribution to force closure of the pelvis. Eur. Spine J. 13 (3), 199.

Verrall, G.M., Slovotinek, J.P., Fon, G.T., 2001. Incidence of pubic bone marrow oedema in Australian rules football players: relation to groin pain. Br. J. Sports Med. 35, 28.

Vicenzino, G., Twomey, L., 1993. Sideflexion induced lumbar spine conjunct rotation and its influencing factors. Aust. Physiother. 39 (4), 299.

Vilensky, J.A., O'Connor, B.L., Fortin, J.D., et al., 2002. Histologic analysis of neural elements in the human sacroiliac joint. Spine 27 (11), 1202.

Vincent-Smith, B., Gibbons, P., 1999. Inter-examiner and intra-examiner reliability of the standing flexion test. Man. Ther. 4 (2), 87.

Vlaeyen, J.W.S., Linton, S.J., 2000. Fear-avoidance and its consequences in chronic musculoskeletal pain: a state of the art. Pain 85, 317.

Vlaeyen, J.W.S., Vancleef, L.M.G., 2007. Behavioral analysis, fear of movement/(re)injury, and cognitive-behavioral management of chronic low back pain. In: Vleeming, A., Mooney, V., Stoeckart, R. (Eds.), Movement, stability and lumbopelvic pain, second ed. Elsevier, Edinburgh, p. 475.

Vleeming, A., Albert, H.B., Ostgaard, H.C., et al., 2007. European guidelines for the diagnosis and treatment of pelvic girdle pain. In: Vleeming, A., Mooney, V., Stoeckart, R. (Eds.), Movement, stability and lumbopelvic pain, second ed. Elsevier, Edinburgh, p. 465.

Vleeming, A., Albert, H.B., Ostgaard, H.C., et al., 2008. European guidelines for the diagnosis and treatment of pelvic girdle pain. Eur. Spine J. 17 (6), 794.

Vleeming, A., Buyruk, H., Stoechart, R., et al., 1992a. An integrated therapy for peripartum pelvic instability: a study of the biomechanical effects of pelvic belts. Am. J. Obstet. Gynecol. 166 (4), 1243.

Vleeming, A., de Vries, H.J., Mens, J.M., et al., 2002. Possible role of the long dorsal sacroiliac ligament in women with peripartum pelvic pain. Acta Obstet. Gynecol. Scand. 81 (5), 430.

Vleeming, A., Mooney, V., Dorman, T., Snijders, C., Stoeckart, R. (Eds.), 1997. Movement, stability and low back pain, the essential role of the pelvis. Churchill Livingstone, Edinburgh.

Vleeming, A., Mooney, V., Snijders, C. et al., 1992b. First interdisciplinary world congress on low back pain and its relation to the sacroiliac joint. San Diego, California.

Vleeming, A., Mooney, V., Stoeckart, R. (Eds.), 2007. Movement, stability and lumbopelvic pain, second ed. Elsevier.

Vleeming, A., Pool-Goudzwaard, A.L., Hammudoghlu, D., et al., 1996. The function of the long dorsal sacroiliac ligament: its implication for understanding low back pain. Spine 21 (5), 556.

Vleeming, A., Pool-Goudzwaard, A.L., Stoeckart, R., et al., 1995a. The posterior layer of the thoracolumbar fascia: its function in load transfer from spine to legs. Spine 20, 753.

Vleeming, A., Snijders, C.J., Stoeckart, R., et al., 1995b. A new light on low back pain. In: Proceedings from the 2nd interdisciplinary world congress on low back pain. San Diego, California.

Vleeming, A., Stoeckart, R., 2007. The role of the pelvic girdle in coupling the spine and the legs: a clinical-anatomical perspective on pelvic stability. In: Vleeming, A., Mooney, V., Stoeckart, R. (Eds.), Movement, stability and lumbopelvic pain, second ed. Elsevier, Edinburgh, p. 113.

Vleeming, A., Stoeckart, R., Snijders, C. J., 1989a. The sacrotuberous ligament: a conceptual approach to its dynamic role in stabilizing the sacroiliac joint. Clin. Biomech. (Bristol, Avon) 4, 201.

Vleeming, A., Stoeckart, R., Volkers, A. C.W., Snijders, C.J., 1990a. Relation between form and function in the sacroiliac joint. 1: Clinical anatomical aspects. Spine 15 (2), 130.

Vleeming, A., van Wingerden, J.P., Dijkstra, P.F., et al., 1992c. Mobility in the SI-joints in old people: a kinematic and radiologic study. Clin. Biomech. (Bristol, Avon) 7, 170.

Vleeming, A., van Wingerden, J.P., Snijders, C.J., et al., 1989b. Load application to the sacrotuberous ligament: influences on sacroiliac joint mechanics. Clin. Biomech. (Bristol, Avon) 4, 204.

Vleeming, A., Volkers, A.C.W., Snijders, C.J., Stoeckart, R., 1990b. Relation between form and function in the sacroiliac joint. 2: Biomechanical aspects. Spine 15 (2), 133.

Vogt, L., Pfeifer, K., Banzer, W., 2003. Neuromuscular control of walking with chronic low-back pain. Man. Ther. 8, 21.

Waddell, G., 2004. The back pain revolution, second ed. Churchill Livingstone, Edinburgh.

Walheim, G.G., Selvik, G., 1984. Mobility of the pubic symphysis. Clin. Orthop. Relat. Res. 191, 129.

Walker, J.M., 1984. Age changes in the sacroiliac joint. In: Proceedings of the 5th International Federation of Orthopaedic Manipulative Therapists, Vancouver, p. 250.

Walker, J.M., 1986. Age-related differences in the human sacroiliac joint: a histological study; implications for therapy. J. Orthop. Sports Phys. Ther. 7, 325.

Weisl, H., 1954. The articular surfaces of the sacro-iliac joint and their relation to the movements of the sacrum. Acta Anat. (Basel) 22, 1.

Weisl, H., 1955. The movements of the sacro-iliac joint. Acta Anat. (Basel) 23, 80.

White, A.A., Panjabi, M.M., 1978. The basic kinematics of the human spine. Spine 3, 12.

WHO Constitution, 1978. www.who.int/governance/eb/constitution/en/index.html.

Wilder, D.G., Pope, M.H., Frymoyer, J.W., 1980. The functional topography of the sacroiliac joint. Spine 5, 575.

Willard, F.H., 1997. The muscular, ligamentous and neural structure of the low back and its relation to back pain. In: Vleeming, A., Mooney, V., Dorman, T., Snijders, C., Stoeckart, R. (Eds.), Movement, stability and low back pain. Churchill Livingstone, Edinburgh, p. 3.

Willard, F.H., 2007. The muscular, ligamentous and neural structure of the low back and its relation to back pain. In: Vleeming, A., Mooney, V., Stoeckart, R. (Eds.), Movement, stability and lumbopelvic pain, second ed. Churchill Livingstone, Edinburgh, p. 5.

Williams, P.L., 1995. Gray's anatomy, thirtyeighth ed. Churchill Livingstone, New York.

Wilson, P.D., Herbison, P., Glazener, C., McGee, M., MacArthur, C., 2002.

Obstetric practice and urinary incontinence 5-7 years after delivery. ICS Proceedings Neurourology and Urodynamics 21 (4), 284.

Wright, A., 2002. Neurophysiology of pain and pain modulation. In: Strong, J., Unruh, M.A., Wright, A., Baxter, G.D. (Eds.), Pain: a textbook for therapists. Churchill Livingstone, Edinburgh.

Wu, W.H., Meijer, O.G., Uegaki, K., et al., 2004. Pregnancy-related pelvic girdle pain (PPP), I: Terminology, clinical presentation, and prevalence. Eur. Spine J. 13 (7), 575.

Wurdinger, S., Humbsch, K., Reichenback, J.R., et al., 2002. MRI of the pelvic ring joints postpartum: normal and pathological findings. J. Magn. Reson. Imaging 15 (3), 324.

Wurff, P., Hagmeijer, R., Meyne, W., 2000. Clinical tests of the sacroiliac joint. A systematic methodological review: part 1: reliability. Man. Ther. 5 (1), 30.

Wyke, B.D., 1981. The neurology of joints: a review of general principles. Clin. Rheum. Dis. 7, 223.

Yahia, L., Rhalmi, S., Newman, N., Isler, M., 1992. Sensory innervation of human thoracolumbar fascia. An immunohistochemical study. Acta Orthop. Scand. 63 (2), 196.

Yamamoto, I., Panjabi, M.M., Oxland, T.R., et al., 1990. The role of the iliolumbar ligament in the lumbosacral junction. Spine 15, 1138.

Young, J., 1940. Relaxation of the pelvic joints in pregnancy: pelvic arthropathy of pregnancy. J. Obstet. Gynecol. 47, 493.

Young, J.Z., 1981. The life of vertebrates, third ed. Clarendon Press, Oxford.

Index

Note: Page numbers followed by "*b*" indicate boxes, "*f*" indicate figures and "*t*" indicate tables.

A

Abdomen, muscle release, 303–312
Abdominal canister, 72*f*
  deep muscle system, 329–352,
    353–355
  regional tests, 232–250
Abdominal wall
  Laura (case report), 277, 278*f*
  muscles, 29–31
  palpation
    assessment, 233–235, 233*f*, 234*f*,
      235*f*, 238*f*, 239*f*
    'waking up', 341, 342, 349
  ultrasound imaging, 227–228, 236*f*
Abductive reasoning, 257
Acetabular labral tears, 124–126, 125*f*
  diagnostic imaging, 126
  history, 124
  treatment, 126
Acetabulum, 26
  adult, 16–17, 16*f*, 17*f*
  comparative anatomy, 7
Acetylcholine, 381
Active release technique, 313
Active straight leg raise (ASLR),
    117–118, 119, 120
  assessment, 206–209, 206*f*, 207*f*,
    208*f*, 248
  Laura (case report), 273
Active system, 131–137, 139
Acute pain, 105–107, 153–155, 156
Adductor magnus (AM), combined
    release, 292*f*
Adjunctive tests, 252
Albinus, Bernhard Siegfried, 8–9

American Medical Association, 163–164
Anatomy, comparative, 6–8, 6*f*
'Anatomy Trains' of myofascial slings,
    83*f*
Ankylosing spondylitis, 253*f*
Anterior compression test, 222, 223*f*
Anterior distraction test, 222, 222*f*
Anterior oblique sling, 81, 82*f*
Anterior superior iliac spine (ASIS), 14
Anteroposterior/posteroanterior
    translation, lumbar spine, 226,
    226*f*
Arcus tendineus fascia pelvis (ATFP),
    40–41, 41*f*
  pregnancy and, 136–137, 136*f*, 137*f*,
    140*f*
Arm
  dissociation, trunk and, 359, 359*f*
  movement, rapid, 77, 78*t*
  one arm fly, 359
Arthrology, pelvic girdle, 17–29
Articular cartilage degeneration, 126–127
  history, 126–127
  treatment, 127
Articular mobilization techniques,
    passive, 265
Articular system, 169–171, 169*t*
  Laura (case report), 275, 280–281
  mobility, 214–218, 215*f*, 218*f*,
    225–226, 225*f*, 229–231, 229*f*
  restraints, 218–219, 218*f*, 219*f*, 220*f*,
    226–227, 226*f*, 231–232, 231*f*
  techniques for mobilizing, 312–320
Articular system impairment, 264–265
ASLR *see* Active straight leg raise (ASLR)

Assessment
  advanced, 368–379
  Clinical Puzzle, 258–259
  see also Objective examination;
    Subjective examination
Attention, focused, 266
Australian Longitudinal Study on
    Women's Health, 130
Awareness, patient
  focused, 266
  hip joint, 291–292, 295
  physical impairment, 285–287
  postural training, 379–381, 380*f*,
    382*f*, 383*f*, 384*b*, 384*f*
  sacroiliac joint (SIJ), 298, 299, 300
  thorax/abdomen, 304, 307, 309,
    310–311, 312
Axial torsion, lumbar segment, 59–60

B

Back muscles, 33–36
Back-gripping, 101, 105, 105*f*, 267, 303*f*
  assessment, 182*f*, 194*f*, 196*f*
Backward bending, 87, 87*f*, 112*f*, 273*f*
  assessment, 187–188, 187*f*, 188*f*,
    191–195
Barral Institute, 138–139
Barral, Jean-Pierre, 320
Barriers, addressing, 261–266, 261*f*
  Laura (case report), 275–276
  patient characteristics, 262–264, 285
  physical impairments, 264–266,
    285–290, 286*f*
  therapist characteristics, 262

Base of support (BOS), centre of mass (COM) over, 378–379, 378f, 390
'Beautiful movement', 371–372, 373f, 385f
  requirements, 83–85
Bending see Backward bending; Forward bending; Lateral bending
Bent knee fall out, 360, 360f
Biceps femoris muscle (BFM), 22–23, 23f
Biomechanics, 85–89, 175–176, 371
Biomedic model of pain, 153
Bladder, 141
  pelvic floor imaging, 339–341, 340f, 342
Bladder neck, stress urinary incontinence (SUI) and, 141
'Blind Man and the Elephant' (Saxe), 47, 47b, 48f, 49
Blood supply
  hip joint, 28–29
  innominate, 17
  sacroiliac joint (SIJ), 24
Body-self neuromatrix concept (Melzack), 165, 367–368, 381
Brain that changes itself (Doidge), 270
Breathing
  expansion, 395
  patterns, 357
Building blocks
  designing, 383–386, 385f, 386f
  for runners, 403–405, 405f, 406f
Burkart, Dr Sandy, 149f
Butt-gripping, 194f, 196f, 268, 324–325, 324f, 328, 329–330, 381
  impairment, 101, 115f, 116f, 121–122, 123, 123f

C

Canadian Academy of Manipulative Therapy, 148, 290
Canadian Physiotherapy Association, 290
Case reports, 270–282
Central nervous system (CNS), 74–81, 157
Centre of mass (COM) over base of support (BOS), 378–379, 378f, 390
Change, facilitating, 260, 262
  see also Barriers, addressing
Chest-gripping, 101, 105, 105f, 312f, 329–330, 330f
Chord cue, finding, 353–355
  clinical examples, 353–354

neural network reinforcement, 354–355, 354f, 355f
Chronic pain, 108–111, 113, 115f, 155, 156, 161f
Clam shell, 361, 361f
Classification of Chronic Pain (Merskey & Bogduk), 155
Clinical expertise, 147–148, 148f, 152, 152f, 162
  clinical reasoning and, 255, 256f, 257–258
Clinical practice, 147–172
  evidence-based practice (EBP), 148–152, 152f, 163b
  integrated systems for optimal health, 163–165
  knowledge, 147–148, 148f
  pain, understanding, 152–158, 152b
  see also Clinical expertise; Integrated Systems Model for Disability and Pain; Pain
Clinical prediction rules (CPRs), 158–163, 289
Clinical Puzzle, 167–171, 167f, 258f
  articular system, 169–171, 169t
  assessment, 258–259
  case report, 271f
  function/performance strategies, 168
  myofascial system, 169–171, 170t
  neural system, 169–171, 170t
  person in middle, 167–168, 174–175, 262–264
  template, 209f
  treatment, components, 260–269, 261f
  visceral system, 169–171, 170t
  see also Objective examination; Subjective examination
Clinical reasoning, 255, 256f, 258–259
  abdominal fascia and, 240–241
  abdominal wall and, 238
  articular system impairment, 216–217
  clinical practice and, 147–148, 148f
  intervertebral lumbar points, 225–226
  lumbar spine, 227, 228
  'on the fly', 209f
  pain provocation and, 223
  sacroiliac joint (SIJ) and, 217, 218, 219
  structural deficit in hamstring, 205
  TrA/dMF palpation, 248
Coccyx
  adult, 12
  anterior aspect, 12f
  posterior aspect, 11f
Cochrane Collaboration, 149f

Cochrane, Professor Archie, 148, 149f
Cognitive dimension, 175, 258, 271b, 285
Communication, methods of, 263
Compensatory strategies, 264–265
Compression
  lumbar segment, 57–59, 59f
  sacroiliac joint (SIJ), 114–117
Com-Pressor belt, 268–269, 269f, 328–329, 329f
Computed tomography (CT) scanning, 253–254, 253f, 254f
Concentration mode, sitting position, 201–202
Congenital anomalies, 98t
  lumbar spine, 253f, 254
Control system, 137–138, 139
Coverroll tape, 269, 269f
Craft knowledge, 162
Critical reflection, 257
Cues, using see Awareness, patient
Cyriax, Dr James, 149f
Cyriax model, 148

D

De Diemerbroeck, 1
Declarative knowledge, 147
Deep fibers of multifidus (dMF)
  coactivation, 353–354
  fractures and, 316f
  palpation, 245–246, 246f, 247–248, 248f, 351, 352
  ultrasound imaging, 246–247, 247f, 351, 352
  unilateral activation, 353
  'waking up', 349–352, 349f, 350f, 351f
Deep muscle systems, 78–81, 79f, 104f
  chord cue, finding, 353–355
  guidelines for training, 338, 338b
  neutral lumbopelvic-hip (LPH) alignment, 353
  release, 294–296
  superficial muscles coordination, 355–365
  'waking up', 268, 276, 326–328, 333–352
Dermatome, 9, 9f
  differentiation and, 9f
  maps, 251, 252f
Descartes, R, 153, 153f
Diaphragm, 42, 43f, 248–249, 249f, 335–337
  function, 72f, 80

lateral costal expansion, 335–337, 336*f*
posterolateral costal expansion, 335–337, 336*f*
Diastasis rectus abdominis (DRA), 131–133, 132*f*
Distraction
lumbar joints, 317, 318–319, 320
sacroiliac joint (SIJ), 314, 315–316, 315*f*, 316*f*
dMF *see* Deep fibers of multifidus (dMF)
Dopamine, 381
Doppler imaging and vibration (DIV) method, 72–73
Drivers
pain, 153, 153*f*
whole body, 368–373, 372*f*
Dry needling/IMS, 290–291, 292
erector spinae (ES), 305–306, 305*f*
internal oblique (IO), 311, 311*f*
principles, 287–288
sacroiliac joint (SIJ), 299, 299*f*, 300, 300*f*
superficial fibers of multifidus (sMF), 301, 301*f*
Dynamic situations, motor control and, 74
Dysesthesia, 174–175

E

Eddy, David, 148
Education, patient, 283, 284, 284*b*, 284*f*, 285*f*, 325–326
Elastic zone of motion, 53–54, 54*f*, 288–289
assessment, 210, 224, 226
Electromyography (EMG), 78–80, 137–138
stress urinary incontinence (SUI) and, 141–143
urinary incontinence (UI) and, 140–141
Elliptical trainer, 280
Emotional states, 85, 127–128, 175, 258, 271*b*, 285
Endopelvic fascia, 40–41, 41*f*, 133–137, 136*f*, 137*f*
ultrasound imaging, 241–242
Equipment, 376–377, 376*f*
Erector spinae (ES), 35, 297, 303–306, 303*f*, 304*f*
Euler model, 50*f*
Evidence-based practice (EBP), 148–152, 152*f*, 163*b*, 255

Exercises
number of, 384
on-field, 386
repetitions, 385–386
Expertise, clinical components, 147–148, 148*f*
see also Clinical expertise
Explain pain (Butler & Moseley), 263–264, 285
External oblique (EO), 30–31, 30*f*
activation, 235, 235*f*
assessment, 233–234, 233*f*
correction responses, 343, 344, 344*f*, 345
hypertonicity, 346*f*
release, 306–308
tears in, 103*f*
ultrasound imaging, 237

F

Failed load transfer (FLT), 164–165
advanced assessment, 368–373, 370*f*, 372*f*, 375*f*
assessment, 177–179
intrapelvic control, 198
pubic symphysis (PS), 220
System-Based Classification for Failed Load Transfer, 164
Fascia, force closure theory, 72–74, 72*f*
Feedback, 381
Femora, adult, 17
Femoral arcuate ligament, 27*f*, 28, 28*f*
Femoral head, 122*f*
backward bending, 187
forward bending, 185, 186*f*
hip extension, 205
intrapelvic control, 196, 199*f*
lateral bending, 189
one leg standing, 190, 191, 191*f*
position, 292, 295, 296
prone knee bend/hip extension, 202, 203*f*, 204
sitting posture, 200, 201*f*
squat, 192, 193*f*
standing posture, 181, 184*f*
Femoral motion, walking, 88–89
Femur
ligaments, 27*f*
osteokinematic motion, 69*f*
squat, 195, 197*f*
'Fin fold' theory, 5
Foot control, one leg standing, 192*f*

Force closure theory, 53, 53*f*, 71–74, 100–104
hip joint, 124, 125–126, 127
lumbar spine, 106–107, 107*f*, 108
sacroiliac joint (SIJ), 116, 121
Form closure theory, 53–71, 53*f*, 54*f*
deficits, 91–100
groin, 99–100, 314
hip joint, 69–70, 69*f*, 99–100, 100*b*, 106, 124, 125–126, 127
ligaments, 70–71, 71*t*
lumbar spine, 54–60, 54*f*, 91–98, 106–107, 107*f*, 108
pelvic girdle, 60–69, 98
sacroiliac joint (SIJ), 116, 121
Forward bending, 86, 86*f*, 116*f*
assessment, 183–187, 185*f*, 186*f*, 187*f*
Laura (case report), 271–272
Fowler, Cliff, 148
Free nerve endings, 45*t*
Function, essential progressions, 397–405
Function/performance strategies, 85, 168, 179–210
general principles, 176–179
key components, 177–179, 178*f*, 179*b*
principles for training, 323–328, 324*b*
see also Integrated Model of Function
Functional tasks, 396–405

G

Gait, 401*f*
Gifford, L, 157
Gillet test *see* One leg standing
Gluteal muscles
dry needling, 293*f*
release of lateral, 295*f*
Gluteus maximus, dry needling, 293*f*
Gluteus medius
combined release, 291*f*
comparative anatomy, 6, 7*f*
dry needling, 293*f*
Gluteus minimus
comparative anatomy, 6, 7*f*
dry needling, 293*f*
Golgi sensory receptor, 45*t*
Gombe Stream Reserve study (Goodall), 7
Greater trochanter, 122*f*
'Gripping', 382*f*
Groin triangle, 103*f*
Gunn, Dr Chan, 287–288, 288*f*

H

Hamstring weakness, 204f
Health, World Health Assembly definition, 163–164
Heel drops, 360, 360f
Heel slides, 360
High acceleration low amplitude thrust (HALAT) techniques
  erector spinae (ES), 304f
  lumbar joints, 318–320, 318f, 319f, 320f
  principles, 289–290
  sacroiliac joint (SIJ), 315–316
Hip joint
  adult, 14, 27f
  articular system restraints, 231f
  blood supply, 28–29
  capsule, 26–27
  clinical presentations, 121–127
  compression and malalignment, 122–124, 123t
  control, extrinsic factors, 200f
  deep muscle release, 294–296, 363–365
  disorders, 100b, 100f
  force closure, 124, 125–126, 127
  form closure, 69–70, 69f, 99–100, 100b, 106, 124, 125–126, 127
  history, 122–123
  kinematics, 69–70
  kinetics, 70, 70f
  ligaments, 26–27
  mobility, 197f
  mobilization technique, 312–313
  motor control, 124, 125–126, 127
  myofascial system influence, 232
  nerve supply, 28
  neural system influence, 232, 363–365, 364f
  regional tests, 228–232
  rotation, 357
  structural changes, 121–122, 124–127
  superficial muscle release, 290–294, 292f, 363–365
  treatment, 124
Hip motion control
  forward bending, 186f
  one leg standing, 191f, 192f
  squat, 193f
  step forward, 199f
Hip region, muscles, 44
Hip-gripping, 101, 121–122, 121f, 123, 123f

Hippocrates, 1
Historical perspective, 1–2, 8–9
Home practice
  deep muscle release, 295, 295f
  diaphragm expansion, 336f
  erector spinae (ES) release, 306, 306f
  external oblique (EO) release, 307–308, 308f, 312f
  hip joint mobilization, 298f, 302f, 313
  internal oblique (IO) release, 309, 311, 311f, 312f
  ischiococcygeus release, 299
  Laura (case report), 279–280, 281–282
  lumbar joints manipulation, 320
  lumbar spine mobilization, 317, 317f
  pelvic alignment, 314f, 321
  piriformis release, 300
  rectus abdominis (RA) release, 312, 312f
  sacroiliac joint (SIJ) mobilization, 314f
  setting, 326
  superficial fibers of multifidus (sMF), 301–302, 302f
  superficial muscle release, 293–294, 295f, 296f, 297f
Hunter, William, 8–9
Hypertonicity, 265–266
  diaphragm, 248–249
  multifidus, 216f
  piriformis muscle, 216, 217f
  sacroiliac joint (SIJ) mobilization, 215–216
Hypothesis development, Laura (case report), 271b, 273b, 274b, 277b
Hypothesis-oriented reasoning, 256–257
Hypothetic-deductive reasoning, 256–257

I

Iliacus, 39f, 42
Iliococcygeus, 38, 39f, 40f
Iliocostalis lumborum pars lumborum, 35, 302
Iliocostalis lumborum pars thoracis, 34f, 35
Iliofemoral ligament, 17f, 27, 27f, 28f
  iliotrochanteric band, 231
  inferior band, 231
Iliolumbar ligament, 17f, 23–24, 23f
Ilium, 12–14
  adult, 14, 16f, 17f
  comparative anatomy, 6
Imagery activates, 379–381
Imaging studies, 175

see also Ultrasound imaging
In Pursuit of Excellence (Orlick), 379–381
Inductive reasoning, 256
Inferior gemelli, release, 300f
Inflammatory disorders, 98t
Injury mechanisms, 153–156
Innominate, 7, 68f, 180
  adult, 14–17
  backward bending, 187, 188f
  blood supply, 17
  comparative anatomy, 6–7, 7f, 8f
  development, 12–14
  forward bending, 185, 187f
  intrapelvic control, 196, 198f
  intrapelvic motion, 65, 67f, 68f
  medial/lateral aspects, 16f
  one leg standing, 190, 190f, 191f
  ossification, 16f
  pelvic position and, 210–211, 211f, 213f
  squat, 192, 193f
  standing posture, 183f
Instability, defined, 94–97, 104
Institute for the Study and Treatment of Pain, 288, 288f
Integrated Model of Function, 52–85, 52f, 53f, 88
  clinical practice, 164–165
  emotional states, 85, 127–128
  see also Force closure theory; Form closure theory; Motor control theory; Posture and movement strategies
Integrated Systems Model for Disability and Pain, 164–171, 173
  underlying constructs, 165–167
  websites, 284
  see also Clinical Puzzle
Integrated systems, optimal health, 163–165
Intercoccygeal joint, 25
Interdisciplinary World Congress on Low Back and Pelvic Pain, 1
  first, 1
  sixth, 47–49
Internal oblique (IO), 30, 30f, 233–234, 234f
  activation, 235, 235f
  correction responses, 343
  release, 308–311
  ultrasound imaging, 236f, 237
International Association for the Study of Pain, 155

International Federation of Orthopaedic
  Manual Therapists (IFOMT), 149*f*
Interosseous ligament, 19*f*, 21, 21*f*
Interpretive reasoning, 257, 258*f*
  Laura (case report), 273*b*
Interstitial sensory receptors, 45*t*
Intervertebral disc, 92*f*
Intervertebral lumbar joints, mobility,
  225–226, 225*f*
Intra-abdominal pressure (IAP), 133
Intramuscular release, 309, 311–312
  combined, 290–294, 291*f*, 292*f*
  psoas, 291*f*
Intramuscular stimulation (IMS),
  287–288, 288*f*
  see also Dry needling/IMS
Intrapelvic control
  backward bending, 188*f*
  forward bending, 187*f*
  squat, 193*f*
Intrapelvic mobility, one leg standing, 190*f*
Intrapelvic motion, kinematics, 61–68
Intrapelvic restraints, 68–69
Intrapelvic torsion (IPT), 111, 115,
  118–120, 180
  backward bending, 187, 187*f*, 273*f*
  forward bending, 185, 186*f*
  lateral bending, 189
  muscle systems and, 324–325, 325*f*
  one leg standing, 189–190
  prone knee bend/hip extension, 202,
    203*f*, 204*f*, 205*f*
  sitting posture, 200, 201*f*
Ischial tuberosities, pelvic position and,
  212, 214*f*
Ischiococcygeus, 39*f*, 42, 42*f*
  compression, 114
  palpation, 216, 217*f*
  release, 295*f*, 297–299, 298*f*, 396*f*
Ischiofemoral ligament, 26–27, 27*f*, 28,
  28*f*, 231–232
Ischium, 12–14, 392*f*
  adult, 16, 16*f*
  comparative anatomy, 7
'Isolation' training, 268

J

Jaeger, Edwin, 318*f*
Joint fibrosis, 264
Joint infection, 98*t*
Joint mobility, influences on, 53–54
Joint mobilization techniques,
  principles, 288–289

K

Kaltenborn model, 148
'Kegel' exercises, 270
Key muscles, 251
Kinematics
  flexion/extension lumbar segment,
    55, 55*f*, 56*f*, 57*f*
  hip, 69–70
  intrapelvic motion, 61–68
  pelvic girdle, 60, 61*f*
  rotation/sideflexion lumbar segment,
    55–57, 58*f*
Kinetics
  axial torsion lumbar segment, 59–60
  hip, 70, 70*f*
  horizontal translation lumbar
    segment, 60, 60*f*
  intrapelvic restraints, 68–69
  vertical compression lumbar segment,
    57–59, 59*f*
Kirkaldy-Willis
  instability, 92*f*, 94–97, 104, 106–107
  stabilization and, 113
  structural changes and, 93–94
Knee
  bent knee fall out, 360, 360*f*
  lunge knee lifts, 400
Knowledge, 147–148, 148*f*
'Knuckle walk', 7
Kyphosis, thoracic, 7

L

Lamb, David, 148
Lateral bending, 87, 88*f*, 188–189, 189*f*
Lateral distraction, hip joint, 312–313,
  313*f*
Laura (case report), 270–282
  articular system, 275
  clinical impression, 275
  Clinical Puzzle, 271*f*
  follow-up action, 276–279, 280–281
  homework practice, 279–280, 281–282
  interpretive reasoning, 273*b*
  myofascial system, 274
  narrative reasoning, 271*b*
  neural system, 274
  reflection/hypothesis, 271*b*, 273*b*,
    274*b*, 277*b*
  reflective reasoning, 279–280,
    281–282
  treatment, 275–276, 279–280,
    281–282, 281*f*

Law of Denervation (Cannon &
  Rosenblueth), 288
Lee, Diane, 2*f*
Leg *see* One leg standing; Trunk and leg
  dissociation
Leisure activities, 175
'Letting go', of old strategy, 267,
  324–325, 381–383
Levator ani, 38–39, 39*f*, 40*f*, 142
'L'Homme de Descartes' (Descartes),
  153*f*
Lifting, 89
Ligaments
  form closure, 70–71, 71*t*
  hip joint, 26–27
  pelvic girdle, 17*f*
  pubic symphysis (PS), 25–26, 25*f*, 26*f*
  sacroiliac joint (SIJ), 17*f*, 20–21
  thoracolumbar fascia, 37*f*
Ligamentum teres, 17*f*, 28
Linea alba, 31, 32*f*, 33*f*
  Laura (case report), 277, 278*f*, 279*f*
  pregnancy and, 131–133, 131*f*, 132*f*
Load effort task analysis, 326
Load transfer tests
  acetabular labral tears, 125
  articular cartilage degeneration, 127
  hip joint, 123–124
  Laura (case report), 278–279, 280
  lumbar dysfunction, 106, 108
  pubic symphysis (PS), 221*f*
  sacroiliac joint (SIJ), 115–116,
    116*f*, 120
Long dorsal sacroiliac ligament, 21–22,
  22*f*
  pain provocation and, 220–222, 222*f*
Longissimus thoracis pars lumborum,
  35, 302
Longissimus thoracis pars thoracis,
  34*f*, 35
Lumbar dysfunction
  acute locked back, 108
  acute pain, stages 1/2, 105–107
  chronic/persistent pain
    stages 1/2, 108–111
    stage 3, 113, 115*f*
  extension control, 109–111, 110*f*
  flexion control, 109, 109*f*, 110*f*
  history, 105, 108
  horizontal translation, 60, 60*f*
  motor control, 106–107, 107*f*, 108
  movement/motion control, 93, 93*f*
  multidirectional control impairment,
    111–113

Lumbar dysfunction (*Continued*)
  rotation control, 111, 112*f*
  treatment, 107, 108, 111
Lumbar joints
  Laura (case report), 275
  manipulation, 318–320, 318*f*, 319*f*,
    320*f*
Lumbar motion
  backward bending, 187, 188*f*
  control, 93, 93*f*
  forward bending, 185, 186*f*
  lateral bending, 189, 189*f*
  walking, 89
Lumbar segment
  extension, 55, 55*f*, 56*f*, 57*f*
  flexion, 55, 55*f*, 56*f*, 57*f*
  sideflexion, 55–57, 58*f*
Lumbar spine
  clinical presentations, 104–113
  force closure, 106–107, 107*f*, 108
  form closure, 54–60, 54*f*, 91–98,
    106–107, 107*f*, 108
  instability, 97*f*
  mobilization, 316–318, 316*f*, 317*f*
  muscle release, 302
  myofascial/neural systems influence,
    227–228, 227*f*
  paraspinal muscles, 225–226, 225*f*
  pathoanatomic changes, 92*f*, 94–97,
    94*f*, 95*f*, 96*f*, 97*f*
  prone knee bend/hip extension, 202,
    203*f*
  range of motion, 301, 305, 307, 317,
    319–320
  regional tests, 224–228
  soft tissue/bony disorders, 92*b*
  structural changes, 93–94, 95*f*
Lumbosacral junction, 59*f*
Lumbosacral multifidus, structural
    changes, 118, 119
Lunges, 400–402, 405*f*
  backward, 400–401
  knee lift, 400
  resistive band, 401
  side/diagonal, 401
  trunk rotation, 401–402
  walking, 400

M

McKenzie, Robin, 149*f*
McKenzie model, 148, 159*t*
McMaster University, 148
Maitland, Geoff, 149*f*

Maitland model, 148
Manubriosternal junction, 387, 387*f*
Massed, focused practice, 266, 267
Mature Organism Model (Gifford),
    156*f*, 157
Meaning perspective, 255–256, 263,
    285, 375
Meaningful tasks, 266–269
  deep/superficial muscle systems, 268
  general principles, 266–268
  Laura (case report), 276
  postural/movement training, 268
  supports, role of, 268–269
  whole body assessment, 373–378,
    374*f*, 375*f*, 376*f*, 377*f*
Mechanical diagnosis and therapy
    (MDT), 148, 159*t*
Mechanoreceptors, 44
Meckel, 8–9
Meisenbach, R.O, 85–86
Melzack, R, 165
Melzack model of pain, 157, 158*f*
  body-self neuromatrix, 165, 367–368,
    381
Mentorship, 148*f*
Metabolic disorders, 98*t*
Metacognitive reflection, 257
Midline anterior abdominal fascia
  palpation, 238, 238*f*, 239*f*
  ultrasound imaging, 238–240, 239*f*
Mixed urinary incontinence (MUI), 139
Mobility tests, 251–252
Mobilization with movement, 313
Motivational interviewing, 263
Motor conduction tests, 251
Motor control impairment, 264–265
Motor control theory, 74–85, 100–104
  beautiful movement requirements,
    83–85
  deep muscles, 78–81, 79*f*
  hip joint, 124, 125–126, 127
  lumbar spine, 106–107, 107*f*, 108
  sacroiliac joint (SIJ), 116, 121
  stability strategies, 74–78, 75*f*, 76*f*, 77*f*
Movement
  building blocks, designing, 383–386,
    385*f*, 386*f*
  control, 355–356
  quality of, 267–268, 325–326
  system impairment, 159*t*
  training, 268
  see also Posture and movement
    strategies
Mulligan mobilization, 313

Multifidus (Mu), 22*f*, 23, 33–35, 34*f*, 79*f*
  palpation, 216*f*
  structural changes, 110–111, 110*f*
  see also Deep fibers of multifidus
    (dMF); Superficial fibers of
    multifidus (sMF)
Muscle energy technique, 304–305, 304*f*
Muscle lengthening
  hip joint, 291*f*, 292, 295–296
  lumbar spine, 305
  sacroiliac joint (SIJ), 299, 300–301
  thorax/abdomen, 305*f*, 307, 308*f*,
    309, 311, 312
Muscle slings, longitudinal/oblique,
    250–251
Muscle spindle sensory receptor, 45*t*
Muscles
  force closure theory, 72–74, 72*f*
  imbalance, 122–124, 211, 212*f*
  specific, 388, 389*f*
  see also Deep muscle systems;
    Superficial muscle systems
Myofascial release techniques, 265
Myofascial slings, 81–82, 82*f*, 83*f*, 399,
    402*f*
  'Anatomy Trains', 83*f*
Myofascial systems, 169–171, 170*t*
  hip joint, 232
  impairments, 265
  Laura (case report), 274, 281
  lumbar spine, 227–228, 227*f*
  pubic symphysis (PS), 220, 221*f*
  sacroiliac joint (SIJ), 219
  techniques for releasing, 290–312
Myofascial trigger point model, 288
Myotome, 9, 9*f*

N

Narrative reasoning, 255–256
  Laura (case report), 271*b*
Nerve supply
  hip joint, 28
  pubic symphysis (PS), 26
  sacroiliac joint (SIJ), 24
Neural network reinforcement,
    354–355, 354*f*, 355*f*
Neural systems, 169–171, 170*t*
  hip joint, 232
  impairment, 264–266
  Laura (case report), 274, 280–281
  lumbar spine, 227–228, 227*f*
  pubic symphysis (PS), 220, 221*f*
  sacroiliac joint (SIJ), 219

techniques for releasing, 290–312
'waking up', 363–365
Neurological conduction status, 111–113, 251–252
Neurology, 44–46, 45*t*
Neuromatrix Theory of Pain (Melzack), 157
Neuromuscular changes, 102, 103*f*
Neuromyofascial forces, pelvic position and, 213*f*
Neuromyofascial imbalance, 211, 213*f*
Neurophysiologic pain model, 159*t*
Neuroplasticity, optimizing, 266, 323
Neurotransmitters, 381
Neutral lumbopelvic-hip (LPH) alignment, 353
   crook lying roll up/down, 332–333, 333*f*, 334*b*, 334*f*
   deep muscle system and, 329–333
   passive positioning
      prone, 332*f*, 357
      sidelying, 331, 332*f*
Neutral spine, defined, 390
Neutral zone of motion, 53–54, 54*f*, 106–107, 107*f*, 116, 288–289
   assessment, 210, 219, 224, 226
Nociceptors, 44
Non-propositional knowledge, 147

O

Objective examination, 175–254, 257, 259, 369–370
   abdominal canister, 232–250
   adjunctive tests, 252
   clinical reflection, 232
   function/performance strategies, 176–179
   hips, 228–232
   longitudinal/oblique muscle slings, 250–251
   lumbar spine, 224–228
   neurological conduction/mobility tests, 251–252
   pelvic girdle, 210–223
   vascular tests, 252
Obturator externus (OE)
   dry needling, 293*f*
   release, 294–295
Obturator internus (OI), 39*f*, 40*f*, 41
   release, 295, 300*f*
Occupation, 175
Oldham, John, 148
One arm fly, 359

One leg standing, 189–191, 190*f*, 192*f*
   hip motion control, 191*f*
   Laura (case report), 272
Osteology, pelvic girdle, 9–17
Overhead flexion, 359
Oxford Centre for Evidence-based Medicine, Levels of Evidence, 149, 150*t*
Oxford grading scale, 134

P

P4 (posterior pelvic pain provocation) test, 222–223, 223*f*
Paccini sensory receptor, 45*t*
Pain, 100–104
   acute, 105–107, 153–155, 156
   algorithm, 104*f*
   centrally mediated, 153, 161–162, 161*f*
   chronic, 108–111, 113, 115*f*, 155, 156, 161*f*
   classification, 153–163, 154*f*, 156*f*, 158*f*, 161*f*
   drivers, 153, 153*f*
   mechanisms, 154*f*, 156–158, 161*f*
   patterns, 153, 154*f*
   peripherally mediated, 153, 161–162, 161*f*
   persistent, 108–111, 113, 115*f*, 155, 156
   pregnancy-related pelvic girdle (PRPGP), 129, 130
   provocation tests, 220–223, 222*f*, 223*f*
   referral, 123*t*
   subjective examination, 174–175
   suppression, 44–45
   understanding, 152–158, 152*b*
   see also Lumbar dysfunction
Panjabi, M.M, 49, 49*f*
   conceptual model, 49*f*, 53–54
Parasagittal abdominal approach, ultrasound imaging, 243, 243*f*
Paraspinal muscles, 225–226, 225*f*
Paravaginal defects, 133–137, 134*f*, 136*f*
Paré, 1
Paris, Dr Stanley, 149*f*
Passive system, 130–131, 139
Pathoanatomic classification, 159*t*
Pathoanatomic model of pain, 153
Patient characteristics, 262–264
Patients
   classification, 159*t*
   education, 267–268

values, 149, 152*f*
   see also Awareness, patient
Patterns
   automatic, 386, 402–403, 405*f*
   recognition, 256, 257–258
   substitution, 264–265
Pelvic alignment, technique for correcting, 321
Pelvic floor, 72*f*, 338–342
   coactivation, 353–354
   Laura (case report), 276–277, 280, 292*f*
   muscles/fascia, 38–41, 39*f*, 80
   stress urinary incontinence (SUI) and, 141–143, 144
   ultrasound imaging, 241–245, 242*f*, 243*f*, 244*f*, 245*f*, 339–341, 340*f*, 342, 342*f*, 352
Pelvic floor Educator, 339, 339*f*
Pelvic girdle
   arthrology, 17–29
   clinical presentations, 114–121
   comparative anatomy, pelvic girdle, 6–8, 6*f*
   evolution, 5–6
   form closure, 60–69, 98–99
   historical perspective, 1–2, 8–9
   human development, 8–46
   kinematics, 60, 61*f*
   ligaments, 17*f*
   motion, 89, 187, 187*f*
   myology, 29–44
   myths and facts, 1
   osteology, 9–17
   pain, pregnancy-related (PRPGP), 129, 130
   regional tests, 210–223
   standing posture, 180
   structural changes, 98–99, 98*t*
'Pelvic rock', 395
'Pelvic Salsa', 197*f*, 302*f*, 313, 317, 320
Pelvis
   deep back wall muscles, 41–42, 42*f*
   pregnancy and, 130–139
   tensegrity model, 83*f*
Perceptual effects, 45–46
Performance
   motor control and, 84–85
   see also Function/performance strategies
Perineal approach, ultrasound imaging and, 244, 244*f*, 245*f*
Peripheral pain generator model, 159*t*
Persistent pain, 108–111, 113, 115*f*, 155, 156

Personal knowledge, 162
Perthes' disease, 100f
Phallic Worshippers, 9
Pharmacology, 163b
Piriformis, 39f, 42, 42f
  compression, 114
  hypertonicity, 216, 217f
  release, 295f, 297, 299–300, 300f
Positional release, 286f
  deep muscles, 295
  erector spinae (ES), 303–304, 304f
  external oblique (EO), 306–307
  internal oblique (IO), 309, 310, 310f
  ischiococcygeus, 297–298
  piriformis, 299
  superficial fibers of multifidus (sMF),
    300
  superficial muscles, 291
Positional tests
  hip joint, 228–229, 228f
  lumbar spine, 224–225, 224f
  pelvic girdle, 210–213, 211f, 212f,
    213f, 214f
Positioning
  active movement, 332–333, 333f,
    334b, 334f
  passive, 331–332, 332f
Positive feedback, 381
Posterior compression test, 222, 222f
Posterior distraction test, 222, 223f
Posterior oblique sling, 81, 82f
Posterior superior iliac spine (PSIS), 14
Postpartum health, 144
Postpartum Health for Moms program,
  144
Postpartum pelvic control impairment,
  case report, 270–282
Posture
  adjustment, rapid arm movements,
    77, 78t
  alignment, 180–183
  comparative, 7–8, 8f
  equilibrium, 177–178
  training, 268
  see also Sitting posture; Standing
    posture
Posture and movement strategies,
  367–408
  advanced assessment, 368–379
  functional/sport specific tasks,
    396–405
  Integrated Systems Model, 367
  static tasks, 389–396, 392f, 394f,
    396f
  tools and techniques, 379–389

Pregnancy complications, 129–146
  pelvis and, 130–139
  postpartum health, 144
  pregnancy-related pelvic girdle pain
    (PRPGP), 129, 130
  urinary incontinence (UI), 129–130,
    139–144
Procedural knowledge, 147
Professional affiliation, 148f
Professional craft knowledge, 147
Progress, plateaus in, 267
Prolotherapy, 265, 365–366
Prone hip extension, 202–205, 204f,
  205f
Prone knee bend, 202–205, 203f, 204f
Propositional knowledge, 147
Psoas, 43–44, 44f
  intramuscular release technique, 291f
  palpation, 249, 250f
  ultrasound imaging, 250, 250f
Psychosocial factors, 375
Psychosocial model, 159t
Pubic symphysis (PS), 387, 387f, 388f
  adult, 25–26, 25f, 26f
  aging and, 26
  anterior aspect, 26f
  compression, insufficient, 117–120
  development, 25
  ligaments, 25–26, 25f, 26f
  myofascial/neural systems influence,
    220, 221f
  nerve supply, 26
  restraints, 219, 220f
  structural changes, 98–99, 98t
  treatment, 120
  vertical control impairment, 119–120
Pubic tubercles, pelvic position and,
  210–211, 211f
Pubis, 12–14, 16f, 17f
Pubococcygeus, 38, 40f, 142
Pubofemoral ligament, 17f, 27–28,
  28f, 231
Puborectalis, 38, 40f, 134, 134f
Pubovisceralis, 39, 40f, 134, 134f
Pyramidalis, 26f, 31

Q

Quadratus femoris, release, 300f
Quadratus lumborum, 35–36, 302

R

RACM see Release, Align, Connect and
  Move (RACM)

Range of motion
  hip joint, 313
  lumbar spine, 301, 305, 307, 317,
    319–320
  sacroiliac joint (SIJ), 299, 301, 314–315
  thorax, 305, 307, 311
Recoil, 304
Rectovaginal fascia, 41f
Rectus abdominis (RA), 26f, 31, 31f, 32f
  correction responses, 343
  release, 311–312
  ultrasound imaging, 240, 241f
Rectus femoris, dry needling, 293f
Rectus sheaths, 32, 32f, 33f
Reflection, 148f, 232, 257–258
  Laura (case report), 271b, 273b,
    274b, 277b
Reflective reasoning, 279–280, 281–282
Reflex effects, 45
Reflex tests, 252
Reiter's disease, 253f
Release, Align, Connect and Move
  (RACM), 354–355, 354f, 355f,
    357
  training and, 381–383, 386, 390,
    407–408
Release with awareness technique,
  285–286, 288, 290–291, 292,
    292f
  external oblique (EO), 307f
  internal oblique (IO), 308, 310f
  ischiococcygeus, 298f
  piriformis, 300f
  principles, 286f, 287
  superficial fibers of multifidus (sMF),
    301f
Release techniques, 265–266, 267
Research evidence, 149, 152f
Resisted movements, 355–356
Rib cage
  anterolateral lower, 388
  palpation, 395
  posterolateral lower, 388
  wiggle, 357
Rigidity, checkpoints for, 357, 357b,
  384, 389
Rotation
  lumbar segment, 55–57, 58f
  lumbar spine, 226, 226f
Ruffini sensory receptor, 45t

S

Sacral thrust test, 223, 223f
Sacrococcygeal joint, 24–25

Sacrococcygeal ligaments, 24–25
Sacroiliac belts, 268, 269f, 328–329, 329f
Sacroiliac joint (SIJ)
  first decade, 18
  second/third decade, 18
  fourth/fifth decade, 18–19
  sixth/seventh decade, 19–20, 19f
  eighth decade, 20, 20f
  acute locked, 120–121
  adult, 20–24, 21f
  anteroposterior plane, neutral zone analysis, 215, 215f
  articular system restraints, 218–219, 218f, 219f
  blood supply, 24
  comparisons, 13f
  compression, 114–120
  craniocaudal plane, neutral zone analysis, 217–218, 218f
  elastic zone analysis, 217
  force closure, 116, 121
  form closure, 116, 121
  historical perspective, 1
  history, 114, 117, 120
  horizontal control impairment, 118–119, 118f
  intrauterine, 17–18, 18f
  Laura (case report), 275
  ligaments, 17f, 20–21
  mobility, 214–218, 215f, 218f, 316
  mobilization technique, 313–315, 314f, 315f
  motor control, 116, 121
  muscle release, 296–302
  myofascial/neural system influence, 219
  nerve supply, 24
  range of motion, 299, 301, 314–315
  structural changes, 98–99, 98t, 99f, 253f
  treatment, 116–117, 118, 119, 121
  vertical control impairment, 117–118, 117f
Sacrospinous ligament, 17f, 23, 23f
Sacrotuberous ligament (STL), 22–23, 22f, 23f
  pain provocation and, 222, 222f
Sacrum
  adult, 10–12
  anterior aspect, 12f
  comparative anatomy, 6
  cranial aspect, 11f
  development, 9–10
  hip extension, 205, 205f

intrapelvic motion, 63, 63f, 64f, 65f, 66f
lateral aspect, 11f
orientation, 14f, 14t
ossification, 10f
pelvic position, 211, 214f
posterior aspect, 11f
prone knee bend/hip extension, 202, 204f
standing posture, 183f
types, 15f
Salsero-chair, 317–318, 318f, 320
Sartorius, dry needling, 293f
Scapula, correction techniques and, 395
Scientific knowledge, 147
Sclerotome, 9, 9f
  differentiation and, 9f
Screening tests, 369–370
Searle, Ian, 149f
Self-release with awareness technique, 288, 289, 381–383, 391
Sensorial dimension, 271b
Sensory conduction tests, 251, 252f
Sensory receptors, 44–46, 45t
Sensory stimulation, 267
Sitting posture, 391–395
  assessment, 200–202, 201f, 202f
  optimal pyramid base, 391
  spinal position, 391–395
Skill acquisition, 148f, 255, 256f
Sleep, 175
Sling squat, 195, 198f
sMF see Superficial fibers of multifidus (sMF)
Specific Theory of Pain (Descartes), 153f
Sport, 175
  specific tasks, 396–405
Squats, 87–88, 88f
  assessment, 191–195, 193f, 194f, 196f, 197f
  awareness and, 382f, 384f
  bilateral, 402, 403f
  Laura (case report), 272–273
  loaded, 389f
  postural training, 383f, 384f, 397–398
  sling, 198f, 398f
  split, 399f
Stability
  defined, 48f, 49–52, 49f, 50f, 51f
  strategies, 74–78, 75f, 76f, 77f
Standing posture
  acetabular labral tears, 124
  articular cartilage degeneration, 127

function/performance tests, 180–183, 181f, 182f, 183f, 184f, 185f
hip malalignment, 123, 123f
Laura (case report), 271–272, 272f, 278
lumbar dysfunction, 105–106, 105f, 108, 112f, 113f
sacroiliac joint (SIJ) disorder, 114–115, 115f, 120
training strategies, 387f, 390–391
Static situations, motor control and, 74
Static tasks, 389–396, 392f, 394f, 396f
Step forward/backward, 195–199, 198f, 199f, 200f, 380f, 398–399
Step up/down, 402, 403f, 405f
Sternum
  lower, 387, 388f
  upper, 387, 388f
Stoddard, Dr Alan, 149f
Strategies
  analysis see Task analysis
  key points of control, 387–389, 389f
  non-optimal, 261–266, 267, 275–276
Stress urinary incontinence (SUI), 135f, 139, 141–144, 143f
  case report, 270–282
Stretch with awareness technique, 288, 289, 292f, 294
  internal oblique (IO), 308, 310f
  ischiococcygeus, 298f
  piriformis, 300f
  principles, 290
  rectus abdominis (RA), 311
  superficial fibers of multifidus (sMF), 301f
  training and, 381–383
Subjective examination, 174–175
  cognitive/emotional states, 175
  general health, 174
  imaging studies, 175
  key questions, 174
  mode of onset, 174
  occupation/leisure, 175
  pain/dysesthesia, 174–175
  sleep, 175
Superficial fibers of multifidus (sMF)
  compression, 114
  release, 297, 300–302
Superficial muscle systems, 81–82, 82f, 83f, 104f
  deep muscles coordination, 355–365, 358b
  release, 290–294, 292f, 296f
  'waking up', 268

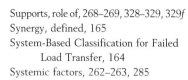

Supports, role of, 268–269, 328–329, 329f
Synergy, defined, 165
System-Based Classification for Failed Load Transfer, 164
Systemic factors, 262–263, 285

T

Talus, standing posture, 181, 185f
Tape (support), 269, 269f, 328–329, 395
Task analysis, 176–179
    key components, 177–179, 178f, 179b
    see also Meaningful tasks
Task-oriented practice, 266
Task-specific postures, 395–396
Tendinopathy, 103f
Tensegrity models, 81–82, 83f, 84f
Tensor fascia latae
    combined release, 291f, 292f
    dry needling, 293f
Theoretical knowledge, 147
Theraband, 379, 383f, 398
Therapists
    characteristics, 262
    role of, 260
Thigh thrust, 222–223, 223f
Thoracic kyphosis, 7
Thoracolumbar fascia, 33f, 36–38
    lamina, 37f, 38f
    ligaments, 37f
    posterior view, 36f
Thoracopelvic orientation, 194f
Thoracopelvic rotation, 197, 200f
    sitting posture, 201, 202f
    step forward, 200f
Thorax
    lateral bending, 188
    muscle release, 303–312
    range of motion, 305, 307, 311
    squat, 192, 194f, 195, 196f
    standing posture, 181, 182f
Timelines, 153–156
Tissue
    healing stages, 153–155, 155t
    mechanisms, pain and, 154f
Toe wiggle, 357
TrA *see* Transversus abdominis (TrA)
Training activities, 381–383
Transverse abdominal approach, ultrasound imaging, 242, 242f

Transverse acetabular ligament, 17f, 27f, 28
Transversus abdominis (TrA), 29, 29f, 79f, 80
    activation, 240
    coactivation, 353–354
    contraction, 309
    non-optimal responses, 235f
    palpation, 234f, 247–248, 248f, 344, 344f, 346, 348, 348f
    pregnancy and, 137–138, 138f, 143f
    tears in, 103f
    ultrasound imaging, 236f, 237, 240, 344–349, 346f, 347f
    unilateral activation, 353, 354f
    'waking up', 326–328, 327f, 342–349, 343f, 345f
Treatment
    compliance to, 373–374
    plans, 259
    principles for evidence-based program, 260
    reassessment, 259
Treatment-based classification system, 159t
Trendelenburg gait, 6, 179–180, 180f
Triceps press, 359, 359f
Trigger points, 288
Trunk and arm dissociation, supine/crook lying, 359, 359f
Trunk and leg dissociation
    crook lying, 359–361, 360f
    hip joint control, 364f, 365
    prone, 362–363, 362f, 363f
    sidelying, 361–362, 361f
Trunk rotation, 402–403, 404f
Trunk-gripping, 101, 105, 105f

U

Ultrasound imaging
    abdominal wall, 227–228, 236f
    midline anterior abdominal fascia, 238–240, 239f
    pelvic floor, 241–245, 242f, 243f, 244f, 245f, 339–341, 340f, 342, 342f, 352
    pelvic organs, 277f
    psoas, 250, 250f
    rectus abdominis (RA), 241f

transversus abdominis (TrA), 344–349, 346f, 347f
Understand pain, live well again (Pearson), 263–264, 285
Urethral sphincter closure system, 140–141
Urethral support system, 139–140, 140f
Urge urinary incontinence (UUI), 139
Urinary incontinence (UI), 139–144
    prevalence, 129–130, 139–144
    urethral sphincter closure system, 140–141
    urethral support system, 139–140, 140f
Urogenital hiatus, 39–40

V

Vascular tests, 252
Vector manipulation, 316, 319, 319f, 320, 320f
Vector mobilization, 313, 314, 317, 317f
Vertebral column, 7, 8f
Vesalius, 1
Virtual body, subjective examination and, 174
Visceral system, 138–139, 169–171, 170t
    impairments, 266
    manipulation, 266
    release, 320
Visualization, 379–381
Vleeming, Andry, 2f
Von Luschka, 8–9

W

Walking, 88–89
    backwards, 398–399
    function/performance tests, 179–180, 180f
    lunges, 400
World Health Assembly, 163–164

Z

Zones of articular motion, 53–54, 54f
Zygapophyseal joint, 92f, 95f
    degeneration, 94f, 97–98
    fracture, 95f, 107, 316f
    posterior, 93, 97–98